Dictionary of DNA and Genome Technology

For Mobby

Dictionary of DNA and Genome Technology

Paul Singleton

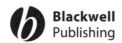

Blackwell Publishing

BLACKWELL PUBLISHING
350 Main Street, Malden, MA 02148-5020, USA
9600 Garsington Road, Oxford OX4 2DQ, UK
550 Swanston Street, Carlton, Victoria 3053, Australia

First published 2008 by Blackwell Publishing Ltd

1   2008

Library of Congress Cataloging-in-Publication Data

Singleton, Paul.
    Dictionary of DNA and genome technology / Paul Singleton.
       p. ; cm.
    Includes bibliographical references.
    ISBN 978-1-4051-5607-3 (hardcover : alk. paper) ISBN 978-1-4051-5608-0 (pbk. : alk. paper)
  1. Genetic engineering—Dictionaries.   2. Genomics—Dictionaries.   3. DNA—Dictionaries.   I. Title.
    [DNLM: 1. Genetic Techniques—Dictionary—English.   2. Genomics—Dictionary—English. QU 13 S617d 2008]
    QH442.S548 2008
    660.6′503—dc22

                                                                                                         2007030247

A catalogue record for this title is available from the British Library.

Set in 8/9 pt Times
by Graphicraft Limited, Hong Kong
Printed and bound in Singapore
by Markono Print Media Pte Ltd

For further information on
Blackwell Publishing, visit our website at
www.blackwellpublishing.com

Contents

Preface

'DNA technology' refers to a variety of procedures – some simple, others extremely complex and sophisticated. At the most basic level they include: isolating and purifying DNA; cutting DNA with specialized enzymes; characterizing, sequencing and expressing DNA; hybridizing, labeling, ligating, staining and quantifying DNA; and amplifying specific regions of DNA. This technology is used in fields such as:

- diagnosis (infectious and hereditary diseases)
- drug development
- epidemiology
- forensic science
- gene therapy
- genetically modified (GM) foods
- industrial enzymes
- oncology
- taxonomy
- vaccine development

Covering much of the established methodology, and some background material, the dictionary also contains many items of new information first reported in mainstream journals within the last 15 months – for example: new methods for amplifying DNA; DFRS plasmids; combined probe–dye monitoring of real-time PCR; binary deoxyribozyme ligase; footprinting *in vivo* with X-radiation; oligonucleotide–peptide conjugation by Diels–Alder chemistry; new notation for DNA; benzylguanine labels for fusion proteins; amplifying damaged DNA; chromosomal *ccdB* gene for plasmid maintenance; and GFP reactivation in methylation analysis.

References to published papers and reviews are cited throughout the dictionary. Some of these are the source(s) of information on which particular entries are based; they can provide further details (e.g. protocols), and they also permit the reader to make his or her own assessment of a given source. Other references are included in order to indicate additional information which is relevant to a given entry.

Some pervasive topics – for example, PCR, gene fusion, forensics, phages, overexpression, typing, retroviruses – are treated more extensively. These essay-style entries are intended to offer the newcomer a broad working knowledge of the area, and such entries may also be of use to the over-specialized researcher.

Commercial systems and materials are widely used in DNA technology, and a number of entries describe these products. This kind of entry may be useful, for example, when a paper offers little information about a given product other than "used according to the manufacturer's instructions" – leaving unanswered questions on the product, the protocol or the principle. Accordingly, these entries give brief overviews of products – and their uses – and in many cases they also cite relevant papers describing work in which a given product has been used. Where the names of products and systems are known to be trademarks this has been indicated.

Notes for the user on the following pages will facilitate use of the dictionary.

Paul Singleton
Clannaborough (UK), 2007

Notes for the user

Alphabetization

The headwords in any dictionary can be listed in either of two distinct ways:

1. According to the way in which the terms are actually written. This approach, called the 'word-by-word' approach, is used in this dictionary.
2. According to the way in which the terms *would* appear if all the spaces and hyphens etc. were deleted. This is the 'letter-by-letter' approach.

The *order* in which headwords are listed depends on the particular approach used; for example:

Approach 1	*Approach 2*
A site	AAS
A-tract	abacavir
AAS	abasic site
abacavir	ABC excinuclease
abasic site	A site
ABC excinuclease	A-tract
bla gene	black–white screening
black–white screening	*bla* gene
blue–white screening	Bluescript®
Bluescript®	blue–white screening
branch migration	branched DNA assay
branched DNA assay	branch migration
col plasmid	colchicine
colchicine	col plasmid
cos site	cosmid
cosmid	*cos* site
Cre–*loxP* system	CREB
CREB	Cre–*loxP* system

Note that a one-letter descriptor (such as the 'A' in 'A site') is treated as a word for the purposes of alphabetization in approach 1.

In practice, neither approach is foolproof. For example, in the first approach, the order in which a given term is listed may depend on whether or not a hyphen is regarded as a necessary part of the term. Thus, on deleting a hyphen – and closing-up the intervening space – the characters on either side of the hyphen become contiguous; in this case, the character following the hyphen becomes important as a primary determinant of alphabetical order. In the second approach, strict adherence to the basic 'letter-by-letter' rule would lead – for example – to the following order:

factor I	(1)
factor II	(2)
factor III	(3)
factor IV	(4)
factor IX	(9)
factor V	(5)
factor VI	(6)
factor VII	(7)
factor VIII	(8)
factor X	(10)

To some readers (and writers) this order may seem reasonable, or even preferable. To others it runs counter to common sense: Roman numerals are generally seen, and used, as the equivalent of numbers – and ought therefore to be arranged in *numerical* order.

When a Greek letter is a significant component of an entry heading – as e.g. in λ phage – it is treated as a word and is listed in the relevant alphabetical position indicated by the English name (i.e. alpha, lambda etc.). However, β-galactosidase and β-lactamases are listed under G and L, respectively; this rule applies also to entry headings starting with letters such as L-, *p*-, *N*-, *O*- etc. which precede the names of certain chemicals. In some cases a headword is given in *both* possible locations (with suitable cross-referencing); this has been done simply in order to assist readers.

Cross references

A word in SMALL CAPITALS refers the reader to an entry elsewhere in the dictionary. Cross references are used e.g. to extend the reader's knowledge into related fields or topics. The cross references may be particularly useful for directing the reader to allied, or parallel, subjects whose relationship to the entry being read may not be immediately obvious.

In some cases a complete understanding of a given entry, or a full appreciation of its context, depends on information contained in other entries – which are indicated by cross reference(s). Dictionaries are often arranged in this way because it avoids the need to repeat information. If it is especially important to follow-up a cross reference, then the cross reference is followed by '(q.v.)'. In other cases, in which the purpose of a cross reference is simply to link one topic with another, the cross reference may be preceded by 'See also . . . .' or 'cf.'.

External references

References to papers, articles or reviews in journals are given in square brackets. The names of journals are abbreviated to save space. The abbreviated journal name is followed by the year of publication, the volume number (and frequently the issue number), and the page number(s). This information is sufficient to enable the reader to obtain any given reference.

Commercial products

Many of the commercial products are listed under their trade names. In general, these products are widely used in studies on all aspects of DNA-based technology and are cited in many research papers. It should be noted that the inclusion of any given product in the dictionary is not based on an evaluation of the product, and implies no comparison of that product with any similar product(s) marketed by other companies. It is obviously not possible to include *every* product currently on the market. Importantly, any details of a product given in the dictionary are those details which are to hand at the time of writing; companies are continually modifying and updating their products, so that the reader should refer to the manufacturer's literature for details of any modifications.

Ready reference

The Greek alphabet

A	α	alpha		N	ν	nu
B	β	beta		Ξ	ξ	xi
Γ	γ	gamma		O	o	omicron
Δ	δ	delta		Π	π	pi
E	ε	epsilon		P	ρ	rho
Z	ζ	zeta		Σ	σ	sigma
H	η	eta		T	τ	tau
Θ	θ	theta		Y	υ	upsilon
I	ι	iota		Φ	φ	phi
K	κ	kappa		X	χ	chi
Λ	λ	lambda		Ψ	ψ	psi
M	μ	mu		Ω	ω	omega

Amino acids

alanine	Ala	A		A	Ala	alanine
arginine	Arg	R		C	Cys	cysteine
asparagine	Asn	N		D	Asp	aspartic acid
aspartic acid	Asp	D		E	Glu	glutamic acid
cysteine	Cys	C		F	Phe	phenylalanine
glutamic acid	Glu	E		G	Gly	glycine
glutamine	Gln	Q		H	His	histidine
glycine	Gly	G		I	Ile	isoleucine
histidine	His	H		K	Lys	lysine
isoleucine	Ile	I		L	Leu	leucine
leucine	Leu	L		M	Met	methionine
lysine	Lys	K		N	Asn	asparagine
methionine	Met	M		P	Pro	proline
phenylalanine	Phe	F		Q	Gln	glutamine
proline	Pro	P		R	Arg	arginine
serine	Ser	S		S	Ser	serine
threonine	Thr	T		T	Thr	threonine
tryptophan	Trp	W		V	Val	valine
tyrosine	Tyr	Y		W	Trp	tryptophan
unknown	Xaa	X		X	Xaa	unknown
valine	Val	V		Y	Tyr	tyrosine

Prefixes used with SI (Système International) units

(prefix, value, symbol)   **(value, prefix, symbol)**

FRACTIONS

atto	10^{-18}	a	10^{-1}	deci	d
centi	10^{-2}	c	10^{-2}	centi	c
deci	10^{-1}	d	10^{-3}	milli	m
femto	10^{-15}	f	10^{-6}	micro	μ
micro	10^{-6}	μ	10^{-9}	nano	n
milli	10^{-3}	m	10^{-12}	pico	p
nano	10^{-9}	n	10^{-15}	femto	f
pico	10^{-12}	p	10^{-18}	atto	a
yocto	10^{-24}	y	10^{-21}	zepto	z
zepto	10^{-21}	z	10^{-24}	yocto	y

MULTIPLES

deca	10	da	10	deca	da
exa	10^{18}	E	10^{2}	hecto	h
giga	10^{9}	G	10^{3}	kilo	k
hecto	10^{2}	h	10^{6}	mega	M
kilo	10^{3}	k	10^{9}	giga	G
mega	10^{6}	M	10^{12}	tera	T
peta	10^{15}	P	10^{15}	peta	P
tera	10^{12}	T	10^{18}	exa	E
yotta	10^{24}	Y	10^{21}	zetta	Z
zetta	10^{21}	Z	10^{24}	yotta	Y

Micro-measurements

1 Å (Ångström unit) = 10^{-1} nm = 10^{-4} μm = 10^{-10} m
1 nm (nanometer) = 10^{-3} μm = 10^{-6} mm = 10^{-9} m
1 μm (micrometer, formerly micron) = 10^{-3} mm = 10^{-6} m
1 mm = 10^{-1} cm = 10^{-3} m = 10^{-6} km

Some restriction enzymes and their cutting sites

ENZYME	CUTTING SITE ($\downarrow$)	NOTES
AluI	AG$\downarrow$CT	Blunt-ended cut
BamHI	G$\downarrow$GATCC	Isoschizomer BstI
BglII	A$\downarrow$GATCT	
BssHI	G$\downarrow$CGCGC	Used e.g. for cutting in CpG islands
DpnI	G(m^{6}A)$\downarrow$TC	Methylation of adenine needed at N6
EcoRI	G$\downarrow$AATTC	No isoschizomers reported
EcoRII	$\downarrow$CCWGG	Needs two recognition sites for activity
HaeIII	GG$\downarrow$CC	
HincII	GTY$\downarrow$RAC	Used in SDA
HindIII	A$\downarrow$AGCTT	
HpaII	C$\downarrow$CGG	Isoschizomer MspI
KpnI	GCTAC$\downarrow$C	
MboI	$\downarrow$GATC	Isoschizomer DpnII
MseI	T$\downarrow$TTA	
MspI	C$\downarrow$CGG	Isoschizomer HpaII
NarI	GG$\downarrow$CGCC	
NcoI	C$\downarrow$CATGG	
NdeI	CA$\downarrow$TATG	
NotI	GC$\downarrow$GGCCGC	Rare-cutting enzyme
PmeI	GTTT$\downarrow$AAAC	
SacI	GAGCT$\downarrow$C	
SalI	G$\downarrow$TCGAC	
SmaI	CCC$\downarrow$GGG	
SpeI	A$\downarrow$CTAGT	
XbaI	T$\downarrow$CTAGA	
XhoI	C$\downarrow$TCGAG	

A

A (1) Adenine (base, nucleoside or nucleotide). (2) L-Alanine (alternative to Ala).

Å Ångström unit, 10^{-10} m; a unit of length used e.g. to indicate intermolecular distances.

A$_{260}$ See ULTRAVIOLET ABSORBANCE.

A-DNA One of the major conformations adopted by dsDNA: a right-handed helix with ~11 base-pairs per turn.

A site (of a ribosome) The aminoacyl or 'acceptor' site at which tRNA molecules carrying the second and subsequent amino acids bind during translation. (cf. P SITE.)

A-tract In genomic DNA: a nucleotide motif associated with regions of the most pronounced curvature of the molecule. In the *Escherichia coli* genome, A-tracts were found to be distributed 'quasi-regularly' throughout, in both coding and noncoding sequences; the A-tracts occur in clusters of ~100 bp in length, with consecutive A-tracts exhibiting a periodicity of 10–12 bp.

It was suggested that the clusters of A-tracts may constitute a form of 'structural code' for the compaction of DNA in the NUCLEOID [Nucleic Acids Res (2005) 33(12):3907–3918].

AAA ATPases 'ATPases associated with diverse cellular activities'. These ATPases occur in various locations – including, for example, in proteasomes and peroxisomes.

AAAVs Avian adeno-associated viruses (see AAVS).

AAS Aminoalkylsilane (3-aminopropyltriethoxysilane; APES): a reagent used e.g. to bind tissue sections to glass (for *in situ* hybridization etc.).

***aat* gene** In *Escherichia coli*: a gene encoding the enzyme that catalyzes the addition of a leucine or phenylalanine residue to the N-terminal of proteins which are synthesized with an N-terminal arginine or lysine residue; such addition facilitates degradation of the protein.

(See also N-END RULE.)

AatII A RESTRICTION ENDONUCLEASE from *Acetobacter aceti*. Recognition sequence/cutting site: GACGT↓C.

AAUAAA In mRNAs: a polyadenylation signal upstream of the site at which the molecule is cut and polyadenylated; the sequence is similar in mRNAs from many organisms.

Other *cis*-acting elements may be involved in regulating the polyadenylation of human mRNAs, including upstream U-rich sequences similar to those identified in yeast and plants [RNA (2005) 11:1485–1493].

AAV Helper-Free System A commercial gene-delivery system (Stratagene, La Jolla CA) in which the genes in two plasmids provide functions necessary for production of infective AAV virions (see AAVS); these virions are used to transfect target cells within which viral DNA, containing the gene of interest, integrates in the host cell's DNA.

Essentially, the gene/fragment of interest is first cloned in a plasmid cloning vector in which the insert is bracketed by a pair of inverted terminal repeats (ITRs) which are necessary for subsequent viral packaging. This plasmid is then used to transfect appropriate cells – which are *co-transfected* with two other plasmids: (i) a plasmid containing the genes that encode viral capsid and replication functions, (ii) a plasmid containing genes that encode the lytic phase of AAV. The resulting infective (*but still replication-deficient*) virions are used to infect the required target cells (in which the gene of interest can be expressed).

[Use of method for genetic modification of cultured human cells: Nucleic Acids Res (2005) 33(18):e158.]

AAVs Adeno-associated viruses (also known as: adeno-satellite viruses): defective viruses that are able to replicate only when certain functions are provided by a co-infecting *helper virus* (adenovirus or herpesvirus) – or, in certain *in vitro* systems, when these functions are provided by plasmid-borne genes (see e.g. AAV HELPER-FREE SYSTEM). (Functions provided by adenovirus type 5 for AAV type 5 include both positive and negative effects; for example, the E4Orf6 function – involved in replication of AAV5 genomic DNA – also (with E1b) acts to degrade AAV5 capsid proteins and Rep52 [J Virol (2007) 81(5):2205–2212].)

The AAVs are parvoviruses in which the genome is linear ssDNA. Positive and negative strands of the viral DNA are encapsidated in separate virions.

It was reported earlier that, in human cells, AAV DNA (in the absence of helper virus) integrates in the genome with an apparent preference for CPG ISLANDS. More recently, AAVs have been reported to integrate, site-specifically, into a locus on chromosome 19, and the occurrence of such integration is apparently influenced by the TRP-185 protein [J Virol (2007) 81(4):1990–2001].

The AAVs infect a wide range of vertebrates. Initial stages of infection, including internalization of DNA, occur without a helper virus.

AAVs are used, for example, in GENE THERAPY. A caprine AAV, resistant to (human) neutralizing antibodies and with a marked tropism for (murine) lung tissue, has been suggested as a vector in CYSTIC FIBROSIS [J Virol (2005) 79:15238–15245].

AAV vectors, encoding genes of the α and the β subunits of hexosaminidase, were used in a mouse model (with intracranial inoculation) to evaluate the potential of gene therapy for the treatment of human GM2 gangliosidoses such as Tay–Sachs disease and Sandhoff disease [Proc Natl Acad Sci USA (2006) 103(27):10373–10378].

[Cloning of an avian AAV – an AAAV – and generation of recombinant AAAV particles: J Virol (2003) 77:6799–6810.]

AB1380 A strain of the yeast *Saccharomyces cerevisiae* (see entry SACCHAROMYCES).

(See also YEAST ARTIFICIAL CHROMOSOME.)

abacavir A NUCLEOSIDE REVERSE TRANSCRIPTASE INHIBITOR used e.g. in antiretroviral therapy; CSF–plasma ratios indicate that it may reach therapeutic levels in the CSF [Antimicrob Agents Chemother (2005) 49(6):2504–2506].

abasic site *Syn.* AP SITE.

ABC excinuclease See UVRABC-MEDIATED REPAIR.

Abelson murine leukemia virus See ABL.

abl (*ABL*) An ONCOGENE first identified in the Abelson murine leukemia virus. The v-*abl* product has TYROSINE KINASE activity. The human homolog of v-*abl*, c-*abl*, is usually present on chromosome 9; however, in the majority of patients with CHRONIC MYELOGENOUS LEUKEMIA it has been translocated to chromosome 22, forming a chimeric gene, known as *bcr-abl*, that encodes a tumor-specific tyrosine kinase (designated P210). Chromosome 22 containing the chimeric *bcr-abl* gene is called the Philadelphia chromosome (also referred to as Ph[1]).

Subcellular localization of c-Abl protein at an early stage in myogenic differentiation was reported to be influenced by its acetylation [EMBO Rep (2006) 7(7):727–733].

abortive transduction TRANSDUCTION in which the transduced DNA persists in a recipient cell as a stable, extrachromosomal but non-replicating molecule; when the recipient divides only one daughter cell receives the DNA fragment.

absorbance (ultraviolet) See ULTRAVIOLET ABSORBANCE.

abzyme *Syn.* CATALYTIC ANTIBODY.

Abzyme® A reagent kit (Abbott Laboratories) used for detecting antibodies in the context of hepatitis B.

acceptor splice site (acceptor splice junction) In pre-mRNA: the splice site (consensus AG) at the 3′ end of an intron.

(cf. DONOR SPLICE SITE.)

accession number (of a gene) A number that refers to the database entry for a specific gene. Some examples: (i) GenBank accession number X17012 refers to data on the gene for rat insulin-like growth factor II (IGF II); (ii) GenBank accession number AY024353 refers to data on the *ftsZ* gene of the bacterium *Sodalis glossinidius*; (iii) GenBank accession number AM160602 refers to data on the mRNA of the gene for cinnamyl alcohol dehydrogenase in the oak species *Quercus ilex*.

AccuPrime™ GC-rich DNA polymerase A DNA polymerase (Invitrogen, Carlsbad CA) optimized for DNA synthesis on difficult-to-amplify templates, including those with a GC content >65%.

AccuProbe® A family of PROBES (Gen-Probe, San Diego CA) used for identifying certain medically important bacteria by detecting specific sequences of nucleotides from lysed cells. The method involves a *hybridization protection assay*. In this assay, an added reagent cleaves the acridinium ester label on all *unbound* probes. Labels on the *bound* probes (which are protected from cleavage by virtue of their position in the probe–target duplex) react with a second reagent, producing a chemiluminescent (light) signal. The light produced by this reaction is measured in RLUs (i.e. relative light units). The threshold value (in RLUs) for a positive result must be carefully examined [see for example: J Clin Microbiol (2005) 43: 3474–3478].

(See also PACE 2C and TMA.)

acetosyringone An agent used e.g. for induction of the *virB* promoter in the plant pathogen *Agrobacterium tumefaciens*.

[Example of use: Infect Immun (2006) 74(1):108–117.]
(See also CROWN GALL.)

N-acetyl-L-cysteine See MUCOLYTIC AGENT.

acetylation (of histones) HISTONE acetylation is regulated e.g. by the opposing effects of: (i) histone deacetylases (HDACs) and (ii) histone acetyltransferases (HATs); (de)acetylation of histones can affect CHROMATIN structure, and may alter the accessibility of DNA for processes such as transcription and repair.

In a genomewide study of HDACs in *Schizosaccharomyces pombe* (a fission yeast), the patterns of histone acetylation, HDAC binding and nucleosome density were compared with gene expression profiles; it was found that different HDACs can have different roles in repression and activation of genes [EMBO J (2005) 24(16):2906–2918].

In (human) nucleosomes, the acetylation of certain lysine residues depends primarily on HATs, but the effect of these enzymes appears to be promoted by binding protein HMGN1 [EMBO J (2005) 24(17):3038–3048].

Acetylation of the histone *chaperone* NUCLEOPHOSMIN, as well as histone acetylation, apparently promotes transcription [Mol Cell Biol (2005) 25(17):7534–7545], while chaperone-stimulated, histone-acetylation-independent transcription has also been reported [Nucleic Acids Res (2007) 35:705–715].

The c-Abl protein (see ABL) has been identified as a substrate for the p300 and other histone acetyltransferases.

(See also TRICHOSTATIN A.)

N-acetylmuramidase See LYSOZYME.

ACF APOBEC-1 complementation factor: see RNA EDITING.

Achilles' heel technique Any technique in which a RESTRICTION ENDONUCLEASE is targeted to one *particular* recognition site when multiple copies of that site are freely available. One method uses a triplex-forming oligonucleotide to mask the required cleavage site. While masked, the remaining sites are methylated in order to inhibit subsequent cleavage; when the triplex is removed specific cleavage can be carried out.

(See also PROGRAMMABLE ENDONUCLEASE.)

aciclovir Alternative spelling for ACYCLOVIR.

acid-fast bacilli Those bacilli (i.e. rod-shaped bacteria) which, when stained with the Ziehl–Neelsen (or similar) stain, resist decolorization with mineral acid or an acid–alcohol mixture. This kind of staining method is used for screening respiratory specimens (such as samples of sputum) for *Mycobacterium tuberculosis* (a so-called acid-fast species).

AcMNPV *Autographa californica* NPV: see NUCLEAR POLYHEDROSIS VIRUSES.

AcNPV *Syn.* AcMNPV – see entry NUCLEAR POLYHEDROSIS VIRUSES.

acridines Heterocyclic, fluorescent compounds which bind to dsDNA (primarily as an INTERCALATING AGENT) and also to single-stranded nucleic acids (and to the backbone chains of double-stranded nucleic acids). Acridines have antimicrobial activity and are mutagenic; they are also used as stains for nucleic acids and can be used for CURING plasmids.

acridinium ester label (on probes) See ACCUPROBE.

acrocentric Refers to a CHROMOSOME in which the CENTROMERE is located close to one end.

acrydite hybridization assay An assay in which molecules of labeled ssDNA or ssRNA, passing through a polyacrylamide gel by electrophoresis, are captured (bound) by complementary oligonucleotides immobilized in a (central) 'capture zone' within the gel; all the molecules of nucleic acid that are *not* complementary to the capture oligos pass through the central capture zone and continue their migration to the end of the gel strip. The complementary oligos are synthesized with a 5′ terminal acrydite group which binds them to the polyacrylamide matrix so that they are immobilized in the gel. (Note that the central region of the gel strip is prepared separately.)

acrylamide A toxic, water-soluble agent (CH_2=CH–CONH$_2$) which can be polymerized to POLYACRYLAMIDE by catalysts such as N,N'-methylene-*bis*-acrylamide ('Bis') which promote cross-linking.

actinomycin C$_1$ *Syn.* ACTINOMYCIN D.

actinomycin D An antibiotic (a substituted phenoxazone linked to two pentapeptide lactone rings) produced by some species of *Streptomyces*; it acts as an INTERCALATING AGENT, binding to DNA and inhibiting DNA-dependent RNA polymerase. The drug has low affinity for AT-rich promoter regions; *initiation* of transcription from such promoters may be little affected by the antibiotic.

activation-induced cytidine deaminase (AID) An enzyme that occurs in germinal center B lymphocytes (B cells) and which is an absolute requirement for affinity maturation and class switching. HYPER-IGM SYNDROME has been associated with a deficiency of AID.
(See also CYTIDINE DEAMINASE and RNA EDITING.)

acyclovir (alternative spelling: aciclovir) 9-(2-hydroxyethoxymethyl) guanine: an antiviral agent which is active against a number of herpesviruses, including herpes simplex. In cells, acyclovir is phosphorylated to the monophosphate by (viral) thymidine kinase; subsequently it is converted to the (active) triphosphate form via host-encoded enzymes. The active drug inhibits *viral* DNA polymerase; the host cell's polymerase is much less sensitive.
In cells that are not virally infected, acyclovir appears not to be significantly phosphorylated.
Acyclovir has been used topically and systemically.

***N*-acyl-homocysteine thiolactone** See QUORUM SENSING.

***N*-acyl-L-homoserine lactone** (AHL) See QUORUM SENSING.

Ada protein (in *Escherichia coli*) See DNA REPAIR.

adaptamer See ORFMER SETS.

adaptive response (to alkylating agents) See DNA REPAIR.

AdEasy™ XL adenoviral vector system A system (Stratagene, La Jolla CA) which can be used for creating adenoviral vectors containing a specific gene/insert of interest.
Initially, the gene/insert is cloned in a small shuttle vector (~7 kb) which includes: (i) the left and right ITRs (inverted terminal repeats) of the adenovirus genome; (ii) two regions homologous to two sequences in another plasmid, pAdEasy-1 (see later), (iii) a gene encoding resistance to kanamycin; and (iv) a recognition site for the restriction endonuclease PmeI. After cloning, the shuttle vector is linearized (by cleavage with PmeI); linearization leaves the two homologous regions (see above) in terminal positions.

The linearized shuttle vector is inserted, by transformation, into a strain of *Escherichia coli*, BJ5183-AD-1, that already contains the (circular) plasmid vector pAdEasy-1. pAdEasy-1 (~33 kb) includes modified genomic DNA of human adenovirus serotype 5 (containing deletions in both the E1 and E3 regions). Homologous recombination occurs (intracellularly) between the linearized shuttle vector and homologous regions in pAdEasy-1; cells containing the recombinant plasmids are selected on kanamycin-containing media.

Recombinant plasmids are cleaved by restriction enzyme PacI, at selected sites, yielding a linear construct with adenoviral terminal sequences. This construct is used to transfect specialized, competent AD-293 cells – within which infective adenovirus virions are produced and released for subsequent use in gene-transfer and gene-expression studies in mammalian cells.

The AdEasy™ vector system has been used e.g. in studies on aptamer-regulated control of intracellular protein activity [Nucleic Acids Res (2006) 34(12):3577–3584].

The underlying principle of the AdEasy™ system has been exploited in the production of oncolytic adenovirus [BMC Biotechnol (2006) 6:36].

adefovir A NUCLEOSIDE REVERSE TRANSCRIPTASE INHIBITOR.

adenine phosphoribosyltransferase An enzyme (EC 2.4.2.7) which forms adenosine monophosphate (AMP) from adenine and 5-phosphoribosyl-1-diphosphate.
In humans, a deficiency of adenine phosphoribosyltransferase (an autosomal recessive disorder) can cause excretion of adenine (in the urine) and the formation of a highly insoluble product, 2,8-dihydroxyadenine, which can give rise to kidney stones and renal failure.

adeno-associated viruses See AAVS.

adeno-satellite viruses See AAVS.

adenosine A riboNUCLEOSIDE.

adenosine deaminase An enzyme (EC 3.5.4.4) which catalyzes the conversion of adenosine to inosine.

adenosine deaminase deficiency The congenital deficiency of a functional adenosine deaminase (EC 3.5.4.4) characterized by lack of normal development of T cells and a (consequent) marked immunodeficiency in which the patient is susceptible to infection by opportunist pathogens. This disorder has been treated successfully by GENE THERAPY.
(See also GENETIC DISEASE (table).)

adenovirus Any member of a family of non-enveloped, icosahedral viruses (genome: linear dsDNA) that infect mammals and birds; each type of adenovirus is commonly specific for one or a limited range of closely related host species.
Adenoviruses are widely used as vectors in various types of investigation, including GENE THERAPY. (See also ADEASY XL ADENOVIRAL VECTOR SYSTEM.) Adenoviruses have also been studied for their oncolytic potential [BMC Biotechnol

(2006) 6:36].

The adenovirus virion is ~70–90 nm in diameter; the capsid encloses a core containing genomic DNA (which is closely associated with an arginine-rich polypeptide). The 5′ end of each strand of the DNA is covalently linked to a hydrophobic 'terminal protein' (TP). The ends of the DNA are characterized by an inverted terminal repeat (ITR) – which varies in length in different types of adenovirus; the 5′ terminal residue is commonly dCMP.

During infection, the core enters the nucleus, releasing viral DNA. Replication of viral DNA involves TP and also a virus-encoded DNA polymerase as well as other virus- and host-encoded proteins. TP, synthesized in precursor form, binds covalently to DNA during replication and is later cleaved to the mature (DNA-bound) TP. A TP-mediated form of DNA replication also occurs in PHAGE φ29 (q.v.).

Expression of late viral genes, encoding structural proteins, is accompanied by the cessation of cellular protein synthesis. Some 10^5 virions may be formed within a single cell.

adenylate cyclase An enzyme (EC 4.6.1.1) which catalyzes the conversion of ATP to CYCLIC AMP.

In *Escherichia coli*, the activity of adenylate cyclase (*cya* gene product) is regulated e.g. via CATABOLITE REPRESSION.

In mammals, the enzyme forms part of a plasma membrane complex and is regulated e.g. via certain G proteins; it is activated by some bacterial exotoxins (e.g. PERTUSSIS TOXIN).

Anthrax toxin (EF component) and *cyclolysin* (a virulence factor synthesized by the Gram-negative bacterial pathogen *Bordetella pertussis*) both have adenylate cyclase activity which is stimulated by CALMODULIN.

adenylate kinase An enzyme (EC 2.7.4.3) which catalyzes the (reversible) conversion of two molecules of ADP to ATP and AMP.

ADP-ribosylation The transfer, to a protein, of an ADP-ribosyl group from NAD^+, mediated by ADP-ribosyltransferase (EC 2.4.2.30). In eukaryotes this can e.g. regulate the properties of HISTONES. In *Escherichia coli*, the RNA polymerase is ADP-ribosylated (with change in activity) following infection with bacteriophage T4.

ADP-ribosylation is an intracellular effect of some bacterial exotoxins (e.g. cholera toxin and PERTUSSIS TOXIN).

Polymerized ADP-ribosyl subunits (up to 50) may be found on certain eukaryotic proteins.

affinity capture electrophoresis Electrophoresis in a medium containing immobilized capture probes; it is used e.g. for the isolation of a given fragment of ssDNA, or a fragment of triplex-forming dsDNA.

(See also ACRYDITE HYBRIDIZATION ASSAY.)

affinity chromatography Chromatography in which specific molecules are isolated (adsorbed) owing to their affinity for an immobilized ligand – any non-specific unbound molecules being removed from the immobilized matrix. This procedure may be used e.g. for isolating/purifing a given type of molecule (see e.g. GENE FUSION (uses)).

Affinity® protein expression and purification A product of Stratagene (La Jolla CA) designed to facilitate the expression and purification of proteins expressed in prokaryotic systems; the product includes various pCAL plasmid vectors, shown in the diagram, each encoding a unique CALMODULIN-binding affinity tag.

Protein expression is maximized by a vector that includes a T7/LacO promoter system. In suitable strains of *Escherichia coli* (e.g. BL21(DE3)), T7 RNA polymerase is expressed in the presence of the inducer IPTG and drives expression from the T7/LacO promoter system on the plasmid. Tight control of expression is achieved with a plasmid-borne copy of *lacI*^{q}. Efficient translation of the protein of interest is promoted by using the strong ribosome-binding site (RBS) of T7 gene 10.

pCAL vectors contain a ColE1 origin of replication and an ampicillin-resistance gene.

All pCAL vectors encode a CALMODULIN-binding peptide (CBP) tag which forms a fusion product with the expressed protein and permits high-level purification following a single passage through CALMODULIN-AFFINITY RESIN. The (small)

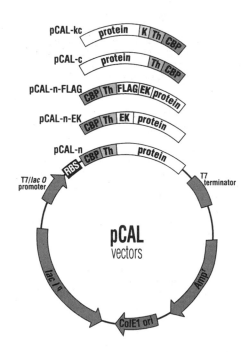

Affinity® PROTEIN EXPRESSION AND PURIFICATION The range of pCAL vectors (see entry for details of the method). CBP (in each vector) refers to calmodulin-binding peptide. EK = enterokinase; K = Kemptide sequence; Th = thrombin proteinase. (See also entry for FLAG.)

Courtesy of Stratagene, La Jolla CA, USA.

size of the CBP tag (about 4 kDa) may be expected to have a smaller effect on the protein of interest compared with larger tags such as 26-kDa glutathione *S*-transferase (GST) affinity tag.

One of the pCAL vectors includes a KEMPTIDE SEQUENCE which can be used e.g. for *in vitro* labeling of the expressed protein with protein kinase A (PKA) and ^{32}P.

All of the pCAL vectors include a cleavage site for enterokinase and/or thrombin proteinase.

One of the pCAL vectors includes a FLAG sequence.

affinity resin See e.g. NICKEL-CHARGED AFFINITY RESIN.

affinity tag *Syn.* AFFINITY TAIL.

affinity tail (affinity tag) That part of a FUSION PROTEIN (sense 2) which facilitates detection/isolation of the protein e.g. by an affinity resin or by AFFINITY CHROMATOGRAPHY.

Some affinity tails are small peptides. One advantage of using a small affinity tail is that it is less likely to interfere with the function of the fusion protein – so that its removal may not be necessary.

(See also FLAG, PESC VECTORS and SIX-HISTIDINE TAG.)

Large (protein) tails, for example glutathione *S*-transferase, may improve the solubility of the fusion protein but they may need subsequent removal in order to avoid interference with the function of the recombinant target protein.

(See also CHAMPION PET SUMO VECTOR.)

A highly temperature-stable affinity tail (a lectin, stable up to 80°C) may be useful for proteins originating from thermophilic organisms; the fusion proteins bind specifically to an agarose matrix containing D-mannose, and the affinity tail can by cleaved by an enterokinase [BioTechniques (2006) 41 (3):327–332].

(See also AFFINITY PROTEIN EXPRESSION AND PURIFICATION.)

aflatoxins Heat-stable toxins produced by certain fungi (strains of *Aspergillus flavus* and *A. parasiticus*); the molecule of an aflatoxin contains a bifuran moiety fused with a substituted coumarin. Aflatoxins have been associated with some cases of hepatocellular carcinoma. Different species may be affected in different ways by these toxins.

Aflatoxins may give rise to errors in DNA replication by reacting with guanine bases.

[Aflatoxin (biosynthesis genes): Appl Environ Microbiol (2005) 71:3192–3198.]

AFLP Either of *two distinct* PCR-based approaches for TYPING bacteria.

One approach ('amplified fragment length polymorphism') includes a number of variant forms of arbitrarily primed PCR (AP-PCR), including e.g. RAPD analysis.

The other approach, outlined here, involves initial digestion of genomic DNA by two types of RESTRICTION ENDONUCLEASE; it is sometimes called 'amplified restriction fragment length polymorphism' but this is incorrect [see original paper: Nucleic Acids Res (1995) 23:4407–4414].

In the digested genome each fragment is flanked by STICKY ENDS produced by one or other of the two types of restriction

enzyme. Two types of adaptor molecule (A, B) are added; the A molecules have *one* sticky end which binds to sites cleaved by one of the restriction enzymes, and B molecules have *one* sticky end that binds to sites cleaved by the other enzyme. A site cleaved by EcoRI (left) and a matching adaptor (right) is shown below:

```
5'-----NNG          AATTGNNNNN-3'
     -----NNCTTAA        CNNNNN
```

Fragment–adaptor binding is followed by ligation – but the cleavage site of EcoRI is *not* regenerated, avoiding repeated restriction. Fragments (with their adaptors) are amplified by PCR; each primer is complementary to a sequence covering part of an adaptor and the (contiguous) restriction site of the fragment. Each primer's 3′ end extends beyond the restriction site for one (or several) nucleotides; thus, a given primer will be extended only if the primer's 3′ terminal 'selective' nucleotide(s) align with *complementary* base(s) in the fragment. In the example given above, one template strand is:

```
5'-----NNGAATTGNNNNN-3'
```

and a primer with a deoxycytidine (C) selective 3′ nucleotide will bind as follows:

```
5'-----NNGAATTGNNNNN-3'
       CCTTAACNNNNN-5'   ← primer
```

The same principle holds for each primer-binding site: only some of the primers will be extended owing to the selective 3′ end. The PCR products undergo gel electrophoresis; bands of products (made visible e.g. by the use of labeled primers) form the *fingerprint*.

AFLP was highly discriminatory e.g. for *Clostridium botulinum* types A, B, E and F [Appl Environ Microbiol (2005) 71:1148–1154] but only limited intraspecies differences were reported in isolates of *Brucella* [J Clin Microbiol (2005) 43: 761–769].

AFM ATOMIC FORCE MICROSCOPY.

agar A complex mixture of galactans obtained from certain red algae (e.g. *Gelidium*); these compounds form part of the cell wall and/or intercellular matrix.

Agar comprises two main components: AGAROSE and agaropectin. Agaropectin is a mixture of sulfated galactans, some of which contain glucuronic acid and/or other constituents.

An agar gel is used as a matrix in many types of solid and semi-solid microbiological medium. This translucent, jelly-like material is prepared by heating a mixture of agar (e.g. 1.5% w/v) and water to >100°C and then cooling it to room temperature; gelling begins at ~40–45°C.

Agar can be an inhibitory factor in PCR (cf. GELLAN GUM).

agarose The major constituent of AGAR: a non-sulfated linear polymer consisting of alternating residues of D-galactose and 3,6-anhydro-L-galactose. Agarose is used e.g. as a medium in

GEL ELECTROPHORESIS for the separation of large fragments of nucleic acid.

(cf. POLYACRYLAMIDE.)

agnoprotein A regulatory protein, encoded by the JC VIRUS, which plays an important role in the infective cycle; it may be involved in facilitating the transport of virions from the nucleus (where virus assembly occurs) to the cytoplasm. It has been found that mutant, phosphorylated forms of agnoprotein are unable to sustain the viral infective cycle [J Virol (2006) 80(8):3893–3903].

Agrobacterium A genus of motile, Gram-negative bacteria that are found primarily in the rhizosphere (root environment of plants). GC% of genomic DNA: 57–63. Optimal temperature for growth: 25–28°C. Various mono- and disaccharides can be metabolized; glucose is metabolized e.g. via the Entner–Doudoroff pathway and the hexose monophosphate pathway.

Colonies which develop on media containing carbohydrates are generally mucilaginous, copious slime being formed.

Most species are pathogenic to plants. *A. tumefaciens* and *A. vitis* are causal agents of CROWN GALL.

(See also BINARY VECTOR SYSTEM.)

agroinfection A method for introducing viral DNA (or cDNA) into plant cells.

In the original procedure, viral DNA is inserted into the T-DNA region of the Ti plasmid of bacterium *Agrobacterium tumefaciens* (see the entry CROWN GALL for details of the Ti plasmid); thus, when infecting a plant, *A. tumefaciens* injects viral DNA (within the T-DNA) into plant cells.

Currently, the commonly used procedure involves the use of a *binary vector* system. In this approach the gene/sequence of interest is inserted into a small (binary) vector in which it is flanked, on each side, by the left border and right border of T-DNA. The binary vector, containing the gene, is inserted into an engineered strain of *Agrobacterium tumefaciens* that contains the *vir* (virulence) region of the Ti plasmid which is concerned with the transfer of DNA into plant cells. This strain is then used to infect a plant. When the *vir* genes are activated, DNA from the *binary vector* (specifically, DNA from the section bracketed by the left and right borders of T-DNA) is transferred into the plant cells, such transfer being mediated by factors encoded by the *vir* region acting in *trans*.

[Example of agroinfection: J Virol (2003) 77:3247–3256.]

In the development of transgenic plants it is desirable to minimize the content of extraneous DNA which is transferred to plant cells through the vector system, particularly when such plants are to be made available in a general agricultural setting; the content of extraneous DNA is covered by certain laws that relate to transgenic plants. To this end, a number of minimal T-DNA vectors have been proposed [BioTechniques (2006) 41(6):708–710].

(See also FLORAL DIP METHOD.)

AGT O^6-alkylguanine-DNA alkyltransferase: see 'Uses of gene fusion' in the entry GENE FUSION.

AHL (*N*-acyl-L-homoserine lactone) See QUORUM SENSING.

ahpC gene See ISONIAZID.

AHT (*N*-acyl-homocysteine thiolactone) See QUORUM SENSING.

AID ACTIVATION-INDUCED CYTIDINE DEAMINASE.

AIDS Acquired immune deficiency syndrome. An HIV$^+$ person with AIDS has counts of CD4$^+$ T cells below a certain level and, additionally, the presence of one or more types of AIDS-defining disease (such as: candidiasis of the *lower* respiratory tract, retinitis with CMV (cytomegalovirus), *extra*pulmonary infection with *Mycobacterium tuberculosis*, pneumonia due to *Pneumocystis carinii* etc.).

alanine scan mutagenesis A method for studying the binding properties (or other characteristics) of particular residues in a protein by replacing them with alanine residues; replacement can be achieved during synthesis of the protein (from a modified mRNA) or by exchanging residues in the protein itself. After insertion of alanine residues the protein is examined for properties/function.

alarmone Any of various low-molecular-weight molecules that are able to mediate some change in cellular metabolism as a response to a particular type of stress. One example is ppGpp which is formed in the stringent response in *Escherichia coli*.

albamycin Syn. NOVOBIOCIN.

(See also ANTIBIOTIC (table).)

AlgZ In *Pseudomonas aeruginosa*: a DNA-binding protein reported to regulate twitching motility (due to type IV fimbriae) as well as alginate biosynthesis [J Bacteriol (2006) 188(1): 132–140].

AlkA protein See DNA REPAIR.

alkaline phosphatase (AP) An enzyme (EC 3.1.3.1; maximum stability at pH ~7.5–9.5) used e.g. for removing 5′ terminal phosphate groups from nucleic acids. When it is bound e.g. to streptavidin, it is also used as a label (see BIOTIN) which can be detected by various types of chromogenic substrate.

(See also CHEMILUMINESCENCE.)

AttoPhos™ is used as a substrate for alkaline phosphatase in a CROSS-LINKING ASSAY.

(See also ELISA.)

alkaline stripping Stripping of hybridized RNA probes from a DNA MICROARRAY by degradation with buffers that contain NaOH (sodium hydroxide) under carefully regulated conditions (e.g. temperatures of 60–62°C). A stripped microarray can be used again, reducing costs, but a microarray cannot be stripped *twice* without loss of quality. Microarrays which had been stripped once gave results similar to those from virgin (non-stripped) arrays [BioTechniques (2005) 38:121–124].

O^6-**alkylguanine-DNA alkyltransferase** (AGT) See 'Uses of gene fusion' in the entry GENE FUSION.

allele (allelomorph) Any one of two or more different versions of a particular GENE; the product or function of a given allele may exhibit qualitative and/or quantitative difference(s) from the product or function of other alleles of that gene.

In a diploid cell or organism, if an allelic pair (i.e. the two alleles of a given gene) consists of two identical alleles then the cell/organism is said to be *homozygous* for that particular gene; if different, the cell/organism is said to be *heterozygous* for the gene.

allele-specific DNA methylation analysis A method, designed for determining allele-specific methylation, which involves PCR-amplification of BISULFITE-treated DNA followed by PYROSEQUENCING of each allele, individually – using allele-specific primers. The method was demonstrated by analyzing methylation of the *H19* gene in which only the paternal allele is usually imprinted [BioTechniques (2006) 41(6):734–739].

allele-specific PCR A variant form of PCR designed to amplify a particular allele of a given gene – but no other allele(s) of that gene. One of the two primers is designed with a 3′ terminal nucleotide that pairs with a *specific* base in the required allele – a base which is known to be different from that in the other allele(s) at this location; this primer can be extended on the required allele, which will be amplified. Other alleles will not be amplified because the mismatch at the primer's 3′ terminal will inhibit extension.

An essential requirement is the use of a polymerase which *lacks* proofreading ability (i.e. one which lacks 3′-to-5′ exonuclease activity); such an enzyme (e.g. the *Taq* polymerase) is not able to remove the primer's terminal nucleotide (i.e. it cannot correct the mismatch) and does not amplify unwanted alleles.

It is also important to carry out the reaction with an appropriate level of stringency.

A modified form of this method is found e.g. in SNP GENOTYPING.

allelic pair See ALLELE.

allelomorph *Syn.* ALLELE.

allolactose β-D-Galactopyranosyl-(1→6)-D-glucopyranose: the natural inducer of the LAC OPERON in *Escherichia coli*; it is formed as a minor product during the cleavage of lactose by β-glucosidase.

(See also IPTG.)

allosteric effect The effect produced when the binding of a ligand to a particular target molecule affects the properties of other site(s) on the same molecule; allosteric effects are due to conformational changes that result from the binding of the ligand.

allosteric nucleic acid enzymes Nucleic acid enzymes (see e.g. APTAZYME) whose function can be subject to regulation e.g. by the activity of a low-molecular-weight molecule – or the activity of an oligonucleotide.

(See BINARY DEOXYRIBOZYME LIGASE and MAXIZYME.)

alpha (α, *Lk*) A symbol for LINKING NUMBER.

alpha peptide (α-peptide) See entry α-PEPTIDE.

alternation of generations See PLOIDY.

alternative splicing SPLICING of a given pre-mRNA which can proceed in at least two different ways; the different modes of splicing produce mRNAs with different sequences.

Alternative splicing is a common (i.e. natural) phenomenon [Nucleic Acids Res (2004) 32(13):3977–3983] which allows a given gene to encode extra information. Thus, e.g. a given gene may encode two mutually antagonistic messages (whose expression must be under appropriate control). Exceptionally,

it is reported that a single gene may potentially give rise to >100 different transcripts.

Events that may occur during alternative splicing include the splicing out (loss) of an exon (*exon skipping*), inclusion of an intron (*intron retention*) and/or splicing at a site *within* an exon.

The regulation of (normal) alternative splicing involves a balance between certain factors which promote or inhibit the use of specific splicing sites in pre-mRNA.

Splicing of pre-mRNA of the *bcl-x* gene can produce a long (anti-apoptotic) mRNA and a short (pro-apoptotic) mRNA; the content of these mRNAs in the cell is a key determinant of cancer progression. Splicing has been modulated, *in vitro* and *in vivo*, by means of a short antisense PNA conjugated to an oligopeptide containing eight serine–arginine repeats (cf. SR PROTEINS); this procedure produced apoptosis in HeLa (cancer) cells [Nucleic Acids Res (2005) 33(20):6547–6554].

In public databases, sequences of many cancer-associated genes are reported to reflect tumor-associated, *atypical* splice forms (rather than normal splice forms) [Nucleic Acids Res (2005) 33(16):5026–5033].

In a comparative study on eight organisms, the extent of alternative splicing was reported to be higher in vertebrates than in invertebrates [Nucleic Acids Res (2007) 35(1):125–131].

(See also EXON TRAPPING.)

Alu sequences (*Alu* sequences) In (at least) some mammalian genomes: a family of related sequences, each typically about 300 nt long and commonly having a recognition site for the RESTRICTION ENDONUCLEASE AluI (AG↓CT); the human genome may contain about one million copies. Alu sequences are RETROTRANSPOSONS; owing to their ability to generate insertional mutations they are regarded as potential factors in genetic disorders.

Alu sequences in the human genome may be undergoing active transposition [amplification of Alu sequences: PLoS Comput Biol (2005) 1(4):e44 and Genome Res (2005) 15(5): 655–664].

(See also SINE and LINE.)

AluI A RESTRICTION ENDONUCLEASE from *Arthrobacter luteus*; recognition site: AG↓CT.

α-amanitin A cyclic peptide which, at low concentrations, can inhibit (eukaryotic) DNA-dependent RNA polymerase II.

amber codon See NONSENSE CODON.

amber mutation A mutation that creates an amber codon (see NONSENSE CODON).

amber suppressor See SUPPRESSOR MUTATION.

ambisense RNA Viral ssRNA in which some gene(s) occur in positive-sense form and other(s) in negative-sense form.

amelogenin A protein associated with dental development. A gene encoding human amelogenin (*AMELX*) occurs on the X chromosome (at location Xp22.3–Xp22.1) and another gene encoding amelogenin (*AMELY*) occurs on the Y chromosome (location Yp11.2).

The amelogenin genes are exploited e.g. in a gender identification assay: see DNA SEX DETERMINATION ASSAY.

AMELX gene   See AMELOGENIN.

AMELY gene   See AMELOGENIN.

Ames strain (of *Bacillus anthracis*)   See BACTERIA (table).

Ames test (Mutatest; *Salmonella*/microsome assay)   A test used to determine whether a given agent is mutagenic (and therefore possibly carcinogenic) by investigating its ability to *reverse* an auxotrophic mutation in *Salmonella typhimurium*; the mutation in *S. typhimurium* makes the organism dependent on an exogenous source of histidine, and reversal of the mutation would allow the organism to synthesize its own histidine (i.e. it would revert to prototrophy). Different strains of *S. typhimurium* may be used, each with a different type of mutation in the histidine operon. Some of these test strains may also contain mutations which make them more permeable to certain chemicals and/or which prevent them from carrying out DNA repair. Moreover, the test strains may contain the plasmid pKM101 which includes genes for so-called error-prone repair and which therefore promotes the mutagenic effects of any DNA-damaging agents present in the reaction.

Because some chemical agents exhibit mutagenic activity only after their metabolic activation, the test system generally includes microsomal enzymes from a liver homogenate (the 9000 *g* supernatant, fraction 'S9') from rats pre-treated with a carcinogen to induce production of the appropriate enzymes.

When performed as a 'plate incorporation test', a culture of *S. typhimurium*, an S9 preparation and the substance under test are mixed with soft agar (which includes a low level of histidine) and this is poured onto a plate of *minimal agar* – which is then incubated at 37°C in the dark. (Minimal agar permits the growth of prototrophs but does not permit growth of the (auxotrophic) test strain of *S. typhimurium*.) The low level of histidine in the soft agar allows (only) limited growth of the (auxotrophic) *S. typhimurium* and this results in a light, confluent growth of this organism in the upper layer of agar (the 'top agar').

If the test substance had caused reversion to prototrophy in any cells of the test strain, those cells (whose growth would not be limited) can grow and form visible colonies.

When interpreting the results, several factors must be borne in mind. An absence of growth in the 'top agar' would suggest that the substance under test has general antibacterial activity, and that any colonies which develop on the plate are unlikely to be true revertants. Again, before drawing conclusions from a number of *apparent* revertant colonies, it is necessary to take into account the known *spontaneous* reversion rate of the particular mutation in the given test strain.

Various modifications of the basic Ames test are used for specific purposes.

[Ames test with a derivative of carbamic acid: Antimicrob Agents Chemother (2005) 49:1160–1168.]

(See also SOS CHROMOTEST.)

amikacin   See AMINOGLYCOSIDE ANTIBIOTICS.

amino acid   A term which, in the present context, usually refers to one of the 20 compounds whose residues are components of oligopeptides, polypeptides and proteins (see table).

Ornithine is just one example of an amino acid which is not represented by a CODON but which is nevertheless found e.g. in certain oligopeptide antibiotics; this kind of oligopeptide is synthesized by a ribosome-free enzyme system (rather than by translation) (see NON-RIBOSOMAL PEPTIDE SYNTHETASE).

aminoglycoside antibiotic   Any of a group of broad-spectrum antibiotics in which the molecular structure typically includes an aminosugar and either 2-deoxystreptamine or streptidine; these antibiotics bind to the bacterial 30S ribosomal subunit and inhibit protein synthesis.

The aminoglycosides include amikacin, framycetin, gentamicin, hygromycin B, kanamycin, neomycin, streptomycin and tobramycin; they are typically bactericidal (at appropriate concentrations) and are active against a wide range of Gram-positive and Gram-negative species.

Resistance to aminoglycosides can arise e.g. by (i) mutation in proteins of the ribosomal 30S subunit (affecting the binding of antibiotics); (ii) inactivation of antibiotics by bacterial enzymes which e.g. carry out *N*-acetylation or *O*-phosphorylation; (iii) decreased uptake by the cell.

(See also G418 SULFATE.)

AMP CT   Amplified *Chlamydia trachomatis* test: a TMA-based assay used for detecting the pathogen *Chlamydia trachomatis* in clinical specimens (Gen-Probe, San Diego CA). One early study [J Clin Microbiol (1997) 35:676–678] examined urine specimens from female patients as a non-invasive method of diagnosing chlamydial infection; both the AMP CT assay and a PCR-based method were found to be sensitive and specific methods for detecting *C. trachomatis* and it was concluded that both methods were suitable screening procedures.

ampholyte   Any electrolyte with both acidic and basic groups.

ampicillin   6(α-aminobenzylamido)-penicillanic acid: a semi-synthetic PENICILLIN used in media e.g. as a selective agent for bacteria containing a vector with an ampicillin-resistance marker gene.

amplicon   (1) A specific (precise) sequence of nucleotides, part of a larger nucleic acid molecule, copied (amplified) by an *in vitro* amplification process such as NASBA or PCR.

(2) One of the copies of a sequence of nucleotides which has been copied (amplified) by methods such as NASBA or PCR.

(3) One of a number of elements of linear DNA (~100 kb) formed in studies on the *JBP1* gene of *Leishmania tarentolae* [term used in: Nucleic Acids Res (2005) 33(5):1699–1709].

(4) *Formerly*: a defective virus vector.

(5) Within a Y chromosome: a region with >99% sequence identity to other region(s) in the same chromosome (hence *adj.* ampliconic). [Use of term: BMC Genet (2007) 8:11.]

amplicon containment   One approach to the minimization of contamination by amplicons from previous assays in methods such as PCR. Essentially, this involves division of the working environment into several dedicated areas, each of which is used for only certain specific stage(s) of the procedure. For example, when working with PCR, it is usual to carry out the thermal cycling and the analysis of products (e.g. electro-

AMINO ACIDS: symbols, molecular weights and codons

Amino acid	1-letter symbol	3-letter symbol	Molecular weight	Codons
Alanine	A	Ala	89	GCA, GCC, GCG, GCU
Arginine	R	Arg	174	AGA, AGG, CGA, CGC, CGG, CGU
Asparagine	N	Asn	150	AAC, AAU
Aspartic acid	D	Asp	133	GAC, GAU
Cysteine	C	Cys	121	UGC, UGU
Glutamic acid	E	Glu	147	GAA, GAG
Glutamine	Q	Gln	146	CAA, CAG
Glycine	G	Gly	75	GGA, GGC, GGG, GGU
Histidine	H	His	155	CAC, CAU
Isoleucine	I	Ile	131	AUA, AUC, AUU
Leucine	L	Leu	131	CUA, CUC, CUG, CUU, UUA, UUG
Lysine	K	Lys	146	AAA, AAG
Methionine	M	Met	149	AUG
Phenylalanine	F	Phe	165	UUC, UUU
Proline	P	Pro	115	CCA, CCC, CCG, CCU
Serine	S	Ser	105	AGC, AGU, UCA, UCC, UCG, UCU
Threonine	T	Thr	119	ACA, ACC, ACG, ACU
Tryptophan	W	Trp	204	UGG
Tyrosine	Y	Tyr	181	UAC, UAU
Valine	V	Val	117	GUA, GUC, GUG, GUU

phoresis) in separate areas, and separate areas may also be specified for extracting target nucleic acid and for preparing reagents.

(See also AMPLICON INACTIVATION.)

amplicon inactivation In PCR: any method which avoids contamination by destroying carry-over amplicons from previous assays. Such contamination can be a major problem e.g. in those clinical laboratories in which specimens are examined routinely for only a small number of target sequences; under these conditions new specimens may risk contamination if amplicons are allowed to build up in the laboratory environment (e.g. in/on equipment or in reagents).

Methods for amplicon inactivation

The uracil-N-glycosylase method. In this method, *all* assays are conducted in the normal way except that deoxythymidine triphosphate (dTTP) is replaced by deoxyuridine triphosphate (dUTP) in the reaction mixture. All amplicons produced in each assay therefore contain dUMP instead of dTMP. These amplicons can be analysed in the normal way by gel electrophoresis etc.

In addition to the use of dUTP, the reaction mixture also includes the enzyme URACIL-N-GLYCOSYLASE (UNG). Thus, if an assay is contaminated with amplicons from a previous assay, these amplicons will act as substrates for the enzyme, uracil being cleaved from each dUMP; this, in itself, does not bring about strand breakage, but the amplicons are degraded to non-amplifiable pieces by the high temperature used for the initial denaturation of target DNA. The high temperature also inactivates UNG; this is necessary in order to avoid degradation of amplicons from the current assay. (The target DNA in the reaction is not affected by UNG as it contains dTMP.)

Normally this method cannot be used in PCR-based studies of DNA methylation in which the sample DNA is treated with BISULFITE; this is because bisulfite treatment converts non-methylated cytosines to uracil, so that the template DNA itself would be subjected to degradation. However, unlike the usual form of bisulfite treatment (in which DNA is sulfonated and is subsequently desulfonated), it has been found that non-desulfonated DNA can be amplified by PCR with the UNG method of decontamination because this (sulfonated) form of DNA is resistant to UNG. Desulfonation of DNA is achieved by a prolonged (30-minute) initial stage of denaturation (at 95°C) [Nucleic Acids Res (2007) 35(1)e4].

The isopsoralen method. In this method isopsoralen is added to the reaction mixture. Isopsoralen is a heterocyclic compound which, when bound to DNA, can form covalent inter-strand crosslinks when photoactivated by ultraviolet radiation (e.g. 365 nm/15 min/4°C); activation of isopsoralen at low temperatures has been reported to be more efficient than at room temperature. Because the (double-stranded) amplicons are covalently crosslinked they cannot be denatured to single strands; this means that they cannot serve as templates, and if they were to contaminate a subsequent assay the outcome would not be affected.

Amplicons produced by this method are suitable for examination by processes such as gel electrophoresis and staining (e.g. for confirming the presence of a given target sequence in the sample DNA). However, they cannot be used for any process (such as SSCP analysis) that requires single-stranded samples.

In a different approach to amplicon inactivation, all the primers have a 5′ tag which incorporates a binding site for a type IIS restriction endonuclease; this enzyme, in the reaction mixture, cleaves any contaminating amplicons and is itself inactivated at the initial high-temperature stage (see APSR).

amplicon primer site restriction   See APSR.

ampliconic   See AMPLICON (sense 5).

amplification (of DNA *in vitro*)   See DNA AMPLIFICATION.

amplification-refractory mutation system   See ARMS.

amplified fragment length polymorphism (AFLP)   See AFLP.

amplified restriction fragment length polymorphism (AFLP)   See AFLP.

Ampligase®   See DNA LIGASE.

amplimer   Any primer used in PCR.

AmpliWax™   See HOT-START PCR.

AMPPD®   A 1,2-dioxetane substrate that emits light when de-phosphorylated by ALKALINE PHOSPHATASE (AP). It is used e.g. for detecting AP-labeled probes.

   (See also CHEMILUMINESCENCE.)

amprenavir   See PROTEASE INHIBITORS.

AMTDT   Amplified *Mycobacterium tuberculosis* direct test: a TMA-based assay for detecting *Mycobacterium tuberculosis* in clinical specimens (Gen-Probe, San Diego CA).

The AMTDT was approved in 1995 by the American FDA (Food and Drug Administration) for use with *smear-positive* respiratory specimens; a smear-positive specimen is one from which a smear showing ACID-FAST BACILLI can be prepared. In the original form of the test, the sample was initially treated with a MUCOLYTIC AGENT, then 'decontaminated' with sodium hydroxide, and finally subjected to sonication to lyse organisms and release nucleic acids. The specimen was then heated (95°C/15 minutes) to remove intra-strand base-pairing in the rRNA.

The reaction mixture contained 45 μL or 50 μL of sample, and amplification (at 42°C) was conducted for 2 hours. The amplification product was detected by the addition of target-specific probes (for details see entry ACCUPROBE).

An attempt was made to adapt AMTDT for the detection of *Mycobacterium tuberculosis* in *non*-respiratory specimens [J Clin Microbiol (1997) 35:307–310], and studies were made to compare the original and subsequent (improved) versions of AMTDT for the detection of *M. tuberculosis* in respiratory and non-respiratory specimens [J Clin Microbiol (1998) 36: 684–689].

The new-format 'enhanced' AMTDT was approved by the FDA in 1998. Among other changes, this version involved the use of a 450 μL aliquot of the sample.

One study reported false-positive results in tests on sputa from patients infected with *Mycobacterium kansasii* and *M. avium*; these species of *Mycobacterium* are not infrequently isolated from infections in immunocompromised patients. The authors of this study suggested a change in the threshold value of luminometer readings considered to be an indication of a positive result [J Clin Microbiol (1999) 37:175–178].

anaerobic respiration   RESPIRATION (q.v.) in the absence of oxygen.

analyte   In a test system: the component whose properties are studied/measured.

anchor primer   A primer that binds to an ANCHOR SEQUENCE.

anchor sequence   Commonly, a sequence of nucleotides, with a known composition, which is present in a given molecule or which is ligated to another sequence (or added by tailing) in order to serve a particular function – e.g. as a primer-binding site. For example, in ANCHORED PCR an anchor sequence is used to provide an otherwise unavailable site for priming the amplification of an unknown sequence.

Certain natural sequences – e.g. the poly(A) tail on many mRNA molecules – are referred to as anchor sequences.

anchored PCR   A form of PCR used for amplifying an unknown sequence of nucleotides adjacent to a known sequence on a fragment of DNA; this approach addresses the problem of the lack of a primer-binding site in the unknown sequence.

To each end of the fragment is ligated a short segment of DNA of known sequence (e.g. a linker). (If the fragment has 3′ or 5′ overhangs then these can be eliminated enzymatically in order to prepare the fragment for blunt-ended ligation to the linkers.) After ligation, the linker contiguous with the unknown region provides an ANCHOR SEQUENCE which can serve as a primer-binding site for one of the PCR primers. The second primer is designed to bind at a site within the known sequence. If PCR is primed in this way, the resulting amplicons will include the unknown sequence and at least part of the known sequence. If the known sequence occurs in the *center* of the fragment, then amplification, as described above, can be carried out for both of the unknown flanking regions.

(See also VECTORETTE PCR.)

anchoring enzyme In SAGE (q.v.): a name sometimes given to the enzyme used for initial cleavage of the cDNAs.

aneuploid Refers to a genome that has one or more chromosomes in excess of, or less than, the number characteristic of the species (see e.g. DOWN'S SYNDROME).

Angelman syndrome A genetically based disorder which may be caused by any of various mechanisms – see table in entry GENETIC DISEASE for further details.

annealing The hybridization of two complementary (or near-complementary) sequences of nucleotides to form a double-stranded molecule or a double-stranded region within a larger molecule (e.g. the binding of primers to primer-binding sites in PCR).

annotation The assignment of a (predicted) function to an uncharacterized gene (and/or attempted characterization of the gene product) based on sequence homology with a gene of known function present in another organism.

antagomir Any of a range of synthetic, chemically engineered oligonucleotides that bind to, and antagonize, specific types of MICRORNA molecule. Intravenous administration (in mice) of antagomirs directed against particular miRNAs resulted in efficient and specific silencing of the given miRNAs [Nature (2005) 438:685–689].

anthrax toxin A toxin, produced by the Gram-positive pathogen *Bacillus anthracis*, which gives rise to the symptoms of anthrax. It comprises three protein components – each, alone, being unable to function as a toxin; these three proteins are encoded by the plasmid pXO1. Another plasmid, pXO2, is needed for the pathogenicity of *B. anthracis*; this encodes an essential anti-phagocytic capsule which protects the organism from the host's immune system.

One component of the toxin localizes in the cell membrane and permits internalization of the other two components – a zinc protease (which disrupts intracellular signaling) and an ADENYLATE CYCLASE (which e.g. promotes edema).

anti Abbreviation for ANTICLINAL.

antibiotic Any of an extensive range of natural, semi-synthetic and fully synthetic compounds which, in low concentrations, are able selectively to inhibit or kill specific types of microorganism and, in some cases, other types of cell – e.g. tumor cells; an antibiotic acts at specific site(s) in a susceptible cell. (Compounds that are active against *viruses* are usually called 'antiviral agents' rather than antibiotics.) Natural antibiotics (see e.g. BACTERIOCIN) have ecological roles. Some types of antibiotic have medical/veterinary uses in the prevention and/or treatment of infectious diseases, while some are used e.g. as food preservatives.

In nucleic-acid-based technology, antibiotics are used in a variety of selective procedures. In one common scenario, the presence of a given antibiotic in a growth medium permits positive selection of cells which are expressing a gene that confers resistance to that particular antibiotic. The gene may be included e.g. in a vector used for the transformation of a population of cells – those cells which internalize the vector (and express the antibiotic-resistance gene) being selected by growth on an antibiotic-containing medium.

Some antibiotics are MICROBICIDAL, others are MICROBISTATIC; a microbicidal antibiotic may behave as a microbistatic antibiotic at lower concentrations.

A mixture of antibiotics may behave synergistically or antagonistically (or may not display either effect).

Synergism is shown when different antibiotics, that are acting simultaneously on a given organism, produce an effect which is greater than the sum of their individual effects. For example, the antibiotics sulfamethoxazole and trimethoprim block different reactions in the same major metabolic pathway: sulfamethoxazole inhibits the formation of dihydrofolic acid (DHF), and trimethoprim inhibits the conversion of DHF to the important coenzyme tetrahydrofolate (THF); these two antibiotics act synergistically and they are used, together, in the therapeutic agent *cotrimoxazole*.

Antagonism, the converse of synergism, can occur in different ways. In one form, an antibiotic that inhibits growth (e.g. CHLORAMPHENICOL) antagonizes those antibiotics (such as the penicillins and other β-lactam antibiotics) whose activity depends on growth in the target cell. In a different form of antagonism, certain antibiotics stimulate cells to produce enzymes that inactivate *other* antibiotics; for example, the β-lactam imipenem (or cefoxitin) induces the synthesis of β-lactamases – enzymes which can inactivate certain other β-lactam antibiotics.

Modes of action

To be effective at all, an antibiotic must be able to enter, or pass through, the cell envelope in order to reach the relevant target site(s). Moreover, an antibiotic can be effective against a given population of cells only if its concentration is above the appropriate minimum level for that agent under the given conditions.

Modes of action include:

● Interference with DNA gyrase (a topoisomerase), with consequent inhibition of DNA synthesis (e.g. novobiocin, quinolone antibiotics).

● Depletion of guanine nucleotides (by inhibiting synthesis of GMP), affecting synthesis of nucleic acids (e.g. mycophenolic acid).

● Binding to ribosomes and inhibiting protein synthesis (e.g. aminoglycoside antibiotics, chloramphenicol, macrolide antibiotics (such as erythromycin), tetracyclines, viomycin).

● Binding to RNA polymerase, inhibiting transcription (e.g. rifamycins).

● Disruption of the bacterial cytoplasmic membrane, altered permeability affecting the cell's integrity (e.g. gramicidins, polymyxins).

● Inhibition of synthesis of the bacterial cell wall polymer peptidoglycan, leading to cell lysis (e.g. β-lactam antibiotics, vancomycin).

● Inhibition of the enzyme dihydrofolate reductase, thereby inhibiting tetrahydrofolate-dependent reactions (that include

ANTIBIOTIC: some antibiotics used in DNA technology (e.g. for marker selection)

Antibiotic	Group	Target organisms	Antibiotic action
Actinomycin D	–	Prokaryotic and eukaryotic	Intercalating agent; inhibits DNA-dependent RNA polymerase
Ampicillin	β-Lactams	Bacteria	Blocks synthesis of cell-wall polymer peptidoglycan
Blasticidin S	Nucleoside	Prokaryotic and eukaryotic	Inhibits protein synthesis by inhibiting the peptidyltransferase-mediated reaction at the ribosome
Carbenicillin	β-Lactams	Bacteria	Blocks synthesis of cell-wall polymer peptidoglycan
Cefotaxime	β-Lactams	Bacteria (mainly Gram-negative)	Blocks synthesis of cell-wall polymer peptidoglycan
Chloramphenicol (= chloromycetin)	–	Bacteria (broad spectrum), some fungi	Binds to prokaryotic and mitochondrial ribosomes; inhibits peptidyltransferase and (hence) protein synthesis
G418 sulfate	Related to gentamicin	Prokaryotes, yeasts, plants, mammalian cells	Inhibits protein synthesis
Gentamicin	Aminoglycosides	Bacteria	Binds to 30S subunit of bacterial ribosomes and inhibits protein synthesis
Hygromycin B	Aminoglycosides	Mammalian and plant cells	Inhibits protein synthesis
Kanamycin	Aminoglycosides	Bacteria	Binds to 30S subunit of bacterial ribosomes and inhibits protein synthesis
Kasugamycin	Aminoglycosides	Bacteria, some fungi	Inhibits polypeptide chain initiation and, hence, protein synthesis
Mycophenolic acid	–	Bacteria (also antitumor agent)	Inhibits synthesis of guanosine monophosphate, inhibiting synthesis of nucleic acids
Nalidixic acid	Quinolones	Bacteria (mainly Gram-negative)	Inhibits function of the A subunit of gyrase; inhibits DNA synthesis
Novobiocin	–	Bacteria	Inhibits binding of ATP to the B subunit of gyrase, inhibiting DNA synthesis
Penicillin G (= benzylpenicillin)	β-Lactams	Bacteria (mainly Gram-positive)	Blocks synthesis of cell-wall polymer peptidoglycan
Polymyxin B	Polymyxins	Bacteria (mainly Gram-negative)	Increases permeability of the cytoplasmic membrane and affects the integrity of the outer membrane
Puromycin	Nucleoside	Prokaryotic and eukaryotic	Inhibits protein synthesis by acting as an analog of part of an aminoacyl-tRNA
Rifampicin	Rifamycins	Bacteria (mainly Gram-positive)	Inhibits DNA-dependent RNA polymerase by binding to the β subunit of the enzyme
Streptomycin	Aminoglycosides	Bacteria, some fungi	Interacts with ribosomes and inhibits protein synthesis
Tetracycline	Tetracyclines	Bacteria	Binds to ribosomes; inhibits protein synthesis by blocking the binding of aminoacyl-tRNAs to the A site
Zeocin™	Bleomycin/ phleomycin	Bacteria, yeast, and mammalian cells	Binds to, and cleaves, DNA

synthesis of deoxythymidine – and, hence, DNA) (e.g. pyrimethamine, trimethoprim).

● Interference with DNA function by intercalating agents (e.g. actinomycin D, quinoxaline antibiotics).

● Interaction with sterols in the cytoplasmic membrane (in e.g. yeasts and other fungi), causing leakage (e.g. polyene antibiotics).

● Inhibition of the enzyme chitin synthase (in certain fungi), affecting cell wall synthesis (e.g. polyoxins).

Mechanisms of bacterial resistance to antibiotics
Resistance to a particular antibiotic is constitutive in those cells which (i) lack the antibiotic's specific target, (ii) have a variant form of the target which is not susceptible to the antibiotic, and (iii) are impermeable to the antibiotic. Examples: (i) *Mycoplasma* is resistant to β-lactam antibiotics because it lacks a cell wall; (ii) strains of *Staphylococcus aureus* known as MRSA (methicillin-resistant *S. aureus*) generally contain a modified target which is not susceptible to methicillin; (iii) typically, Gram-negative bacteria are insensitive to penicillin G (a β-lactam antibiotic) because this antibiotic is not able to penetrate the outer membrane of Gram-negative bacteria.

As well as constitutive resistance (see above) resistance can also be acquired e.g. by mutation or by the acquisition of plasmid or transposon gene(s) specifying resistance to one or more antibiotics. Examples include:

● Due to mutation, the target of a given antibiotic may be altered so that it fails to bind the antibiotic; consequently, the target (e.g. an enzyme) is not affected by otherwise inhibitory concentrations of that antibiotic. Thus, a mutant form of the ribosomal protein L22 in *Staphylococcus aureus* confers resistance to quinupristin/dalfopristin (Synercid®), a streptogramin, and in *Mycobacterium tuberculosis* point mutations in the *rpoB* gene (encoding the β subunit of RNA polymerase) can confer resistance to rifamycins (such as rifampin) for which RNA polymerase is the target.

● Transposon Tn*10* encodes an inducible efflux system that enables certain Gram-negative bacteria to externalize tetracycline via an 'efflux pump' located in the cell envelope.

● Mutant forms of some envelope proteins are associated with decreased permeability. For example, alteration in outer membrane porins in *Enterobacter aerogenes* increases resistance to certain antibiotics, and in *Pseudomonas aeruginosa* resistance to the aminoglycosides and other antibiotics can be determined through membrane permeability controlled by a TWO-COMPONENT REGULATORY SYSTEM.

● Degradation of antibiotics by plasmid-encoded or chromosome-encoded enzymes. Such enzymes include the inducible and constitutive β-lactamases that cleave the β-lactam ring in, and hence inactivate, β-lactam antibiotics such as penicillins and cephalosporins. The enzyme chloramphenicol acetyltransferase (which degrades CHLORAMPHENICOL) is another example – as are the acetyltransferases, adenylyltransferases and phosphotransferases that inactivate aminoglycoside antibiotics.

● Increased production of an affected metabolite. Thus, for example, synthesis of higher levels of *p*-aminobenzoic acid (PABA) may overcome the effect of competitive inhibition by sulfonamides.

antibody-labeling reagents See e.g. ZENON ANTIBODY LABELING REAGENTS.

anticlinal (*anti*) Of a nucleotide: the conformation in which the oxygen atom within the sugar ring (–O–) is the maximum distance from the 6-position of a purine (or the 2-position of a pyrimidine). (cf. SYNCLINAL.)

anticoagulant (*DNA technol.*) A term that usually refers to an agent which inhibits the coagulation (i.e. clotting) of blood.

The anticoagulants include sodium citrate, sodium oxalate, heparin and sodium polyanetholesulfonate (SPS); the latter two agents can inhibit PCR.

anticodon Three consecutive bases in a tRNA molecule complementary to a CODON which specifies the particular amino acid carried by that tRNA.

An anticodon is written in the 5′-to-3′ direction – as is a codon.

anti-downstream box (*or* antidownstream box) See DOWNSTREAM BOX.

antigenic variation Successive changes in surface antigens exhibited by certain types of microorganism (e.g. *Trypanosoma*). There are at least two distinct mechanisms: (i) the alternative antigens are transcribed from specific, *pre-existing* genes (see PHASE VARIATION), and (ii) the alternative antigens arise by ongoing recombinational events – i.e. they are encoded by newly formed, rather than pre-existing, genes. An example of the second mechanism is the formation of new versions of a subunit in the fimbriae of *Neisseria gonorrhoeae*; variant forms of this subunit arise through repeated recombination between the chromosomal subunit gene, *pilE*, and another chromosomal gene, *pilS*, as well as between *pilE* and any homologous DNA received e.g. by transformation.

Antigenic variation apparently helps a pathogen to evade a host's immunologic defense mechanisms.

antimutator gene Any gene whose activity reduces the rate of spontaneous mutation in a cell. For example, some strains of *Escherichia coli*, with a mutant form of DNA polymerase, have mutation rates below those of wild-type strains; in this case the antimutator activity presumably involves improved fidelity/proof-reading.

antiparallel (of strands in dsDNA) The (usual) arrangement in which a 5′-to-3′ strand is hybridized to a 3′-to-5′ strand, i.e. each end of a double-stranded DNA molecule has a 5′ terminal and a 3′ terminal.

(See also DNA.)

antiretroviral agents Agents with activity against retroviruses; some are useful e.g. in chemotherapy against AIDS. See e.g. NON-NUCLEOSIDE REVERSE TRANSCRIPTASE INHIBITORS, NUCLEOSIDE REVERSE TRANSCRIPTASE INHIBITORS and PROTEASE INHIBITORS.

anti-reverse cap analog (ARCA) A chemically modified form of CAP ANALOG (Ambion, Austin TX) designed to maximize the efficiency of *in vitro* translation by ensuring that the cap analog is incorporated in the transcript in the correct orientation (a cap analog incorporated in the reverse orientation does not support translation).

[Example of use of anti-reverse cap analog: Nucleic Acids Res (2005) 33(9):e86.]

antisense gene In a genetically engineered cell: any gene, inserted into the cell, whose presence is intended to inhibit or block the expression of an endogenous gene.

antisense RNA Any natural or synthetic RNA whose sequence permits interaction with a given sense sequence, in RNA or DNA, and which can affect the activity/expression of the target molecule (see FINOP SYSTEM, MICRORNA, MULTICOPY INHIBITION, POST-SEGREGATIONAL KILLING, R1 PLASMID, RNA INTERFERENCE).

While usually forming double-stranded structures, ssRNA can also form triple-stranded structures with dsDNA (see also TRIPLEX DNA), and may bind to ssDNA during transcription; in either case, transcription may be affected.

The search for antisense RNAs may be hindered e.g. by their relatively small size and because their sequences may not exactly match those of their target molecules; moreover, in at least some cases a given antisense molecule may have more than one target. [Detection of 5′- and 3′-UTR-derived small RNAs and *cis*-encoded antisense RNAs in *Escherichia coli*: Nucleic Acids Res (2005) 33(3):1040–1050.]

antisense strand (of DNA) The non-CODING STRAND.

antizyme Any of a group of proteins associated with regulation of ornithine decarboxylase (ODC) – which is involved in biosynthesis of polyamines. In eukaryotes functional antizyme is expressed in the presence of increased levels of polyamines, antizyme 1 promoting UBIQUITIN-dependent degradation of ODC via the 26S PROTEASOME; antizymes are regulated by antizyme inhibitor [Biochem J (2005) 385(1):21–28].

[Antizyme in prokaryotes: BMC Biochem (2007) 8:1.]

AOX1 In the (methylotrophic) yeast *Pichia pastoris*: a highly regulated, inducible gene which encodes alcohol oxidase – a peroxisomal enzyme involved in the metabolism of methanol.

(See also PPICZ VECTOR.)

AP ALKALINE PHOSPHATASE.

AP endonuclease Any enzyme with endonuclease activity that is involved in the excision of apurinic/apyrimidinic nucleotide residues (see e.g. BASE EXCISION REPAIR).

AP-PCR Arbitrarily primed PCR: any form of PCR which uses primers of arbitrary sequence and which amplifies random, but discrete, sequences of chromosomal DNA; AP-PCR has been used for TYPING bacteria.

PCR is initially carried out under low stringency, and the primers bind at various sites to each strand of heat-denatured chromosomal DNA; the binding of primers occurs at 'best-fit' sequences, and may include mismatches. In some cases two primers bind with relative efficiency, on opposite strands, at locations separated by a few hundred bases. If synthesis can occur normally from these two primers, a further round of cycling under low-stringency conditions, followed by many cycles under high-stringency conditions, may produce copies of an amplicon delimited by the two best-fit sequences. In the phase of high-stringency cycling not all the primers will bind to their best-fit sequences – so that only a proportion of the amplicons produced under low-stringency conditions will be amplified in the high-stringency phase.

The amplicons from a given sample are subjected to gel electrophoresis, and the stained bands of amplicons form the fingerprint. Strains are compared and classified on the basis of their fingerprints.

One advantage of this approach is that there is no need for prior knowledge of the genome sequence; there is no need to design specific primers, and any isolate is potentially typable.

Results are generally reproducible under standardized conditions in a given laboratory, but comparable results will not necessarily be obtained in other laboratories unless the procedures are *identical*; reproducibility of results depends not only on the primer sequence but also e.g. on the particular type of polymerase used and on the initial procedure used for preparing the sample DNA.

Some other named methods are based on the same principle – RAPD (random amplified polymorphic DNA) analysis and DAF (direct amplification fingerprinting). These methods may differ e.g. in the length of the primers used, annealing temperature for the primers, and the type of gel used for electrophoresis. The original AP-PCR employed primers of 20–50 nucleotides, with an annealing temperature of about 40°C, and used an agarose gel. In RAPD the primers are typically 10–20 nt, the annealing temperature is ~36°C, and products are separated in an agarose gel. DAF uses short primers (5–8 nt) at an annealing temperature of ~30°C; because there are many more, smaller products, electrophoresis is carried out in a polyacrylamide gel, and silver staining is used to detect bands in the fingerprint.

AP site (abasic site) In a nucleotide sequence: a site at which the base (purine or pyrimidine) is missing – the remainder of the nucleotide (sugar, phosphate) being present. (cf. GAP.)

APES See AAS.

aphidicolin A tetracyclic diterpenoid, isolated from a fungus, which strongly inhibits the eukaryotic α DNA polymerase. Bacterial DNA polymerases are unaffected, but aphidicolin was reported to inhibit DNA synthesis in at least some members of the domain ARCHAEA (e.g. some methanogens).

APOBEC-1 See CYTIDINE DEAMINASE and RNA EDITING.

apolipoprotein B See RNA EDITING.

APSR (amplicon primer site restriction) In PCR, a method for preventing the contamination of a reaction mixture with amplicons from previous assays. In APSR, *all* the assays are conducted with primers whose 5′ ends carry a recognition site for a (type IIS) RESTRICTION ENDONUCLEASE which cleaves both strands 3′ of its binding site. In a reaction mixture, the (added) restriction enzyme will cut any carry-over amplicons but will not cleave the template DNA (unless, by chance, it contains the given recognition site); the restriction enzyme is inactivated during PCR temperature cycling.

14

[Method: BioTechniques (2005) 39:69–73.]

(See also AMPLICON INACTIVATION.)

APT paper See SOUTHERN BLOTTING.

aptamer (1) Any of a large number of synthetic oligonucleotides which can adopt a three-dimensional structure and bind with high specificity to a given ligand. (See also INTRAMER.)

Selection of an RNA aptamer for a given target molecule can be achieved by SELEX (systematic evolution of ligands by exponential enrichment). Briefly, in SELEX, the immobilized target ligand (for example, a protein) is exposed to a large and diverse population of oligonucleotides synthesized with random sequences. After removal of unbound oligos, the relatively few bound oligos are eluted and then converted to cDNAs. The cDNAs are amplified by PCR using primers that incorporate a promoter; the resulting amplicons are transcribed, and the transcripts are used in another round of selection with the target molecule. The cycle is repeated, with target–RNA binding becoming more specific at each round; the range and affinity of selected aptamers can be determined e.g. by regulating the buffer conditions at the binding stage. (A principle similar to this is found in PHAGE DISPLAY.)

In general, SELEX is useful for analyzing protein–nucleic acid binding and e.g. interactions between RNA and various low-molecular-weight molecules.

An aptamer–shRNA fusion transcript has been used to regulate gene expression in mammalian cells; in this system, the activity of the shRNA moiety was controlled by interaction between the aptamer and its ligand – theophylline (1,3-dimethylxanthine) [RNA (2006) 12:710–716].

An aptamer – known to bind to prostate tumor cells – has been conjugated to an siRNA via a streptavidin bridge; on addition to cells, this conjugate was internalized, and the siRNA was able to inhibit gene expression as efficiently as when it was internalized by a lipid-based method [Nucleic Acids Res (2006) 34(10):e73.

(See also APTAZYME.)

[Aptamer database: Nucleic Acids Res (2004) 32(Database issue):D95–D100; online: http://aptamer.icmb.utexas.edu/]

(2) A *natural* sequence within a RIBOSWITCH.

aptazyme A composite APTAMER–RIBOZYME; the aptamer can bind certain molecules that may modify/regulate the activity of the ribozyme.

apurinic Lacking a purine residue: see AP SITE.

apyrase A nucleotide-degrading enzyme (EC 3.6.1.5) with various applications in technology (see e.g. PYROSEQUENCING).

apyrimidinic Lacking a pyrimidine residue: see AP SITE.

araBAD **operon** See OPERON.

Arabidopsis thaliana A small cruciferous plant commonly used in plant genetics owing to its simple genome and its short generation time. [Genome of *A. thaliana*: Nature (2000) 408: 791–826.]

(See also FLORAL DIP METHOD.)

araC See OPERON.

Aranesp® See BIOPHARMACEUTICAL (table).

arbitrarily primed PCR See AP-PCR.

ARCA See ANTI-REVERSE CAP ANALOG.

Archaea One of the two domains of prokaryotic organisms, the other being Bacteria. Organisms in these two domains differ e.g. in 16S rRNA sequences, composition of cell wall macromolecules, composition of cytoplasmic membrane lipids and flagellar structure. The general features of gene expression in the two domains are also dissimilar.

(See also PROKARYOTE.)

archaean (*syn.* archaeon) An organism within the (prokaryotic) domain ARCHAEA.

Archaebacteria A now-obsolete kingdom of prokaryotes; the organisms formerly placed in this taxon are currently classified in the domain ARCHAEA.

ArchaeMaxx™ A polymerase-enhancing factor, marketed by Stratagene (La Jolla CA), which is designed to overcome the so-called DUTP POISONING effect.

This factor is used e.g. in association with the *PfuTurbo®* and Herculase® DNA polymerases (also marketed by Stratagene).

[Example of use: PLoS Biol (2006) 4(3):e73.]

archaeon See ARCHAEAN.

ARES™ See PROBE LABELING.

Argonaute 2 See RNA INTERFERENCE.

ARMS Amplification-refractory mutation system: a procedure used e.g. for demonstrating or detecting a point mutation *at a specific site* in DNA whose wild-type (non-mutant) sequence is known.

Essentially, use is made of a primer in which the 3′-terminal nucleotide is complementary to the *mutant* base at the given site. After hybridization, extension of the primer by a polymerase signals the presence of the mutation at that site, while the absence of extension indicates the presence of a wild-type (or other) nucleotide.

armyworm The insect *Spodoptera frugiperda*. Cell cultures of this organism are used e.g. for the synthesis of recombinant proteins encoded by baculovirus vectors.

(See also SF9 CELLS.)

aRNA Antisense RNA; for example of use see MESSAGEAMP ARNA AMPLIFICATION KIT.

array Often: a shortened version of MICROARRAY; also used to refer to other oligonucleotide- or tissue-based arrangements etc. with analogous or distinct uses.

ARS Autonomously replicating sequence: a genomic sequence which, if linked to a non-replicative fragment of DNA, promotes the ability of that fragment to replicate independently (extrachromosomally) in the cell. ARSs were first reported in the yeast *Saccharomyces cerevisiae*; this organism contains, on average, one ARS in every ~40 kb of genomic DNA, and these elements are also found in at least some yeast plasmids. Apparently some ARSs are active chromosomal origins while others are *silent origins*; some of the silent origins (and some active ones) may function as transcription silencers.

[Genome-wide hierarchy of replication origin usage in the yeast *Saccharomyces cerevisiae*: PLoS Genetics (2006) 2(9): e141.]

Factors reported to contribute to the efficient replication of ARS-containing plasmids in yeast cells include (i) the CEN (centromere) element and (ii) minichromosome maintenance protein 1 (Mcm1).

The circular dsDNA genome of human papillomavirus type 16 can replicate stably in *S. cerevisiae* independently of ARS or CEN; sequences in the viral DNA can substitute for both ARS and CEN [J Virol (2005) 79(10):5933–5942].

ARSs have also been described in species of the ARCHAEA [e.g. J Bacteriol (2003) 185(20):5959–5966].

(See also SIDD and YEAST ARTIFICIAL CHROMOSOME.)

ascospores See SACCHAROMYCES.

ascus See SACCHAROMYCES.

aseptic technique Measures taken to avoid contamination of cultures, sterile media etc. – and/or contamination of persons, animals or plants – by microorganisms that are present in the environment (e.g. in the air) and that may be associated with particular source(s).

In this approach, the vessels used for media etc. must be sterile before use (e.g. pre-sterilized Petri dishes), and sterile material should not be exposed to any non-sterile conditions before use.

The working surfaces of forceps and other types of metal instrument (such as bacteriological loops etc.) are sterilized by 'flaming' before use, and the rims of bottles etc. used for dispensing sterile (non-flammable) materials are also flamed.

Benches are regularly treated with disinfectants and/or with ULTRAVIOLET RADIATION (UVR). The so-called 'germicidal' lamps, which may emit UVR at ~254 nm, are used e.g. for the disinfection of air and exposed surfaces in enclosed areas. In general, UVR has rather poor powers of penetration, and its effects on microorganisms may be reversible by certain DNA repair processes (see e.g. UVRABC-MEDIATED REPAIR).

Some procedures, e.g. handling specimens likely to contain certain pathogens (such as *Mycobacterium tuberculosis*, or certain highly hazardous viruses such as Ebola virus or Lassa fever virus), are carried out in a SAFETY CABINET.

ASP APOBEC-1-stimulating protein: see RNA EDITING.

aspart See INSULIN ASPART.

asymmetric PCR A form of PCR in which the concentration of *one* of the primers is much lower than that of the other (e.g. a ratio of 1:50); during temperature cycling, this primer will be quickly used up – so that only one strand of the target sequence will be significantly amplified.

Uses of asymmetric PCR include the preparation of probes and the preparation of single-stranded DNA for sequencing.

ssDNA products from PCR can also be obtained in a different way. One of the two types of primer can be labeled with BIOTIN and the reaction carried out with both primers in their normal concentrations. At the end of the reaction, STREPT-AVIDIN is added, and this binds only to the biotin-labeled strands; subsequent gel electrophoresis (in a denaturing gel) separates the two types of strand because the mobility of the streptavidin-bound strand is much lower. (The biotinylated primer forms the strand which is *not* required.)

AT type See BASE RATIO.

ATMS *p*-Aminophenyltrimethoxysilane: a reagent used for covalently binding DNA probes to a solid support when preparing a MICROARRAY. (In an earlier procedure, DNA was bound *non*-covalently to glass slides by the reagent poly-L-lysine.) [Method: Nucleic Acids Res (2001) 29:e107.]

(See also DENDRICHIP.)

atomic force microscopy (AFM; scanning force microscopy) A method for imaging *surfaces*, including those of molecules and of (living) cells, in e.g. air or liquid, at nanometer-scale resolution. Essentially, the object's surface is scanned in a raster pattern with a fine probe located underneath a traveling cantilever; a laser, reflected from the cantilever (and thus incorporating information on the cantilever's movements) is detected by a photodiode assembly, and the incoming signals are converted by computer into a surface profile.

att **sites** Sites involved in the SITE-SPECIFIC RECOMBINATION that occurs e.g. when the PHAGE LAMBDA genome integrates into a bacterial chromosome.

Lambda *att* sites are used in commercial DNA technology systems: see e.g. GATEWAY SITE-SPECIFIC RECOMBINATION SYSTEM, MULTISITE GATEWAY TECHNOLOGY, BP CLONASE, LR CLONASE.

In addition to their commercial exploitation, *att* sites have been used e.g. for the production of excisable cassettes which (it has been suggested) may provide a new approach to the functional analysis of the genome of the Gram-positive bacterium *Streptomyces* [Appl Environ Microbiol (2006) 72(7): 4839–4844].

attaching and effacing lesion See PATHOGENICITY ISLAND.

*att***B,** *att***P** See PHAGE LAMBDA.

(See also ATT SITES.)

attenuator control See OPERON.

*att***L,** *att***R** See PHAGE LAMBDA.

(See also ATT SITES.)

atto- Prefix meaning 10^{-18}.

AttoPhos™ A commercial reagent (Promega) which can be cleaved by ALKALINE PHOSPHATASE to yield a fluorescent product. It has been used e.g. in a CROSS-LINKING ASSAY.

*att***Tn7** See TN7.

autoactivation (*syn.* self-activation) (two-hybrid systems) See e.g. BACTERIOMATCH TWO-HYBRID SYSTEM.

autocatalytic splicing See SPLICING.

autoclave An apparatus within which objects and/or materials are sterilized by saturated (air-free) steam under pressure; the conditions within a working autoclave are typically in the range 115°C (~69 kPa; 10 lb/inch²) to 134°C (~207 kPa; 30 lb/inch²).

STERILIZATION in an autoclave is carried out e.g. when preparing certain types of media. Heat-labile constituents of a medium (e.g. a solution of an antibiotic) may be membrane-filtered before being added to a sterile (autoclaved) medium.

Some steam-impermeable items that cannot be sterilized by autoclaving may be sterilized e.g. in a hot-air oven at ~160–170°C for ~1 hour.

autoclave tape   A paper strip (usually self-adhesive) which is included with the objects being sterilized in an autoclave; it exhibits a visible change (e.g. in color) when it is subjected to appropriate sterilizing conditions, and can therefore act as a check on the correct operation of the autoclave.

Autographa californica **NPV**   See NUCLEAR POLYHEDROSIS VIRUSES.

autoinducer (in quorum sensing)   See QUORUM SENSING.

automated sequencing (of DNA)   A method used for rapidly sequencing DNA fragments of up to ~500 nt. Essentially, the process involves conventional chain-termination (i.e. Sanger) sequencing (see DIDEOXY METHOD) with fluorophore-labeled ddNTPs – each type of ddNTP (A, G, C, T) being labeled with a fluorophore that emits a distinctive color on excitation. The sequencing products are separated by polyacrylamide gel electrophoresis and the bands of products are scanned by laser; the positions of individual nucleotides, identified by the color of the fluorescence, are recorded automatically.

(See also DNA SEQUENCING and PYROSEQUENCING.)

autonomously replicating sequence   See ARS.

autoplast   A PROTOPLAST or SPHEROPLAST which develops as a result of activity of the organism's own autolytic enzymes.

autoradiography   A procedure in which a radioactive source is detected or quantitated by its effect on a photographic film; a film is exposed to the radioactive source, in the dark, and for an appropriate period of time, and is subsequently processed.

Autoradiography is used e.g. for investigating intracellular processes (radioactive isotopes being incorporated into biomolecules) and also e.g. for detecting bands of products (such as isotopically labeled fragments of DNA), *in situ*, after gel electrophoresis.

In general, optimal resolution may require the use of those isotopes which have relatively low-energy emission (such as tritium, ^{3}H) rather than those (such as ^{32}P) which have high-energy emission.

autosomal dominant disorder   Refers to a genetic disorder in which the phenotypic manifestation arising from expression of an abnormal autosomic allele occurs in the presence of the corresponding normal allele – that is, the influence of the abnormal allele overrides that of the normal allele. This type of disorder tends to exhibit a so-called *vertical* pattern of transmission from one generation to the next; in such cases, an abnormal trait is more likely (than in an autosomal recessive condition) to affect each successive generation.

Both males and females can be affected – and, unlike the situation in X-linked dominant disorders, father-to-son transmission can occur.

One example of this type of disorder: AXENFELD–RIEGER SYNDROME; another example is PEUTZ–JEGHERS SYNDROME. (See also CHARCOT–MARIE–TOOTH DISEASE.)

(cf. AUTOSOMAL RECESSIVE DISORDER and X-LINKED DISORDER.)

autosomal recessive disorder   Refers to a genetic disorder in which manifestation of the abnormal phenotype is exhibited when the abnormal allele is not accompanied by the presence of the corresponding normal, wild-type allele; heterozygous individuals with one normal allele do not usually exhibit the abnormal phenotype.

Both males and females can be affected.

Only when mating occurs between two (homozygously) affected individuals will the trait necessarily appear in all the offspring; mating between two heterozygous individuals, or between one heterozygous and one normal individual, tends to spare some of the offspring, so that an autosomal recessive disorder may miss generation(s) and is said to exhibit a *horizontal* mode of transmission.

(cf. AUTOSOMAL DOMINANT DISORDER and X-LINKED DISORDER.)

autosome   Any chromosome other than a HETEROSOME.

autotransporter   See OMPT GENE.

auxins   Phytohormones (plant hormones) which promote stem elongation and other aspects of plant development; the auxins are derivatives of tryptophan. Indole 3-acetic acid (IAA; also called 'auxin' or 'heteroauxin') is a major auxin; it is synthesized from the precursor indole 3-acetonitrile (IAN).

Abnormally high levels of auxins (*hyperauxiny*) are found in some plant diseases (e.g. CROWN GALL).

auxotrophic mutant   Any microorganism which, as a result of a mutation, is unable to synthesize an essential nutrient and which therefore can grow only if provided with an exogenous source of that nutrient. (An organism which does *not* contain such a mutation, and which can synthesize all of its essential nutrients, is called a *prototroph*.)

One example of an auxotrophic mutant is mentioned in the entry AMES TEST.

Isolation of auxotrophic mutant bacteria

The usual (selective) procedures cannot be used to isolate auxotrophic bacteria from a mixture of prototrophs and auxotrophs because the requirements of auxotrophs are in excess of those of prototrophs.

The *limited enrichment* method uses an agar-based *minimal medium* enriched with *small* amounts of nutrients. A minimal medium is one which supports the growth of prototrophs but – because it lacks one or more essential nutrients – does not support the growth of auxotrophs. Any colony of auxotrophic cells will quickly exhaust the nutrients in its vicinity – so that the colony remains small; however, the unrestricted growth of prototrophs means that the colonies of prototrophs will be larger than those of auxotrophs. Hence, the small colonies indicate presumptive auxotrophs.

The *delayed enrichment* technique employs an agar-based minimal medium for initial growth, so that prototrophs (only) form colonies in the initial incubation. Complete medium is then poured onto the plate and allowed to set; the nutrients in this medium diffuse into the minimal medium below, allowing the growth of auxotrophs. Again, small colonies indicate presumptive auxotrophs.

For (penicillin-sensitive) bacteria, auxotrophic mutants can be isolated by virtue of their inability to grow in a (penicillin-containing) minimal medium; penicillin is an antibiotic that acts only on *growing* cells. In this approach, a well-washed population of bacteria (that includes auxotrophs) is exposed to penicillin in a minimal medium; the prototrophs (which can grow) are killed by the penicillin. The remaining cells are washed and re-plated on a complete medium to recover any auxotrophs. It's important to note that, if the auxotrophs had developed through an *in vitro* process of mutagenization, it is essential that the cells be allowed to grow for several generations in complete medium prior to exposure to penicillin; this is because newly mutated cells contain a full complement of (prototrophic) enzymes, and the auxotrophic phenotype develops only after several rounds of cell division – during which the prototrophic enzymes are 'diluted out'. A further requirement in this method is that only a low concentration of cells be used; this is because auxotrophs should not be allowed to grow on nutrients released by lysed prototrophs – as this would render them susceptible to lysis by the penicillin. For this reason, STREPTOZOTOCIN may be used in place of penicillin.

Auxotrophs may also be isolated by REPLICA PLATING.

avian erythroblastosis virus See ERB.

avirulence gene See GENE-FOR-GENE CONCEPT.

Axenfeld–Rieger syndrome An autosomal dominant disorder involving eye defects and certain systemic abnormalities. The syndrome has been associated with mutations in the *PITX2* gene (which encodes a transcription factor). In some patients the disorder is reported to involve aberrant splicing of pre-RNA; it has been suggested that variability in the extent of the splicing fault may be reflected in the observed variability of phenotypic manifestations [BMC Med Genet (2006) 7:59].

5-aza-2′-deoxycytidine A cell-permeant agent used e.g. for studying DEMETHYLATION.

[Example of use: BioTechniques (2006) 41(4):461–466.]

azaserine (*O*-diazoacetyl-L-serine) An agent with antimicrobial and antitumor activity produced by *Streptomyces* sp (a Gram-positive bacterium). Azaserine inhibits the activity of certain enzymes, including phosphoribosylformylglycinamidine synthetase – thus inhibiting biosynthesis of purines and, hence, nucleotides.

(cf. DON; see also HADACIDIN.)

AZT See ZIDOVUDINE.

B

B A specific indicator of ambiguity in the recognition site of a RESTRICTION ENDONUCLEASE or in another nucleic acid sequence; 'B' indicates C or G or T in DNA, C or G or U in RNA.

B-DNA The form of DNA that appears to be the most common type found *in vivo* (and on which is based the Watson–Crick model, the so-called 'double helix'): a right-handed double-helix of ~10.4 base pairs/turn and a diameter of ~20Å.

(See also RIGHT-HANDED HELIX.)

Bac-to-Bac® A BACULOVIRUS EXPRESSION SYSTEM, marketed by Invitrogen (Carlsbad CA), in which a recombinant baculo-virus genome – containing the gene of interest – is generated within specialized cells of *Escherichia coli* by site-specific transposition.

The strain of *E. coli* used in this system (DH10Bac™) contains a BACMID into which the gene of interest is inserted (to form an *expression bacmid*).

Initially, the gene of interest is inserted into the polylinker of a small (4.8 kb) pFastBac™ plasmid. Within this vector, the inserted gene is positioned downstream of the (strong) promoter of the baculovirus polyhedrin gene; the expression cassette within the pFastBac vector is flanked by the terminal sequences, Tn7L and Tn7R, of transposon Tn7. The vector, containing the gene of interest, is then transfected into cells of the DH10Bac strain of *E. coli*, within which the expression cassette is transferred from the vector to the bacmid by site-specific transposition.

The recombinant bacmid, containing the gene of interest, is isolated from *E. coli* and is then transfected into insect cells for the production of extracellular recombinant baculovirus.

The Bac-to-Bac system has been used e.g. in studies on the capsid protein of the beak-and-feather-disease virus (BFDV) [J Virol (2006) 80(14):7219–7225] and for studying the conformational states of a SARS virus protein [J Virol (2006) 80 (14):6794–6800].

(See also PFASTBAC DUAL VECTOR KIT.)

Bacillus anthracis A species of Gram-positive, spore-forming, typically square-ended rod-shaped bacteria, virulent strains of which form anthrax toxin (encoded by plasmid pXO1) and a poly-D-glutamic acid capsule (encoded by plasmid pXO2). *B. anthracis* grows on nutient agar; in biochemical tests it gives results similar to those from *Bacillus cereus*. *B. anthracis* is susceptible to the γ phage (gamma phage).

The Sterne strain of *B. anthracis* forms anthrax toxin but lacks the capsule – lack of the capsule permitting elimination of the pathogen by phagocytosis.

Ames strain: see entry BACTERIA (table).

Disease similar to anthrax has been reported to be caused e.g. by strains of *Bacillus cereus* [see PLoS Pathogens (2006) 2(11):e122].

(See also SORTASE.)

back mutation (reverse mutation) (1) Following a given (primary) mutation: a mutation that restores the original nucleotide sequence.

(2) An *intragenic* SUPPRESSOR MUTATION.

bacmid A replicon, first constructed in the 1990s, which can replicate as a plasmid in *Escherichia coli* and can be used to transfect (susceptible) insect cells.

A bacmid consists of a recombinant baculovirus genome (see BACULOVIRIDAE) which includes a plasmid origin of replication and also a target (insertion) site for transposon Tn7 (*att*Tn7).

If a bacmid is present in *E. coli*, a gene cassette – flanked by the two terminal parts of Tn7 – can be transposed into the *att*Tn7 site in the bacmid by site-specific transposition, given that the functions for transposition are provided in *trans* from a helper plasmid in the bacterium.

bacteria A term used to refer to some or all organisms of the domain BACTERIA. Note that this term has a lower-case 'b'; an upper-case 'B' is used for the *domain* Bacteria because this is the name of a *taxon* (a specific taxonomic category).

Bacteria One of the two domains of prokaryotic organisms – the other being ARCHAEA. Organisms in these two domains differ e.g. in their 16S rRNA, in the composition of their cell-wall macromolecules, in the composition of their membrane lipids and also in flagellar structure; moreover, in general, gene expression in the Archaea (in terms of transcription and translation) appears to resemble the eukaryotic mode of expression more closely than the bacterial mode.

The *typical* bacterial genome is a circular chromosome (i.e. ccc dsDNA). Cells may contain a single chromosome or may contain more than one copy per cell (the number depending on species and on growth conditions).

In some species of bacteria the genome is *linear* dsDNA: see e.g. BORRELIA BURGDORFERI. (A linear chromosome is also present e.g. in a species with one of the largest genomes sequenced thus far in bacteria (~9.7 Mbp): *Rhodococcus* sp RHA1 [Proc Natl Acad Sci USA (2006) 103:15582–15587].)

In general, only one *type* of chromosome is found in the cells of a given species. In *Vibrio cholerae* each cell contains two types of chromosome – one (chromosome I) being larger than the other (chromosome II); jointly, these two chromosomes form the genome of *V. cholerae*.

Bacterial chromosomes are extensively folded into compact bodies. (See also NUCLEOID.)

The size of the genome varies among different species. In a number of cases the genome has been completely sequenced. The table lists the approximate size of the genome in various species and includes sources of information on sequences.

In addition to chromosome(s), many bacteria contain one or more types of PLASMID; however, plasmids are not normally present in certain bacteria (e.g. *Brucella* and *Rickettsia*). In *Rhodococcus* sp RHA1 the large (~9.7 Mbp) genome consists of a linear chromosome and three linear plasmids.

Bacteria are commonly susceptible to one or more types of BACTERIOPHAGE, and a lysogenic strain of bacteria contains the phage genome (the *prophage*) in addition to the cell's

19

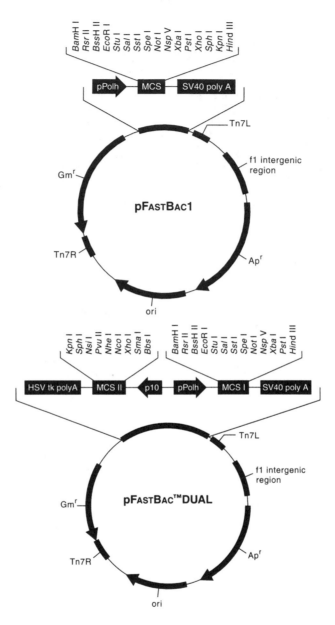

Bac-to-Bac® VECTORS *Above.* The basic pFastBac™1 vector. See entry for details of the method. *Below.* The pFastBac™ Dual vector into which two DNA sequences can be inserted and expressed simultaneously.

Courtesy of Invitrogen, Carlsbad CA, USA.

BACTERIAL GENOMES: examples of size and sources of information

Species	Genome (~Mbp)[a]	Reference
Gram-positive		
Bacillus anthracis (Ames strain)	5.2	Nature (2003) 423:81–86
Bacillus subtilis	4.2	Nature (1997) 390:249–256
Bacteroides thetaiotaomicron	6.3	Science (2003) 299:2074–2076
Clostridium perfringens	3.0	PNAS[b] (2002) 99(2):996–1001
Lactobacillus acidophilus NCFM	2.0	PNAS[b] (2005) 102(11):3906–3912
Lactobacillus plantarum	3.3	PNAS[b] (2003) 100:1900–1995
Listeria welshimeri	2.8	J Bacteriol (2006) 188:7405–7415
Mycobacterium avium subsp *paratuberculosis*	4.8	PNAS[b] (2005) 102(35):12344–12349
Mycobacterium leprae	3.3	Nature (2001) 409:1007–1011
Mycobacterium tuberculosis	4.4	Nature (1998) 393:537–544
Rhodococcus sp RHA1	9.7	PNAS[b] (2006) 103:15582–15587
Streptococcus pneumoniae	2.1	Science (2001) 293:498–506
Streptococcus pyogenes	1.9	PNAS[b] (2001) 98:4656–4663
Tropheryma whipplei	0.9	Lancet (2003) 361:637–644
Gram-negative		
Aeromonas hydrophila	4.7	J Bacteriol (2006) 188(3):8272–8282
Borrelia burgdorferi	0.9	Nature (1997) 390:580–586
Caulobacter crescentus	4.0	PNAS[b] (2001) 98(7):4136–4141
Chlamydia trachomatis	1.0	Science (1998) 282:754–759
Coxiella burnetii	2.0	PNAS[b] (2003) 100(9):5455–5460
Escherichia coli	5.0[c]	Science (1997) 277:1453–1474
Escherichia coli O157:H7	5.5	Nature (2001) 409:529–533; erratum (2001) 410:240
Helicobacter pylori	1.6	Nature (1997) 388:539–547
Helicobacter pylori (HPAG1)	1.6	PNAS[b] (2006) 103(26):9999–10004
Neisseria meningitidis	2.2	Nature (2000) 404:502–506
Pasteurella multocida	2.2	PNAS[b] (2001) 98:3460–3465
Pseudomonas syringae pv. tomato	6.5	PNAS[b] (2003) 100(18):10181–10186
Rhizobium leguminosarum	7.7	Genome Biol (2006) 7(4):R34
Rickettsia typhi	1.1	J Bacteriol (2004) 186(17):5842–5855
Shigella flexneri 5b	4.5	BMC Genomics (2006) 7:62
Thiomicrospira crunogena	2.4	PLoS Biol (2006) 4(12):e383
Vibrio cholerae	4.0[d]	Nature (2000) 406:477–483

[a]Approximate genome size in Mbp (bp × 10^6). Variation in genome size can occur within a given species.
[b]Proc Natl Acad Sci USA.
[c]Values of ~4.7–5.5 have been reported for different strains.
[d]*Vibrio cholerae* chromosome I ~3.0 Mbp, chromosome II ~1.0 Mbp (genome size: ~4.0 Mbp).

own genome. In some cases the prophage confers important characteristics on the host cell – e.g. the CTXΦ prophage (which encodes cholera toxin) is the major virulence factor in cholera-causing strains of *Vibrio cholerae*. Commonly, the prophage integrates in the bacterial chromosome; this is not the case, however, in e.g. phage P1.

Bacteria are used frequently in recombinant technology for a variety of reasons which include: (i) typically, rapid growth and division, (ii) ease of manipulation and mutagenesis, (iii) ease of storage, and (iv) (compared with eukaryotic cells)

cellular processes which are relatively easy to manage. In particular, *Escherichia coli* has been extensively used as an experimental organism. (Other bacteria that have been widely used as experimental organisms include e.g. *Bacillus subtilis* (Gram-positive), *Pseudomonas aeruginosa* (Gram-negative), and *Salmonella typhimurium* (Gram-negative).) Moreover, some bacterial *components* (e.g. plasmids and RESTRICTION ENDONUCLEASES) are invaluable in this area of study.

Before the 1980s, bacterial taxonomy was based on various phenotypic characteristics (including e.g. reaction to certain dyes). Modern bacterial taxonomy is based primarily on the comparison of nucleic acids. Most TYPING methods are also genotypic (an important exception being PHAGE TYPING).

bacterial two-hybrid system See e.g. BACTERIOMATCH TWO-HYBRID SYSTEM.

bacteriocin Any of a variety of (typically) protein or peptide factors, produced by certain bacteria (including both Gram-negative and Gram-positive species), which kill or inhibit other bacteria – frequently closely related species; they range from high-molecular-weight proteins and short peptides to a simple modified amino acid (microcin A15). (The activity of some bacteriocins requires post-translational modification.)

Analogous agents are produced by members of the Archaea (e.g. the *halocins* of halobacteria) but their amino acid sequences are apparently not homologous to those of their bacterial counterparts.

Bacteriocins are of various distinct types: see e.g. COLICIN, LANTIBIOTIC and MICROCIN.

Most bacteriocins are encoded by genes in conjugative or non-conjugative plasmids. Chromosomally encoded bacteriocins include some of those formed by lactic acid bacteria and e.g. 'bacteriocin 28b' (a colicin from *Serratia marcescens*).

Bacteriocins act in characteristic ways. Some (e.g. microcin B17) inhibit DNA gyrase; some (e.g. cloacin DF13) cleave 16S rRNA; and some form pores in the bacterial cytoplasmic membrane.

BacterioMatch® two-hybrid system A system (Stratagene, La Jolla CA) for detecting interaction between two proteins in a bacterial cell. The proteins (*bait* and *target*) correspond to the 'bait' and 'prey' proteins in the YEAST TWO-HYBRID SYSTEM (q.v. for basic information on two-hybrid systems). Each of these proteins is encoded in a separate expression vector – in which the protein-encoding sequence is part of a fusion gene; the two vectors, pBT and pTRG, are introduced into a bacterial cell and expressed in the cell. [Use (e.g.): Appl Environ Microbiol (2007) 73(4):1320–1331.]

The bait vector contains the gene of the bait protein fused to the gene of the cI protein of PHAGE LAMBDA. The (DNA-binding) fusion protein (which is expressed in the cell) has a region that can bind to a λ operator sequence located a short distance upstream of the promoter of a reporter gene.

In the target vector, the gene of the target protein is fused to a sequence encoding the N-terminal region of the (bacterial) RNA polymerase α-subunit; the fusion protein is expressed in the cell.

Within the (engineered) reporter cell, interaction between bait and target proteins results in the recruitment of a functional RNA polymerase to the (nearby) downstream promoter, thus initiating transcription of the reporter gene.

The reporter gene encodes resistance to ampicillin; this allows the positive selection of cells in which protein–protein interaction has occurred (because these cells are able to grow on ampicillin-containing media). Another reporter gene, *lacZ* (encoding β-galactosidase), is transcribed in series with the Amp^r gene; it can be used to validate interaction between the two proteins.

In *any* bacterial two-hybrid system (and in the yeast two-hybrid system), one problem is *self-activation* – in which e.g. a bait protein may activate the reporter system without first interacting with the target protein – leading to a false-positive result. This problem was addressed, in one approach, by a counter-selective procedure designed for use specifically in bacteria; this is based on the URA3/5-FOA mechanism (see YEAST TWO-HYBRID SYSTEM) which is modified for use in *Escherichia coli*. In *E. coli*, the *pyrF* gene is homologous to *URA3*, and a Δ*pyrF* strain of *E. coli* (in which the *pyrF* gene is inactivated) can be complemented by an introduced copy of the gene *URA3*. In this counter-selective system, *URA3* is introduced on a plasmid and is used as the reporter gene in a *one-hybrid arrangement*: transcription of *URA3* depends on interaction between the DNA-binding domain, DBD, and a specific binding sequence upstream of the *URA3* reporter. As the DBD *in this counter-selective system* is covalently bound to the α subunit of RNA polymerase, an interaction between DBD and the specific binding site can recruit a functional RNA polymerase and promote transcription of *URA3* – with the formation of a suicide substrate in the presence of 5-FOA. Accordingly, cells in which this occurs fail to grow. [Method: BioTechniques (2006) 40(2):179–184.]

bacteriophage (phage) Any virus that infects *bacteria*; many (perhaps most, or all) bacteria are susceptible to one or more types of phage. (See entries under PHAGE for some specific examples.)

A given phage may specifically infect bacteria of only one species or strain, or it may have a wider host range. Certain phages are specific for conjugative *donor* cells (i.e. 'male' cells), in which the PILUS forms the site of initial attachment. (See also FEMALE-SPECIFIC PHAGES.)

Phages are often said to be *virulent* or *temperate*. A virulent phage lyses (kills) the bacterial host cell. A temperate phage can form a more or less stable relationship with a bacterium; in most cases the phage genome (the *prophage*) integrates in the bacterial chromosome, but in some cases (e.g. phage P1) it remains a circular, extrachromosomal 'plasmid'. (See also PHAGE N15.)

Under certain conditions a temperate phage may be induced to enter the lytic cycle – in which case virions are formed and cell lysis occurs; thus, a prophage may retain the potential for virulence, and in a population of *lysogenic* bacteria (i.e. bacteria which are hosts to a temperate phage), spontaneous induction may occur in a small number of cells.

Phages of the family Inoviridae (e.g. phages f1, fd, M13 in enterobacteria; Pf1 in *Pseudomonas*; Xf in *Xanthomonas*; v6 in *Vibrio*) are long filamentous phages which, in most or all cases, infect only 'male' (conjugative donor) cells. Although these phages replicate (and form virions) within the host cells they do not cause lysis: the virions are extruded through the cell envelope of the (living) host cells.

Phages commonly consist of nucleic acid enclosed within a protein coat called a *capsid*. However, certain phages contain

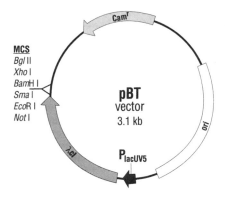

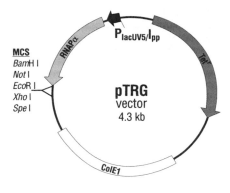

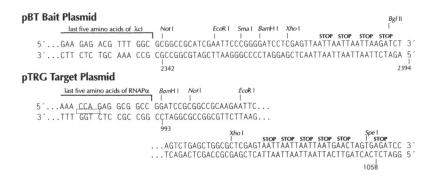

BacterioMatch® VECTORS The 'bait' and 'target' vectors (pBT and pTRG, respectively) of the BacterioMatch® two-hybrid system. See entry for details of the method. λcI refers to the gene of the cI protein of bacteriophage lambda (λ). MCS = multiple cloning site (polylinker); P = promoter; ColE1 = origin of replication of the ColE1 plasmid; RNAPα = a region encoding the N-terminal sequence of the α subunit of (bacterial) RNA polymerase; Tet^r = resistance to the antibiotic tetracycline; Cam^r = resistance to the antibiotic chloramphenicol.

Courtesy of Stratagene, La Jolla CA, USA.

lipid, either within the virion (for example, phage PM2 in *Alteromonas espejiana*) or as an outer *envelope* (e.g. phage φ6 in *Pseudomonas syringae* p.v. *phaseolicola*), and certain phages contain components such as fucose or spermidine.

The phages vary greatly in shape and size. Many have a roughly spherical or icosahedral protein *head* (containing the genome) which carries a thin, elongated, contractile or non-contractile *tail* involved in attachment to the host cell. Some are small icosahedral virions which lack a tail, some have a complex, irregular shape, and some (as mentioned above) are long filaments.

In size, phages range from ~25 nm in diameter (e.g. φX174, Qβ – both tail-less, icosahedral phages) to ~200 nm (e.g. λ, T4 – both tailed phages), while filamentous phages (e.g. f1, M13) can be >750 nm in length, although they are only ~6 nm in width.

Genome

Depending on phage, the genome may be linear dsDNA (e.g. phages λ, P1, P2, P22, φ29, T4, T7); ccc dsDNA (e.g. PM2); ccc ssDNA (e.g. f1, φX174); ssRNA (e.g. MS2, Qβ) – or dsRNA (e.g. φ6).

Phage φ6 is unusual in that it has a SEGMENTED GENOME.

Phages in DNA technology

Phages, their components and/or the enzymes they encode are widely used in DNA technology (see the table for some examples).

Phages as potential therapeutic agents

Many studies have been carried out to investigate the use of phages against the bacteria that cause certain human diseases [see e.g. Antimicrob Agents Chemother (2001) 45:649–659]. Phage-encoded endolysins (enzymes that cleave the bacterial cell-wall polymer peptidoglycan) have also been considered

BACTERIOPHAGE: some uses of phages in DNA technology

Bacteriophage	Genome	Uses (e.g.)
f1	ccc ssDNA	• Replication origin used in pBluescript® phagemids • PHAGE DISPLAY technology
λ (lambda)	linear dsDNA	• cI protein gene used in bacterial two-hybrid system (see BACTERIOMATCH TWO-HYBRID SYSTEM) • *cos* site used in cosmids and phasmids (see COSMID, PHASMID) • Derivatives used as cloning vectors (see e.g. ZAP EXPRESS VECTOR) • λ Red recombination system used for *in vivo* recombination (see the entry LAMBDA (λ) RED RECOMBINATION) • Constituents used in a range of GATEWAY SITE-SPECIFIC RECOMBINATION systems
M13	ccc ssDNA	• Used for making single-stranded copies of DNA target sequences for site-specific mutagenesis or sequencing etc. • Helper phage for phagemids, including e.g. gene-delivery phagemid particle vectors for eukaryotic cells (see entry GENE THERAPY)
N15	linear dsDNA	• Derivative used as a linear cloning vector in the BigEasy™ linear cloning system (q.v.)
P1	linear dsDNA	• Cre–*loxP* site-specific recombination system used e.g. in cassette-exchange mechanisms (e.g. RECOMBINASE-MEDIATED CASSETTE EXCHANGE)
φ29 (phi 29)	linear dsDNA	• MULTIPLE DISPLACEMENT AMPLIFICATION
T3	linear dsDNA	• RNA polymerase used for *in vitro* transcription • RNA polymerase used for incorporation of labeled nucleotides
T4	linear dsDNA	• DNA polymerase used for incorporation of digoxigenin-labeled nucleotides • DNA ligase used for closing nicks • UvsX recombinase used for the (isothermal) recombinase polymerase amplification of DNA (see entry RPA, sense 1)
T7	linear dsDNA	• As for T3 • Eberwine technique • DNA polymerase (Sequenase®), helicase and single-strand binding protein (gp2.5) used in circular helicase-dependent amplification of plasmids (see entry CHDA)

as therapeutic agents [Exp Biol Med (2006) 231:366–377].

In an entirely different approach, a number of studies have assessed phages, or phagemid particles, for gene delivery in the genetic modification of mammalian cells and, hence, their possible use in GENE THERAPY; in this context, an engineered helper phage has been developed to enable phagemid particles to incorporate a specific, helper-encoded peptide ligand in order to facilitate binding to target cells [BioTechniques (2005) 39:493–497].

Phage delivery vehicles were also used for DNA vaccines [see e.g. Infect Immun (2006) 74(1):167–174].

bacteriophage conversion See LYSOGENY.

bacteroid A term used to refer to certain forms of bacteria that are distinct (e.g. morphologically) from related, normal wild-type cells – e.g. the bacterial nitrogen-fixing cells found in root nodules of leguminous plants.

BaculoDirect™ A BACULOVIRUS EXPRESSION SYSTEM (Invitrogen, Carlsbad CA) in which a gene/fragment of interest is inserted into a modified, linearized baculovirus genome in a 1-hour *in vitro* step – following which the recombinant genome can be transfected directly into insect cells (such as Sf21 cells). After 72 hours, the supernatant (containing extracellular virions) can be used to infect a fresh batch of insect cells.

Insertion of a gene of interest into the baculovirus genome is carried out by a technique involving the GATEWAY SITE-SPECIFIC RECOMBINATION SYSTEM: the baculovirus genome includes a pair of *att*R sites into which the *att*L-flanked target DNA can be inserted by the activity of LR Clonase.

In the LR Clonase reaction – in which the target DNA is inserted – part of the linearized baculovirus genome, which contains a *lacZ* gene, is excised and forms a by-product. Subsequent staining of the baculovirus-infected cells to detect the *absence* of *lacZ* can be used to check that the cells do not contain non-recombinant baculovirus vectors.

In the recombinant baculovirus vector, the target DNA is

driven by a strong promoter (the promoter of the polyhedrin gene), and the vector encodes a V5-His tag (see also NICKEL-CHARGED AFFINITY RESIN) to facilitate purification of the product.

One version of this vector contains a sequence encoding the MELITTIN peptide which is intended to promote secretion of the expressed protein.

The expression of heterologous proteins in insect cells can also be carried out in a baculovirus-independent manner by using simpler vector systems (including Gateway® and topo-type systems) in *Drosophila* Schneider S2 cells: see DES.

Baculoviridae A family of enveloped viruses that infect a wide range of arthropods – including members of the Coleoptera (beetles), Diptera (flies), Hymenoptera (ants, bees etc.) and Lepidoptera (butterflies, moths).

The baculovirus genome consists of ccc dsDNA and ranges from ~80 kbp to ~200 kbp, according to virus.

In DNA technology, these viruses are exploited e.g. in the BACULOVIRUS EXPRESSION SYSTEMS used for the expression of recombinant proteins.

The baculoviruses include two major groups: the NUCLEAR POLYHEDROSIS VIRUSES (NPVs) and GRANULOSIS VIRUSES (GVs).

OBs, ODVs

Very late in the phase of infection, in the cell's nucleus, the replicated viral nucleocapsids are enclosed within envelopes. They are subsequently embedded in a crystalline matrix that is composed of a virus-encoded protein, forming so-called *occlusion bodies* (OBs); the viruses occluded within these bodies are called *occlusion-derived virions* (ODVs).

The OBs of the nuclear polyhedrosis viruses (also referred to as *polyhedra*, owing to their shape) contain multiple enveloped particles, each of which contains either a single nucleocapsid or multiple nucleocapsids, according to virus. On the other hand, in granulosis viruses, each of the OBs contains a single enveloped particle containing a single nucleocapsid or, rarely, two nucleocapsids.

In the NPVs the crystalline matrix of the occlusion body is composed of the protein *polyhedrin*. In the granulosis viruses the matrix protein is *granulin*.

The OBs serve as disseminative units: when the host dies, and OBs are ingested by a new, susceptible host, infectious virions are released in the midgut of the new host and initiate infection.

BVs

Baculoviruses also form so-called *budded virions* (BVs). The BVs are formed when nucleocapsids are transported to the cell's plasma membrane and then bud from the surface into the extracellular environment to produce enveloped virions (BVs). The BVs spread the infection to other cells in the host.

Baculovirus genes/gene products

Baculovirus genes/gene products referred to in the literature include e.g. *ie-1* (encoding a transregulatory protein activator of transcription of both early and late genes); the *lef* genes (late expression factor genes, encoding e.g. a primase and its accessory factor); gene *gp64* (encoding a low-pH-dependent protein, GP64, involved in virion attachment to the host cell membrane); and *p143* (a helicase).

The gene encoding very late expression factor 1 (VLF-1) is apparently present in the genomes of all baculoviruses. The product, VLF-1, is reported to have homology with members of the tyrosine recombinase family; however, a function unrelated to recombinase action (in which VLF-1 is involved in the production of normal capsid particles) has been reported for this product [J Virol (2006) 80(4):1724–1733].

Biological control

In addition to their uses in DNA technology, baculoviruses have been widely used for the biological control of various insect pests; they are regarded as particularly suitable for this purpose because of their apparent lack of relationship to the animal and plant viruses. The baculoviruses have been used e.g. to control the European pine sawfly (*Neodiprion sertifer*) and the European spruce sawfly (*Gilpinia hercyniae*) as well as the Small White Butterfly (*Artogeia rapae*).

baculovirus Any virus of the family BACULOVIRIDAE.

baculovirus expression systems Systems in which vectors that are based on the baculovirus genome (see BACULOVIRIDAE) are used for the expression of recombinant proteins in insect cells (or, more recently, in the cells of vertebrates). The use of baculovirus vectors for this purpose was suggested by the large quantities of matrix protein that are produced in insect cells infected with these viruses; as early as the 1980s, human interferon was produced in this kind of system.

Advantages of baculovirus expression systems

The advantages claimed for these systems include:

● High-level expression of recombinant proteins. Given the use of strong promoters to drive recombinant genes, yields of recombinant protein have been reported to reach up to ~500 mg/L (up to ~50% of total cell protein).

● Unlike prokaryotic cells, insect cells can carry out various post-translational modifications of expressed proteins similar to those carried out in mammalian cells.

● Procedures for growing (culturing) insect cells are simpler than those involved in the growth of mammalian cells – e.g. relatively simple, serum-free media can be used, and there is no requirement for CO_2.

● High-density suspension culture can be employed.

● Protein expression can be easily scaled-up.

● Insect cells are characteristically refractory to infection by human viruses – so that recombinant proteins are unlikely to be contaminated by viral pathogens.

Baculovirus expression systems have been used e.g. for the production of veterinary products which include a vaccine against swine fever.

Disadvantages of baculovirus expression systems

These expression systems have several disadvantages:

● Some of the required post-translational modifications are poorly represented, or lacking, in insect cells. For example, patterns of glycosylation may be significantly different from those that characterize human glycoproteins. To combat this, genetically modified cells (see e.g. MIMIC SF9 INSECT CELLS) can be used; these cells are designed to express stably various mammalian glycosyltransferases.

● Recombinant proteins expressed in insect cells may remain largely intracellular. This is contrary to the general requirements of a production process – in which the formation of extracellular (i.e. secreted) protein facilitates the downstream processing of the product. In some systems, the gene of the recombinant protein is fused with a tag (e.g. a tag encoding multiple histidine residues – see NICKEL-CHARGED AFFINITY RESIN) which can facilitate detection/isolation/purification of the product following cell lysis.

Development of baculovirus expression systems

Early procedures used for inserting a foreign gene into the baculovirus genome depended initially on homologous recombination – insect cells were co-transfected with (i) baculovirus DNA and (ii) the gene of interest, present in a separate vector and flanked by (non-essential) baculovirus DNA (e.g. sequences from the polyhedrin gene). If the gene of interest inserts into the polyhedrin gene (homologous recombination), the plaque morphology of the resulting recombinant baculovirus will be altered, thus allowing identification of recombinant viruses (and, hence, separation from the background of non-recombinant viruses). This approach, however, was found to yield only a low proportion (<1%) of recombinant viruses.

Improved recovery of recombinant viruses was achieved by using linearized viral genomes, and a further improvement resulted from the prior removal from the viral genome of an essential sequence, ORF 1629; in this case, a functional viral genome is produced only if recombination occurs with the experimental DNA – which includes ORF 1629 as well as the target sequence.

A rapid, commercial system produces recombinant baculovirus genomes by a 1-hour procedure involving *in vitro* site-specific (*att*-mediated) recombination between a linearized, modified baculovirus genome and the cloned gene of interest: see BACULODIRECT.

(See also BAC-TO-BAC and PFASTBAC DUAL VECTOR KIT.)

A convenient method for producing recombinant baculoviruses involves the (directional) insertion of target DNA via a simplified, low-cost technique which employs a restriction enzyme (Bsu36I) and the T4 DNA polymerase and T4 DNA ligase [see BioTechniques (2006) 41(4):453–458].

In some cases, expression of recombinant proteins has been achieved in whole (live) insects. For example, production of the veterinary product Vibragen Omega (used therapeutically for canine parvovirus infection) is carried out in silkworms; in this process, insects are infected with a recombinant polyhedrosis virus containing a sequence encoding recombinant feline interferon omega.

BaeI A type IIB RESTRICTION ENDONUCLEASE from *Bacillus sphaericus*.

bait protein See YEAST TWO-HYBRID SYSTEM and BACTERIOMATCH TWO-HYBRID SYSTEM.

BALB/c mice An inbred, laboratory strain of mice prone to the development of myelomas following certain stimuli.

barcoding See MOLECULAR INVERSION PROBE GENOTYPING.

Bardet–Biedl syndrome A genetically heterogeneous disorder involving a range of chromosomes (2, 3, 4, 7, 9, 11, 12, 14, 15, 16, 20) and exhibiting various phenotypic manifestations, including renal and retinal abnormalities.

barnase A bacterial endoribonuclease, produced by *Bacillus amyloliquefaciens*, which forms cyclic products.

Barr body (chromatin body; sex chromatin; X chromatin) A small, discrete body of CHROMATIN which can be seen in the nucleus in stained, interphase cells from female mammals. A Barr body is derived from an inactivated X CHROMOSOME (see X-INACTIVATION); hence, cells from a (normal) female contain one Barr body per nucleus, while cells from a normal male contain none.

In those individuals with atypical genotypes – such as XXX (superfemale) or XO (Turner's syndrome) – the number of Barr bodies per nucleus is also atypical (respectively, two and zero in the superfemale and in individuals with Turner's syndrome).

base composition See BASE RATIO.

base excision repair A DNA repair system, found in organisms ranging from bacteria to humans, that deals with chemically induced damage, including damage caused by reactive oxygen species.

The excision of an aberrant, chemically modified base is catalyzed by a DNA glycosylase. (See also 8-OXOG.) The phosphodiester bond on one side of the AP site is then cut by an AP endonuclease – e.g. exonuclease III in *Escherichia coli* (an enzyme which has exonuclease and apurinic/apyrimidinic endonuclease activity). Replacement of the damaged nucleotide (and apparently of several adjacent nucleotides) is then effected by a DNA polymerase.

(See also MISMATCH REPAIR.)

base J β-D-glucosylhydroxymethyluracil: an unusual base in the nuclear DNA of kinetoplastid protozoans and in *Euglena*.

In trypanosomatids, base J appears to replace a proportion of thymine residues and is found e.g. in the telomere region.

Attempts were made to obtain a null mutation in the gene of the base J-binding protein JBP1 but were not successful [Nucleic Acids Res (2005) 33(5):1699–1709].

base pairing (in double-stranded DNA and RNA) The pairing (i.e. binding, annealing, hybridization) of each base in one of the strands with a particular, *complementary* base in the other strand; such *complementarity* depends on the specificity of binding between cytosine and guanine, and between thymine (or uracil in RNA) and adenine.

base ratio (base composition; dissymmetry ratio) In DNA, the ratio:

$$[A+T]/[G+C]$$

in which A, T, G and C are relative molar amounts of the four types of nucleotide. Microbes with a base ratio of >1 are sometimes called *AT types*; those with a base ratio <1 are *GC types*.

(cf. GC%.)

BCIP 5-Bromo-4-chloro-3-indolyl phosphate: a substrate for the enzyme alkaline phosphatase used in PROBE LABELING.

bcr-abl (*BCR-ABL*) See ABL.

bDNA assay Branched DNA assay: a method for quantitation of a specific DNA or RNA target sequence. Based on SIGNAL AMPLIFICATION, it avoids a major problem associated with TARGET AMPLIFICATION methods such as PCR, i.e. potential contamination of apparatus and environment with amplicons from previous assays.

Essentially, a bDNA assay involves: (i) a target-specific PROBE that immobilizes target sequences on a solid support, and (ii) a second type of probe which links each immobilized target to a synthetic, multi-*branched* molecule of DNA (so-called bDNA) – which, in turn, binds many enzyme-linked probes; using a dioxetane substrate, the enzyme generates an amplified chemiluminescent signal whose intensity is related to the number of target sequences in the sample.

bDNA kits (Quantiplex™; Bayer Diagnostics, Leverkusen) have been used e.g. for assaying viruses such as HIV (the human immunodeficiency virus) [J Clin Microbiol (2003) 41:3361–3367; J Clin Microbiol (2004) 42:3012–3016] and the simian immunodeficiency virus [J Virol (2004) 78:5324–5337].

Beijing/W See W-BEIJING STRAIN.

BENA435 A cell-permeant DNA-staining fluorophore, with absorption and emission maxima at 435 nm and 484 nm respectively (when complexed with DNA), which is reported to be non-toxic and photoactivated *in vivo*. The compound is apparently an intercalating agent; fluorescence is reported to be stronger with dA/dT homopolymers than with dG/dC homopolymers.

It appears that BENA435 is not related to any other DNA-staining agent.

[BENA435: Nucleic Acids Res (2006) 34(5):e43.]

(See also DNA STAINING.)

Benefix® A recombinant form of blood-clotting factor IX used for the management of hemophilia B.

benzene-1,3,5-triacetic acid See BTA.

***O*^{6}-benzylguanine labels** See GENE FUSION (uses).

benzylpenicillin *Syn.* Penicillin G (see also table in the entry ANTIBIOTIC).

Bernard–Soulier syndrome (hemorrhagiparous thrombocytic dystrophy) A rare autosomal recessive condition characterized by a tendency for abnormal/excessive bleeding. Genetic lesions associated with this condition – on chromosomes 3, 17 and 22 – affect genes encoding subunits of a multi-subunit receptor for the von Willebrand factor.

[Bernard–Soulier syndrome: Orphanet J Rare Dis (2006) 1: 46.]

BEVS Baculovirus expression vector system(s) (see BACULO-VIRUS EXPRESSION SYSTEMS).

***bgl* operon** See CATABOLITE REPRESSION.

BglF See CATABOLITE REPRESSION.

BglG See CATABOLITE REPRESSION.

BHK cells Cells derived from baby hamster kidney.

BiFC BIMOLECULAR FLUORESCENCE COMPLEMENTATION.

bifunctional intercalating agent See INTERCALATING AGENT.

bifunctional vector *Syn.* SHUTTLE VECTOR.

BigEasy™ linear cloning system A cloning system (Lucigen Corporation, Middleton WI) which involves a *linear* plasmid vector (pJAZZ-KA) derived from the linear dsDNA genome of coliphage N15. (See PHAGE N15.) The prophage of phage N15 does not integrate into the bacterial chromosome but replicates as an extrachromosomal 'plasmid'. The mechanism of replication in N15 has features in common with replication in some other (linear genome) phages (e.g. φKO2) and with replication in the bacterium *Borrelia burgdorferi* (which also has a linear genome); see BORRELIA BURGDORFERI for more details.

Advantages of a linear vector system include the ability to clone sequences (e.g. inverted repeats, AT-rich regions) that may exhibit instability when cloned in circular, supercoiled plasmid vectors.

bimolecular fluorescence complementation (BiFC) A method used for the detection of protein–protein interaction *in vivo*; in this method, the two proteins of interest are each tagged with a (non-fluorescent) fragment of a fluorophore (such as YELLOW FLUORESCENT PROTEIN) so that interaction between the two proteins *in vivo* may result in juxtaposition of the two parts of the fluorophore – with consequent production of a fluorescent signal on appropriate excitation.

In the procedure called extended BiFC (exBiFC), the pair of proteins whose interaction is being studied are each tagged with a *constitutively* fluorescent domain (a different fluorophore for each protein) in addition to the fragment of fluorophore used for the basic BiFC reaction. This enables the researcher to follow both (i) the expression of each protein and (ii) the localization of each of the proteins; it also permits normalization of the BiFC signal in relation to the levels of expression of the two proteins.

[exBiFC (e.g.): BioTechniques (2006) 41(6):688–692.]

[BiFC fragments: BioTechniques (2006) 40(1):61–66.]

BiFC for demonstrating protein interaction in *Arabidopsis* [Plant Physiol (2007) 143(2):650–660] and *Saccharomyces cerevisiae* [Eukaryotic Cell (2007) 6(3):378–387].

binary deoxyribozyme ligase A type of engineered DEOXY-RIBOZYME which can be used to re-code sequence information [Nucleic Acids Res (2006) 34(8):2166–2172].

Based on the MAXIZYME principle, this ligase consists of two (ssDNA) 'half deoxyribozymes' which can be activated to become a functional enzyme by the binding of a sequence-specific 'bridging oligonucleotide'. In the active enzyme, the two 'half-deoxyribozymes' are base-paired in their central regions to form a (dsDNA) stem; at *each* end of this stem the pair of single strands – one from each 'half-deoxyribozyme' – can act as recognition sequences. At each end of the stem, i.e. at the junction between double-stranded and single-stranded regions, is a catalytic (ligase) domain.

When a single *effector* strand of DNA is hybridized to both of the recognition sequences at *one* end of the stem (acting as a 'bridging oligonucleotide' across the two sequences), the enzyme is stimulated to carry out ligation of two separate DNA strands which have bound to the recognition sequences at the *other* end of the stem. Hence, it is possible to ligate two *specified* sequences to form a new sequence, i.e. to 'write' a new sequence.

binary probe　A composite PROBE that consists of two single-stranded oligonucleotides designed to hybridize to the target sequence in an end-to-end fashion – with the (labeled) 5′ end of one oligo juxtaposed to the (labeled) 3′ end of the other. *Correct* hybridization of *both* probes to the target sequence can be indicated in two main ways.

In one approach, the 5′ and 3′ labels are a compatible pair of fluorophores which, when closely juxtaposed in a correctly hybridized probe, exhibit so-called fluorescence resonance energy transfer (see FRET; see also LIGHTCYCLER).

In a different approach, both of the oligos are labeled with a pyrene molecule. The rationale is that the emission maxima of pyrene on free (unbound) oligos are significantly different from those of two juxtaposed pyrene molecules on a bound probe (an excited dimer, or so-called *excimer*).

(See also PYRENE BINARY PROBE.)

binary vector system　A vector system in which a given event or function requires the co-ordinated activity of two separate components.

A binary vector system is used, for example, in the method with which plants are genetically modified by the activity of the plant-pathogenic bacterium *Agrobacterium tumefaciens*. This method exploits the ability of *A. tumefaciens* to transfer DNA to plant cells – as occurs when it causes CROWN GALL (q.v.). Genetic modification of plants by this method involves specialized, engineered strains of *A. tumefaciens* which retain the *vir* (virulence) function, i.e. they are able to promote the transfer of T-DNA – or of DNA which is flanked by the end-sequences of T-DNA – into plant cells. The given DNA to be inserted into plant cells (e.g. viral DNA) is first inserted, *in vitro*, into a small vector molecule at a location flanked by T-DNA border sequences. This vector is then inserted into one of the engineered strains of *A. tumefaciens*, forming a binary vector system; thus, when the (Ti-dependent) *vir* function is activated in the bacterium, the T-DNA-flanked target DNA is transferred from the small vector into plant cells.

The design of the small vector (i.e. the one carrying the T-DNA-flanked target sequence) is particularly important if the genetically modified plant is subsequently to enter the general agricultural environment. These vectors should exclude extraneous DNA, and various minimal T-DNA vectors have been proposed [e.g. BioTechniques (2006) 41(6):708–710].

BioEase™　The designation of several expression vectors (from Invitrogen, Carlsbad CA) which encode a 72-amino-acid tag that directs IN VIVO BIOTINYLATION of a protein–tag fusion product; biotinylation can be achieved in bacterial, insect and mammalian cells.

Biotinylated proteins can be detected and purified *in vitro* with STREPTAVIDIN-based systems.

(See also destination vectors pcDNA™6/BioEase™-DEST and pMT/BioEase™-DEST in entry GATEWAY SITE-SPECIFIC RECOMBINATION SYSTEM (table).)

bioinformatics　A computer-based approach to storing, organizing, making accessible and analyzing the vast amounts of information derived primarily from studies on genomes and proteins.

Much of the information consists of sequences of nucleotide residues (from DNA and RNA) and amino acid residues (from proteins) that are stored in databases (see DATABASE). Such stored information can be used, for example, to infer the function/activity of a newly identified gene or protein by comparing its sequence with sequences of existing (known) genes or proteins.

Analysis of the sequence data (by a process referred to as *computational biology*) has a number of aims. In the context of nucleic acids, one of the requirements is to identify genes among the long, continuous sequences of nucleotide residues. A further aim is to develop approaches that enable prediction of the three-dimensional structure and function of molecules of RNA and protein.

An overarching aim is to classify data into categories which reflect evolutionary relationships.

Desktop facilities for studies in bioinformatics include e.g. the VECTOR NTI ADVANCE 9.1.

[Online bioinformatics resources collection (the University of Pittsburgh Health Sciences Library System) – a one-stop gateway to online bioinformatics databases/software tools: Nucleic Acids Res (2006) published online November 15: doi: 10.1093/nar/gkl781.]

biolistic method　A form of 'bombardment' used for inserting DNA into certain types of cell; the DNA is coated onto μm-scale gold particles and fired into the cells.

[Example: Mol Biol Cell (2007) 18(2):369–379.]

biological containment　A safety-orientated approach to experimentation with genetically engineered, or other, organisms or entities in which e.g. a 'limited life' or 'self-destruct' mechanism is brought into operation automatically when the function of the organism or entity has been completed.

(See also AMPLICON CONTAINMENT.)

bioluminescence　Light generated within living organisms, or in systems obtained from living organisms, that is derived from a chemical reaction. (See also the entry for (engineered) IN VIVO BIOLUMINESCENCE.) (cf. CHEMILUMINESCENCE.)

Bioluminescence is exhibited by some bacteria (e.g. species of *Alteromonas*, *Vibrio* (*Photobacterium*) and *Xenorhabdus*), fungi (e.g. *Armillaria mellea*, species of *Mycena*), dinoflagellates (e.g. *Gonyaulax*, *Noctiluca*, *Pyrocystis*, *Pyrodinium*) and fireflies (*Photinus pyralis*).

All organisms that exhibit bioluminescence use a (species-specific) thiol-containing oxidoreductase involved in excitation of the light-emitting entity; the generic term for this enzyme is LUCIFERASE (q.v.).

The light-emitting entity from different species is referred to by the generic term *luciferin*. In the firefly, luciferin is 4,5-dihydro-2-(6-hydroxy-2-benzothiazolyl)-4-thiazolecarboxylic acid.

Production of bioluminescence depends on the presence of free oxygen – although only very low levels may be required. The source of energy in bioluminescence depends on species; for example, the firefly uses ATP, but bacteria use NAD and FMN.

Different organisms emit light of different wavelengths; for example, the light from fireflies is ~560 nm while that from bacteria is ~475–505 nm. Some dinoflagellates emit light of ~480 nm in pulses of ~0.1 second duration.

Applications of bioluminescence

The luciferase–luciferin system of the firefly is employed e.g. for detecting ATP in PYROSEQUENCING, and a luciferase reporter has been used in a wide range of studies – e.g. for studying promoter function [Appl Environ Microbiol (2005) 71:1356–1363].

A bioluminescent system has been used e.g. to detect ATP in certain products (such as UHT milk), the presence of ATP in samples of these products being used as an indication of metabolism by contaminating organisms.

(See also BRET, and *Vibrio* in the entry QUORUM SENSING.)

bioluminescence resonance energy transfer See BRET.

biomagnetic separation See DYNABEADS.

biopanning See PHAGE DISPLAY.

biopharmaceutical Any of a wide category of products (which include nucleic-acid-based and protein-based agents) that are used therapeutically, or as *in vivo* diagnostics, and which are prepared by procedures other than simple extraction of pre-existing compounds from natural, non-engineered organisms.

The biopharmaceuticals include a number of products that depend on recombinant DNA technology. In some cases (see e.g. INSULINS) a recombinant protein is largely based on, and is designed to mimic, a natural protein, but may act over a different time-scale. In other cases (for example, the fusion protein etanercept – see accompanying table) the product is an artificial construct which has no natural counterpart.

A number of allied products are manufactured specifically for research, and are not intended for therapeutic, diagnostic or other clinical purposes. They include various products that are used in cell/tissue-culture studies – e.g. basic fibroblast growth factor (bFGF), acidic fibroblast growth factor (aFGF), glial-derived neurotrophic factor (GDNF) and insulin-like growth factor-1 (IGF-1); all of these are recombinant human proteins which are synthesized in *Escherichia coli*.

The manufacture of proteins that are active in a medical or veterinary setting requires not only the correct formulation of nucleic acid coding sequences but also synthesis of proteins which, for correct activity, have the appropriate type of post-translational modification, e.g. specific patterns of glycosylation. This requirement may preclude the use of cells which are unable to carry out a specific type of post-translational modification; for example, bacteria typically do not carry out the type of glycosylation required in a number of mammalian proteins. Nevertheless, in some cases, such a facility may be incorporated in cells in which it is normally lacking (see e.g. MIMIC SF9 INSECT CELLS).

The table shows only a limited selection of the wide range of products that have been produced on a commercial basis.

biotin (coenzyme R, vitamin H) A cofactor which, *in vivo*, is involved in various types of carboxylation reaction; in these reactions biotin binds (via its carboxyl group) to the ε-amino group of a lysine residue in the enzyme.

(See also IN VIVO BIOTINYLATION.)

Biotin is used e.g. for labeling PROBES. For this purpose it can be linked, covalently, to nucleoside triphosphate molecules (e.g. dATP) through an allylamine *spacer arm* that may contain e.g. a chain of 10 or more carbon atoms. Biotinylated nucleoside triphosphates can be incorporated into DNA e.g. by 3′ END LABELING or by NICK TRANSLATION.

Biotin can be used to label DNA or RNA. For example, in one commercial product, biotin is linked via a 14-C spacer arm to the 6-position of dATP; this labeled nucleotide can be incorporated efficiently into DNA by nick translation in the presence of dCTP, dGTP and dTTP. CTP labeled at the N4-position via a 14-C spacer arm can be incorporated efficiently into transcripts (e.g. with T7 or T3 RNA polymerase) in the presence of the template and ATP, GTP and UTP.

Site-specific biotinylation of RNA may be achieved during transcription (with T7 RNA polymerase) by the use of special engineered bases, one of which can carry a biotin (or other) residue [Nucleic Acids Res (2005) 33(15):e129].

A biotinylated label may be detected e.g. with a STREPTAVIDIN-bound fluorophore or enzyme; as the biotin molecule is tethered to its nucleotide via the (long) allylamine chain, biotin–streptavidin binding can occur freely (i.e. unhindered by the nucleic acid molecule).

biotin ligase See IN VIVO BIOTINYLATION (engineered).

biotin ligase recognition peptide (BLRP) See IN VIVO BIOTINYLATION (engineered).

biotinylation *in vivo* (engineered) See entry IN VIVO BIOTINYLATION (engineered).

BirA The protein–biotin ligase of *Escherichia coli* (encoded by gene *birA*). (See IN VIVO BIOTINYLATION (engineered).)

Bis A shorthand form for *N,N′*-methylene-bis-acrylamide, a catalyst used for cross-linking ACRYLAMIDE in the preparation of POLYACRYLAMIDE.

bisulfite (action on DNA) Bisulfite can deaminate cytosine to uracil in single-stranded DNA; subsequent replication leads to a GC to AT change. *Methylated* cytosines are refractory to this treatment.

Bisulfite can also cause cross-linking between nucleic acids and proteins.

[Bisulfite in assays of genomic methylation: BioTechniques (2005) 38:354–358; BioTechniques (2006) 41(6):734–739.]

(See also COBRA, HEADLOOP SUPPRESSION PCR, METHYLATION-SPECIFIC PCR, METHYLATION-SPECIFIC SINGLE-BASE

BIOPHARMACEUTICAL: examples of some commercial products whose production involves recombinant DNA technology

Product (Company)	Function/use
Aranesp® (Amgen) (darbepoietin-α)	An erythropoietic protein which stimulates production of erythrocytes (red blood cells). This recombinant protein is produced in a mammalian cell line. Aranesp® is used e.g. for the treatment of anemia associated with chronic renal disease, a condition in which the body's natural erythropoietic system is impaired
Benefix® (Genetics Institute)	A recombinant form of blood-clotting factor IX, produced in Chinese hamster ovary (CHO) cells, which is used in the management of hemophilia B
Enbrel® (Amgen) (etanercept)	A soluble fusion protein combining the extracellular domain of the p75 cell-surface receptor of tumor necrosis factor (TNF) with the Fc portion of immunoglobulin IgG. By sequestering TNF, this agent inhibits the binding of TNF (a pro-inflammatory cytokine) to its natural cell-surface receptor. (The Fc moiety, which has a binding site on macrophages, may facilitate the removal of complexed TNF via phagocytosis.) The product has been used successfully in rheumatoid arthritis to reduce pain and inflammation, an effect which is associated with a fall in the level of TNF
EPOGEN® (Amgen)	A recombinant form of the natural agent erythropoietin (involved in stimulating production of red blood cells) which is produced in a mammalian cell line. It is used in some cases of anemia
Fabrazyme® (Genzyme)	A recombinant form of the enzyme α-galactosidase A (prepared in Chinese hamster ovary (CHO) cells). The product is used for treating Fabry disease (see entry), a condition characterized by a deficiency in α-galactosidase A activity
INTRON® A (Schering-Plough)	Recombinant interferon α-2b. This agent is intended for use in a range of conditions, including e.g. malignant melanoma, chronic hepatitis C and AIDS-related Kaposi sarcoma
Kepivance® (Amgen) (palifermin)	A recombinant form of the human keratinocyte growth factor (KGF). This agent is used in severe oral mucositis, in which cells of the mouth and throat surfaces have been damaged by cancer chemotherapy or by other treatments; it helps to protect the existing cells and stimulates growth/development of new cells
Kineret® (Amgen)	A recombinant form of the interleukin-1 (IL-1) receptor antagonist (IL-1ra) which is produced in *Escherichia coli*. IL-1 is formed in excess in patients with rheumatoid arthritis; by inhibiting the activity of IL-1 in the body, this agent is able to reduce the inflammatory response in the disease. (Other products synthesized in *E. coli* include e.g. Neupogen® (see below); see also entry GLYCOSYLATION.)
Kogenate® (Bayer)	A recombinant form of human factor VIII which is produced in BHK (baby hamster kidney) cells. It is used therapeutically in cases of hemophilia A
Lantus® (Sanofi-Aventis)	INSULIN GLARGINE: a long-acting recombinant form of human insulin used for the treatment of diabetics. (See also NovoRapid®, below.)
Nespo® (Dompé Biotec)	A product in the same category as Aranesp® (see above)
Neulasta® (Amgen) (PEGfilgrastim)	A longer-acting form of Neupogen® (see below)
Neupogen® (Amgen) (filgrastim)	A recombinant form of G-CSF (granulocyte colony-stimulating factor) (produced in *Escherichia coli*). This agent stimulates the production of neutrophils (infection-fighting white blood cells) which are depleted in neutropenia. The recombinant product is not glycosylated (unlike the natural protein) but its biological activity is equivalent to that of the natural G-CSF
NovoRapid® (Novo Nordisk)	A short-acting, recombinant form of insulin: insulin aspart (see entry INSULINS) used for the treatment of diabetics. (See also Lantus®, above.)
NovoSeven® (Novo Nordisk)	A recombinant form of factor VIIa (produced in baby hamster kidney (BHK) cells). This agent permits the coagulation of blood in the absence of factors VIII and IX (although it does not replace factors VIII and IX). It is used e.g. for the prevention of bleeding during surgery in hemophiliac patients
Refludan® (Hoechst) (lepirudin)	A recombinant form of the thrombin-inhibitor hirudin (produced in the yeast *Saccharomyces cerevisiae*). This product is used e.g. as an anticoagulant
Vitravene® (ISIS)	An antisense oligonucleotide (21 nucleotides in length) used for the treatment of CMV (cytomegalovirus) retinitis in AIDS patients. This agent is injected directly into the eye and inhibits viral replication by interfering with the function of certain viral mRNAs

EXTENSION.)

(See also the note on bisulfite-treated (sulfonated) DNA in the entry AMPLICON INACTIVATION.)

BK virus A polyomavirus (genome: ccc dsDNA) which infects humans and other mammals. It is related to JC VIRUS (q.v.).

BL21-CodonPlus® See CODON BIAS.

BL21 Star™ Strains of *Escherichia coli* (Invitrogen, Carlsbad CA) used e.g. for T7-promoter-based protein expression. The strains have a mutation, *rne131*, in the gene encoding RNase E; the resulting decrease in RNase activity in these strains is reported to result in an improvement in the stability of transcripts and an increase the yield of protein.

bla gene A gene encoding a β-LACTAMASE.

black–white screening A method of screening for recombinants in which the host cells contain the same indicator system (β-galactosidase and α-peptide genes) as that used in *blue–white screening* (see PBLUESCRIPT for details) but in which a different chromogenic reagent (Sgal) is used. In this system, the presence of an insert (recombinants: no β-galactosidase activity) is indicated by the development of white colonies, while cells lacking an insert (β-galactosidase activity) cleave Sgal to products that form a black compound with (added) ferric chloride (and hence form black colonies).

BLAST Basic local alignment search tool (a program used for comparing sequences):

http://www.ncbi.nlm.nih.gov/BLAST/

Using this search tool, it is possible to make the following comparisons:

1. Nucleotide query sequence compared with nucleotide database.

2. Products of the six possible reading frames of a nucleotide query sequence (three reading frames per strand) compared with a protein database.

3. Six possible reading frames of a nucleotide query sequence compared with six reading frames in a nucleotide database.

4. A polypeptide or protein query sequence compared with a protein database.

5. A polypeptide/protein query sequence compared with the products of all six reading frames of a nucleotide database.

Analysis of BLAST alignment reports may be facilitated by web-based interface SEQUEROME [BioTechniques (2005) 39(2):186–188].

blasticidin S An antibiotic which inhibits protein synthesis by inhibiting the peptidyltransferase reaction during translation in both prokaryotic and eukaryotic cells.

Examples of use of blasticidin S in mammalian cells (at 6 μg/mL) [PLoS Medicine (2006) 3(10):e420], and in fungal cells (at 300 μg/mL) [Eukaryotic Cell (2006) 5(6):896–904].

bleomycin A structurally complex, glycoprotein, DNA-binding anticancer agent, produced by *Streptomyces verticillus*, that causes single-strand and double-strand cleavage of DNA in the presence of Fe^{2+} and oxygen.

blocked reading frame See OPEN READING FRAME.

blood RNA isolation kit See e.g. PAXGENE BLOOD RNA KIT.

blotting Any of various procedures in which molecules or frag-

ments are transferred from a gel (following electrophoresis) to a nitrocellulose or other matrix.

(See SOUTHERN BLOTTING, NORTHERN BLOTTING, WESTERN BLOTTING, IMMUNOBLOTTING.)

BLRP Biotin ligase recognition peptide: see IN VIVO BIOTINYLATION.

blue-green algae The former name of the CYANOBACTERIA; they were called 'blue-green algae' because of their ability to carry out photosynthesis in the oxygenic manner, i.e. a mode similar to that found in algae and higher plants.

blue–white screening See PBLUESCRIPT.

(cf. BLACK–WHITE SCREENING.)

Bluescript® See PBLUESCRIPT.

blunt-end ligation Ligation of two blunt-ended molecules of nucleic acid using e.g. the (ATP-dependent) T4 DNA ligase.

(See also POLISHING.)

blunt-ended DNA Double-stranded DNA which has no 5′ or 3′ single-stranded overhangs. A pair of blunt-ended termini is generated by cleavage with *certain* types of RESTRICTION ENDONUCLEASE (e.g. HpaI) that make a 'blunt-ended cut'. (Compare with STICKY ENDS.)

(See also END-IT DNA END-REPAIR KIT and POLISHING.)

Bluo-gal See X-GAL.

BmSNPV See NUCLEAR POLYHEDROSIS VIRUSES.

BODIPY The trade name of a range of fluorophores based on a substituted tricyclic indacene core. Some of the dyes are used e.g. in the automated sequencing of DNA and for the labeling of probes etc.

BODIPY dyes are designated systematically on the basis of their approximate absorption/emission maxima (nm), as determined in methanol.

***Bombyx mori* NPV** See NUCLEAR POLYHEDROSIS VIRUSES.

Borrelia burgdorferi A species of Gram-negative bacteria in which the genome consists of *linear* double-stranded DNA. In this organism the terminal regions of the chromosome are closed (hairpin) structures called *telomeres*.

Chromosomal replication in *B. burgdorferi* is initiated bidirectionally from an internal origin. Replication involves an intermediate circular molecule which consists of a chromosome dimer in a head-to-head, tail-to-tail arrangement. The junctions between the individual chromosomes are processed by a breakage-and-reunion mechanism (*telomere resolution*) to form the closed (hairpin) termini in each daughter chromosome; telomere resolution is catalysed by an enzyme called PROTELOMERASE.

Features of this type of genome replication are also shown by certain phages (e.g. N15, φKO2).

B. burgdorferi (*sensu lato*) is the causal agent of the tick-borne infection Lyme disease.

bovine syncytial virus See SPUMAVIRINAE.

BOX element A type of repetitive intergenic sequence which occurs in the genomes of certain bacteria (e.g. *Streptococcus pneumoniae*) and which has been used in one form of REP-PCR.

In *S. pneumoniae* the genome is reported to contain more

31

than 100 BOX elements; these elements have been found to affect the expression of neighboring genes, and there is also evidence that they are mobile [J Bacteriol (2006) 188(23): 8307–8312].

BOXTO A fluorescent cyanine dye which (bound to dsDNA) has an emission maximum at 552 nm on excitation at 515 nm; it was reported to show preferential binding in the minor groove [Nucleic Acids Res (2003) 31(21):6227–6234].

This dye was used in combination with a target-specific probe in real-time PCR [BioTechniques (2006) 40(3):315–319].

bp Base pairs: see KB.

BP Clonase™ An enzyme used in the GATEWAY SITE-SPECIFIC RECOMBINATION SYSTEM. It can mediate *in vitro* exchange between a segment flanked by *att*B sites (e.g. a linear dsDNA PCR-generated amplicon) and a segment flanked by *att*P sites (e.g. in a circular vector molecule); the PCR amplicon can be generated by using primers that incorporate 5′ *att*B sites.

BP Clonase™ is used, for example, for generating an *entry clone* which can be subsequently expressed in a destination vector (for examples of destination vectors see the table in GATEWAY SITE-SPECIFIC RECOMBINATION SYSTEM).

(cf. LR CLONASE.)

branch migration See HOLLIDAY JUNCTION.

branched DNA assay See BDNA ASSAY.

BRCA Breast cancer gene: either of two genes, referred to as *BRCA1* and *BRCA2*; inherited mutations in these genes are associated with a risk for breast cancer and ovarian cancer.

One study found that weight loss in early adulthood (18–30 years) may reduce the risk of early-onset BRCA-associated breast cancers [Breast Cancer Res (2005) 7(5):R833–R843].

BrdU *Syn.* BUDR.

BRE Transcription factor IIB recognition element: a eukaryotic promoter sequence that recognizes transcription factor IIB.

breast cancer (associated topics) See, for example, the entries BRCA, EPSTEIN–BARR VIRUS and EPIDERMAL GROWTH FACTOR RECEPTOR FAMILY.

breast cancer genes See BRCA.

BRET Bioluminescence resonance energy transfer: the phenomenon, analogous to FRET, in which the donor is a molecule that exhibits chemiluminescence when supplied with a suitable substrate; under these conditions, the acceptor molecule – in close proximity to the donor – is activated to produce a fluorescent signal.

One advantage of BRET, compared with FRET, is that, owing to the absence of external excitation, it offers a higher signal-to-background ratio and is therefore particularly well suited to conditions in which low-level signals are produced *within* experimental animals.

[Example of use: Mol Endocrinol (2006) 20(3):661–674.]

brlf-1 gene See ZEBRA.

broad-range primer ('universal' primer) Any PRIMER whose target sequence is a conserved sequence of nucleotides that occurs in a wide range of species. Thus, for example, certain sequences in the bacterial 16S rRNA gene are common to all species of bacteria. Primers that are complementary to these sequences have various uses. Broad-range primers have been used e.g. as a control in PCR-based assays of species-specific targets in bacterial genomic DNA; in such an assay, failure to amplify a conserved sequence with the broad-range primers may indicate e.g. a failure of the DNA extraction process or failure of the particular PCR protocol used to amplify target sequences.

Another use of broad-range primers in PCR is the detection of PCR-inhibitory substances in test samples; thus, inhibitors may be suspected if a sample containing bacterial genomic DNA yields no products when assayed by PCR with broad-range primers.

5-bromouracil (BU) A mutagenic analog of thymine. The *keto* tautomer pairs with adenine, but the *enol* tautomer pairs with cytosine; if present in the *enol* form during DNA replication it can cause an AT→GC mutation.

BssHII A type IIP RESTRICTION ENDONUCLEASE produced by *Bacillus stearothermophilus*; recognition site: G↓CGCGC. It forms fragments with a 5′ overhang. BssHII is useful e.g. for the preferential cutting of genomic DNA at (GC-rich) sites in CPG ISLANDS.

BTA Benzene-1,3,5-triacetic acid: an agent used e.g. for attaching 5′-aminated oligonucleotides to an aminosilanized glass surface [Nucleic Acids Res (2006) 34(3):e22].

BU BROMOURACIL.

bubble-linker PCR *Syn.* VECTORETTE PCR.

buccal cell sampling Collection of cells from inside the cheek as a source of DNA for analysis (e.g. DNA profiling); a swab or filter-paper device is commonly used. The yield of DNA per sample varies considerably between individuals – as does the ratio of human to non-human (e.g. bacterial) DNA in the sample. Using a filter-paper device, the (total) DNA yield per sample may be within the range 20–500 ng [BioTechniques (2005) 39:257–261].

Double-stranded DNA in solution can be quantitated e.g. by the PICOGREEN ASSAY.

(See also FORENSIC APPLICATIONS.)

Analogous procedures are employed for collecting DNA samples from animals (mammals). Among *non*-mammalian species, efficient buccal swabbing for DNA samples has been reported for the sunfish (*Lepomis*) [BioTechniques (2005) 38: 188–192].

budded virions (BVs) See BACULOVIRIDAE.

BUdR (BrdU) 5-Bromo-2′-deoxyuridine: a mutagenic analog of thymine which can be phosphorylated by thymidine kinase and incorporated into DNA during replication.

buffy coat The thin layer of white cells on top of the packed red cells in a sample of centrifuged unclotted blood.

bumper primer See STRAND DISPLACEMENT.

BVs (budded virions) See BACULOVIRIDAE.

Bxb1 See PHAGE BXB1.

bZIP Basic zipper: a feature of certain proteins consisting of a basic region and a LEUCINE ZIPPER.

bzlf-1 gene See ZEBRA.

C

C L-Cysteine (alternative to Cys).

c-*myc* See MYC.

(See also GELDANAMYCIN.)

c-*onc* A *cellular* ONCOGENE.

C value (*C*-value etc.) The quantity of DNA in a *haploid* genome measured in e.g. picograms or number of kilobase-pairs.

cadang-cadang viroid COCONUT CADANG-CADANG VIROID.

Caenorhabditis elegans A small (~1 mm) transparent nematode worm used in genetic studies. The genome of *C. elegans* is not typically eukaryotic because many of the genes are found in *operons* (clusters of contiguous genes typical of bacterial genomic organization); polycistronic transcripts derived from these operons are processed by TRANS SPLICING.

caged DNA DNA that is transcriptionally inactivated (or partly so) by covalent modification with certain photolabile compounds; it can be inserted into cells and then 'uncaged' (i.e. made transcriptionally active) by a short burst of ultraviolet radiation (e.g. λ 360 nm) – which does not damage the cells. A similar procedure can be used with individual nucleotides, including ATP. Caging is used e.g. for studying intracellular events with a precise control of timing.

caged luciferin A form of inactive luciferin that can be inserted into cells (across the cytoplasmic membrane) and then activated intracellularly as and when required.

(See also BIOLUMINESCENCE.)

Within cells, luciferin can be activated instantaneously by a pulse of ultraviolet radiation, or alternatively, active luciferin can be released – over time – by the action of endogenous esterases on the caged luciferin, thus allowing measurements to be made over extended periods.

Caged luciferin is available commercially.

(See also LUCIFERASE.)

caged nucleotide See CAGED DNA.

call rate (in SNP genotyping) See SNP GENOTYPING.

calmodulin A ~17-kDa heat-stable, acid-stable protein which, when activated by calcium ions, stimulates various enzymes, including certain bacterial exotoxins which have ADENYLATE CYCLASE activity.

(See also AFFINITY PROTEIN EXPRESSION AND PURIFICATION.)

calmodulin affinity resin A product that binds CALMODULIN-binding peptide tag (see AFFINITY PROTEIN EXPRESSION AND PURIFICATION) in the presence of low concentrations of Ca^{2+}; elution is achieved in the presence of 2 mM EGTA at pH 7.

calreticulin A 46 kDa Ca^{2+}-binding protein, associated (e.g.) with the endoplasmic reticulum, which has role(s) in antigen presentation. Complexes formed with peptides, *in vitro*, can induce a peptide-specific T cell response.

A DNA VACCINE that also encoded calreticulin elicited a better immune response [J Virol (2004) 78(16):8468–8476].

Calreticulin has been implicated as a cell-surface ligand in adiponectin-mediated phagocytosis of apoptotic cells [J Clin Invest (2007) 117(2):375–386].

CAM (1) CALMODULIN.

(2) Cell adhesion molecule.

(3) Chorioallantoic membrane.

CAM plasmid A large *Pseudomonas* plasmid which encodes functions for the degradation of camphor.

Cambridge Reference Sequence A sequence of mitochondrial DNA (mtDNA) used as a standard against which individual mtDNA profiles are defined in the US government's mtDNA Popstats Population Database (see FORENSIC APPLICATIONS).

cAMP CYCLIC AMP.

cAMP phosphodiesterase See CYCLIC AMP.

cAMP receptor protein (CRP) See CATABOLITE REPRESSION.

Campbell model An early model, proposed by Campbell in the 1960s, for the integration of a circular plasmid or phage into a bacterial chromosome by a single cross-over.

Campylobacter A genus of Gram-negative, motile, respiratory (oxidative), oxidase-positive bacteria that metabolize amino acids and TCA cycle intermediates; the cells, spirally curved rods, are often 1–5 μm in length.

The GC% of the genomic DNA is 30–38. The type species is *C. fetus*.

Campylobacter spp are found as parasites and pathogens in man and other animals. *C. jejuni* and *C. coli* can cause e.g. food-borne infections in man. *C. fetus* can cause abortion in sheep. *C. sputorum* can cause enteric disease in hogs (pigs).

cancer (UV-induced) See ULTRAVIOLET RADIATION.

cap (in mRNA) In most eukaryotic (and some viral) mRNAs: the 5′ terminal region consisting of:

$$5'\text{-}m^7G^{5'}ppp^{5'}N^{3'}p^{5'}N^{3'}p\ldots\ldots3'$$

which is added shortly after the start of transcription. The guanosine residue is linked 5′-to-5′ to the 5′-triphosphate end of the growing transcript by the enzyme guanylyl transferase and this residue is subsequently methylated by a specific 7-methyltransferase. The methylguanosine residue appears to facilitate translation by binding to *cap-binding proteins* in the 40S ribosomal subunit.

Cap-independent translation of proteins can be achieved, *in vitro* and *in vivo*, e.g. by using an internal ribosomal entry site (see IRES).

The cap also appears to inhibit exonucleolytic degradation of the mRNA.

The cap structure is recognized by (eukaryotic) eIF4E (part of the translation initiation complex).

A (5′) 2,2,7-trimethylguanosine cap is found on snRNAs.

(See also CAPFINDER and CAPSELECT; cf. CAP ANALOG.)

CAP Catabolite activator protein (see CATABOLITE REPRESSION).

cap analog Any of various synthetic sequences of nucleotides – based on the CAP sequence and its natural variant forms – that are used for preparing transcripts for *in vitro* translation reactions. (See also IRES.)

Various types of cap analog can be obtained commercially (from e.g. Ambion, Austin TX).

[Novel cap analogs for *in vitro* synthesis of mRNAs with high translational efficiency: RNA (2004) 10(9):1479–1487.]

(See also ANTI-REVERSE CAP ANALOG.)

cap-binding proteins See CAP (in mRNA).

CapFinder A technique used for facilitating the preparation of *full-length* cDNAs. Essentially, when synthesis of the FIRST STRAND has copied the 5′ CAP region on the mRNA template strand, the MMLV reverse transcriptase adds several deoxycytidines to the 3′ end of the newly formed first strand; this addition appears to occur preferentially when the first strand has *completely* copied the capped mRNA. The reaction mixture includes copies of a short oligonucleotide (the so-called *T-S oligo*) whose 3′ end consists of several guanosine residues. This oligo binds to the short chain of terminal deoxycytidines in the first strand. The enzyme reverse transcriptase then *switches template* from the mRNA template to the T-S oligo template and, as synthesis continues, a complementary copy of the 5′ end of the T-S oligo is added to the 3′ end of the first strand. Consequently, the T-S oligo is able to prime synthesis of the second strand.

One problem with this scheme is that the 3′ end of the T-S oligo may bind to any complementary sequence(s) available in the mixture; hence, were the T-S oligo to be used as a PCR primer in a subsequent round of amplification there might be heavy contamination with random products.

The problem of contamination was addressed by a protocol which combines the template-switching effect of CapFinder with INVERSE PCR. In this approach, the cDNA, prepared as described above, was first amplified by PCR using the oligo d(T) and T-S oligo primers. Products from the PCR reaction were phosphorylated and then self-ligated (i.e. circularized). The circularized products were used as templates for inverse PCR – in which both primers were complementary to *known* (internal) sequences within the double-stranded cDNA; any random (non-specific) products would not be amplified by these primers because such products would lack the specific primer-binding sites. In this method, therefore, the products of inverse PCR include both the 5′ and the 3′ end-sequences of the (full-length) cDNA [BioTechniques (2006) 40(2):187–189].

(See also CAPSELECT.)

CAPS Cleaved amplified polymorphic sequences: a method which has been used e.g. for typing isolates of bacteria and for detecting polymorphisms. The principle underlying CAPS relates to the ability of a polymorphism (such as an SNP) to create or destroy the recognition sequence of a RESTRICTION ENDONUCLEASE; in either case (i.e. whether a restriction site is created or destroyed) the relevant site may be scored as a CAPS marker. An SNP that gives rise to a CAPS marker has been termed a SNIP-SNP.

In one study, a CAPS approach was examined for its ability to type strains of *Staphylococcus epidermidis*. Initially, to identify CAPS markers (for comparing strains), a selection of genomic target sequences were chosen and the corresponding sequences from each strain were amplified by PCR; each type of amplicon from each strain was then subjected to a panel of restriction enzymes. The results showed that most strains (33 out of 35) could be classified into five categories (referred to as CAPS types A–E) on the basis of CAPS markers detected in the amplicons.

As SNPs may produce CAPS markers it has been suggested that the latter may be useful as indicators for detecting SNPs.

capsduction Transfer of random sequences of (chromosomal or plasmid) linear dsDNA between strains of *Rhodobacter capsulatus* (*Rhodopseudomonas capsulata*) by a phage-like particle (*gene transfer agent*; GTA). No phage-specific DNA has been identified. Some strains of *R. capsulatus* can apparently receive DNA by capsduction without themselves becoming donors of GTAs.

A similar process was reported in *Methanococcus voltae* (an archaean) [J Bacteriol (1999) 181(10):2992–3002].

CapSelect A technique used for facilitating the preparation of *full-length* cDNAs from mRNAs [first described in: Nucleic Acids Res (1999) 27(21):e31]. As in the CAPFINDER method (q.v.), a short chain of deoxycytidines is added to the 3′ end of the growing FIRST STRAND after synthesis has passed the cap region on the (mRNA) template. However, a template-switching mechanism (as used in CapFinder) is not involved. Instead, the 3′ end of the first strand (which consists of the short chain of deoxycytidines) is extended by controlled ribonucleotide tailing with rATP; hence, the 3′ end of the first strand is modified to:

$$3'\text{-rA.rA...dC.dC...}$$

The modified 3′ end of the first strand is then ligated to a dsDNA adaptor which contains the 3′ overhang:

$$\text{dT.dT...dG.dG...}3'$$

in which the strand containing the overhang forms the primer for second-strand synthesis.

capsid The protein *coat* or *shell* surrounding the nucleic acid genome (or surrounding the nucleoprotein core) of a virion; in some viruses the proteins of the capsid are arranged with icosahedral symmetry. In some viruses there is an outer (lipid or lipoprotein) *envelope* (*peplos*) that surrounds the capsid; the lipid components are apparently always derived from the host cell's membranes.

carbon source responsive element See CSRE.

carcinogen Any cancer-inducing agent. Carcinogens include various types of low-molecular-weight chemical MUTAGENS, complex substances (e.g. asbestos in mesothelioma), physical agents such as ULTRAVIOLET RADIATION and X-rays, and some viruses (e.g. Epstein–Barr virus in Burkitt's lymphoma, hepatitis B virus in hepatocellular carcinoma).

(See also AMES TEST.)

CARD Catalyzed reporter deposition: see TYRAMIDE SIGNAL

AMPLIFICATION.

carrier DNA   DNA included in TRANSFORMATION experiments (i.e. in addition to 'experimental' DNA) in order to improve the efficiency of uptake.

carrier gene   See GENE FUSION.

Cascade™ expression system   A system (Active Motif) which is designed to provide tightly regulated expression of proteins in *Escherichia coli*, with low basal levels of expression prior to induction; the latter feature is important e.g. for producing toxic proteins (i.e. proteins that are toxic to the cells in which they are synthesized).

The system involves *two* transcriptional regulators, NahR and XylS2, which act sequentially. The initial induction of the system is achieved with salicylate – NahR then initiating transcription of XylS2. When produced, XylS2 is activated by the salicylate and it then induces transcription of the gene of interest.

In this system, the genes for NahR and XylS2 are located in the chromosome of an *ad hoc* expression strain of *E. coli*; the gene of interest can be either plasmid-borne or chromosomal.

Advantages of this system include e.g. tightly controlled expression, minimal background expression, and an inducer (salicylate) which is much cheaper than e.g. IPTG (used for inducing *lac*-based systems) – so that large-scale work can be carried out more economically.

cassette (gene cassette)   A DNA segment (usually encoding one or more genes) that behaves as a single unit when inserting into, or being excised from, a larger molecule.

CAT   Chloramphenicol acetyltransferase (see REPORTER GENE).

catabolite activator protein   See CATABOLITE REPRESSION.

catabolite control protein A   See CATABOLITE REPRESSION.

catabolite repression   In (Gram-negative and Gram-positive) bacteria: a phenomenon in which certain substrates (sources of carbon/energy) are used in preference to other substrates, even when the latter are freely available. For example, in *Escherichia coli*, the LAC OPERON is not induced (i.e. lactose is not utilized) – even in the presence of lactose – if glucose is available; this so-called *glucose effect* is also seen with other operons (e.g. the *ara* operon, involved in metabolism of the sugar arabinose).

Catabolite repression can operate by at least two distinct mechanisms – one characteristic of *E. coli* (and other Gram-negative, enteric bacteria) and one that has been found almost exclusively in Gram-positive species of bacteria. Both of these mechanisms are regulated by signals derived from the phosphoenolpyruvate-dependent phosphotransferase system (see PTS), a transport system used by various Gram-positive and Gram-negative bacteria for the uptake (internalization) of a range of substrates.

Gram-negative, enteric bacteria

In these bacteria the key regulator molecule is a cytoplasmic protein: the IIA component of the *glucose permease* complex (see PTS). When glucose is absent, IIA~P (the phosphorylated form of IIA) remains phosphorylated and, in this state, it activates the enzyme adenylate cyclase; this stimulates the synthesis of cyclic AMP (cAMP). cAMP forms a complex with the *cAMP-receptor protein* (CRP; = *catabolite activator protein*, CAP). This complex (cAMP-CRP) acts as a transcriptional activator, binding to the promoters of e.g. the *ara*, *lac* and other operons, permitting expression of these operons in the presence of their respective inducers.

When glucose is *present*, the *un*phosphorylated form of IIA binds to the (membrane-associated) permeases of lactose and certain other sugars; this inhibits uptake of the corresponding sugars. Because these sugars act as inducers of their respective operons, this phenomenon has been referred to as *inducer exclusion*.

Gram-positive bacteria

Certain operons in these bacteria are controlled by *operon-specific* regulator proteins. According to one scheme, the activity of these proteins depends not only on whether or not they are phosphorylated but also on *which* PTS protein was involved in their phosphorylation. In each regulator protein there are two copies of a specific phosphorylation site, each copy being designated a PRD (for PTS regulation domain).

A given PRD may be phosphorylated either by the phosphorylated IIB (IIB~P) component *of the relevant permease* or by HPr~P (both intermediates in the PTS). Phosphorylation by IIB~P is inhibitory (causing the regulator to inhibit expression of the corresponding operon). Phosphorylation by HPr~P tends to promote expression of the relevant operon.

In this model, an operon is expressed when its regulator is phosphorylated *only* by HPr~P, i.e. in the absence of glucose (and in the presence of the specific inducer). An operon stays inactive if one of the PRD sites is phosphorylated by HPr~P and the other is phosphorylated by IIB~P (i.e. in the absence of both glucose and inducer). The rationale for this is that, for the permease controlling the uptake of a given substrate, the *absence* of the substrate (i.e. inducer) leaves IIB phosphorylated and therefore able to phophorylate a PRD site – thus inhibiting the corresponding operon; this is appropriate as, in the absence of the inducer (substrate) there is no need for the given operon to be active. When the inducer is present, IIB is dephosphorylated by the inducer and so cannot phosphorylate a PRD site; if, concurrently, *glucose is absent*, HPr~P will be available to phosphorylate a PRD, thus promoting expression of the relevant operon.

In certain Gram-positive bacteria catabolite repression may involve an additional mechanism in which an ATP-dependent enzyme, *HPr kinase*, mediates the phosphorylation of IIPr. HPr~P produced by HPr kinase-mediated phosphorylation is able to form a complex with the *catabolite control protein A* (CcpA); this complex is able to inhibit transcription in target operons by binding to the appropriate regulatory site. In the species *Staphylococcus xylosus*, inactivation of *hprK* (which encodes HPr kinase) was found to abolish repression in three of the species' catabolic enzyme systems [J Bacteriol (2000) 182:1895–1902].

The *bgl* operon in (Gram-negative) *E. coli*, which encodes a catabolic system involved e.g. in the metabolism of salicin, is regulated by a PRD-containing protein designated BglG. In the absence of a β-glucoside (e.g. salicin) BglG is phosphorylated by the IIB component of β-glucoside permease (BglF), thus blocking transcription of the *bgl* operon.

(See also CSRE.)

catalytic antibody (abzyme) Any antibody which has catalytic activity.

[Example of use: Proc Natl Acad Sci USA (2005) 102 (11): 4109–4113.]

catalyzed reporter deposition See TYRAMIDE SIGNAL AMPLIFICATION.

catenane A complex consisting of two or more circular molecules of nucleic acid interlocked like the links in a chain.

(cf. CONCATEMER, CONCATENATE.)

CBP (1) CRE-binding protein: see CREB PROTEIN.

(2) CALMODULIN-binding peptide: a feature of the AFFINITY PROTEIN EXPRESSION AND PURIFICATION system (q.v.).

CBPs Cap-binding proteins: see CAP.

cccDNA Covalently closed circular DNA – i.e. DNA (either single-stranded or double-stranded) which has no free 5′ or 3′ ends.

***ccd* mechanism** One form of POST-SEGREGATIONAL KILLING, encoded by the F PLASMID, that promotes stable maintenance of the plasmid in a bacterial population. The genes *ccdB* (previously named *letB*) and *ccdA* (*letA*) encode a lethal toxin (CcdB) and its antidote (CcdA), respectively. CcdB is stable, but CcdA is slowly degraded by the Lon protease of the host cell; hence, CcdA can protect against CcdB only when it is being synthesized in (plasmid-containing) cells. Plasmid-free daughter cells are killed by CcdB (derived from the parent cell) because they lack the (plasmid-borne) *ccdA* gene from which the antidote can be synthesized.

The designation *ccd* is derived from 'coupled cell division' or from 'control of cell death' (according to different authors).

If used *in vitro* for ensuring the continued presence of the F plasmid in a bacterial strain, the *ccd* mechanism is reported to break down eventually, yielding plasmid-free cells. To avoid this problem of plasmid instability, the *ccd* system has been engineered so that the gene encoding the toxin resides on the *bacterial chromosome*, while the antidote-encoding gene remains in the plasmid. With this arrangement, plasmid-less cells are automatically killed by the toxin [BioTechniques (2005) 38(5):775–781].

CCF2 substrate See FRET.

CcpA See CATABOLITE REPRESSION.

***ccr* genes** (in *Staphylococcus aureus*) See SCCMEC.

CCR5 (in HIV-1 infection) See HIV-1.

CD11a/CD18 (leukocyte function-associated antigen, LFA-1) A cell-surface molecule of the β_2 INTEGRIN group which occurs on leukocytes. On activation, during inflammation, this molecule binds strongly to ligands, such as ICAM-1, on vascular endothelium. Individuals with leukocyte adhesion deficiency, an autosomal recessive disorder, are characterized by inadequate β_2 integrins and an abnormal susceptibility to certain infectious diseases.

CD11b/CD18 (CR3; Mac-1) A cell-surface molecule of the β_2 INTEGRIN group which occurs on certain leukocytes and is involved e.g. in adhesion reactions. The expression of Mac-1 on neutrophils seems to be a contributory factor in the phagocytosis of *Bordetella pertussis* (causal agent of whooping cough) [Infect Immun (2005) 73(11):7317–7323].

CD11c/CD18 (CR4) A cell-surface protein of the β_2 INTEGRIN group found e.g. on macrophages and neutrophils; it binds components of the complement system.

CD11d/CD18 A protein of the β_2 INTEGRIN group, found e.g. on macrophage foam cells, which is reported to bind multiple ligands [Blood (2006) 107(4):1643–1650].

CD21 A cell-surface molecule found e.g. on epithelial cells of the human oropharynx and on B lymphocytes (B cells). The molecule acts as a receptor for the EPSTEIN–BARR VIRUS.

CD27 A cell-surface molecule which is used as a marker for (human) memory B lymphocytes (memory B cells).

CD34 A cell-surface antigen on hemopoietic stem cells.

(See also GENE THERAPY.)

CD40 A cell-surface molecule on B lymphocytes (B cells) that interacts with the CD40L ligand on T cells, thus triggering an important phase of development in the B cell.

(See also CD40L and HYPER-IGM SYNDROME.)

CD40L CD40 ligand: a cell-surface molecule on T lymphocytes (T cells) that interacts with CD40 on B cells; such interaction promotes development of a normal antibody response in the B cells and is also a factor in the development of the T cells.

(See also CD40 and HYPER-IGM SYNDROME.)

CD81 A cell-surface protein (of the tetraspanin family) found in human cells. CD81 acts as a receptor for the E2 envelope glycoprotein of hepatitis C virus.

Factors other than CD81 are apparently also required for infection by the hepatitis C virus [J Virol 2006) 80(10):4940–4948].

CD209 *Syn.* DC-SIGN (q.v.).

CD209L (L-SIGN) A C-type lectin reported to act as a receptor for the SARS virus.

CdC6 protein See DNAA GENE.

cdc25 (in *Saccharomyces cerevisiae*) See e.g. CYTOTRAP TWO-HYBRID SYSTEM.

cDNA Copy DNA (sometimes called complementary DNA): a dsDNA or ssDNA copy of an RNA molecule – commonly a mature, poly(A)-tailed mRNA (see also FIRST STRAND).

Note. C-DNA refers to a particular conformation of DNA; it is unrelated to cDNA.

Some methods for producing cDNA can be inefficient. One problem is that reverse transcriptase may have exonuclease activity (i.e. it may degrade a newly synthesized strand); this problem may be overcome by using a recombinant form of the Moloney murine leukemia virus (MMLV) reverse transcriptase which has no exonuclease activity.

In some methods, priming of the second strand depends on the 3′ end of the first strand folding back on itself (to form a hairpin structure); the 3′ end is then extended – using the first strand as template. Because the hairpin's (single-stranded) loop has to be enzymatically removed (e.g. with endonuclease S_1), this inevitably leads to a loss of part of the 5′ sequence of the mRNA.

Full-length cDNAs (i.e. those containing the *entire* coding sequence) are an important requirement for the preparation of adequate cDNA libraries. Because the (5′) CAP sequence of a eukaryotic mRNA is a good marker for the presence of the 5′ end of the coding region, various methods have been devised which depend on copying this structure during the synthesis of (full-length) cDNAs: see e.g. CAPFINDER and CAPSELECT.

In a different approach, the proportion of full-length cDNA molecules was reported to be increased by excluding *non-full-length* copies.

If only a *small* amount of mRNA is available, one approach is to use a protocol that includes two rounds of amplification of cRNA and subsequent plasmid-mediated cloning of cDNA [BioTechniques (2005) 38(3):451–458].

cDNA library   See LIBRARY.

CDP™   A CHEMILUMINESCENCE-generating substrate which is cleaved by ALKALINE PHOSPHATASE.

cefepime   See CEPHALOSPORINS.

cefoxitin   See CEPHAMYCINS.

ceftazidime   See CEPHALOSPORINS.

ceftriaxone   See CEPHALOSPORINS.

CEL I   A member of the SINGLE-STRAND-SPECIFIC NUCLEASE group.

cell-free protein synthesis (coupled transcription–translation)   Any of various forms of *in vitro* (i.e. cell-free) system used for the transcription and translation of a given recombinant protein from a specific template introduced into the system.

Commonly used commercial and non-commercial systems are based on lysates of *Escherichia coli* which contain all the molecular machinery needed for the transcription and translation of a linear or circular template added to the system.

A cell-free system necessarily includes components such as ribosomes, tRNAs and transcription factors, and it commonly includes RNA polymerase from bacteriophage T7; the gene/fragment of interest is accordingly flanked by a T7 promoter and a terminator sequence.

Yields of up to several grams/liter of protein are reported to be obtained under optimal conditions from cell-free systems.

Quantitative studies on polysomes in cell-free protein synthesis systems have indicated that the rates of synthesis could be improved e.g. by adding purified elongation factors to the reaction mixture [Biotechnol Bioeng (2005) 91(4):425–435].

Advantages of cell-free protein synthesis
● Speed. There is no requirement for initial transfection and selection, cell culture etc.
● Potential to focus the synthetic capacity of the system on the target template.
● Ability to experiment more freely with conditions and e.g. to use amino acid analogs.
● Ability to synthesize proteins which would be toxic/lethal if produced intracellularly.

Commercial systems for cell-free protein synthesis include the Expressway™ Plus Expression System from Invitrogen (Carlsbad CA) that uses pEXP-DEST vectors; these plasmids contain *att* sites and are accordingly accessible as destination vectors within the GATEWAY SITE-SPECIFIC RECOMBINATION SYSTEM. The vectors include a T7 promoter and terminator; they also contain sequences encoding tags, e.g. XPRESS, SIX-HISTIDINE TAG, which facilitate purification of the expressed protein.

The pEXP3-DEST vector (4.6 kb) includes a sequence that encodes a LUMIO tag which – when used with the Lumio™ detection reagent – permits real-time detection of protein synthesis in the cell-free system. The specialized lysate used with this vector is derived from a *slyD* mutant of *Escherichia coli*; this avoids non-specific binding of the Lumio™ reagent to the cell's SlyD protein – and, hence, optimizes background (by reducing background signal) for detecting the required tag–protein fusion product.

The activity (functionality) of proteins produced in cell-free systems may be suboptimal, and it was hypothesized that this may be caused e.g. by poor coupling between transcription and translation due to the rapid activity of the T7 polymerase (as compared with the native bacterial enzyme). The situation was found to be improved by using a slower T7 enzyme or carrying out the process at 20°C [Nucleic Acids Res (2006) 34(19):e135].

(See also POLYSOME.)

cell fusion (somatic cell hybridization)   *In vitro* coalescence of cells, forming a single hybrid cell in which the nuclear and cytoplasmic contents of both cells are enclosed by a single cytoplasmic membrane.

In one method, populations of both types of cell are mixed and centrifuged. The pellet is then exposed briefly to an agent (*fusogen*) such as polyethylene glycol (PEG) which promotes cell fusion. (Lysophosphatidylcholine or inactivated Sendai virus may be used in place of PEG.) Free fusogen is removed by dilution, and the cells are resuspended in growth medium and incubated.

Cell fusion is used e.g. in the preparation of a HYBRIDOMA.

cell wall sorting signal   See SORTASE.

CENP-A, CENP-B etc.   See KINETOCHORE.

centiMorgan (cM)   A unit of distance on a chromosome: the distance between two loci when there is a 1% probability of those loci being separated by recombination during meiosis.

(See also MAP UNIT.)

centromere   The region in which two CHROMATIDS are joined.

(See also KINETOCHORE.)

cephalosporins   A category of β-LACTAM ANTIBIOTICS. They include e.g. cefepime, cefixime, ceftazidime, ceftriaxone and cephalothin.

(See also CEPHAMYCINS.)

cephalothin   See CEPHALOSPORINS.

cephamycins   A category of β-LACTAM ANTIBIOTICS: the 7-α-methoxycephalosporins; compared with the cephalosporins, cephamycins (e.g. cefoxitin) tend to have better penetration of the Gram-negative outer membrane and to have increased resistance to some β-lactamases.

c-*erbB* See EPIDERMAL GROWTH FACTOR RECEPTOR FAMILY.

CFLP analysis CLEAVASE FRAGMENT LENGTH POLYMORPHISM ANALYSIS.

CFP-10 See ESAT-6.

CFPS CELL-FREE PROTEIN SYNTHESIS.

CFTR CYSTIC FIBROSIS transmembrane conductance regulator.

CGH COMPARATIVE GENOMIC HYBRIDIZATION.

chain-terminating codon See NONSENSE CODON.

chain-termination method (DNA sequencing) See DIDEOXY METHOD.

Champion™ pET SUMO vector A 5.6-kb expression vector (Invitrogen, Carlsbad CA) designed for high-level expression of recombinant proteins in *Escherichia coli*. It includes a sequence encoding an 11-kDa solubility-enhancing SUMO protein which forms a fusion product with the target protein; following expression, the fusion protein can be cleaved at the C-terminal of the SUMO moiety by a SUMO protease (a recombinant form of the Ulp1 SUMO protease). (See the entry SUMOYLATION for the background on SUMO technology.) Cleavage of the fusion protein with this SUMO protease is effective except for those proteins whose terminal residue is leucine, lysine, proline or valine.

The plasmid vector also includes a T7 promoter and a tag encoding a series of six (consecutive) histidine residues; this tag facilitates purification of the target protein (see NICKEL-CHARGED AFFINITY RESIN for a rationale). The (linearized) vector has single-nucleotide (thymidine) 3′ overhangs for use with *Taq* DNA polymerase-generated PCR fragments (see EXTENDASE ACTIVITY for a rationale).

Champion™ pET104-DEST vector A destination vector in the GATEWAY SITE-SPECIFIC RECOMBINATION SYSTEM (see table in entry).

chaotrope Any agent that affects interactions between water molecules and which is able to promote the transfer of non-polar substances to a hydrophilic medium. The chaotropes include thiocyanide, iodide, bromide and chloride ions, and also certain compounds (such as urea); they are frequently used for disrupting cell membranes, solubilizing proteins and denaturing nucleic acids.

chaperone (*DNA technol.*) See OVEREXPRESSION (in section: *Inclusion bodies*).

Charcot–Marie–Tooth disease (CMT disease) Any of a group of heterogeneous inherited neuropathies which include both demyelinating and axonal types; autosomal dominant, autosomal recessive and X-linked cases are recognized.

Type 1A demyelinating CMT is associated with abnormality of the gene encoding peripheral myelin protein-22 located at 17p11.2, while type 1B demyelinating disease is associated with mutation in the gene for myelin protein zero at 1q22. X-linked CMT disease (CMTX) is reported to exhibit features of both the demyelinating and axonal types.

The type 2A disease has been associated with mutations in the mitofusin 2 gene (*MFN2*). More recently, new mutations

have been detected in this gene [BMC Med Genet (2006) 7: 53].

ChargeSwitch® technology A method used for isolating and purifying DNA (Invitrogen, Carlsbad CA). When released from the sample, DNA binds to minute, charged beads. This binding occurs because DNA carries a negative charge and the beads develop a positive charge when the pH (buffer) is <6.5. After two washes in a water-based buffer (during which time the beads are held by magnetic force) DNA is released from the beads by elution buffer (pH 8.5) which abolishes the mutual attraction between beads and DNA.

The ChargeSwitch® forensic DNA purification kit was reported to have recovered ~50–150 ng of DNA (quantitated by PICOGREEN and fluorometric analyses) from 48 specimen cigarette butts. (See also FORENSIC APPLICATIONS.)

charomid A COSMID containing a dispensable sequence (the 'stuffer') which differs in length in different charomids. A POLYLINKER permits the insertion of various lengths of target DNA (for cloning) such that the total length [stuffer + target DNA] is within the upper and lower limits for *in vitro* packaging.

Charon vector A CLONING VECTOR, derived from the phage λ genome, which lacks the ability to establish lysogeny.

(See also ZAP EXPRESS VECTOR.)

cHDA Circular helicase-dependent amplification: an isothermal method of NUCLEIC ACID AMPLIFICATION in which strand separation in a *circular* dsDNA template is achieved by the highly processive helicase of bacteriophage T7, extension of sequence-specific primers by a ROLLING CIRCLE mechanism resulting in concatemeric products. cHDA also exploits the DNA polymerase of phage T7 (Sequenase®) and the phage's single-strand binding protein (gp2.5).

Amplification, reported to be up to 10000-fold, is achieved at 25°C. The procedure may be used e.g. with a purified preparation of plasmids or a crude cell lysate.

[Method: Nucleic Acids Res (2006) 34(13):e98.]

CHEF See PFGE.

chemical cleavage method (of DNA sequencing) See MAXAM–GILBERT METHOD.

chemiluminescence Light produced from a chemical reaction. One example is BIOLUMINESCENCE; other examples include light generated from certain types of *in vitro* reaction which involve enzymic cleavage of chemicals of non-living origin.

Chemiluminescence can be exploited in reporter systems in place of fluorescence (in various applications). The principle underlying all of these chemiluminescent reporter systems is the enzyme-mediated decomposition of certain types of substrate which, when cleaved, emit light. A high signal-to-noise ratio can be achieved owing to the low background. (See also CHEMILUMINESCENCE ENHANCEMENT.)

On membranes, chemiluminescence can be used for detecting specific biomolecules. For example, a nucleic acid PROBE which is labeled with BIOTIN (q.v.) can be detected (following hybridization to its target sequence) by incubating the membrane with a conjugate that consists of STREPTAVIDIN bound to ALKALINE PHOSPHATASE; the addition of a chemiluminescent substrate then yields a light signal at the location of the probe, thus indicating the specific target biomolecule.

Alternatively, a probe can be labeled with DIGOXIGENIN; detection is then achieved with a conjugate consisting of anti-DIG (antibody to digoxigenin) bound to alkaline phosphatase and subsequent exposure of the membrane to a chemiluminescent substrate.

A probe may also be labeled directly with alkaline phosphatase.

In DNA SEQUENCING, use can be made of biotinylated sequencing primers; following gel electrophoresis, the fragments are transferred to a nylon membrane and then visualized by a streptavidin–AP conjugate and a chemiluminescent substrate.

Substrates that emit light when cleaved by AP include the 1,2-dioxetanes CSPD®, AMPPD® and CDP™.

Enzymes other than AP are also used in chemiluminescent reactions. The reporter enzyme β-galactosidase is detected in cell extracts by using the substrate Galacton™.

The reporter enzyme β-glucuronidase can be detected in cell extracts by using the substrate Glucuron™.

Chemiluminescent reporting can also be used for proteins on Western blots. For example, a given target protein can be initially bound by its antibody – which, in turn, is bound by an anti-Ig (anti-immunoglobulin) antibody conjugated to AP and exposed e.g. to CSPD®.

Examples of the use of chemiluminescent systems include studies on varicella-zoster virus involving DIG-labeled riboprobes detected with an anti-DIG–AP conjugate and CSPD® [J Virol (2006) 80(7):3238–3248], and the detection of target protein with primary antibody, an AP-conjugated secondary antibody, and CSPD® [BMC Cancer (2006) 6:75].

(See also FLASH CHEMILUMINESCENT GENE MAPPING KIT.)

chemiluminescence enhancement   A decrease in the (water-mediated) quenching of a chemiluminescent signal by the addition of certain macromolecules ('enhancers') that effectively shield the site of chemiluminescence from water molecules. Enhancers can also shift the wavelength of the emitted light.

[Use of Sapphire-II™ chemiluminescence enhancer: BMC Genetics (2006) 7:18.]

chi (χ) site   See e.g. HOMOLOGOUS RECOMBINATION.

chimera (chimaera)   Any *hybrid* individual, cell or construct – formed from at least two genetically distinct sources.

A chimeric gene may be constructed e.g. by joining two components with the SEAMLESS CLONING KIT.

chimeraplast (RDO: RNA–DNA chimeric oligonucleotide)   A double-stranded nucleic acid structure, containing two hairpin ends, which develops by the folding (self-hybridization) of a single strand that includes stretches of RNA and DNA. Chimeraplasts have been used for inducing single-base-pair changes at specified sites in the genomes of e.g. mammalian and plant cells.

Each chimeraplast includes a sequence which – except for a single mismatch – is homologous to the target sequence in the given genome. When a chimeraplast aligns with its target sequence, an endogenous repair process takes place at the site of the mismatch, leading to a single base change in the genomic DNA. It has been suggested that such a system may have potential use in GENE THERAPY for correcting deleterious point mutations.

[Sequence details of a chimeraplast (example): see Figure 4 in Reprod Biol Endocrinol (2003) 1:83.]

chip (DNA chip)   A small piece of glass (or other material) on which the components of a MICROARRAY or other test system are immobilized; the immobilized components may consist of e.g. oligonucleotides, strands of PNA or sections of tissue. (See MICROARRAY for a description of some immobilization procedures; see also DENDRICHIP.)

ChIP   CHROMATIN IMMUNOPRECIPITATION.

Chlamydia   A genus of Gram-negative, obligately intracellular parasitic/pathogenic bacteria found in man and other animals; species of *Chlamydia* give rise to diseases such as inclusion conjunctivitis and trachoma in man, and enteric diseases in young domestic animals. These bacteria are usually sensitive to tetracyclines.

The cells are non-motile and coccoid, ranging in size from about 0.2 μm to 1.5 μm – depending on the stage within the developmental cycle (see below). The cell envelope appears to contain little or no peptidoglycan but does include an outer membrane similar to that of other Gram-negative bacteria.

The GC% of the genomic DNA is 41–44. (See also pCT in the table for the entry PLASMID.)

The type species of the genus is *C. trachomatis*.

Chlamydia cannot be grown in the usual laboratory media; these organisms are grown in animals, in the chick embryo (yolk sac), and in cell cultures.

Chlamydia undergoes a development cycle. The form of the organism which is infectious for host cells is called the *elementary body* (EB); this is a small (~0.2–0.4 μm) cell that does not divide and which has few ribosomes. Much of the cell's interior consists of condensed nuclear material. The EB binds to a host cell and is taken up by endocytosis; phagosomes containing EBs do not fuse with lysosomes. EBs later differentiate to become so-called *reticulate bodies* (RBs); the RBs are larger (~0.6–1.5 μm), are metabolically more active, and they contain more ribosomes. Some 10 hours after initial infection RBs undergo binary fission; cell division continues, and from ~20 hours after the initial infection the RBs start to give rise to EBs. The cycle is complete by about 48–72 hours – when each infected host cell contains a population of EBs that constitutes a so-called *inclusion* that may occupy a major part of the cell's interior.

Chlamydophila pneumoniae   See NASBA (uses).

chloramphenicol (chloromycetin)   A broad-spectrum antibiotic produced by the bacterium *Streptomyces venezuelae* and also prepared synthetically; it binds to prokaryotic and mitochondrial ribosomes, inhibiting the activity of peptidyltransferase and, hence, inhibiting protein synthesis. Chloramphenicol is bacteriostatic for a wide range of bacteria (Gram-positive and

Gram-negative), and this antibiotic can also inhibit vegetative growth in some fungi.

Bacterial resistance to chloramphenicol is often due to the expression of a plasmid-encoded enzyme, chloramphenicol acetyltransferase (CAT), which catalyzes acetylation of the antibiotic in an acetyl-CoA-dependent way. Plasmid-encoded CAT is typically produced constitutively in Gram-negative bacteria but is inducible e.g. in species of the (Gram-positive) bacteria *Staphylococcus* and *Streptococcus*.

The pathogen *Pseudomonas aeruginosa* is innately resistant to chloramphenicol.

Chloramphenicol behaves antagonistically towards those antibiotics, such as penicillins, which are active against only growing and dividing bacteria.

chloramphenicol acetyltransferase　See CHLORAMPHENICOL and REPORTER GENE.

chloromycetin　*Syn.* CHLORAMPHENICOL.

***p*-chlorophenylalanine**　A lethal substrate which has been used e.g. for the elimination of a SUICIDE VECTOR (q.v.).

CHO cells　Cells derived from Chinese hamster ovary.

Christmas factor　Blood-clotting factor IX; a deficiency in this factor is a (less common) cause of hemophilia (hemophilia B) (see also 'Hemophilia' in the entry GENETIC DISEASE (table)).

The product Benefix® is a recombinant form of factor IX used for the management of this condition; this protein is produced in Chinese hamster ovary (CHO) cells.

(See also PYROPHOSPHOROLYSIS-ACTIVATED POLYMERIZ-ATION.)

chromatid　Either of the two products formed when a (eukaryotic) chromosome replicates. *Sister* chromatids, derived from the same chromosome, are connected at the centromere.

(See also KINETOCHORE.)

ChromaTide™ nucleotides　See PROBE LABELING.

chromatin　In a eukaryotic nucleus: the nucleoprotein complex which includes DNA, histones and non-histone proteins. The following is a generalized account.

Fully unraveled, chromatin is seen as fibers of DNA (~10 nm diam.) with a regular beaded appearance. The beads are *nucleosomes*. Each nucleosome has a *core* consisting of two of *each* of the following types of HISTONE: H2A, H2B, H3 and H4; this structure is encircled by several turns of DNA (~146 bp). The DNA enters and exits each nucleosome via histone H1. The nucleosomes are connected by *linker DNA* of variable length. (If treated with endonuclease, the beaded fibers yield *chromatosomes*, each consisting of a nucleosome together with histone H1 and some associated DNA.)

In vivo, the beaded (nucleosomal) fibers form superhelical chains: 30 nm fibers (*solenoids*) whose stabilization involves histone H1. Looped structures of nucleosomal and solenoidal DNA are anchored at intranuclear attachment sites.

For transcription, replication and repair, the DNA must be accessible to enzymes and binding proteins etc., so that the highly condensed chromatin structure must regularly undergo modification or *remodeling*. Some reported mechanisms are as follows. The properties of histones may be modified, post-translationally, by e.g. ACETYLATION, ADP-RIBOSYLATION, phosphorylation or ubiquitylation. Mechanical displacement of nucleosomes along the DNA (relocation) may be carried out by (ATP-dependent) remodeling complexes [Curr Opin Genetics Dev (2004) 14(2):165–173]. Incorporation of *variant* forms of HISTONES (q.v.) may modulate the properties of nucleosomes [Genes Dev (2005) 19(3):295–316].

The *accessibility*, in chromatin, of three members of a gene family (immunoglobulin $V_H S107$ family) was quantified by using a combination of LIGATION-MEDIATED PCR and real-time PCR [BioTechniques (2006) 41(4):404–408].

chromatin body　*Syn.* BARR BODY.

chromatin immunoprecipitation (ChIP)　A procedure used for investigating protein–DNA interactions. Initially, a formalin-based protein–DNA cross-linking procedure is carried out with the sample of DNA, and this is followed by sonication of the DNA into fragments of several hundred base-pairs in length. Antibodies, specific to the protein of interest, are then used for the selective precipitation of the given protein with its associated DNA. When isolated from protein, the DNA fragment can be amplified and sequenced.

[Examples of use: BioTechniques (2005) 39(5):715–725]; J Virol (2006) 80(5):2243–2256; J Virol (2006) 80(5):2358–2368; Mol Cell Biol (2006) 26(1):169–181; Mol Biol Cell (2006) 17(2):585–597.]

The sensitivity of ChIP is reported to be improved by biotinylating the target proteins *in vivo*, i.e. prior to cell lysis, in a protocol in which formalinization was carried out before extraction of chromatin. Because biotinylated proteins can be captured and held securely by a STREPTAVIDIN-based system, biotinylation of target proteins permitted stringent washing conditions which lead to an improved signal-to-noise ratio [Nucleic Acids Res (2006) 34(4):e33]. The biotinylation procedure is outlined in the entry IN VIVO BIOTINYLATION.

The commonly used agent for DNA–protein cross-linking, formaldehyde, is appropriate for investigating proteins that are bound directly to DNA (such as histones and transcription factors) but may not be as effective for investigating those proteins which are indirectly associated with DNA (such as transcriptional co-activators). Studies on various compounds have found that ethylene glycol-bis-(succinimidyl succinate) (EGS) – which has a long 'spacer arm' – is an effective cross-linking agent; an investigation using both EGS and formaldehyde reported sequential cross-linking by these two agents, enabling analysis of multiple transcriptional cofactors that cannot be investigated satisfactorily by the (conventional) use of formaldehyde as the sole agent [BioTechniques (2006) 41 (6):694–698].

(See also SOUTHWESTERN BLOTTING.)

chromatin insulator　A sequence of DNA, present in diverse species, which acts as a boundary between chromosomal loci that are subject to different patterns of regulation; insulators are believed to prevent the regulatory influence that affects a given locus from affecting adjacent loci.

chromatosome　See CHROMATIN.

Chromobacterium violaceum (CV026) (as biosensor in quorum sensing)   See QUORUM SENSING.

chromosome   A structure which contains part or all of a cell's genetic information; chromosomes consist essentially of DNA associated with certain proteins. (See also CHROMATIN; cf. GENOME.) The term 'chromosome' is generally not applied to the genetic material of either RNA or DNA viruses.

In prokaryotes (i.e. bacteria, archaeans) chromosome(s) and cytoplasm are in direct contact. (See also NUCLEOID.) In cells which lack extrachromosomal elements (such as a PLASMID) the chromosomes contain the entire genetic complement of the cell.

In a eukaryotic cell, all the chromosomes occur within the space enclosed by the nuclear membrane, and they are thus separated from the extranuclear region by this (permeable) barrier. The nuclear membrane must be permeable and be able to support two-way traffic; for example, transcripts of polypeptide-encoding genes must be able to leave the nucleus in order to undergo translation on the ribosomes. Chromosomes contain most of the genetic complement in eukaryotic cells; some of the DNA is found in mitochondria (see also MITOCHONDRIAL DNA) and (in photosynthetic species) in chloroplasts. (See also KINETOPLAST.)

Circular and linear chromosomes

Most (not all) of the prokaryotic chromosomes studied contain a covalently-closed circular (ccc) dsDNA molecule. Size varies with species; for example, *Buchnera* (an intracellular parasite of aphids) has a rather small chromosome (~640 kb), while the *Escherichia coli* chromosome is ~5 Mbp.

Linear DNA is found in the chromosomes of e.g. the Gram-negative bacterium BORRELIA BURGDORFERI and the Gram-positive bacterium *Streptomyces*. A large (~9.7 Mbp) genome consisting of a linear chromosome and three linear plasmids is found in *Rhodococcus* sp RHA1 [Proc Natl Acad Sci USA (2006) 103:15582–15587].

Eukaryotic chromosomes are structurally distinct. The ends of each linear dsDNA molecule include specialized sites that are involved in maintaining the integrity of the molecule: see TELOMERE. Moreover, the involvement of processes such as mitosis in cell division requires that these chromosomes contain specialized and structurally complex regions in order to permit their mechanical movement within the cell: see e.g. KINETOCHORE.

Number of chromosomes per cell

In prokaryotic cells, the number of chromosomes per cell is determined by (i) species and also by (ii) growth conditions. For example, while (slow-growing) cells of *Escherichia coli* contain one chromosome, a minimum of about four occur in *Deinococcus radiodurans*, and more than ten may be found in *Desulfovibrio gigas*.

In prokaryotes, it is generally assumed that when chromosomes occur in multiple copies in a cell then those chromosomes will be similar or identical to each other. Atypically, in e.g. the Gram-negative pathogen *Vibrio cholerae*, each cell contains *two dissimilar types* of chromosome – one ~3 Mbp, the other ~1 Mbp.

In *E. coli*, growth rate affects the chromosome complement of the cell; thus, according to the Helmstetter–Cooper model, during rapid growth a new round of DNA replication (i.e. chromosomal replication) begins before the existing round has been completed, leading to an increased chromosomal complement in rapidly growing cells.

Eukaryotic cells contain a species-dependent complement of chromosomes. Thus, cells of the slime mold *Dictyostelium* have six chromosomes (chromosome 2 containing about 25% of the genome), while the (somatic) cells of humans normally contain 46: 22 homologous pairs of autosomes and two so-called sex chromosomes (XX in females and XY in males). (See also X CHROMOSOME.)

In the human population, atypical, i.e. abnormal, numbers of chromosomes are found in some individuals – e.g. XXX in superfemales and XYY in some males (see also e.g. DOWN'S SYNDROME).

Variation in the normal number of X chromosomes may be determined e.g. by examining the number of Barr bodies (see BARR BODY) in a stained preparation.

Nomenclature (human chromosomes)

A particular location on a given chromosome can be indicated with reference to a chromosome map. In this system, the location is indicated by (i) the chromosome number (i.e. a number from 1 to 22), or a letter (X or Y), followed by (ii) 'p' (the *short* arm of the chromosome) or 'q' (the *long* arm), and then (iii) a number that refers to a particular *band*, the bands reflecting the reaction of chromosomes to certain dyes. Thus, using this system, a location may be given as e.g. 14q32.1 or Xp22.

Examples of some chromosomal locations are given in the table for the entry GENETIC DISEASE.

chromosome aberration   Any abnormality in the structure or number of a cell's chromosomes. Thus, e.g. a HETEROPLOID cell may lack a single chromosome from a (normal) diploid set, i.e. one of the chromosomes is unpaired; such a cell is referred to as *monosomic*. A diploid cell which has one extra chromosome (i.e. three copies of one particular chromosome) is *trisomic*.

(See also EUPLOID.)

chromosome banding   A banding pattern seen when chromosomes are stained with certain dyes that bind preferentially to AT-rich regions in DNA.

chromosome painting   A procedure in which a library of fluorescently labeled fragments of chromosome-specific DNA are used as PROBES e.g. to examine a preparation of immobilized metaphase chromosomes or particular individual chromosome(s); the fragments are differentially labeled such that the emission spectrum from a given fragment correlates with the particular chromosome for which that fragment is specific.

In the context of pathology, this procedure is able to reveal chromosome aberrations such as aneuploidy and the kinds of rearrangement/translocation which are found in the chromosomes of some tumor cells; thus, for example, a translocation would be indicated if fragments specific to a given chromosome (identified by the emission spectrum of the fluorescent label) bind to a different chromosome.

chromosome walking A procedure used e.g. to assemble sequences of DNA, from a genomic library, into a series of *overlapping* fragments (i.e. to prepare a 'clone contig'). This is a preliminary step in the preparation of a physical map of the given genome. Once a contig has been established it is then possible to sequence each of the fragments of cloned DNA and arrive at a defined sequence of nucleotides for the entire segment of genomic DNA covered by the contig.

Initially, one of the cloned sequences in the genomic library is chosen as the starting clone; this sequence may e.g. contain a known gene. An *end* fragment of this sequence is then prepared, labeled, and used as an *end probe* to probe the other sequences in the library. Sequence(s) that are bound by the end probe are taken to be sequences that overlap the starting clone; these seqences, in turn, are used for the preparation of end probes for detecting *their* overlapping sequences, and so on.

Chromosome walking can proceed in both directions from the starting clone.

(cf. COSMID WALKING.)

chronic myelogenous leukemia (chronic myeloid leukemia) A disease affecting hematopoietic stem cells; the chronic phase of the disease can develop to blast crisis via an incompletely understood mode of progression. (See also ABL.)

chylomicron See e.g. RNA EDITING.

CIB protein (in platelets) See WISKOTT–ALDRICH SYNDROME.

cinoxacin See QUINOLONE ANTIBIOTICS.

ciprofloxacin See QUINOLONE ANTIBIOTICS.

(See also SOS SYSTEM (*Staphylococcus aureus*).)

circular helicase-dependent amplification See CHDA.

circularization The formation of a covalent linkage between the two ends of a linear (single-stranded or double-stranded) molecule of nucleic acid involving the joining of 3'-hydroxyl to 5'- phosphate; it requires the activity of a LIGASE.

circularly permuted Refers to molecules of nucleic acid which have different terminal nucleotides but whose nucleotides are in the same consecutive order, for example 5'-ABCDEFG, 5'-GABCDEF, 5'-FGABCDE.

***cis*-acting element** A discrete sequence of nucleotides (such as a promoter) whose influence is limited to other regions of the *same molecule* of nucleic acid. A *cis*-acting protein acts on the molecule which encoded that protein.

(cf. TRANS-ACTING ELEMENT.)

cisplatin *cis*-Diaminedichloroplatinum: an agent which forms DNA adducts that cause cell-cycle arrest, blocking of DNA replication and apoptosis.

Cisplatin has been used for treating some types of cancer (e.g. ovarian and testicular cancers).

citrullinemia A disorder caused by a deficiency in the enzyme arginosuccinate synthetase (EC 6.3.4.5) – which catalyzes the reaction between citrulline and aspartate (resulting in arginosuccinate). Patients suffering from citrullinemia accumulate citrulline and ammonia in their plasma and they often have a damaged nervous system.

Classic (type I) citrullinemia results from mutation in the gene encoding arginosuccinate synthetase.

Adult-onset (type II) citrullinemia is an autosomal recessive disorder resulting from mutation in the *SLC25A13* gene (that encodes citrin); a deficiency in citrin leads to a deficiency in arginosuccinate synthetase.

(See also GENETIC DISEASE (table).)

clamping (PCR) See PCR CLAMPING.

class I transposon See TRANSPOSON.

class II transposon See TRANSPOSON.

class switching (in B cells) See e.g. HYPER-IGM SYNDROME.

clavulanic acid See β-LACTAMASES.

clean-up resin (for DNA) See e.g. STRATACLEAN RESIN.

cleared lysate The supernatant obtained after lysis of a suspension of bacteria and ultracentrifugation; given appropriate methodology, a cleared lysate may contain e.g. plasmids (if present in the original cells) but should be free of cell debris and of (unsheared) chromosomal DNA.

Cleavase® A structure-dependent endonuclease (Third Wave Technologies Inc., Madison WI) which cleaves at junctions between single- and double-stranded regions of DNA. Thus, for example, in a single strand of DNA which has been heat-treated and subsequently cooled, this enzyme recognizes and cleaves sites where (double-stranded) regions are contiguous with the intervening single-stranded regions; this activity is the basis of e.g. the typing/subtyping procedure CLEAVASE FRAGMENT LENGTH POLYMORPHISM ANALYSIS.

cleavase fragment length polymorphism analysis A form of TYPING/subtyping in which single-stranded samples of the DNA under test are first heat-denatured and then cooled to a temperature at which secondary structures (e.g. hairpins) are formed; the samples are then subjected to CLEAVASE and the resulting fragments are analysed. The sample strands of DNA are end-labeled, prior to enzymic cleavage, and the fragments resulting from Cleavase® action are examined by gel electrophoresis.

As well as typing/subtyping, this approach has been used e.g. for investigating mutations and polymorphisms in PCR products.

cleaved amplified polymorphic sequences See CAPS.

Cleland's reagent DITHIOTHREITOL.

cloacin DF13 A plasmid-encoded COLICIN produced e.g. by *Enterobacter cloacae*.

(See also IUTA GENE.)

Clonase™ An enzyme used in the GATEWAY SITE-SPECIFIC RECOMBINATION SYSTEM: see BP CLONASE and LR CLONASE (enzymes active at different types of *att* site).

clone contig See CONTIG.

cloning (DNA cloning, gene cloning, genomic cloning, molecular cloning) A procedure used for producing millions of copies of a given sequence of nucleic acid (commonly a gene or restriction fragment) – copies which can be used e.g. for sequencing or for subsequently expressing a product encoded by the gene etc.

Note. This process is distinct from *whole-animal* cloning: see next entry.

The term 'cloning' is generally understood to refer specifically to those procedures in which the target gene or fragment is inserted into a *vector* molecule – see CLONING VECTOR – which is then replicated in bacteria, or in eukaryotic cells, the number of target sequences increasing progressively as the vector molecules continue to replicate; however, in principle, a method such as PCR could be considered to be a cloning procedure. (Note that the expression 'PCR cloning' has been used to refer to a procedure in which the amplicons produced by PCR are inserted into vector molecules – which are then replicated in cells.)

The type of vector used for cloning depends e.g. on the size of the gene/insert to be cloned. Inserts up to ~10 kb may be cloned in small, high-copy-number bacterial plasmid vectors or e.g. in the INSERTION VECTORS based on phage lambda. Inserts of ~9–23 kb can be cloned in lambda REPLACEMENT VECTORS such as the LAMBDA FIX II VECTOR. Inserts of ~40 kb can be cloned in COSMIDS. Inserts of up to ~300 kb can be cloned in bacterial artificial chromosomes (that are based on the F PLASMID), and inserts of up to ~1 Mb can be cloned in YEAST ARTIFICIAL CHROMOSOMES.

The type of vector used for cloning can also be influenced by the source of the target sequence. For example, when the target sequence is produced by a PCR reaction in which the *Taq* DNA polymerase is used, the amplicons commonly have 3′ single-nucleotide adenosine overhangs due to EXTENDASE ACTIVITY; this feature is reflected in the use of vectors which have 3′ single-nucleotide thymidine overhangs to facilitate ligation of such amplicons (see e.g. TOPO TA CLONING KIT).

Various commercial products offer a range of facilities for cloning. For example, advantages of phage-mediated cloning (e.g. avoiding the need for transformation or electroporation) are available in lambda-based vectors (such as LAMBDA FIX II VECTOR). Cloning of AT-rich sequences (or other sequences which may be unstable within circular, supercoiled plasmid vectors) may be facilitated in linear vectors (see e.g. BIGEASY LINEAR CLONING SYSTEM). Transfer of a gene/insert between different vectors may be facilitated e.g. with the GATEWAY SITE-SPECIFIC RECOMBINATION SYSTEM, and cassette-based changing of markers can be facilitated with the EXCHANGER SYSTEM.

(See also the SEAMLESS CLONING KIT, TOPOISOMERASE I CLONING, USER CLONING and ZAP EXPRESS VECTOR.)

Linguistic note

A gene can be inserted *into* a vector and is cloned *in* a vector. The widely used phrase *cloned into* apparently results from thoughtless repetition.

cloning (whole-animal cloning) A procedure that involves the replacement of chromosomes in an (unfertilized) oocyte with chromosomes from a somatic cell – the engineered oocyte then being allowed to develop, in a surrogate mother, into a live animal.

(See also SCNT.)

cloning site In general, in a CLONING VECTOR: the recognition sequence of a given RESTRICTION ENDONUCLEASE; when cut by the particular restriction endonuclease the site generally provides STICKY ENDS which can be used for the insertion of a sample fragment which is flanked by the same sticky ends. This kind of procedure (i.e. the use of a single cloning site) does not permit control of the orientation of the insert within the vector.

To promote flexibility, and to permit control of the orientation of the insert, vectors commonly include a region which contains a multiple cloning site (MCS), i.e. a POLYLINKER.

In TOPO TA CLONING KITS the (linearized) vector contains 3′ single-nucleotide thymine overhangs which allow insertion of the (PCR-generated) fragment by topoisomerase activity – i.e. without the involvement of a restriction endonuclease.

cloning vector A VECTOR, capable of independent replication in a host cell, which is used for CLONING a given fragment of DNA (or gene) in order to produce sufficient material for use e.g. in mapping or sequencing. (cf. EXPRESSION VECTOR.)

Many cloning vectors are small (~3 kb) plasmids designed for replication in bacteria; they typically include a POLYLINKER (or ample restriction sites for inserting target DNA) and at least one marker/selection gene (e.g. a gene encoding antibiotic resistance) – but see REPRESSOR TITRATION. (See also PBR322 and PUC PLASMIDS.)

While cloning vectors are typically circular molecules, the BIGEASY LINEAR CLONING SYSTEM employs a *linear* plasmid vector.

A particular strand of the target DNA can be cloned e.g. in a PHAGEMID (see also PBLUESCRIPT).

Cloning vectors derived from bacteriophage λ (Stratagene, La Jolla CA) include INSERTION VECTORS (inserts up to 12 kb) and also REPLACEMENT VECTORS (inserts ~9–23 kb) – see e.g. LAMBDA FIX II VECTOR. These vectors have several advantages; for example, they avoid the requirement for processes such as transformation and electroporation, and they do not suffer from the kind of size bias seen with plasmids. (See also ZAP EXPRESS VECTOR.)

The (3128-bp) cloning vector pJET1/blunt (marketed by Fermentas) provides a positive selection system for cloning blunt-ended PCR products. A pJET1/blunt plasmid containing the required insert (ligated into the multiple cloning site) is replicated following insertion into *Escherichia coli* cells by transformation; following transformation, any recircularized plasmid which lacks the insert expresses a restriction endonuclease which kills the host cell.

Some cloning vectors permit *expression* of the cloned gene or fragment.

cluster (of genes) Any group of genes (in a given genome) that have a similar or identical pattern of expression.

cM CENTIMORGAN.

CML CHRONIC MYELOGENOUS LEUKEMIA.

(See also ABL.)

CMTX X-linked CHARCOT–MARIE–TOOTH DISEASE.

coa gene   A gene which encodes the (plasma-clotting) enzyme coagulase and which has been widely used as a marker for the Gram-positive bacterium *Staphylococcus aureus*.

coat protein (*virol.*)   See CAPSID.

COBRA   Combined bisulfite restriction analysis: a method for detecting and/or quantitating methylation of cytosine bases in a given (known) sequence of genomic DNA [seminal paper: Nucleic Acids Res (1997) 25(12):2532–2534]. An aliquot of the sample DNA is initially treated with BISULFITE, and the (bisulfite-modified) DNA is subsequently amplified by PCR. [Primer design for PCR on bisulfite-treated genomes: Nucleic Acids Res (2005) 33(1):e9.]

The products of PCR reflect any changes (due to bisulfite treatment) at positions occupied by cytosine in the original, untreated sample. Thus, for example, if a particular cytosine had been converted to uracil, the PCR product would contain *thymine* in place of the original cytosine.

The PCR products are digested with a RESTRICTION ENDO-NUCLEASE whose recognition sequence includes a particular cytosine of interest. If (due to bisulfite treatment) the given cytosine is represented as a thymine in the PCR amplicons, then restriction will not occur at this site – and this can be observed when the restriction fragments are examined by gel electrophoresis. Had the given cytosine *not* been converted to uracil when treated with bisulfite it would remain as cytosine in the PCR amplicons and restriction would occur at the site; hence, the restriction fragments can indicate whether or not a given cytosine was unmethylated or methylated in the original sample of DNA.

The relative amounts of digested and undigested products of PCR in a sample of DNA can therefore give an estimate of the overall level of methylation in the original sample DNA.

Instead of depending on visual inspection of the restriction patterns, greater accuracy in quantitation can be achieved by using appropriate instrumentation [Nucleic Acids Res (2006) 34(3):e17].

Cockayne syndrome   A disorder that is characterized by poor development, photosensitivity and, usually, failure to survive beyond early adulthood. The two categories of the condition, A and B, are associated with mutations in genes encoding DNA-repair proteins CSA and CSB – chromosome locations of the genes 5q12, 10q11, respectively. It was reported that CSB is degraded in a CSA-dependent way via the ubiquitin–proteasome pathway [Genes Dev (2006) 20(11):1429–1434].

coconut cadang-cadang viroid (CCCV)   A VIROID (q.v.) that has caused severe economic losses of coconut palm (e.g. in the Philippines).

coding region (in dsDNA)   (1) Any region encoding product(s), part(s) of products, or function(s).

(2) An exon or, collectively, all the exons, in a given gene.

coding strand (of a gene)   That strand which is homologous to – rather than complementary to – the corresponding mRNA. This appears to be the current (consensus) view. Earlier, the opposite view was held by many, i.e. the coding strand was regarded as the strand *on which* mRNA is trans-cribed, i.e. a strand complementary to mRNA.

The coding strand is also referred to as the *plus strand* or *sense strand*.

The *non-coding strand* (= *minus strand* or *antisense strand*) is that strand which is complementary to the coding strand, i.e. the *template strand* on which mRNA is transcribed.

(See also FORWARD PRIMER.)

CODIS   Combined DNA Index System: a database of human DNA profiles used by the FBI (i.e. Federal Bureau of Invest-igation) in the USA. Profiling may be achievable with only a small amount of DNA (e.g. ~1 ng) and may be possible even with damaged or degraded samples.

An individual's DNA profile is obtained by analyzing each of 13 *short tandem repeats* (see STR), found at specific chro-mosomal loci, and determining the number of repeat units in each of these STRs. The number of repeats in a given STR is recorded, and this is compared with the number of repeats, in the same STR, in other members of the database population. When all 13 STRs are analyzed (completing the profile), the 'uniqueness' of a given sample of DNA can be calculated by combining the probabilities determined for each STR site; the *random match probability* of a given DNA sample may be as low as ~1 in 10^{14} or ~1 in 10^{15}.

In the analysis, MULTIPLEX PCR is used for simultaneous amplification of multiple loci. The number of repeats in a given STR is indicated by the *length* of the amplicons: for each extra repeat unit the length increases by a fixed number of bases.

The use of small quantities of degraded DNA for analysis of STRs is reported to be possible by pre-amplification with a form of isothermal whole-genome amplification based on the use of bioinformatically optimized primers [DNA Res (2006) 13(2):77–88].

codominant gene   Any gene which, when present with other gene(s), contributes to a phenotype distinct from that specif-ied by any of the gene(s) individually.

codon   A triplet of consecutive bases in a nucleic acid molecule encoding a given amino acid or one of the three termination signals (see NONSENSE CODON).

(cf. ANTICODON.)

Codons are written in the 5′-to-3′ direction.

There are 64 possible triplets (from the four bases). Each of the two amino acids methionine and tryptophan is specified by a single codon (AUG and UGG respectively). Each of the remaining amino acids is specified by more than one codon; the existence of multiple (*synonymous*) codons for each of these amino acids is referred to by saying that the genetic code is *degenerate*. *Degeneracy* is a factor in the formulation of DEGENERATE PRIMERS.

(See also WOBBLE HYPOTHESIS.)

When comparing codon usage in different species it has been found that, for a given amino acid, different synonym-ous codons may be used preferentially by different organ-isms; even in a given organism, a particular amino acid may be specified by different codons in different genes – see

CODON BIAS (sense 3).

codon bias (1) (*technol.*) During the expression of a heterologous ('foreign') gene, e.g. a mammalian gene in bacteria: an *effect* due to the presence of certain codon(s) in the gene for which the expressing organism has an insufficient number of tRNAs; for example, if a gene with a high frequency of the arginine codon AGG, or the proline codon CCC, is expressed in *Escherichia coli*, translation is likely to be inefficient, or aborted, because these codons are much less common in the genes of *E. coli*.

One solution is to express heterologous genes in cells that are supplemented with extra copies of the given tRNAs (for example, encoded by plasmid genes). *Escherichia coli* BL21-CodonPlus® (Stratagene, La Jolla CA) carries extra copies of *argU* and other tRNA-encoding genes; one strain is suitable for high-AT genes, another for high-GC genes.

Another solution is to adapt the target gene so that its tRNA requirements match more closely those of the expressing organism. JCat (Java codon adaptation tool) is a program designed to facilitate such adaptation [Nucleic Acids Res (2005) 33: W526–W531].

(See also CODON OPTIMIZATION.)

(2) An *attribute*, of a given organism, involving a difference in codon usage compared with other (specified) organism(s). [Example of use: J Virol (2004) 74(10):4839–4852.]

(3) (*general biol.*) The *observation* that a given amino acid can be specified, preferentially, by different codons in different species – and also by different codons in different genes within the same organism.

In the bacterial chromosome it has been reported that genes exhibiting similar codon usage tend to be located close to each other in the genome and that (in at least some species) a number of 'codon usage domains' can be identified in the chromosome [PLoS Comput Biol (2006) 2(4):e37]

codon optimization The (pre-use) modification of a transgene in order e.g. to exclude codons that are rarely used by the expressing organism; such codons, which are normal for the species of origin, are replaced by codons that are commonly used in the transgenic cell or organism – leading to enhanced expression of the given gene.

(See also CODON BIAS sense 1.)

When codons in a mycobacterial gene were optimized for expression in mammalian cells, a DNA VACCINE encoding the given gene exhibited an enhanced immune response within BALB/c mice [Infect Immun (2005) 73(9):5666–5674].

Replacement of a rare codon for leucine by a common codon in the gene encoding mono-oxygenase resulted in greater enzymic activity in the bacterial strain expressing this gene [Appl Environ Microbiol (2005) 71(11):6977–6985].

codon usage domain See CODON BIAS (sense 3).

coenzyme I See NAD.

coenzyme R *Syn.* BIOTIN.

cohesive ends *Syn.* STICKY ENDS.

cointegrate The (circular) product formed by the fusion of two circular replicons – e.g. during *replicative* transposition: see

TRANSPOSABLE ELEMENT (figure and figure legend).

col plasmid COLICIN PLASMID.

colchicine A tricyclic alkaloid, from e.g. *Colchicum autumnale*, whose molecule includes a tropolone ring. Colchicine binds to tubulin and inhibits polymerization – blocking mitosis and e.g. promoting polyploidy in some types of cell.

The *in vitro* effect of colchicine can be terminated e.g. by using ultraviolet radiation; radiation converts colchicine to an inactive derivative: *lumicolchicine*.

ColE1 plasmid A small, non-conjugative, multi-copy PLASMID which is present in cells (strains of enterobacteria) typically at a copy number of about 10–30; it encodes a pore-forming COLICIN of the E category.

The GC% of ColE1 DNA is ~50.

The initiation of replication of ColE1 DNA is regulated at the level of primer formation. A plasmid-encoded molecule of RNA (RNA II) is transcribed on a particular strand from a site upstream of the origin of replication. This transcript has the potential to develop into a primer from which DNA synthesis may ensue. Another plasmid-encoded molecule (RNA I), also transcribed from a site upstream of the origin (but on the other strand), has a regulatory role: it represses RNAII's function by base-pairing with it. Thus, whether or not a given initiation event takes place will depend on the outcome of the interaction between RNA II and RNA I.

The concentration of RNA I may be limited by the activity of an RNase when the copy number of ColE1 is submaximal; this, in turn, affects the freedom of the RNA II transcript to initiate replication.

A further regulatory influence on RNA II is the (plasmid-encoded) Rop protein (sometimes called Rom) which appears to promote the hybridization of RNA I and RNA II.

In *Escherichia coli*, mutation in the *pcnB* gene can affect the frequency of initiation of replication of ColE1 DNA. This gene encodes poly(A)polymerase I, an enzyme which adds a poly(A) tail to certain transcripts, including RNA I. The poly-(A) tail which is normally present on RNA I facilitates its degradation. Hence, a non-functional poly(A)polymerase that prevents poly(A) tailing of RNA I will enhance the stability of this molecule and therefore serve to enhance its inhibitory action on RNA II.

(See also MULTICOPY PLASMID.)

In DNA technology the origin of replication of ColE1 is widely used in various types of vector molecule.

colicin Any of various high-molecular-weight, mostly plasmid-encoded BACTERIOCINS formed by enterobacteria. [Biology: Microbiol Mol Biol Rev (2007) 71(1):158–229.]

Three genes are associated with a given colicin: the genes encoding (i) the colicin itself; (ii) an *immunity protein* (which protects against the *same* colicin produced by nearby cells); and (iii) a *lysis protein* (which promotes release of the colicin from the producing cell). The immunity gene is expressed constitutively.

Synthesis of colicins (in *colicinogenic* cells) is triggered by the so-called SOS response, which is activated by damage to

DNA.

Some colicins (e.g. E6, DF13) have RNase activity; some (e.g. E2, E8) have DNase activity; some (e.g. E1, A, N, B, Ia, Ib) are pore-formers, and others (e.g. M) inhibit synthesis of the bacterial cell wall polymer peptidoglycan.

colicin factor An early name for a COLICIN PLASMID.

colicin plasmid Any plasmid encoding one or more COLICINS; they include small multicopy plasmids and large low-copy-number plasmids (and both conjugative and non-conjugative plasmids).

Repression of transcription of colicin genes by LexA (see SOS SYSTEM) is abolished during the response to damaged DNA, i.e. agents which trigger the SOS response promote colicin synthesis.

(See also COLE1 PLASMID.)

coliphage Any bacteriophage which can infect *Escherichia coli* (*E. coli* is a species of *coliform* bacteria).

colony hybridization (modified Grunstein–Hogness procedure) A method for selecting colonies of recombinant bacteria that contain a *particular* sequence of DNA. When a population of bacteria is transformed with a genomic LIBRARY, and then plated on a growth medium, *each* colony formed on the plate typically consists of bacteria containing *one* of the fragments from the library. To select colonies that contain a *particular* fragment, the original plate (= *master plate*) is replica plated (see REPLICA PLATING) to a nitrocellulose filter; cells from each colony adhere to the filter – which is then treated with alkali to (i) lyse the cells and (ii) denature DNA to the single-stranded state. The alkali is neutralized, and any protein is digested with proteinase. The filter is baked (70–80°C) under vacuum, to bind ssDNA to the filter, and is then exposed to labeled probes (see PROBE) to detect any DNA (and hence any colony) that contains the required sequence; this information is used to identify relevant colonies on the master plate.

Other methods for screening a genomic library include the REACTIVE system.

combination probe test Any test in which a PROBE is used to detect two or more target sequences simultaneously, i.e. in the same assay – see e.g. PACE 2C.

combinatorial (of oligonucleotides, oligopeptides etc.) Refers to a collection or library of oligonucleotides or oligopeptides etc. in which the constituent subunits (nucleotides and amino acid residues in these cases) in the individual members of the collection are arranged in many different combinations, such combinations sometimes covering all possible permutations of the subunits.

combined bisulfite restriction analysis See COBRA.

Combined DNA Index System See CODIS.

combined gold standard See GOLD STANDARD.

combing (of DNA) See DNA COMBING.

comparative DNA cleavage See e.g. CPNPG SITES.

comparative genomic hybridization (CGH) A technique for detecting changes (e.g. losses or gains) in particular chromosomes, or regions of a chromosome, in a sample of genomic DNA. Essentially, fragmented whole-genome preparations of sample DNA and normal DNA, each labeled with a different fluorescent dye, are allowed to hybridize simultaneously with a spread of *normal* metaphase chromosomes. The loss or gain of a chromosome, or sequence, in the sample DNA is detected by measuring the ratio of fluorescence intensities of the two fluorophores at various locations along the length of the metaphase chromosomes. If a given sequence in a particular metaphase chromosome hybridizes with normal DNA but not with sample DNA (shown by the absence of fluorescence from the *sample's* dye) this would indicate a deletion in the corresponding sequence of that chromosome in the sample DNA.

CGH has been used e.g. to detect aneuploidy (as in DOWN'S SYNDROME).

(cf. MULTIPLEX LIGATION-DEPENDENT PROBE AMPLIFICATION.)

compatible sticky ends See STICKY ENDS.

competence (in transformation) See TRANSFORMATION.

competent cells (*DNA technol.*) Cells selected, or engineered, for specific uses.

Cells which have 'extra' functions include e.g. *Escherichia coli* supplemented with an inducible gene for tyrosine kinase; unlike wild-type cells of *E. coli*, these cells can synthesize tyrosine-phosphorylated proteins.

(See also CODON BIAS.)

Cells with defective functions include e.g. METHYLATION-DEFICIENT CELLS (q.v.). Cells which contain an error-prone DNA polymerase (such as Mutazyme®; Stratagene, La Jolla CA) are used for MUTAGENESIS. Extra-permeable cells (e.g. ElectroTenBlue®; Stratagene) are used for ELECTROPORATION. Cells of *E. coli* with a *lacZ∆M15* mutation permit blue–white color screening for recombinant phagemids when used e.g. for replicating pBluescript® vectors (see PBLUESCRIPT).

(See the table in the entry ESCHERICHIA COLI for examples of various other modifications made to host cells for specific uses in recombinant DNA technology.)

competimer A PRIMER which has a non-extendable 3′ terminus but which competes with another primer for binding sites – thereby reducing the level of synthesis from the given binding site.

Competimers are used e.g. in quantitative RT-PCR when an 18S rRNA target is used as an internal control. As 18S rRNA is usually present in relatively large quantities, amplification of this target may go beyond the exponential phase in only a small number of cycles of PCR so that the internal control is not able to fulfill its function. To maintain a balance between levels of amplification of the internal control and the mRNA of interest, the reaction mixture can be supplemented with a proportion of competimers, thereby reducing amplification of the internal control; with an appropriate ratio of competimers to primers it is possible to reduce synthesis of the control sequence to the required level.

Competimers are obtainable commercially (Competimer™, Ambion). [Uses (e.g.): Plant Physiol (2004) 135:2230–2240; Proc Natl Acad Sci USA (2007) 104(6):1766–1770.]

In an analogous context, dominant *DNA* templates may be dealt with by techniques such as PCR CLAMPING and SUICIDE POLYMERASE ENDONUCLEASE RESTRICTION.

competitive clamping   See PCR CLAMPING.

competitive RT-PCR   A form of QUANTITATIVE PCR used for assessing the absolute number of specific target sequences in a given sample.

Essentially, the target is co-amplified with an (exogenous) 'competitor RNA' using a single pair of primers for both target and competitor. The assay is carried out with a range of concentrations of the competitor. If, in a given reaction, the amount of product from the target matches that from the competitor then this is taken to indicate that the target and competitor were present in equal amounts at the start of that reaction.

For meaningful results, the competitor should be amplified with an efficiency similar to that of the target, and it should also yield a product distinguishable from that of the target sequence.

complementarity   See BASE PAIRING.

complementary DNA (cDNA)   See CDNA.

α-complementation   A procedure involved in the blue–white screening method: see α-PEPTIDE.

complete medium   Any medium which supports the growth of a given AUXOTROPHIC MUTANT (q.v.).

complete transduction   See TRANSDUCTION.

composite transposon (class I transposon)   See TRANSPOSON.

computational biology   See BIOINFORMATICS.

ComX   See TRANSFORMATION.

concatemer   Two or more identical, linear molecules of nucleic acid covalently linked, end to end, in the same orientation. The term CONCATENATE has been used as a synonym. (cf. CATENANE.)

concatenate   A term which has been used as a synonym of both CATENANE and CONCATEMER.

conjugation (*bacteriol.*)   A natural process in which DNA is transferred from one cell (the *donor* or 'male') bacterium to another (*recipient* or 'female') bacterium while the cells are in physical contact. A bacterium which has received DNA in this process is termed a *transconjugant*. (See also RETRO-TRANSFER.) In many cases the donor phenotype is conferred by the intracellular presence of a conjugative PLASMID; in other cases, conjugation is mediated by a TRANSPOSON (and may be regarded as intercellular transposition – see the entry CONJUGATIVE TRANSPOSITION). The following account is concerned specifically with plasmid-mediated conjugation.

Plasmid-mediated DNA transfer can occur between Gram-negative species and it can also occur between Gram-positive species. The way in which the cells establish contact differs mechanistically in Gram-negative and Gram-positive species; however, there are similarities between Gram-negative and (some) Gram-positive species in the mechanism(s) involved in mobilization and transfer of DNA.

Conjugation in Gram-negative bacteria

The feature that distinguishes conjugation in Gram-negative species is the PILUS; pili appear to be essential for the establishment of conjugative cell–cell contact in these species but, thus far, they have not been detected in any Gram-positive species.

Much of the published information on Gram-negative conjugation has been obtained from studies on the conjugative transfer of the F PLASMID, and of related plasmids, between strains of enterobacteria (such as *Escherichia coli*). However, the general features of the F plasmid–*E. coli* transfer system are not common to all forms of conjugative transfer in Gram-negative bacteria; for example, the type of pilus differs markedly in some other systems, and the *tra* (i.e. transfer) operon (which is constitutively de-repressed in the F plasmid – see FINOP SYSTEM) is often repressed in other types of plasmid.

Moreover, the type of pilus expressed by a donor influences the physicochemical conditions under which conjugation can take place. For example, the F pilus (and similar types of pili) can mediate conjugation when cells are freely suspended in a liquid medium, while other types of pili (e.g. those specified by IncN plasmids) mediate so-called *surface-obligatory* conjugation which occurs *only* when bacteria are located on an appropriate surface. (Early studies on IncN-mediated conjugation reported that donor–recipient contact appears to need, or to be assisted by, surface tension.)

In at least some cases, initial donor–recipient contact, via the pilus, is followed by pilus retraction and the subsequent establishment of wall-to-wall contact between the conjugants. Some authors have reported an (electron-dense) *conjugative junction* at the region of cell–cell contact. Effective cell–cell contact precedes the *mobilization* and transfer of DNA from the donor. In the F plasmid, a specific site (in the *T strand*) at the origin of transfer (*oriT*) is nicked, and a single strand of DNA (5′-end leading) is transferred to the recipient. Nicking is carried out by an endonuclease (*traI* gene product) which forms part of the so-called *relaxosome* complex. It is possible that the subsequent unwinding of the transferred strand may provide energy for the transfer process.

Within the recipient, a complementary strand is synthesized on the transferred strand, forming a circularized molecule of dsDNA – a process termed *replication*.

Within the donor, a complementary strand is synthesized on the non-transmitted strand, reconstituting the plasmid; this process, which may occur by a ROLLING CIRCLE mechanism is referred to as *donor conjugal DNA synthesis* (DCDS).

In conjugation, *mobilization* can also refer to those cases in which DNA that is covalently continuous with a conjugative plasmid (e.g. a fused non-conjugative plasmid, or a bacterial genome which contains an integrated conjugative plasmid) is transferred to a recipient.

Conjugation in Gram-positive bacteria

Conjugation can occur in various Gram-positive bacteria, e.g. species of *Bacillus*, *Enterococcus* and *Staphylococcus* as well as the mycelial organism *Streptomyces*; in no case have pili been demonstrated.

Pheromone-mediated conjugation occurs in certain Gram-positive species. In this context, pheromones are small, linear peptides that are secreted by *potential recipients* of certain plasmids; a particular pheromone can act on a potential donor of the given plasmid – causing the donor to synthesize a cell-surface 'aggregation substance' which promotes adhesion between the potential conjugants. When a recipient receives the plasmid it stops secreting the particular pheromone – but may continue to secrete other pheromones corresponding to other plasmids.

Pheromone-mediated conjugation occurs e.g. within liquid cultures of certain strains of *Enterococcus faecalis*; plasmids which mediate such transfer often contain genes encoding resistance to particular antibiotic(s). In some cases a plasmid also encodes a peptide which antagonizes the corresponding pheromone; the function of this peptide may be to ensure that a mating response is not triggered in the donor cell unless the pheromone has reached a certain critical concentration – i.e. conditions under which there is a good chance of a random collision between potential conjugants.

Some strains of e.g. *Staphylococcus* and *Streptococcus* can carry out pheromone-independent conjugation on surfaces (rather than in free suspension); the plasmids encoding this type of transfer are often >15 kb in size.

A recent survey of plasmid-mediated conjugation in Gram-positive species proposed that there are two distinct mechanisms. The mechanism operating in unicellular species is seen as functionally similar (in terms of DNA mobilization etc.) to the Gram-negative model. A different mechanism operates in the multicellular Gram-positive species; this process appears to be characterized by the transfer of *double*-stranded DNA.

conjugative pilus *Syn.* PILUS.

conjugative plasmid See PLASMID.

conjugative transposition In bacteria: a plasmid-independent process – mediated by a *conjugative transposon* – in which DNA is transferred from a donor cell to a recipient cell while the cells are in physical contact. Conjugative transposition is known to occur between Gram-positive bacteria and between Gram-negative bacteria; it may also be able to mediate gene transfer between Gram-positive and Gram-negative bacteria.

Conjugative transposons resemble 'classic' transposons in that e.g. they can move from one DNA duplex to another and can occur in chromosomes and plasmids. Unlike most classic TRANSPOSABLE ELEMENTS they usually excise before transfer and they do not duplicate the target site when inserting in the recipient cell. The smallest of the conjugative transposons include Tn*916* (also referred to as CTn*916*; 18 kb), while the largest conjugative transposons are >50 kb.

Most or all conjugative transposons carry at least one gene that encodes antibiotic-resistance. Typically, the conjugative transposons are resistant to degradation by host cell restriction enzymes.

In one early model for conjugative transposition between Gram-positive bacteria, excision of the transposon is triggered by donor–recipient contact and it involves a transposon-encoded recombinase (*int* gene product). The excised trans-

poson circularizes, and a single strand may be transferred to the recipient cell; synthesis of a complementary strand (in the recipient) is followed by insertion into the target site.

In the (Gram-negative) bacterium *Bacteroides* it has been reported that transfer of *part* of the conjugative transposon CTnERL can occur in an excision-deficient strain, transfer apparently involving an 'Hfr-type' mechanism [J Bacteriol (2006) 188(3):1169–1174].

conjugative transposon See CONJUGATIVE TRANSPOSITION.

consensus sequence (in nucleic acids) In a particular genetic element (for example, a given type of promoter): an actual or theoretical sequence of nucleotides in which each specified nucleotide is the one found most often, at that location, in the variant forms of the element which have been determined for different organisms or strains.

constitutive gene *Syn.* HOUSEKEEPING GENE.

contig A word which has been used with various, incompatible meanings. When first used [see Nucleic Acids Res (1980) 8: 3673–3694] *contig* referred to '. . . *a set* of gel [electrophoresis] readings that are related to one another by overlap of their sequences.'. In the *Oxford Dictionary of Biochemistry and Molecular Biology* (revised edition, 2000), contig is defined as: 'one of a set of overlapping clones that represent a continuous region of DNA. Each contig is a genomic clone. . . .'. Other uses of the term contig refer to a continuous sequence of DNA 'assembled' or 'constructed' from overlapping clones.

The current consensus view appears to be that a *contig* is a linear series of sequences that mutually overlap, throughout, and which, collectively, span a large, continuous sequence; the phrase *clone contig* has been used for a series of cloned DNA sequences with these properties.

contig mapping An approach used for the physical mapping of genomic DNA. Essentially, the DNA is cut, by restriction endonucleases, into fragments that are cloned and sequenced. A computer-based search for overlapping regions permits the fragments to be assembled into the correct overall sequence.

contour-clamped homogeneous electric field electrophoresis (CHEF) See PFGE.

Cooley's anemia *Syn.* THALASSEMIA.

copA See R1 PLASMID.

CopB See R1 PLASMID.

copia element In *Drosophila*: any of a category of transposable elements, each ~5 kb in length and present in a copy number of ~50; each element is bracketed by long terminal repeats (LTRs) of ~280 nt, and the coding region specifies products analogous to those of RETROVIRUSES.

copy DNA (cDNA) See CDNA.

copy mutant See COPY NUMBER.

copy number (1) (of bacterial plasmids) The number of copies of a given plasmid, per chromosome, in a bacterial cell. The copy number is characteristic for a given plasmid in a host cell growing exponentially; the F PLASMID is an example of a low-copy-number plasmid, while pBR322 is an example of a multicopy plasmid.

Copy number is determined e.g. by the replication-control

system; different control systems occur in different plasmids. Mutations can give rise to a *copy mutant* in which the copy number differs from that of the wild-type plasmid.

(2) The number of copies of a given gene, per cell, or e.g. the number of copies of a gene product per gene or per cell.

cordycepin 3′-Deoxyadenosine: a nucleoside analog used e.g. to block RNA synthesis and polyadenylation.

core promoter (promoter core) Regions of a promoter that are essential for initiation of transcription of the given gene; they are involved in the assembly of the transcriptional machinery at the initiation site. For example, sequences found in at least some RNA polymerase II promoters include: a TATA box (*Goldberg–Hogness box, Hogness box*), an AT-rich sequence about 30 nt upstream of the start site; a TFIIB recognition element; an initiator; a DOWNSTREAM PROMOTER ELEMENT (DPE). All of these are sequences which act as binding sites for transcription-related factors. Not all of these sequences may be present in the same promoter; for example, some core promoters have a DPE and lack a TATA box.

***cos* site** In PHAGE LAMBDA: the 12-nt 5′ STICKY ENDS which form the terminal parts of the genome in the phage virion; when injected into a host cell the genome circularizes via the sticky ends.

In DNA technology, *cos* sites are exploited e.g. in various constructs (see e.g. COSMID).

cosmid A plasmid containing the (double-stranded) 12-bp *cos* site of PHAGE LAMBDA; cosmids have been widely used e.g. as cloning vectors for preparing genomic libraries.

(See also COSMID WALKING.)

Linearized cosmids (with a *non*-terminal *cos* site) can be mixed with DNA fragments of various lengths prepared with the same restriction enzyme as that used for linearizing the cosmid. Some fragments will bind a cosmid at both ends; if the *cos*-to-*cos* distance is about 40–50 kb (depending on the given fragment), the *cos*–*cos* sequence is of the correct size for packaging into the head of phage λ. *Cos* sites are cleaved enzymically, and packaging (*in vitro*) occurs in the presence of phage components. Once assembled, the phage virions can inject their recombinant DNA into appropriate bacteria.

Several improvements can be made to this basic protocol. For example, the sample fragments (derived e.g. by digestion of genomic DNA with restriction endonucleases) can be size-fractionated prior to mixing with the cosmids; in this way the reaction can be enriched with fragments of appropriate length (i.e. fragments which, when flanked by cosmids, will be suit-able, in size, for packaging).

One problem with the basic scheme is that many of the cos-mids may bind to one another and form multimers. This can be prevented by cleaving the terminal 5′-phosphate from both strands of the cosmid (e.g. with ALKALINE PHOSPHATASE). In this case the terminal 5′-phosphate groups on the inserts will permit ligation to cosmids and subsequent packaging.

(See also SUPERCOS I VECTOR.)

Products for packaging are available commercially: see e.g. GIGAPACK.

cosmid walking A procedure, similar to CHROMOSOME WALK-ING (q.v.), in which a clone contig is prepared from a COS-MID library. Because the inserts in cosmids are not too long, it is possible to use the entire sequence as a probe – thereby avoiding the need to prepare end probes (as is necessary in chromosome walking).

co-suppression See PTGS.

cotrimoxazole See ANTIBIOTIC (synergism).

counterselection *Syn.* NEGATIVE SELECTION.

coupled transcription–translation (*in vitro*) See CELL-FREE PROTEIN SYNTHESIS.

cozymase See NAD.

CPD Cyclobutyl pyrimidine dimer (see THYMINE DIMER).

CpG island One of a number of regions in genomic DNA that contains a high frequency of the dinucleotide 5′-CpG-3′. CpG islands (stretches of ~0.5–4 kb) are often associated with the 5′ end (promoter region) of genes, and in these locations the cytosines are typically unmethylated; the significance of this is that aberrant methylation of cytosines in these regions has been associated with the silencing of genes (which may lead e.g. to tumor development if the inactivated gene is a tumor suppressor).

Observations on (human) lymphocytes suggested that the composition of DNA in CpG islands (in terms of sequence, repeats, structure) has a significant role in predisposing CpG islands to methylation [PLoS Genet (2006) 2(3):e26].

The DNA in a CpG island typically has a GC% greater than ~60.

Elsewhere in the genome the CpG dinucleotides are often methylated. Methylated cytosines are particularly susceptible to mutation because the spontaneous deamination of methyl-cytosine residues yields the (normal) base thymine, which is not a target for DNA repair mechanisms.

(See also METHYLATION.)

[CpG Analyzer (a Windows-based program for the study of DNA methylation): BioTechniques (2005) 39(5):656–662.]

(Other relevant entries: AAVS, BSSHII, ISLAND RESCUE PCR, KAISO PROTEIN, MBD PROTEINS, SSSI, TAGM.)

One novel technique for the detection of methyl-CpGs is based on the construction of a multimeric form of a naturally occurring methyl-CpG-binding domain (MBD) that is found in a family of proteins associated e.g. with the repression of transcription. These synthetic poly-MBD proteins were found to be sensitive reagents for detecting DNA methylation levels in isolated DNA – as well as for the cytological detection of CpG methylation in chromosomes [Nucleic Acids Res (2006) 34(13):e96].

Detection of 5′-methylated cytosine residues, without using bisulfite treatment or DNA amplification, was reported with monoclonal antibodies (mAbs) that bind specifically to 5′-methylated cytosines in strands base-paired to oligonucleotide probes; mAbs bound to the target (5′-methylated) cytosines were detected by secondary antibodies (dye-conjugated anti-immunoglobulin antibodies) that are visualized via the dye's fluorescence. In this method, probe sequences were designed on the basis of analysis of predicted promoter sequences for possible methylation sites. [Method: DNA Res (2006) 13(1): 37–42.]

Changes in CpG methylation are detected by methods such as (methylation-specific) MULTIPLEX LIGATION-DEPENDENT PROBE AMPLIFICATION and RESTRICTION LANDMARK GENOMIC SCANNING.

(See also COBRA and METHYL-BINDING PCR.)

CpG methylation is also monitored by direct sequencing of BISULFITE-treated DNA. When using PYROSEQUENCING for quantitative analysis of CpG methylation, one approach is to re-use the sequencing template so that different sets of CpG sites can be monitored by the consecutive binding of different sequencing primers to a given template strand. The bisulfite-treated target sequence is initially copied by PCR using a BIOTINylated reverse primer; the biotinylated strand of the resulting amplicon is then separated from its complementary strand and subsequently used as the sequencing template. A Pyrosequencing™ primer is annealed to this template and is extended in the first sequencing run. The newly synthesized strand is stripped from the template, and the purified template strand is used again with a different Pyrosequencing primer in order to assay a different set of CpGs on the template. (Up to seven uses of a given template strand are reported to be possible without loss of accuracy.) Manipulation of the (biotinylated) sequencing template is facilitated, throughout the procedure, by using streptavidin-coated Sepharose™ beads. [Method: Biotechniques (2006) 40:721–726.]

CpGV *Cydia pomonella* GV: see GRANULOSIS VIRUSES.

CpNpG sites In the genomes of mammalian (and other) cells: sites in DNA at which, in at least some cases, methylation of cytosine has important physiologic effects.

The methylation pattern in the sequence CC(A/T)GG may be determined e.g. by carrying out comparative (differential) DNA cleavage with methylation-resistant and methylation-sensitive restriction endonucleases. The activity of restriction enzyme BstNI is not affected by methylation of the internal cytosine, and BstNI may be used as the methylation-resistant endonuclease.

EcoRII recognizes this site, and is sensitive to methylation; however, as it is a type IIE RESTRICTION ENDONUCLEASE, it requires *two* copies of the recognition site for activity. To be useful in comparative DNA cleavage (for detecting methylation at CpNpG sites) the methylation-sensitive enzyme must be able to act on *single* copies of the recognition sequence; this need has been met by an engineered version of EcoRII (designated EcoRII-C) which is able to cleave at a single site in a methylation-sensitive manner [BioTechniques (2005) 38: 855–856].

CR3 *Syn.* CD11b/CD18 (q.v.).

CR4 *Syn.* CD11c/CD18 (q.v.).

Cre–*loxP* system A recombinase (product of gene *cre*) and its corresponding recognition site (*loxP*) derived from PHAGE P1.

A sequence of DNA flanked by two *loxP* sites (both in the same orientation) can be excised from a larger molecule, and circularized, by Cre. With an inducible *cre*, the Cre-mediated excision of a *loxP*–DNA–*loxP* sequence can be achieved *in vivo* (within cells). For example, in one study, transposons containing *loxP*-flanked selective markers were inserted (*in vitro*) into gene-targeting vectors; following internalization of the vectors, the markers were excised inside the transfected cells [Nucleic Acids Res (2005) 33(5):e52].

Cre–*loxP* can also mediate the *exchange* of a sequence in a circular vector molecule with a sequence in genomic DNA; for this purpose, each of the sequences is flanked by a pair of *loxP* sites (in the same orientation). Dissimilar *loxP* sites (e.g. one wild-type and one modified) can be used to bracket each sequence; this promotes exchange such that the sequences are inserted in a known orientation within their respective molecules.

(cf. RECOMBINASE-MEDIATED CASSETTE EXCHANGE.)

DNA flanked by a pair of *loxP* sites in opposite orientation can be inverted by Cre.

The Cre–*loxP* system can also mediate the insertion of one vector into another, e.g. the integration of two circular molecules to form a single circular molecule; for this purpose, each molecule contains a single *loxP* site. This approach has been exploited in a method for expressing transfected genes in plant cells [BioTechniques (2005) 39(3):301–304].

In the bacterium *Streptomyces coelicolor* the Cre–*loxP* system has been used for the removal of a *loxP*-flanked marker by exploiting *transient* infection by a phage which expresses the Cre recombinase [Nucleic Acids Res (2006) 34 (3):e20].

[Use of the Cre–*loxP* system for making deletions in the bacterium *Lactobacillus plantarum*: Appl Environ Microbiol (2007) 73(4):1126–1135.]

[Cryptic *loxP* sites reported in the mouse genome: Nucleic Acids Res (2007) 35(5):1402–1410.]

Peptides which inhibit Cre have been reported from studies on the HOLLIDAY JUNCTION (q.v.). (See also DAM GENE.)

[*loxP* sites used for efficient generation of random chromosome deletions: BioTechniques (2007) 42(5):572–576.]

(See also FLP.)

CREB protein Cyclic AMP (cAMP) response element binding protein: a protein which acts as a transcription factor when it is phosphorylated by an appropriate enzyme at the serine-133 residue; when the CREB protein is thus activated, it binds to its target sequence – the response element 5′-TGACGTCA-3′ (CRE) – which is involved in the regulation of various genes. The phosphorylation of CREB can be carried out by a variety of kinases, including PKA, PKC, mitogen-activated protein kinases (MAPKs) and calcium/calmodulin-dependent protein kinases.

(See also PATHDETECT SYSTEMS.)

CRM1 See KARYOPHERINS.

cRNA A sense strand of RNA transcribed from a molecule of double-stranded cDNA.

cross-linking assay (photo-cross-linking assay) A probe-based assay that was used originally for detecting/quantitating DNA from the hepatitis B virus (HBV) in samples of serum.

Initially, the samples are incubated (65°C/30 minutes) with a lysis reagent that includes proteinase K and sodium dodecyl sulfate in order to release viral DNA. The viral DNA is then denatured by heat at an alkaline pH. Following cooling and centrifugation, the supernatant is neutralized and an aliquot is used for the assay: probes are added and hybridization carried out at 45°C/20 minutes.

The probes are of two types, each type being targeted to its complementary sequence in the HBV DNA.

Each *capture probe* has a BIOTINylated tag.

Each *reporter probe* carries a number of fluorescein molecules.

Both types of probe incorporate a cross-linking agent (a derivative of 7-hydroxycoumarin) which can be activated by exposure to ultraviolet radiation; when this agent is activated, the bound probe becomes covalently linked to its target sequence.

Following the hybridization stage, the reaction mixture is exposed to ultraviolet radiation for 30 minutes. Subsequently, streptavidin-coated DYNABEADS are added, and these bind to the capture probes (via their biotinylated tags) – thereby also binding the target DNA and the (covalently linked) reporter probes. The beads are washed (while retained by a magnetic field) and then incubated with an antifluorescein antibody–alkaline phosphatase (AP) conjugate; this conjugate binds to reporter probes via their fluorescein tags. The washed preparation is then incubated with ATTOPHOS, at 37°/60 minutes, and the fluorescent product detected by a microplate reader. For quantitation, the mean signal (from repeat tests) is interpreted against a standard curve.

The original assay [J Clin Microbiol (1999) 37:161–164] was improved by a modified arrangement that was reported to give a ~10-fold increase in sensitivity when used to detect Factor V Leiden mutations in clinical samples [Clin Chem (2004) 50:296–305].

An advantage of a cross-linking assay is that manipulation/ washing etc. can be carried out under conditions that would be likely to denature conventional probe–target complexes.

crossing over   Recombination involving breakage of strands in each of two juxtaposed DNA duplexes, cross-wise exchange of ends, and ligation. Crossing over occurs e.g. between non-sister chromatids during meiosis.

(See also RECOMBINASE.)

crown gall   A PLASMID-mediated plant neoplasm that is found typically at the crown (i.e. stem–root junction), primarily in a range of gymnosperms and dicotyledonous angiosperms.

Development of the neoplasm follows infection of a wound by a virulent (plasmid-containing) strain of certain species of the bacterium *Agrobacterium*, commonly *A. tumefaciens* (but crown gall in the grape is caused by *A. vitis*). Crown gall may cause stunting/death of affected plants; important economic losses have been caused (e.g. in stone-fruit trees and vines) in e.g. Europe, the USA and Australia.

In crown gall, bacterial virulence (the ability to promote tumorigenesis) is conferred by a large plasmid called the Ti (tumor-inducing) plasmid. The genes directly responsible for tumorigenesis are in a subregion of the plasmid referred to as T-DNA; during infection of the plant, a single-stranded form of T-DNA is transferred from the bacterium to the plant.

Some ~25 of the Ti genes (in regions outside T-DNA) are needed for transfer of T-DNA to the plant. Certain of these genes encode elements of a TWO-COMPONENT REGULATORY SYSTEM: VirA (the sensor) and VirG (response regulator). VirA seems to respond to certain phenolic compounds (e.g. acetosyringone) that occur in plant wounds; variant forms of VirA may respond to sensor-specific plant signals.

When activated, VirG promotes transcription of a number of plasmid genes, some of which encode a site-specific endonuclease complex which nicks one strand of the Ti plasmid at unique sites in a pair of 24-bp direct repeats flanking T-DNA. The ssDNA copy of T-DNA, with a protein (VirD2) linked covalently to the 5′ end, is transferred from the bacterium to the plant cell nucleus.

In the plant cell, T-DNA inserts into nuclear DNA. T-DNA encodes certain phytohormones (e.g. AUXINS, CYTOKININS) that are considered to be responsible for tumorigenesis.

The tumor cells produce certain T-DNA-encoded products (*opines*) which (according to the strain of *Agrobacterium*) may be compounds of the *octopine* family or of the *nopaline* family. Opines produced by the tumor cells can be used as the sole source of carbon and nitrogen by the particular strain of *Agrobacterium* infecting the plant; the Ti plasmid (in the bacterium) encodes enzymes which degrade the opines that are encoded by the T-DNA.

Transfer of the Ti plasmid from Ti⁺ strains to Ti⁻ strains of agrobacteria (enlarging the pathogen population) is regulated e.g. by a QUORUM SENSING mechanism in which activation of transfer ability depends on the population density of *donor* cells. As in various other Gram-negative bacteria, the agents which mediate quorum sensing (*autoinducers*) are *N*-acyl-L-homoserine lactones (AHLs). In at least certain strains of *Agrobacterium* the quorum sensing system is dependent on the presence of opines, formed by the tumor cells, that are needed for activation of the system.

The ability of *A. tumefaciens* to promote transfer of DNA into plant cells has been exploited in a widely-used BINARY VECTOR SYSTEM for introducing viral DNA (or cDNA) into plants.

(See also AGROINFECTION.)

CRP   cAMP-receptor protein: see CATABOLITE REPRESSION.

cruciform (*DNA technol.*)   See e.g. PALINDROMIC SEQUENCE.

cryptic plasmid   Any plasmid which has no known phenotypic effects.

cryptic splicing   An aberrant form of SPLICING which occurs when a sequence in the pre-mRNA, *resembling* a true splice site, is used in the splicing process as though it were a genuine splice site.

cryptic viruses   Virus-like particles seen in various (symptomless) plants. Some (e.g. beet cryptic viruses) contain dsRNA.

CspD   In *Escherichia coli*: a protein which can be induced by nutrient deprivation; it also appears in the stationary phase of growth at 37°C. CspD is also included within the category of cold-shock proteins.

CSPD® A 1,2-dioxetane substrate that emits light ($\lambda = 477$ nm) when dephosphorylated by ALKALINE PHOSPHATASE. It is used e.g. to detect enzyme-labeled probes.

(See also CHEMILUMINESCENCE.)

CSRE Carbon source responsive element (in *Saccharomyces cerevisiae*): a consensus sequence in the promoters of certain genes (e.g. genes involved in gluconeogenesis); if cells are supplied with glucose, CSRE elements mediate repression of the corresponding genes.

(See also CATABOLITE REPRESSION.)

C_t (threshold cycle) See REAL-TIME PCR.

CTn*916* See CONJUGATIVE TRANSPOSITION.

CTnERL See CONJUGATIVE TRANSPOSITION.

cullin-RING complexes A large group of ubiquitin ligases (see PROTEASOME).

[Review: Nature Rev Mol Cell Biol (2005) 6(1):9–20.]

Curie point pyrolysis PYROLYSIS involving a *ferromagnetic* wire which is heated inductively, i.e. within a high-frequency alternating magnetic field. Rapidly (e.g. in 0.1 second) the temperature of the wire reaches the Curie point: a temperature which is maintained by the alternating magnetic field – but which cannot be exceeded because, above a certain temperature, the wire is no longer susceptible to inductive heating. The Curie point varies with the chemical composition of the wire; iron–nickel wires often have a Curie point of 510°C.

curing (of bacterial plasmids) Loss of plasmid(s) from bacteria, which retain viability. Spontaneous curing may occur e.g. if the plasmid's partition system is defective. Experimentally, it can be achieved e.g. by the use of sublethal doses of certain INTERCALATING AGENTS which inhibit plasmid replication; increasing numbers of plasmid-free cells are produced when a growing population of bacteria is exposed to such agents. Thus, curing may be carried out e.g. with certain acridines or (in *Pseudomonas*) with mitomycin C.

Some (temperature-sensitive) plasmids can be cured simply by growing the host cells at a non-permissive temperature. For example, the derivative plasmid pWV01 was stable at 30°C but lost by growth at or above 37°C [FEMS Microbiol Lett (2005) 245(2):315–319].

(See also SUICIDE VECTOR.)

cut-and-paste mechanism (in transposable elements) See TRANSPOSABLE ELEMENT (figure and legend).

CXCR4 (in HIV-1 infection) See HIV-1.

cya gene In *Escherichia coli*: the gene encoding ADENYLATE CYCLASE.

cyanobacteria ('blue-green algae') A (non-taxonomic) category of heterogeneous bacteria characterized by the ability to carry out oxygenic (oxygen-producing) photosynthesis, i.e. a mode of photosynthesis similar to that found in eukaryotes (such as algae) – and unlike the anoxygenic photosynthesis carried out (anaerobically) by some other bacteria. The organisms range from unicellular to filamentous and complex forms, with var-

ious types of pigmentation. The cell envelope is essentially of the Gram-negative type, although features of Gram-positive organization can be seen in some species. Flagella are absent, but some strains can move e.g. by a so-called *gliding motility*.

The cyanobacteria are widespread in nature, in both aquatic and non-aquatic habitats and also in a wide range of climatic conditions.

cybrid A cell prepared by transferring mitochondria, or mitochondrial DNA (mtDNA), from a given type of cell to a RHO-ZERO CELL. Cybrids are prepared e.g. in order to investigate the effects of mutations in mtDNA on various functions, such as oxidative phosphorylation and cell growth.

[Examples of use: Biochem Biophys Res Commun (2005) 328(2):491–498; Proc Natl Acad Sci USA (2005) 102(52): 19126–19131.]

[Production of *trans*mitochondrial cybrids containing naturally occuring pathogenic mtDNA variants: Nucleic Acids Res (2006) 34(13):e95.]

cyclic AMP (cAMP) Adenosine 3′,5′-monophosphate, in which phosphate links the 3′ and 5′ positions of the sugar residue. cAMP is synthesized from ATP by ADENYLATE CYCLASE.

cAMP is a key regulatory molecule in both eukaryotes and prokaryotes; it is involved e.g. in signal transduction pathways and, in prokaryotes, in CATABOLITE REPRESSION.

cAMP is converted to AMP by cAMP phosphodiesterase (EC 3.1.4.17).

cyclic AMP response element binding protein See CREB.

cyclobutyl thymine dimer See e.g. THYMINE DIMER.

cycloheximide An antibiotic produced e.g. by certain strains of *Streptomyces griseus*: β-[2-(3,5-dimethyl-2-oxocyclohexyl)-2-hydroxyethyl]-glutarimide. Cycloheximide is active against various fungi and other eukaryotes; it binds to the 60S ribosomal subunit and blocks translocation.

Cycloheximide has been used e.g. in TOEPRINTING.

cyclolysin See ADENYLATE CYCLASE.

cystic fibrosis A congenital disorder that typically involves a defective membrane protein (*cystic fibrosis transmembrane conductance regulator*, CFTR). The disorder is characterized by abnormal secretion, most notably in the respiratory tract; CFTR is apparently an ABC transporter (an ATP-energized transport protein) associated with transmembrane transport of chloride (Cl⁻). Infections (e.g. with alginate-producing strains of *Pseudomonas aeruginosa*) can be refractory to antibiotic treatment.

(See also GENE THERAPY and *Pandoraea apista* in entry REP-PCR.)

cytidine A riboNUCLEOSIDE.

cytidine deaminase Any enzyme which deaminates cytidine to uridine.

One example is APOBEC-1, part of an RNA editing complex which acts on transcripts of apolioprotein B (see RNA EDITING).

Another example is AID (ACTIVATION-INDUCED CYTIDINE DEAMINASE), which may also be involved in RNA editing.

APOBEC-1 and AID were found to have distinct functional

properties when examined in an experimental yeast system [Mol Immunol (2006) 43(4):295–307].

cytogenetics A branch of science in which cellular features, e.g. structure and function of the chromosomes, are studied in the context of inheritance.

cytokinins (phytokinins) Phytohormones (plant hormones) that stimulate metabolism and cell division; they are substituted adenines synthesized mainly at the root apex.

(See also AUXINS and CROWN GALL.)

cytoplasmic genes (extrachromosomal genes; also extranuclear genes) Genes other than those which occur in a prokaryotic chromosome or in the eukaryotic nucleus. In prokaryotes, the term commonly refers to genes in an autonomously replicating PLASMID, while in eukaryotes it generally refers e.g. to genes in mitochondria and chloroplasts.

cytoplasmic inheritance (extrachromosomal inheritance or non-Mendelian inheritance) Inheritance that involves factors such as CYTOPLASMIC GENES, i.e. inheritance unrelated to nuclear or chromosomal genes and not subject to Mendelian laws.

(See also MATERNAL INHERITANCE.)

CytoTrap™ two-hybrid system A two-hybrid system (Stratagene, La Jolla CA) for detecting protein–protein interaction within the *cytoplasm* of the yeast *Saccharomyces cerevisiae*; this approach is therefore distinct from those systems (e.g. YEAST TWO-HYBRID SYSTEM) which detect protein–protein interaction by assaying for transcriptional activation in the nucleus.

As in other two-hybrid systems, the 'bait' protein forms part of a fusion protein encoded by a plasmid vector. The target protein (one of various proteins to be assayed) also forms part of a fusion protein encoded by a separate plasmid vector.

Both plasmid vectors include sequences that encode factors required for gene expression in *S. cerevisiae*; both vectors are introduced into *S. cerevisiae* by an appropriate method.

The pMyr vector includes the gene of the target protein that is fused to a sequence encoding the *myristylation membrane localization signal*; when expressed in the yeast host cell, the localization signal becomes anchored to the cell membrane – together with the target protein, which is therefore accessible in the cytoplasm.

The pSos vector contains the gene of the bait protein fused to a sequence from the gene of the human Sos protein, hSos. hSos is a *guanosine nucleotide exchange factor* which, when brought into close proximity to a membrane-associated Ras protein by bait–target binding, can activate Ras by promoting the exchange of bound GDP for GTP; when activated in this way, Ras initiates intracellular signaling, leading to growth of the cell.

The strain of *S. cerevisiae* used as host cell has a mutation in the cdc25 gene (the homolog of the gene encoding hSos). This makes the host cell temperature-sensitive: growth occurs at 25°C but not at 37°C. However, when hSos is internalized, and activating Ras, it can complement the defect in cdc25 – so that growth can occur at 37°C. Hence, growth of the host cell at 37°C is used as an indicator of bait–target interaction.

The CytoTrap™ two-hybrid system has been used e.g. for studies on the association of heat-shock transcription factor 4b with a kinase and a tyrosine phosphatase [Mol Cell Biol (2006) 26(8):3282–3294], and for studying the regulation of apoptosis by the p8/prothymosin α complex [Proc Natl Acad Sci USA (2006) 103(8):2671–2676].

D

D (1) A specific indicator of ambiguity in the recognition site of a RESTRICTION ENDONUCLEASE or in another nucleic acid sequence; for example, in the recognition site GDGCH↓C (enzyme SduI) the 'D' indicates A or G or T. (In RNA 'D' indicates A or G or U.) In the example, 'H' is A or C or T. (2) L-Aspartic acid (an alternative to Asp).

D loop (displacement loop)   A loop of ssDNA that is formed, for example, when a short ssDNA fragment hybridizes with a complementary sequence in one of the strands of dsDNA; the displaced, homologous strand is the D loop. (A D loop can be used e.g. for bisulfite-mediated site-directed mutagenesis.)

Formation of a D loop can be demonstrated *in vitro* with a negatively supercoiled ccc dsDNA molecule. A D loop forms spontaneously as the resulting structure is more relaxed. D loops are promoted e.g. by the RecA protein.

If a short *ssRNA* fragment hybridizes in this way, the resulting loop of ssDNA is called an *R loop*. If the ssRNA is a *mature* mRNA transcribed from a SPLIT GENE, then, when it binds to the gene, R loops will be formed at the exons; intron regions (which have no homologous sequences in the mature mRNA) form loops of dsDNA.

DAB   3,3′-diaminobenzidine: a substrate for HORSERADISH PEROXIDASE.

dabcyl   4-((4-(dimethylamino)phenyl)azo) benzoic acid: a non-fluorescent quenches of fluorescence which is used e.g. as a FRET acceptor molecule; dabcyl appears to act as a universal quenches, i.e. it quenches the emission from a wide range of fluorophores regardless of their emission profile.

(cf. DABSYL CHLORIDE.)

dabsyl chloride   4-dimethylaminobenzene-4′-sulfonyl chloride: a reagent used e.g. for labeling peptides and proteins.

(cf. DABCYL.)

DAF (direct amplification fingerprinting)   See AP-PCR.

Dam-directed mismatch repair   See MISMATCH REPAIR.

dam **gene**   In various prokaryotes, including *Escherichia coli*: a gene encoding the enzyme Dam methylase which methylates DNA at the N-6 position of adenine within the sequence 5′-GATC-3′ (a so-called 'Dam site'); during DNA replication the daughter strand is methylated soon after its synthesis. Inactivation of the *dam* gene blocks methylation at Dam sites.

In *E. coli*, Dam methylation is a factor in the MISMATCH REPAIR system and is involved in the regulation of certain genes that have Dam sites in their promoters. In transposon Tn*10*, for example, transposition is inhibited by Dam methylation within the promoter of the transposase gene; inhibition is due to a reduction in transposase activity. Transposition may occur during DNA synthesis when the replication fork has passed the Dam site but before the occurrence of Dam methylation at this site.

Other genes affected by Dam methylation include the *cre* gene of phage P1 (see CRE–LOXP SYSTEM) and the *trpR* gene of *E. coli*.

In *E. coli*, the chromosomal origin of replication, *oriC*, contains a number of Dam sites.

(See also DCM GENE.)

Dam methylase   See DAM GENE.

Dam methylation   See DAM GENE.

Dam site   See DAM GENE.

damaged DNA   See CODIS, FORENSIC APPLICATIONS, WHOLE-GENOME AMPLIFICATION and Y FAMILY DNA POLYMERASES.

DAPI   4′,6-Diamidino-2-phenylindole dihydrochloride: a fluorescent stain for dsDNA which binds preferentially to AT-rich regions. DAPI binds to RNA with lower affinity; moreover, the fluorescence emission maximum of a DAPI–RNA complex (~500 nm) differs from that of a DAPI–dsDNA complex (~460 nm).

On binding to dsDNA the fluorescence of DAPI is reported to be enhanced by about 20-fold.

darbepoietin-α   See BIOPHARMACEUTICAL (table).

dark quenching   A FRET-type technique which has been used to study the mechanism of homologous recombination – specifically, separation of the two strands of the target duplex prior to hybridization of the presynaptic filament with one of the strands. In this study the fluorophore FAM was used to 5′-end-label one strand of the target duplex, and the quenches DABCYL was used to 3′-end-label the other strand; hence, prior to separation of the two strands there was no fluorescent signal. On strand separation the fluorophore is unquenched – so that a fluorescent signal is produced.

The advantage of this procedure is that it achieves a signal-to-background ratio approximately 5- to 10-fold higher than that obtained with the use of a conventional FRET arrangement [BioTechniques (2006) 40:736–738].

DASH   DYNAMIC ALLELE-SPECIFIC HYBRIDIZATION.

database   In the present context: any organized and retrievable collection of data on particular sequences of nucleic acid or whole-genome sequences (see e.g. INTERNATIONAL NUCLEOTIDE SEQUENCE DATABASE COLLABORATION and TIGR MICROBIAL DATABASE); polypeptide sequences; gene expression profiles; specific genomic features (see e.g. CODIS) etc. or data on particular types of enzyme (e.g. RESTRICTION ENDONUCLEASES: see e.g. REBASE).

(See also ONLINE MENDELIAN INHERITANCE IN MAN and the databases mentioned in entries MITOCHONDRIAL DNA, P53, QUADRUPLEX DNA, RNA MODIFICATION PATHWAYS, SPOLIGOTYPING and STR.)

The phrase DNA DATABASE frequently refers to a database, maintained e.g. by a government/law-enforcement agency, which contains a record of the DNA sequences of specific individuals.

There are also *collections* of databases [e.g. The Molecular Biology Database Collection (2006 update): Nucleic Acids Res (2006) 34(Database issue):D3–D5].

Some databases have limited access; others are available to the public.

Reliability of databases

The reliability of some public databases has been questioned. For example, significant discrepancies have been noticed in the genome sequences of different strains of (the prokaryote) *Pyrococcus furiosus* [see J Bacteriol (2005) 187:7325–7332]. Among human SNP databases, it was suggested that some of the reported SNPs may be associated with *editing* sites rather than representing actual SNPs [Nucleic Acids Res (2005) 33 (14):4612–4617]. Moreover, the database sequences of many cancer-associated genes may reflect atypical splice forms of the type found in tumor cells [see Nucleic Acids Res (2005) 33(16):5026–5033].

dATPαS Deoxyadenosine α-thiotriphosphate (α-thiophosphoryl dATP).

This modified nucleotide is used in various types of method (see e.g. PYROSEQUENCING and SDA).

DC-SIGN (CD209) DC-specific ICAM3-grabbing nonintegrin: a cell-surface receptor molecule (a C-type lectin) that occurs on dendritic cells (and also on other types of cell); it binds to the envelope glycoprotein gp120 of HIV-1 (human immunodeficiency virus), and is reported to act as a receptor for e.g. cytomegalovirus (CMV), the Ebola virus and the bacterium *Mycobacterium tuberculosis*.

Expression of DC-SIGN on a subset of B lymphocytes (B cells) was increased, *in vitro*, on stimulation with interleukin 4 (IL-4) and the CD40 ligand. Activated B cells bound and internalized certain strains of HIV-1 and were able to mediate infection of T cells with the virus [PLoS Pathogens (2006) 2(7):e70].

It appears that DC-SIGN is involved in some of the cases in which dendritic cells promote the infection of CD4+ T cells with HIV-1 [J Virol (2007) 81(5):2497–2507; J Virol (2007) 81(5):2519–2523].

DCDS Donor conjugal DNA synthesis: see CONJUGATION.

dcm **gene** In *Escherichia coli*: a gene encoding an enzyme that methylates DNA at the C-5 position in the (second) cytosine residue within the sequence 5′-CCA/TGG-3′. Inactivation of the gene blocks methylation at these sites.

dda **gene** (of phage T4) See HELICASE.

DDBJ DNA DataBank of Japan.

ddF DIDEOXY FINGERPRINTING.

DDMR Dam-directed mismatch repair: see MISMATCH REPAIR.

ddNTP 2′,3′-Dideoxyribonucleoside triphosphate: any of the (synthetic) nucleoside triphosphates used e.g. for chain termination in the DIDEOXY METHOD OF DNA SEQUENCING.

DEAD-box proteins Various types of protein which have the motif: Asp-Glu-Ala-Asp ('DEAD' by the single-letter designations of the amino acids); they include eIF4A (a eukaryotic initiation factor in protein synthesis) and certain proteins involved in the SPLICING of pre-mRNA.

decoyinine See PSICOFURANINE.

defective interfering particle (DI particle) A defective derivative of a normal, non-defective (*standard*) virus; the presence of the standard virus is needed for replication of the DI particle, but this lowers the yield of the standard virus. In cell cultures, and in experimental animals, at least some types of DI particle have been reported to attenuate the pathogenic effects of a virulent standard virus.

degeneracy (of the genetic code) See CODON.

degenerate primer One of a set of primers used to amplify a particular region of DNA whose sequence has been predicted e.g. on the basis of the amino acid sequence of an encoded protein. Because, as a result of the degeneracy of the genetic code, an amino acid may be specified by more than one type of CODON, the nucleotide sequence of the coding region of the given protein could be any of various combinations of nucleotides; hence, a number of different primers (referred to as degenerate primers) may be used in an attempt to find one primer complementary to the *actual* sequence of nucleotides that encodes the protein.

(cf. DEGENERATE PROBE.)

degenerate probe One of a set of probes that are designed to be complementary to each of various possible (predicted) variant forms of a given target sequence. A set of degenerate probes is used e.g. when the target sequence is not completely known.

(cf. DEGENERATE PRIMER.)

degradosome (RNA degradosome) A multi-component complex, e.g. in *Escherichia coli*, that processes/degrades RNA molecules; it includes RNase E, polynucleotide phosphorylase, Rh1B helicase [Proc Natl Acad Sci USA (2005) 102(46): 16590–16595], polynucleotide phosphate kinase, DnaK and GroEL. The complex degrades *some* types of mRNA [Proc Natl Acad Sci USA (2004) 101:2758–2763], and also e.g. mediates formation of the 5S rRNA ribosomal component.

degron See N-END RULE.

delavirdine A NON-NUCLEOSIDE REVERSE TRANSCRIPTASE INHIBITOR.

delayed enrichment method See AUXOTROPHIC MUTANT.

deletions (nested) See NESTED DELETIONS.

Δ*lon* (delta *lon*) See entry ESCHERICHIA COLI (table).

demethylation (of DNA) Removal of the methyl group (–CH₃) from bases in DNA. Methods involving demethylation and methylation-inhibition have been used e.g. for investigating methylation-based GENE SILENCING.

The methods employed include the use of certain chemical agents (such as 5-aza-2′-deoxycytidine) which inhibit *in vivo* methylation, and direct inhibition of DNA methyltransferase 1 by RNAi or other means. The agent 5-aza-2′-deoxycytidine is incorporated into the DNA of actively dividing cells – after which it binds and inactivates DNA methyltransferase 1; this causes a generalized fall in the maintenance methyltransferase activity in the cell, leading to a global demethylation or under-methylation.

One problem associated with drug-induced demethylation (e.g. with 5-aza-2′-deoxycytidine) is that, in a given culture, cells in different stages of the cell cycle may respond differently (e.g. by exhibiting different levels of demethylation) on exposure to the drug. Moreover, cells which are not actively dividing will be unaffected by the treatment. Consequently, a drug-treated culture may consist of a mixed population in which demethylation has occurred to varying degrees among the cells.

Problems associated with methods that involve *direct* inactivation of the Dnmt1 gene include failure of the intervention in a proportion of the cells, again resulting in heterogeneity in demethylation among the population of cells in a culture.

Drug-mediated DNA demethylation is reported to be facilitated by the GFP REACTIVATION TECHNIQUE.

denaturing-gradient gel electrophoresis See DGGE.

dendrichip A MICROARRAY prepared by covalently binding NH_2-modified DNA probes (via their 5′ termini) to dendrimer-activated glass slides (*dendrislides*); each dendrimer is a nanometric spherical structure (a polyfunctional polymer) which links the probe to the slide. These dendrimers can be prepared with various reactive surface groups such as aldehyde, thiol, epoxy. [For background information see: Nucleic Acids Res (2003) 31(16):e88.]

DNA dendrimers (three-dimensional, branched structures with ssDNA arms which can carry various types of functional molecule) have been used e.g. for the enzymatic detection of microRNA in microtiter plates [BioTechniques (2006) 41(4): 420–424].

dendrimer See DENDRICHIP.

deoxyadenosine α-thiotriphosphate (dATPαS) The modified, synthetic form of dATP in which sulfur replaces phosphorus at the α position. dATPαS is used, for example, in the PYROSEQUENCING procedure and in SDA.

deoxyribonuclease See DNASE.

deoxyribozyme (DNA enzyme, DNAzyme) Any molecule of DNA which has catalytic activity, typically for a nucleic acid substrate.

[*In vitro* selection, characterization and application of deoxyribozymes that cleave RNA substrates: Nucleic Acids Res (2005) 33(19):6151–6163.]

Certain Zn^{2+}-dependent deoxyribozymes were reported to ligate molecules of RNA [Biochemistry (2005) 44(25):9217–9231].

(See also BINARY DEOXYRIBOZYME LIGASE.)

(cf. RIBOZYME.)

DEPC DIETHYLPYROCARBONATE.

derepressed Refers e.g. to a gene or operon which, formerly inactive (i.e. repressed), is being expressed – or to a gene or operon which is not subject to the repression that is normal for related molecules (see e.g. F PLASMID).

DES® The *Drosophila* expression system (Invitrogen, Carlsbad CA): a system designed for the expression of recombinant proteins from simple types of vector in *Drosophila* Schneider S2 cells. (Expression of heterologous proteins in insect cells can also be achieved in a baculovirus-mediated format: see e.g. BACULODIRECT.)

The pMT/V5-His vector permits expression of recombinant proteins regulated by the *Drosophila* copper-sulfate-inducible metallothionein gene promoter. Purification of the expressed protein is facilitated by a SIX-HISTIDINE TAG. An alternative version of this vector includes the N-terminal signal sequence

of the BiP gene (which promotes secretion of the expressed recombinant protein).

The pMT-DEST48 vector permits expression of a gene or sequence received from a Gateway® entry clone (see table in entry GATEWAY SITE-SPECIFIC RECOMBINATION SYSTEM for details).

The linearized pMT/V5-His-TOPO® vector (3.6 kb) allows expression of a gene or sequence prepared as a *Taq*-created PCR product (see TOPOISOMERASE I CLONING).

destination vector In the GATEWAY SITE-SPECIFIC RECOMBINATION SYSTEM: any vector which is able to receive a gene or insert from an entry clone. (See table in the entry GATEWAY SITE-SPECIFIC RECOMBINATION SYSTEM for some examples of destination vectors.)

desumoylation See SUMOYLATION.

DFRS plasmid Dual-fluorescence reporter/sensor plasmid: a plasmid that contains sequences which encode two different fluorophores – one of the fluorophores being used to signal the intracellular presence of the plasmid, the other being used to detect the presence or absence of a specific intracellular target sequence; DFRS plasmids were used e.g. for monitoring the dynamics of specific types of microRNA (miRNA; see MICRORNA) within individual living cells of the zebrafish (*Danio rerio*) and mouse (*Mus* sp) [BioTechniques (2006) 41 (6):727–732].

In the above study, the GREEN FLUORESCENT PROTEIN was used as reporter; MONOMERIC RED FLUORESCENT PROTEIN was used as the sensor. Both genes were under the regulation of identical constitutive promoters. The 3′ untranslated region of the mRFP mRNA contained a tandem cassette which was complementary to the particular miRNA studied. Given the *absence* of the target species of miRNA, the mRNA of mRFP is translated – and this is detected by red fluorescence. In the presence of the target miRNA, hybridization occurs between the miRNA and the complementary sequence in the mRNA of mRFP, inhibiting translation of mRFP; this is detected by an absence of red fluorescence.

DGGE Denaturing-gradient gel electrophoresis: a method used for comparing *related*, *double-stranded*, PCR-generated fragments of DNA (or fragments of DNA generated by restriction endonucleases).

(cf. SSCP ANALYSIS.)

The method involves two-dimensional electrophoresis. In the first phase, fragments are separated, by size, in a routine form of GEL ELECTROPHORESIS.

In the second phase, electrophoretic movement of the fragments occurs in a direction perpendicular (at right-angles) to the original path. During the second phase, fragments move into an increasing gradient of DNA-denaturing agents (such as urea + formamide). Hence, at given levels in the gradient, the dsDNA fragments will exhibit *sequence-dependent* melting (i.e. strand separation) – and this will affect their speed of movement through the gel; different fragments, with different sequences, are likely to have different melting characteristics under these conditions, and this can result in the separation of fragments through differential changes in their rates of movement in the gel. (Note that base-pairing is stronger in GC-rich regions of a fragment; strand separation in such regions will occur less readily than strand separation in AT-rich regions. Thus, for example, an AT→CG mutation in a given fragment is likely to affect the ease of strand separation in the fragment and, hence, to affect the electrophoretic mobility of that fragment.)

In some protocols, the PCR primers used to prepare sample fragments are modified with GC-rich tags at the 5′ end; this is useful e.g. in that it avoids the *complete* denaturation of fragments in the higher concentrations of denaturing agent – thus avoiding complex and unwanted patterns of movement in at least some of the fragments.

Fluorophore-labeled primers have been reported to improve the sensitivity of DGGE [Appl Environ Microbiol (2005) 71 (8):4893–4896].

DGGE has been useful e.g. for studying *pncA* mutations in *Mycobacterium tuberculosis* associated with resistance to the drug pyrazinamide (used in anti-tuberculosis chemotherapy) [Antimicrob Agents Chemother (2005) 49:2210–2217].

DGGE has also been useful for TYPING various species of bacteria (for example, differentiating isolates of *Escherichia coli* by analysis of the 16S–23S intergenic spacers in the RRN OPERON).

A method related to DGGE uses an ongoing rise in temperature (instead of a chemical gradient) in the second phase of electrophoresis; this procedure is referred to as temporal temperature-gradient gel electrophoresis: see TTGE.

DHPA   (*S*)-9-(2,3-dihydroxypropyl)adenine: an analog of adenosine which has antiviral activity (against e.g. herpes simplex and varicella–zoster viruses).

DHPG   9-(1,3-dihydroxy-2-propoxymethyl)guanine: an antiviral agent which has activity against e.g. herpes simplex virus. The mode of action resembles that of ACYCLOVIR.

DI particle   See DEFECTIVE INTERFERING PARTICLE.

diagnostic tag   See SAGE.

diamidines   Compounds that have two amidine [$NH_2.C(=NH)–$] groups. Some aromatic diamidines can bind to KINETOPLAST DNA, and such binding may contribute to their trypanocidal properties.

6-diazo-5-oxo-L-norleucine   See DON.

diazomethane   See STREPTOZOTOCIN.

Dicer (DICER)   An RNase-III-like enzyme involved in various types of post-transcriptional gene silencing (see PTGS). The enzyme cleaves double-stranded RNA (dsRNA) into pieces of regular size, reported to be within the range 21–28 nucleotides in length in individual cases; in at least some cases these fragments have characteristic 2-nucleotide 3′ overhangs.

Dicer is widespread in eukaryotic organisms, and it appears to have an important role in gene expression; for example, a deficiency of the enzyme is reported to compromise proliferation of murine embryonic stem cells [Proc Natl Acad Sci USA (2005) 102(34):12135–12140].

The enzyme contains a number of domains which include a C-terminal dsRNA-binding domain, an N-terminal DEAD-box helicase domain and two RNase III-like domains.

[Contribution of the dsRNA structure to Dicer specificity and efficiency: RNA (2005) 11(5):674–682.]

Bacterial RNASE III and also recombinant forms of Dicer are used in experimental RNAi.

dichroic beamsplitter   In fluorescence microscopy: a filter, interposed between the eyepiece and objective which (i) transmits light emitted from the fluorophore, but (ii) *reflects* the (shorter-wavelength) light from the excitation filter onto the sample.

didanosine   See NUCLEOSIDE REVERSE TRANSCRIPTASE INHIBITORS.

dideoxy fingerprinting (ddF)   An early method which has been used e.g. for detecting resistance to an anti-tuberculosis drug, rifampicin, in *Mycobacterium tuberculosis*.

In this method, resistance to rifampicin is detected by demonstrating the presence of certain mutations in the *rpoB* gene; *rpoB* encodes the β subunit of the enzyme RNA polymerase, the target of rifampicin.

Dideoxy fingerprinting involves an initial amplification, by PCR, of the target sequence (in *rpoB*). The resulting (dsDNA) amplicons are then used as templates in a modified form of the DIDEOXY METHOD of sequencing involving temperature cycling (as in PCR); temperature cycling permits the use of double-stranded DNA amplicons, avoiding e.g. the need for ssDNA templates (which are required, for example, in SSCP). In contrast to the standard procedure for dideoxy sequencing, only one type of dideoxyribonucleotide is used; this ddNTP is used for each strain being tested so that the results can be compared. The products of the sequencing reaction are examined by electrophoresis in a *non*-denaturing gel.

Mutations may be detected e.g. by changes in the mobility of full-length and/or chain-terminated products, such changes being due to alterations in intra-strand base-pairing resulting from mutation(s). Mutations can also be indicated by changes in the *number* of chain-terminated products in a given reaction; the number of products can change when mutation(s) increase or decrease the number of chain-terminating sites in the template strand, a chain-terminating site being a base that is complementary to the particular ddNTP being used in a given reaction.

Interpretation of the results from dideoxy fingerprinting is facilitated by a knowledge of common resistance-conferring mutations in *rpoB* (i.e. base change and location); these have been mapped.

dideoxy method (DNA sequencing) (Sanger's method, or chain-termination method)   A method of DNA SEQUENCING (q.v.) which is widely used for sequencing templates of up to ~500 nucleotides; longer templates can be sequenced in stages.

The method is shown diagrammatically in the figure.

dideoxyribonucleoside triphosphate   See DDNTP.

Diels–Alder reaction   A reaction that creates a six-membered ring structure as a result of interaction between a dienophile and a 1,3-diene. The Diels–Alder reaction has been exploited

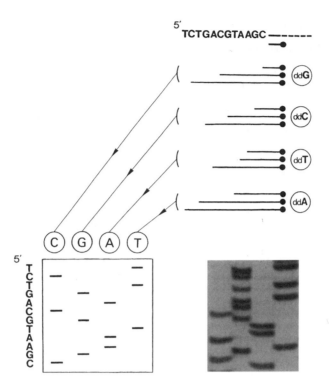

DIDEOXY METHOD (DNA sequencing) The fragment to be sequenced is first obtained in single-stranded form. This can be achieved e.g. by cloning in a phage M13 vector or by asymmetric PCR. Either strand can be sequenced; for increased accuracy both strands are sequenced (in separate sequencing reactions).

In this example the unknown sequence is 5′-TCT.....AGC-3′ (*top*). Regardless of the method used for obtaining single-stranded templates, the unknown sequence will be flanked on its 3′ side by a known sequence of nucleotides; this permits the design of a primer which can bind next to the unknown sequence such that the first nucleotide to be added to the primer will pair with the first 3′ nucleotide of the unknown sequence. In the diagram, a primer (*short line*), carrying a label (*black disk*), has bound at a site flanking the 3′ end of the unknown sequence (*top*).

DNA synthesis *in vitro* is usually carried out with a reaction mixture that includes: (i) templates (in this case, single-stranded fragments that include the unknown sequence); (ii) primers; (iii) the four types of deoxyribonucleoside triphosphate (dNTP) – i.e. dATP, dCTP, dGTP and dTTP; and (iv) DNA polymerase. When base-paired to the template strand, the primer is extended (5′→3′) by the sequential addition of nucleotides, as dictated by the template.

For sequencing, there are four separate reactions. A given reaction determines each of the sites at which *one* of the four types of nucleotide (A, C, G or T) occurs in the unknown sequence. Each of the four reactions contains all of the constituents mentioned above (including many copies of the template, and of the primer). Additionally, each of the reaction mixtures contains *one* type of *di*deoxyribonucleoside triphosphate (ddNTP) – that is, ddT, ddG, ddC or ddA.

When a dideoxyribonucleotide is added to a growing strand of DNA it prevents the addition of the *next* nucleotide; this is because a dideoxyribonucleotide lacks the 3′-OH group which is necessary for making the next phosphodiester bond. Hence, extension of the primer will stop (= chain termination) at any position where a dideoxyribonucleotide has been incorporated. In a given reaction mixture, the concentration of the ddNTP is such that, in most growing strands, synthesis will be stopped – at some stage – by the incorporation of a dideoxyribonucleotide. Because a given type of ddNTP molecule can pair with its complementary base wherever it occurs in the template strand, chain termination can occur at different sites on different copies of the template strand – so that, in a given reaction, in the preparation of peptide–oligonucleotide conjugates; this has been achieved by interacting diene-modified oligonucleotides and maleimide-derivatized peptides [Nucleic Acids Res (2006) 34(3):e24].

This procedure may be used e.g. for conjugating antisense oligonucleotides to appropriate peptides in order to facilitate their uptake by target cells.

diethylpyrocarbonate (DEPC) $C_2H_5.O.CO.O.CO.C_2H_5$ – an inactivator of RNases used e.g. for treating glassware etc. in order to avoid loss of sample RNA through exogenous RNase activity; autoclaving, after treatment, is used to remove any remaining DEPC.

DEPC can also modify the exposed N-7 position of an unpaired adenine in RNA or DNA.

(See also RNALATER.)

differential DNA cleavage See e.g. CPNPG SITES.

differential display A method which is used e.g. for detecting genes that are expressed in a given type of cell only under certain circumstances.

Essentially, this method compares mRNAs isolated from two or more populations of the given cell which are expected to reveal differential expression of genes. *Selected* mRNAs from each population being studied are initially converted to cDNAs by reverse transcription; selection is achieved by the use of primers having a 3′ terminal base complementary to only a proportion of the mRNAs from a given population. The resulting cDNAs are amplified by PCR using the original ('selective') primer and a primer of arbitrary sequence; the products of PCR therefore represent the 3′ ends of selected mRNA molecules.

The amplicons from each population are subjected to gel electrophoresis in separate lanes, and the fingerprints of the different populations are compared. Any band of interest (e.g. one present in a given fingerprint but absent in others) can be extracted from the gel and amplified (using the same primers) prior to e.g. sequencing.

Differential display was used e.g. to study gene expression during the development of different zones of the neural tube in the chick embryo [BMC Dev Biol (2006) 6:9].

digoxigenin (DIG) A steroid (from the plant *Digitalis*) used e.g. for labeling PROBES. DIG-labeled RNA probes are made e.g. by *in vitro* transcription on a DNA target sequence using labeled nucleotides.

DIG-dUTP can be incorporated into DNA probes during synthesis by various types of DNA polymerase – including *Taq* polymerase, phage T4 polymerase, Klenow fragment and

---

DIDEOXY METHOD (DNA sequencing) (*continued*) product strands of different lengths will be formed. For example, with ddG (see diagram) the three products are of different lengths because, during extension of primers, ddG has paired with a cytosine residue at three different locations in the template; note that, in this case, *the length of a given product strand is related to the location of a particular cytosine residue in the unknown sequence*. Analogous comments apply to reaction mixtures containing the other types of ddNTP.

At the end of the reaction, new product strands are separated from templates by formamide. Each of the four reaction mixtures is then subjected to electrophoresis in a separate lane of a polyacrylamide gel. During electrophoresis, small products move further than larger ones, in a given time; products that differ in length by only one nucleotide can be distinguished in this way – the shorter product moving just a little further.

The gel used for electrophoresis contains a denaturing agent which inhibits intra-strand base-pairing. This is essential: in order to be able to deduce the locations of a given base in the template strand it is necessary to compare the *lengths* of all the product strands (by comparing their positions within the gel), and this requires proportionality between strand length and electrophoretic mobility, i.e. between the length of a given strand and the position of its band in the gel. Were intra-strand base-pairing to occur, there would be no fixed relationship between a product's length and the position of its band in the gel.

After electrophoresis, bands in the gel may be revealed by autoradiography (if the primers had been labeled e.g. with ^{32}P) or by exposure to ultraviolet radiation (if the primers had been labeled with a fluorophore).

An alternative approach to detecting the bands of products exploits chemiluminescence (see entry) and uses e.g. biotin-labeled primers; after electrophoresis, bands in the gel are transferred to a membrane – which is exposed to a streptavidin–alkaline phosphatase conjugate and a substrate (such as CSPD®) which generates a light signal.

The locations of the bands in the gel (*bottom, left*) indicate the relative lengths of the product strands – the shorter products having moved further along the gel (from top to bottom in the diagram). Note that the first unknown 3′ nucleotide (C) is identified by (i) the shortest product strand (which has moved the furthest), and (ii) the fact that this product came from the ddG reaction mixture, indicating a base that pairs with G, i.e. C. Similarly, the next unknown nucleotide (G) is indicated by the next shortest product strand – which came from the ddC reaction mixture, thus indicating G in the template. The whole of the unknown sequence can be deduced in this way.

Bottom, right. Part of an autoradiograph of a sequencing gel (courtesy of Joop Gaken, Molecular Medicine Unit, King's College, London).

Figure reproduced from *Bacteria in Biology, Biotechnology and Medicine*, 6th edition, Figure 8.23, pages 260–261, Paul Singleton (2004) John Wiley & Sons Ltd, UK [ISBN 0-470-09027-8] with permission from the publisher.

at least some types of reverse transcriptase.

Detection of DIG-labeled probes can be achieved with anti-digoxigenin antibodies covalently linked to a fluorophore or linked to an enzyme such as alkaline phosphatase that gives a chromogenic reaction with appropriate substrates.

(See also EMEA.)

7,8-dihydro-8-oxoguanine See 8-OXOG.

dikaryon (1) A cell with two genetically dissimilar (haploid) nuclei, or a (fungal) mycelium comprising such cells.

(2) A pair of nuclei that may be genetically dissimilar.

dinB **gene** See DNA POLYMERASE IV.

dioecism See HETEROTHALLISM.

diphosphate See PYROPHOSPHATE.

diphosphopyridine nucleotide See NAD.

diploid See PLOIDY.

direct amplification fingerprinting (DAF) See AP-PCR.

direct repeat (DR) One of two (or more) identical or closely similar sequences, in a given molecule of nucleic acid, which have the same polarity and orientation. Repeats may or may not be contiguous. An example:

```
5′.....GCCTA.....GCCTA.....3′
3′.....CGGAT.....CGGAT.....5′
```

The direct repeat sequences in the genome of *Mycobacterium tuberculosis* and related bacteria have been used in SPOLIGO-TYPING.

(See also ITERON and TANDEM REPEAT.)

direct repeat (DR) locus (of *Mycobacterium tuberculosis*) A distinct region of the chromosome, found in members of the *M. tuberculosis* complex, consisting of a number of highly conserved 36-bp direct repeats (DRs) which are interspersed with spacers of 34–41 bp. The number of repeats, as well as the presence/length of the spacers, are strain-dependent characteristics; such variation may have arisen through intramolecular homologous recombination and/or integration of an insertion sequence.

Variability in the DR locus has been exploited in SPOLIGO-TYPING.

direct selection *Syn.* POSITIVE SELECTION.

directed evolution Any technique whose object is, effectively, to enact a rapid evolutionary process in the laboratory with the object of selecting molecules with certain desired characteristics; this approach can be used e.g. with nucleic acids and proteins.

[Laboratory-directed protein evolution: Microbiol Mol Biol Rev (2005) 69(3):373–392.]

(See also DNA SHUFFLING and HOMING ENDONUCLEASE.)

directional cloning *Syn.* FORCED CLONING.

directional TOPO® pENTR™ vectors Vectors (Invitrogen, Carlsbad CA) used for cloning an insert, in a specific orientation, using the TOPOISOMERASE I CLONING approach.

Directional insertion of a fragment is achieved by using an asymmetric arrangement in which one end of the (linearized) vector is blunt-ended and the other end has a four-nucleotide overhang; as in other forms of topo cloning the enzyme topo-isomerase I is bound to phosphate at each end of the vector – on opposite strands – and carries out the same function.

These vectors include *att* sequences, permitting recombination with any of a range of Gateway® destination vectors – see the table in GATEWAY SITE-SPECIFIC RECOMBINATION SYSTEM; they also include sites suitable for sequencing.

disjunction Separation of chromosomes during the process of nuclear division.

displacement loop (D loop) See D LOOP.

dissymmetry ratio *Syn.* BASE RATIO.

distal box See RNASE III.

ditag See SAGE.

dithiothreitol (DDT, Cleland's reagent) A reagent used e.g. to reduce disulfides to thiols and to maintain thiol groups in the reduced state. High concentrations of dithiothreitol facilitate denaturation of proteins by chaotropes and detergents.

In DNA technology, the reagent has also been used e.g. as a mucolytic agent for the treatment of mucoid specimens of sputum prior to examination by nucleic-acid-based tests for *Mycobacterium tuberculosis*.

divergent transcription Transcription from two closely adjacent promoters, in opposite directions.

DNA Deoxyribonucleic acid: typically, a double-stranded (i.e. 'duplex') molecule or a single-stranded molecule – referred to as dsDNA and ssDNA, respectively – that consists of linearly polymerized deoxyribonucleotides, with adjacent nucleotides linked by a *phosphodiester bond*. The major bases found in the nucleotides of DNA are adenine, guanine, cytosine and thymine; this differs from RNA (ribonucleic acid) – in which the major bases are adenine, guanine, cytosine and uracil.

(See also TRIPLEX DNA and QUADRUPLEX DNA.)

DNA encodes the genetic information in cells and in some types of virus. In prokaryotes, DNA is found in the nucleoid (see also PLASMID), while in eukaryotes it occurs primarily in the nucleus, in mitochondria and (in photosynthetic species) in chloroplasts.

In linear molecules of DNA each strand has *polarity*: a 5′ end and a 3′ end. At one end of a strand, 5′ refers to the 5′ carbon atom in a ribose residue which is *not* linked to another nucleotide, while 3′ at the other end of the strand refers to the 3′ carbon atom in the ribose residue which, similarly, is *not* linked to another nucleotide.

In linear dsDNA molecules the two strands are arranged in an *antiparallel* mode: a 5′-to-3′ strand is bound to a 3′-to-5′ strand. The hybridization (binding) between the two strands involves hydrogen bonding between the bases in opposite strands. Hydrogen bonding occurs between specific pairs of bases: adenine base-pairs with thymine, while cytosine base-pairs with guanine; adenine and thymine are *complementary* bases, as are cytosine and guanine. One strand of the duplex is said to be complementary to the other (when all the bases are correctly paired).

In so-called 'circular' molecules of dsDNA the polymer is continuous, i.e. there are no free 5′ and 3′ ends. Such molecules may be in either a relaxed or a supercoiled state. (See also TOPOISOMERASE.) ssDNA can also occur as a circular molecule. (See also DNA NANOCIRCLE.)

(See also PNA.)

DNA amplification (*in vitro*) Any of various procedures in which, typically, a defined sequence of nucleotides in DNA is replicated – often with the production of a large number of copies.

(See also NUCLEIC ACID AMPLIFICATION and cf. WHOLE-GENOME AMPLIFICATION.)

Isothermal amplification (amplification at a fixed temperature) can be carried out by methods such as strand displacement amplification (see SDA). (cf. NASBA.)

Other methods, such as the LIGASE CHAIN REACTION and the polymerase chain reaction (see PCR), involve repetitive temperature cycling (e.g. for ~25–40 cycles). Temperatures used in such processes include an initial high temperature (e.g. 94°C) that is designed to separate the strands of dsDNA in order to expose target sequence(s). These methods require the use of thermostable enzymes (e.g. a thermostable ligase in LCR and a thermostable polymerase in PCR).

All of these methods may yield false-positive and/or false-negative results under inappropriate conditions. In particular, contamination by extraneous nucleic acids must be rigorously excluded (see e.g. AMPLICON CONTAINMENT and AMPLICON INACTIVATION).

The methods mentioned above are well established and have been available for some years. More recent methods are HELICASE-DEPENDENT AMPLIFICATION and the MOLECULAR ZIPPER.

Recombinase polymerase amplification is a method which combines recombinase-mediated binding of primers with the strand-displacement synthesis of DNA: see RPA.

(See also *in situ* solid-phase DNA amplification in SOLID-PHASE PCR.)

DNA-binding proteins (in assays) See CHROMATIN IMMUNO-PRECIPITATION, EMSA, FOOTPRINTING and SCINTILLATION PROXIMITY ASSAY.

DNA caging See CAGED DNA.

DNA chip See CHIP; see also MICROARRAY.

DNA clean-up resin See e.g. STRATACLEAN RESIN.

DNA cloning See CLONING.

DNA combing Any procedure used for preparing DNA in a condition in which individual molecules are made available for analysis (e.g. fluoroscopic analysis) in a *stretched* state. In some methods, the molecules of DNA are anchored at one end to a solid (e.g. glass) surface, and stretching is carried out e.g. by the forces present in a receding meniscus.

[Simple method for stretching linear DNA molecules (of up to 18 kb) for fluorescent imaging: Nucleic Acids Res (2006) 34(17):e113.]

DNA database A phrase that frequently refers to a DATABASE containing a record of the DNA sequences from a number of individuals; such databases are often maintained e.g. by law-enforcement agencies.

(See also CODIS and FORENSIC APPLICATIONS.)

DNA delay mutant (of phage T4) A strain with mutation(s) in topoisomerase-encoding gene(s) which exhibits delayed synthesis of DNA and a smaller burst size. For replication, a T4 DNA delay mutant depends on a functional gyrase in the host cell.

DNA demethylation See DEMETHYLATION.

DNA dendrimer See DENDRICHIP.

DNA-dependent DNA polymerase (DNA polymerase) Any enzyme which polymerizes dNTPs (deoxyribonucleoside triphosphates) in the 5′-to-3′ direction on a DNA template, with elimination of pyrophosphate.

Escherichia coli encodes two main DNA polymerases that are designated I and III. (See also DNA POLYMERASE II, DNA POLYMERASE IV and DNA POLYMERASE V.)

Eukaryotes typically have a number of different DNA polymerases which include separate enzymes for replicating mitochondrial and nuclear DNA. Nuclear polymerases include DNA polymerases α and δ (see also OKAZAKI FRAGMENT).

(See also Y FAMILY.)

There is an extensive range of commercial DNA polymerases, many of which are thermostable enzymes intended for use in PCR (see e.g. ACCUPRIME GC-RICH DNA POLYMERASE, PFUTURBO, PLATINUM TAQ DNA POLYMERASE and RTTH DNA POLYMERASE).

Various forms of the well-known TAQ DNA POLYMERASE (including recombinant forms) are available.

An *error-prone* DNA polymerase (Mutazyme™) is used for generating random mutations during PCR (in the GENE-MORPH PCR MUTAGENESIS KIT).

DNA-dependent RNA polymerase See RNA POLYMERASE.

DNA DIRECT™ See DYNABEADS.

DNA enzyme See DEOXYRIBOZYME.

DNA extraction See DNA ISOLATION.

DNA fingerprinting (restriction enzyme analysis) A method used e.g. for TYPING bacteria. In the original method, the genomic DNA from a test strain is cleaved by certain restriction endonucleases and the resulting fragments separated by gel electrophoresis. The bands of fragments are stained *in situ* or, alternatively, denatured in the gel and blotted onto a membrane before staining. The pattern of bands in the gel, or on the membrane, is the *fingerprint*; strains are compared and classified on the basis of similarities and differences in their fingerprints.

One disadvantage of this method is that it may generate too many fragments and thus make a complex fingerprint which is difficult to interpret. Fewer, larger fragments are generated if a so-called 'rare-cutting' restriction enzyme is used for the initial restriction. These large fragments can be separated by PFGE, although this procedure requires 2–3 days and may be susceptible to endogenous nucleases.

The problem of too many fragments can also be addressed by using a labeled probe which binds only to those fragments that contain the probe's target sequence; in this case, only fragments which bind the probe are visible in the gel – so that the fingerprint consists of only a limited number of bands. This principle is exploited in RIBOTYPING.

DNA-free cell A cell, modified *in vitro*, in which the chromosomal DNA has undergone cleavage and extensive degradation. This can be achieved in at least two ways. First, treatment of certain types of cell with ULTRAVIOLET RADIATION (see e.g. MAXICELL). Second, treatment of *dam* mutants of *Escherichia coli* with 2-aminopurine, resulting in mismatch repair-related degradation of the chromosome [see J Bacteriol (2006) 188(1):339–342].

DNA glycosylase Any enzyme which cleaves an aberrant base from a nucleotide in DNA; DNA glycosylases are active in the BASE EXCISION REPAIR pathway.

(See also 8-OXOG.)

DNA glycosylase I (in *Escherichia coli*) *Syn.* Tag protein (see DNA REPAIR).

DNA glycosylase II (in *Escherichia coli*) *Syn.* AlkA (see DNA REPAIR).

DNA helicase See HELICASE.

DNA identification tag See IDENTIFIER DNA.

DNA isolation (DNA extraction) Any procedure for removing and concentrating DNA from cells/tissues. The methods are influenced by factors such as the type of DNA sought (genomic, plasmid DNA etc.), the required quality of DNA, amount of sample available, and nature of sample (e.g. fungal, bacterial, mammalian cells). [Isolation of *ancient* DNA (optimization of procedures): BioTechniques (2007) 42(3):343–352.]

(See also entry NUCLEIC ACID ISOLATION.)

Protocols include a wide range of *ad hoc* in-house methods and commercial systems.

For 'difficult' tissues (such as skin) the method may include an initial stage of mechanical disaggregation of the tissue followed by digestion with a proteinase; DNA may then be recovered by phenol–chloroform extraction and precipitated by ethanol (or e.g. isopropanol).

DNA can be extracted from some tissues (e.g. brain, liver) without organic solvents. The RecoverEase™ DNA isolation procedure (Stratagene, La Jolla CA) employs an initial stage of physical disaggregation and coarse filtration. The nuclei are separated by centrifugation. Incubation with proteinase K is continued overnight within a dialysis cup, yielding purified high-molecular-weight DNA.

DNA from whole blood can be obtained rapidly e.g. with the QIAamp® blood kit (QIAGEN, Hilden, Germany). After buffer-mediated lysis, the lysate is loaded into a spin column. On centrifugation, lysate passes through a specialized membrane to which DNA is adsorbed. Following spin washes, the DNA can be eluted from the membrane. This system can be used with blood containing common anticoagulants such as citrate and heparin. (Other types of QIAamp kit are available for different sources of DNA.)

Plasmid DNA may be recovered from bacteria e.g. with the QIAGEN® plasmid mini kit. The starting point is a pellet of cells of (e.g.) *Escherichia coli*. The pellet is resuspended in a buffer which disrupts the bacterial outer membrane. The use of controlled alkaline lysis with NaOH and the detergent

DNA ISOLATION: some common problems and their possible causes

Problem	Possible cause(s)
Low yield	Failure to ensure adequate lysis of cells, preventing release of cellular genomic DNA
Low yield	In spin columns: use of buffers which have incorrect pH or incorrect electrolyte concentration
Low yield	Pellet over-dried, causing incomplete re-suspension in buffer
Low yield of supercoiled plasmid DNA	Prolonged exposure to alkaline lysis buffer, resulting in denaturation and anomalous migration in gel electrophoresis
No yield (in gels)	Bands of *small* fragments migrated to full length of gel – avoided by use of lower voltage or shorter run
Quality (plasmid DNA) poor	Effect of endogenous nucleases. High-level activity of endonucleases is common in some bacteria
Quality (plasmid DNA) poor	Over-vigorous pipeting or vortexing, resulting in shearing
Contamination of plasmid DNA with chromosomal DNA	In controlled lysis methods: over-vigorous agitation of the lysate, with escape of both genomic and plasmid DNA – instead of only plasmid DNA
Contamination with RNA	A routine finding in some procedures; the RNA can be eliminated with RNase
Smeared bands in gel electrophoresis	Assuming correct conditions for electrophoresis: possible degradation of DNA via contamination with nucleases, or loading of gel with excess DNA; electrolyte levels in the DNA may be incorrect

sodium dodecyl sulfate (SDS) then releases soluble proteins, RNA and plasmids from the cells. The RNA is degraded by RNase A. Conditions are optimized for maximum release of plasmid DNA without release of the chromosomal DNA; the protocol is also designed to avoid irreversible denaturation of plasmid DNA. Neutralization by a high-salt buffer (pH 5.5) precipitates the SDS; proteins are entrapped in the salt–SDS complexes – but plasmids renature and remain in solution. Centrifugation removes the proteins etc., leaving plasmids in the supernatant. The supernatant is then passed through a QIAGEN anion-exchange resin; given the pH and electrolyte concentration of the supernatant, plasmid DNA is retained by the resin. After washing, the plasmid DNA is eluted in buffer containing 1.25 M NaCl (pH 8.5), desalted, and concentrated by precipitation with isopropanol.

Some of the problems (and possible causes) experienced in DNA isolation are listed in the table.

DNA ladder See GEL ELECTROPHORESIS.

DNA ligase Any LIGASE which can catalyze a phosphodiester bond between the 3′-OH terminal of a strand of DNA and the correctly juxtaposed 5′-phosphate terminal of the same strand or of a different strand.

A thermostable ligase, Ampligase®, from a thermophilic prokaryote, has uses which include e.g. the LIGASE CHAIN REACTION and REPEAT-EXPANSION DETECTION; however, it is not used for blunt-ended ligation.

The phage T4 DNA ligase (EC 6.5.1.1) and the (NAD$^+$-dependent) *Escherichia coli* DNA ligase (EC 6.5.1.2) are used e.g for closing nicks.

DNA looping See LOOPING.

DNA melting See MELTING.

DNA methylation See METHYLATION.

DNA methyltransferase (MTase) Any enzyme that catalyzes the METHYLATION of (specific) bases in DNA.

One example of a prokaryotic methyltransferase is M.SssI, an enzyme that carries out SYMMETRIC METHYLATION at the 5-position in the cytosine residues in the sequence 5′-CG-3′.

Many prokaryotic RESTRICTION ENDONUCLEASES carry out specific methylation as well as restriction.

The primary role of methylation in prokaryotes is generally taken to be the protection of genomic DNA from the cell's own restriction enzymes (enzymes which degrade DNA, e.g. 'foreign' DNA lacking the particular pattern of methylation characteristic of the cell's own DNA).

[Use of prokaryotic DNA methyltransferases as analytical and experimental tools in biology: Anal Biochem (2005) 338 (1):1–11.]

Mammals have a range of DNA methyltransferases, and it appears that the activities of these enzymes are essential for normal function or survival. The mammalian DNA methyltransferases are apparently involved in maintaining an overall pattern of methylation that determines the normal functioning of cells. The dysregulation of methylation – either aberrant demethylation or aberrant hyper-methylation – can cause disorders or death; thus, for example, mutation in *DNMT3B*, the

gene encoding DNA methyltransferase 3B (Dnmt3B), results in the disorder ICF SYNDROME.

Methyltransferases Dnmt3A and Dnmt3B appear to be required for *de novo* methylation; Dnmt1 is generally viewed as a 'maintenance' enzyme.

[Methyltransferases of mammals: Hum Mol Genet (2000) 9(16):2395–2402.]

(See also DEMETHYLATION and TAGM.)

DNA nanocircle A small, synthetic circular ssDNA molecule (up to ~120 nt) which can be transcribed *in vitro* or in bacteria (after insertion by heat shock); RNA synthesis occurs by the ROLLING CIRCLE mechanism. RNA polymerase may be able to initiate transcription with GTP at any cytosine residue in the circle, although the conformation of the template can strongly inhibit or promote transcription.

A nanocircle containing an optimized promoter sequence, and encoding a self-cleaving monomeric hammerhead RIBOZYME, was able to express the active ribozyme in cells of *Escherichia coli* [Proc Natl Acad Sci USA (2002) 99(1):54–59].

DNA notation See e.g. DNA SKYLINE.

DNA-only transposon Any TRANSPOSABLE ELEMENT that can transpose without the involvement of an RNA intermediate. (cf. RETROTRANSPOSON.)

DNA photolyase See PHOTOLYASE.

DNA polymerase See DNA-DEPENDENT DNA POLYMERASE for a definition and for some commercial examples.

DNA polymerase I (Kornberg enzyme) In *Escherichia coli*, the DNA-DEPENDENT DNA POLYMERASE which is involved e.g. in EXCISION REPAIR and in the degradation of RNA primers during DNA replication; it has proof-reading (3′-to-5′ exonuclease) and 5′-to-3′ exonuclease activities. It can also act as a reverse transcriptase, but with low efficiency.

Proteolytic cleavage of the polymerase (e.g. with subtilisin) gives rise to the 75-kDa *Klenow fragment*, an enzyme with polymerase and proof-reading activities but lacking the 5′ exonuclease activity. It is used, for example, in the Sanger (chain-termination) method of DNA sequencing and for 3′-end-labeling of dsDNA, second-strand synthesis of cDNA, and filling in 5′ overhangs; its strand-displacement activity can be employed in SDA.

(See also EXO KLENOW FRAGMENT.)

DNA polymerase II In *Escherichia coli*, a DNA-DEPENDENT DNA POLYMERASE that is induced following damage to DNA or inhibition of replication (in the so-called SOS response).

(See also DNA POLYMERASE IV.)

DNA polymerase III In *Escherichia coli*, the major DNA-DEPENDENT DNA POLYMERASE which is used e.g. in chromosomal replication; it has both 3′ and 5′ exonuclease activities.

DNA polymerase IV In *Escherichia coli*, a DNA polymerase (product of the *dinB* gene) involved in mutagenesis when induced in the SOS response.

(See also DNA POLYMERASE II and DNA POLYMERASE V.)

In *recA730* strains of *Escherichia coli*, constitutive expression of the SOS SYSTEM produces a mutator phenotype in which DNA polymerase IV is reported to contribute significantly [J Bacteriol (2006) 188(22):7977–7980].

(See also Y FAMILY.)

DNA polymerase V In *Escherichia coli*, a DNA polymerase consisting of two UmuD' proteins and one UmuC protein (products of the *umuD* and *umuC* genes respectively), which is involved in error-prone repair of DNA (TRANSLESION SYNTHESIS) when induced in the SOS response.

(See also DNA POLYMERASE IV, Y FAMILY, TOL PLASMID.)

DNA Polymorphism Discovery Resource A collection of 450 samples of DNA from US residents, with ancestry from all major regions of the world, intended for studies to facilitate discovery of human genetic variation [Genome Res (1998) 8(12):1229–1231; erratum: Genome Res (1999) 9(2):210].

[Example of use of resource (discovery of rare nucleotide polymorphisms): Nucleic Acids Res (2006) 34(13):e99.]

DNA profile Data specific to the DNA of a given individual. For example, a profile may consist of details of the number of short tandem repeats at given genomic loci (e.g. CODIS).

DNA quadruplex See QUADRUPLEX DNA.

DNA repair Any of various (normal) physiological processes which recognize and repair damaged/abnormal DNA.

Some repair processes remove the damaged (or abnormal) part of a strand and replace it by synthesis (see e.g. EXCISION REPAIR).

By contrast, direct reversal of damage caused by a methylating agent in *Escherichia coli* can be carried out by the Ada protein; this protein is a bifunctional methyltransferase which can transfer a methyl group from e.g. O^6-methylguanine to a cysteine residue on the Ada protein itself. Methylation of a phosphodiester bond can also be reversed by Ada: the methyl group is transferred to a different cysteine residue on the Ada protein.

Some repair systems are constitutive (i.e. usually present in the cell). By contrast, the Ada protein is part of an inducible repair system (the so-called 'adaptive response') produced in *E. coli* in response to the presence of low levels of certain alkylating agents (e.g. *N*-methyl-*N'*-nitro-*N*-nitrosoguanidine (MNNG) and *N*-methyl-*N*-nitrosourea (MNU)). Another enzyme produced in the adaptive response is 3-methyladenine DNA glycosylase II (the AlkA protein) which can cleave the methylated bases from N^3-methyladenine, N^3-methylguanine and N^7-methylguanine as well as from O^2-methylcytosine.

The Tag (TAG) protein (*tag* gene product) is a constitutive glycosylase that specifically cleaves N^3-methyladenine. [Activity of Tag: EMBO J (2007) 26:2411–2420.]

(See also BASE EXCISION REPAIR.)

The DNA repair enzyme O^6-alkylguanine-DNA alkyltransferase (AGT) is used as a partner in certain fusion proteins (see GENE FUSION (uses)).

DNA sampling See, for example, BUCCAL CELL SAMPLING and FORENSIC APPLICATIONS.

DNA sequencing Determining the identity and position of each of the constituent nucleotides in a molecule or fragment of DNA. Sequencing provides definitive information on a given

molecule or fragment; such information is required e.g. for identification, characterization and taxonomic studies.

Once determined, the sequence of nucleotides in a given sample of DNA may or may not give a direct indication of the composition of any protein(s) encoded by the DNA; this is because the actual sequence of amino acid residues in a protein can be influenced by factors such as INTRONS and by events such as FRAMESHIFTING during translation – that is, a given sequence of nucleotides in genomic DNA does not necessarily indicate a series of codons (see CODON).

As the strands in duplex DNA are normally complementary (so that the sequence of one strand can be deduced from the sequence of the other), it might be supposed that sequencing of only one strand would be adequate; however, sequencing of both strands increases the level of accuracy.

Single-stranded templates (of the sample to be sequenced) may be prepared e.g. by asymmetric PCR or by cloning in a filamentous phage (such as phage M13).

Methods used for sequencing DNA

A commonly used procedure is the DIDEOXY METHOD (q.v.) which can be used for sequencing templates of up to ~500 nt in length. Longer templates may be sequenced by using a solid-phase approach (see PRIMER WALKING). The dideoxy method can be automated (see AUTOMATED SEQUENCING).

The MAXAM–GILBERT METHOD (= the chemical cleavage method) is a mechanistically distinct approach involving the base-specific cleavage of end-labeled fragments and analysis of the resulting products.

Visualization of sequencing products in gels (which originally involved the use of radioactive labels) can be achieved with e.g. fluorescent labels; alternatively, use can be made of CHEMILUMINESCENCE systems.

Pyrosequencing™ (see PYROSEQUENCING) can be used for relatively short templates (e.g. ~40 nt).

HYBRIDIZATION-BASED SEQUENCING is a further option.

DNA sequencing has been reported with a MALDI-TOF-based approach [Nucleic Acids Res (2007) 35(8):e62].

An approach to sequencing that may be possible in the future depends on translocation of DNA molecules through nanopores under conditions which allow the identification of individual nucleotides in transit [see e.g. Biophys J (2004) 87 (3):2086–2097].

DNA sex determination assay Any DNA-based assay used to determine the gender of the individual from which a given sample has been obtained.

One widely used assay (e.g. in archeological and forensic work) involves amplification of a specific sequence in each of the two genes encoding AMELOGENIN (q.v.). In each of the genes, a sequence in the region of the first intron is targeted by a pair of PCR primers; the targets are chosen so that easily distinguishable products of different sizes and sequences are obtained from the X and Y chromosomes. With this arrangement, the formation of products of one type only (from the X chromosome) generally indicates a female source – products of two types (from the X and Y chromosomes) indicating a

DNA SEQUENCING (summary of methods)[a]

Method	Features
Dideoxy (chain-termination) method (Sanger's method)	Labeled primers are extended on template strands in a reaction mixture which includes a proportion of dideoxyribonucleoside triphosphates (of one type), resulting in chain-terminated products of various lengths (corresponding to locations of the complementary nucleotide within the template). A similar reaction is carried out for each of the four types of nucleotide. Products from each of the four reactions are examined (in separate lanes) by gel electrophoresis, the location of each band in the gel indicating the identity of the nucleotide at a particular location within the sequence. (See entry DIDEOXY METHOD.)
Hybridization-based sequencing	Sample strands are hybridized to an array of oligonucleotides which, collectively, represent all possible combinations of nucleotides; the particular oligonucleotides to which the sample strands bind are analysed by computer and these data are used to indicate the sequence of the sample DNA. (See entry HYBRIDIZATION-BASED SEQUENCING.)
Maxam–Gilbert (chemical cleavage) method	End-labeled strands of sample DNA are cleaved (ideally at only one location in each strand) by a base-specific chemical agent, resulting in products of various lengths (as different strands are cut at different locations of the given base within the strand). A similar reaction is carried out for each of the four types of nucleotide, using a different base-specific agent in each reaction. Products from each of the four reactions are examined by gel electrophoresis to identify the nucleotides at specific locations. (See entry MAXAM–GILBERT METHOD.)
Nanopore-based sequencing	A possible future method based on translocation of DNA molecules through a nanopore with the identification of each nucleotide in transit
Pyrosequencing™	A primer, bound to the template strand, is extended by the sequential addition of each of the four types of dNTP (dATPαS being used in place of dATP – see entry). The addition of a nucleotide to the primer releases pyrophosphate which is converted, enzymatically, to ATP. The ATP generates a light signal, via the luciferase system, thus indicating the identity of the nucleotide incorporated at a given location. (See entry PYROSEQUENCING.)
Solid-phase sequencing	End-bound sample strands are sequenced by a series of primers, each primer being extended over a different region of the strand. (See entry PRIMER WALKING.)

[a]See separate entries for further details.

male source.

Various commercial assay kits are available, and different sets of primers are used, but the same principle applies in all of the assays.

Failures in accuracy of the amelogenin assay can occur as a result of mutation. For example, mutation in the Y allele, blocking amplification of the specific sequence from the Y chromosome, could cause misinterpretation of the result (i.e. products from only the X chromosome) as an indication of a female source.

Failures in the amelogenin assay may be affected by ethnic group/geographical location. Thus, in one study on an Indian population, relevant deletions were observed in the Y copy of the amelogenin gene in 10 of 4257 males [BMC Med Genet (2006) 7:37].

(See also FORENSIC APPLICATIONS.)

DNA shuffling (gene shuffling; sometimes referred to as 'sexual PCR') A technique in which the properties of a given protein can be modified by extensive *in vitro* recombination between the encoding gene and a number of allelic or related forms of that gene.

The isolated genes are initially cleaved by DNase I to form fragments of ~50 bp. The fragments from all of these genes are then used in a primer-less form of PCR in which *the fragments prime each other*; fragment–fragment binding occurs owing to high-level homology among the genes. During this process there is frequent switching of templates (successive priming of different fragments), giving rise to a wide range of chimeric genes. These chimeric genes are then amplified by conventional PCR, and the resulting library of recombinant genes can be screened for those products with the desired characteristics.

One or more further rounds of shuffling can be carried out if required.

(See also PSEUDORECOMBINATION.)

DNA Skyline A form of notation in which a sequence of

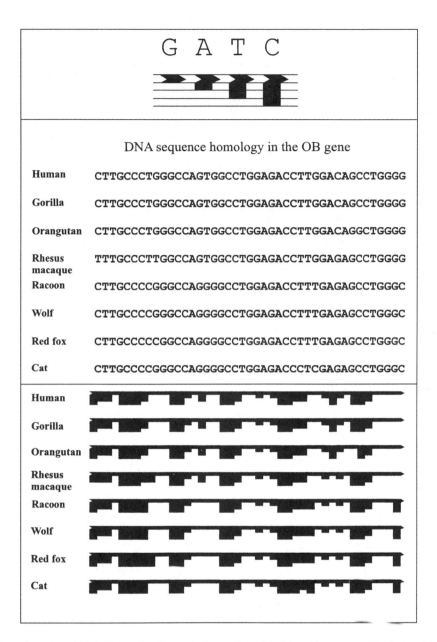

DNA Skyline: a form of notation which facilitates visual inspection/comparison of nucleic acid sequences. The design of the Skyline GATC font is shown in the top panel. The center panel shows a sequence of nucleotides in the obesity (OB) gene from different species of mammal. In the lower panel the nucleotides shown in the center panel are displayed in the GATC version of the Skyline font.

Figure reproduced, with permission, from 'DNA Skyline: fonts to facilitate visual inspection of nucleic acid sequences' by Jonas Jarvius and Ulf Landegren, *BioTechniques* (2006) 40:740.

nucleotides is shown as a series of symbols – rather than by a series of the letters A, C, G and T; in this system, the bases adenine, cytosine, guanine and thymine are represented by four symbols of different height, and these symbols are used instead of the usual letters (see figure). Skyline was designed to facilitate *visual* comparison of strand complementarity and conserved motifs etc. [BioTechniques (2006) 40:740].

DNA staining A procedure in which a dye, often a fluorophore, is bound to DNA. Such binding may be non-covalent – for example, by INTERCALATING AGENTS such as ETHIDIUM BROMIDE, or by minor-groove-binding agents such as DAPI and Hoechst 33342 (see also BOXTO) – or covalent (e.g. following amine modification: see PROBE LABELING).

DNA may be stained e.g. to detect bands of amplification products in gel electrophoresis strips, to study preparations of chromosomes or *in situ* genomes, to demonstrate chromosome banding, to facilitate flow cytometry and to distinguish between living and dead cells; the latter role depends on the ability of some dyes to penetrate the cell membrane in living cells (and of other dyes to be excluded): see e.g. LIVE/DEAD BACLIGHT BACTERIAL VIABILITY KIT.

The (many) DNA-staining dyes include e.g. ACRIDINES, BENA435, BOXTO, DAPI, ETHIDIUM BROMIDE and ETHIDIUM MONOAZIDE, HEXIDIUM IODIDE, PROPIDIUM IODIDE, QUINACRINE, SYBR GREEN I and various SYTO DYES.

ssDNA may be quantitated e.g. with OLIGREEN.

(See also ULTRAVIOLET ABSORBANCE.)

DNA stretching *Syn.* DNA COMBING.

DNA thermal cycler *Syn.* THERMOCYCLER.

DNA toroid A highly compacted form of DNA found e.g. in the nucleoid of the bacterium *Deinococcus radiodurans* and in bacterial endospores. The toroidal structure may contribute to the resistance of *D. radiodurans* (and of endospores) to DNA-damaging agents such as certain types of radiation; it may facilitate the repair of double-stranded breaks in DNA in a template-independent, RecA-independent way [J Bacteriol (2004) 186:5973–5977].

The DNA in human sperm cells occurs in nucleoprotamine toroids [DNA structure in human sperm cells: J Cell Sci (2005) 118(19):4541–4550].

DNA unwinding protein See HELICASE.

DNA uptake site See TRANSFORMATION.

DNA vaccine Any parenterally administered vaccine containing DNA encoding specific antigen(s) that are synthesized in the vaccinated individual; the object of such vaccination is to induce humoral (that is, antibody) and cell-mediated immune responses to given antigen(s). (See also pVAX™200-DEST in the table of destination vectors in GATEWAY SITE-SPECIFIC RECOMBINATION SYSTEM.)

A DNA vaccine may be administered intradermally by a biolistic approach (see also GENE GUN). Administration may also be achieved by intramuscular injection, by aerosol, or by intravenous delivery.

The efficacy/immunogenicity of a vaccine can be improved e.g. by optimization of codon usage [Infect Immun (2005)

73(9):5666–5674] and by the use of a DNA vector encoding certain proteins *in addition to* the target antigen(s) – e.g. CALRETICULIN [J Virol (2004) 78(16):8468–8476] or VP22 protein of bovine herpesvirus 1 [J Virol (2005) 79(3):1948–1953].

The effective induction of specific antibodies in laboratory animals has been achieved by the intravenous delivery of an antibody-specifying plasmid [BioTechniques (2006) 40(2): 199–208]. [See also J Virol (2007) 81(13):6879–6889.]

Bacteriophages have been used as vehicles for the delivery of DNA vaccines in a mammalian setting [e.g. Infect Immun (2006) 74(1):167–174].

(See also GENE THERAPY.)

***dnaA* gene** (*Escherichia coli*) A gene whose product (DnaA) is required for DNA replication. During initiation of replication, copies of DnaA bind to so-called 'DnaA boxes' located in the origin or replication (*oriC*); this is a prelude to strand separation ('melting'), an essential feature of the replication process. The Orc1–6 proteins provide a similar function in eukaryotic cells, while in archaeans the function involves the Orc1 and CdC6 proteins.

Some early reports indicated that DnaA may be needed for the replication of certain plasmids (including pSC101), but it now appears that this is not the case.

***dnaB* gene** (*Escherichia coli*) See HELICASE.

***dnaF* gene** (*Escherichia coli*) *Syn.* NRDA GENE.

***dnaG* gene** (*Escherichia coli*) See RNA POLYMERASE.

DNase (deoxyribonuclease) Any enzyme that cleaves phosphodiester bonds in DNA. An *exo*deoxyribonuclease is a DNase that cleaves terminal bonds, while an *endo*deoxyribonuclease is a DNase that cleaves internal bonds. A few examples of DNases: DNASE I, DNASE II, ENDONUCLEASE S1, EXONUCLEASE III, EXONUCLEASE IV.

DNases are produced by various microorganisms and e.g. by the human pancreas.

Microbial DNases include e.g. the staphylococcal 'thermonuclease' – a Ca^+-dependent thermostable enzyme with both exonuclease and endonuclease activity.

(See also STREPTODORNASE.)

To detect DNase production by bacteria, the test strain is plated on an agar medium that contains DNA and a calcium salt. Following development of colonies, the plate is flooded with hydrochloric acid (1 N HCl) to precipitate non-degraded DNA; any DNase-producing colonies are surrounded by a clear halo in which the DNA has been degraded.

DNase I A DNASE whose products have 5′-phosphate terminal groups (compare DNASE II). This enzyme is EC 3.1.21.1.

(See also STREPTODORNASE.)

DNase II A DNASE whose products have 3′-phosphate terminal groups (compare DNASE I). This enzyme is EC 3.1.22.1.

DNAzyme *Syn.* DEOXYRIBOZYME.

Dnmt1 (DNMT1) DNA METHYLTRANSFERASE 1.

(See also DEMETHYLATION.)

DNMT3B The gene encoding (mammalian) DNA methyltransferase 3B.

dominant templates   Those templates, present in great excess, which may, as a result of their dominance, interfere e.g. with the amplification of rare or low-copy-number templates.

For approaches to dealing with dominant templates see e.g. PCR CLAMPING and SUICIDE POLYMERASE ENDONUCLEASE RESTRICTION for DNA templates and COMPETIMER for RNA templates.

DON (6-diazo-5-oxo-L-norleucine)   A compound which acts as an analog of L-glutamine and interferes with the biosynthesis of purines (and, hence, nucleotides); DON is produced by the Gram-positive bacterium *Streptomyces*.

DON has antimicrobial and antitumor activity.

(cf. AZASERINE; see also HADACIDIN.)

donor (conjugative)   See F PLASMID and CONJUGATION.

donor conjugal DNA synthesis (DCDS)   See CONJUGATION.

donor splice site (donor splice junction)   In pre-mRNA: the splice site (consensus GU) at the 5′ end of an intron.

(cf. ACCEPTOR SPLICE SITE.)

dot blot   A simple PROBE-based method for detecting and/or quantitating a given sequence of nucleotides in a sample. A drop of the sample, on a membrane, is treated so that all the nucleic acid molecules are released and bound to the membrane in single-stranded form. Target-specific probes are then used to detect the given sequence; the probes are usually labeled with e.g. DIGOXIGENIN or BIOTIN. For quantitation of the target, the sample can be diluted serially and each dilution probed in the way described; quantity is estimated by comparing the strength of label from one or more dilutions of the sample with the strength of label from control(s) of known concentration.

Slot blot is a similar method involving elongated (rather than dot-like) inoculations of sample on the membrane.

double helix   See B-DNA.

double inhomogeneous field electrophoresis   See PFGE.

down mutation (down-promoter mutation)   Any mutation in a promoter sequence resulting in decreased transcription from that promoter.

Down's syndrome (detection)   Down's syndrome is commonly associated with trisomy (three copies of chromosome 21). This (and other forms of aneuploidy) can be detected e.g. by methods such as COMPARATIVE GENOMIC HYBRIDIZATION; FISH (hybridization of fluorophore-labeled probes to metaphase chromosome spreads); and also MULTIPLEX LIGATION-DEPENDENT PROBE AMPLIFICATION.

downstream   Refers e.g. to the direction in which a strand of nucleic acid is synthesized. The converse is *upstream*.

downstream box   In some prokaryotic and phage genes: a DNA sequence, downstream of the transcription start site, which is associated with enhancement of translation; it was suggested that this sequence may bind to certain bases in the 30S ribosomal subunit (the *anti-downstream box*) but this notion has been questioned [J Bacteriol (2001) 183(11):3499–3505].

downstream promoter element (DPE)   In certain eukaryotic genes: a region of the CORE PROMOTER located about 30 nt downstream of the start site. It binds an initiation factor and is apparently functionally analogous to the TATA box. The DPE mediates efficient initiation of transcription in at least some TATA-less promoters.

DPE   DOWNSTREAM PROMOTER ELEMENT.

DPN   See NAD.

DR   DIRECT REPEAT.

DR locus   In members of the *Mycobacterium tuberculosis* complex: a distinct genomic region consisting of a number of highly conserved 36-bp direct repeats which are interspersed with spacers of 34–41 bp. The number of direct repeats varies between strains, and the presence/absence/length of spacers also varies; such variation is the basis of SPOLIGOTYPING.

drd **plasmid**   A conjugative plasmid whose transfer operon is permanently DEREPRESSED.

Drosha   See MICRORNAS.

Drosophila **expression system**   See DES.

Drosophila melanogaster   A species of fruitfly much studied in classical genetics and also used e.g. for studying POLYTENE CHROMOSOMES. The P ELEMENT facilitates mutagenesis in *D. melanogaster*.

[Genome sequence of *Drosophila melanogaster*: Science (2000) 287:2185–2195.]

Drosophila Schneider S2 cells are used e.g. in a system for expressing recombinant proteins: see DES.

A useful source of information: www.fruitfly.org

DSB   Double-strand break: referring to cleavage of both strands at a given site in a duplex molecule of nucleic acid.

dsDNA   Double-stranded DNA.

DsRed   A red fluorescent protein from the reef coral *Discosoma* which forms tetramers. (cf. MONOMERIC RED FLUORESCENT PROTEIN; see also entries for GREEN FLUORESCENT PROTEIN and for YELLOW FLUORESCENT PROTEIN.) [Example of use: BioTechniques (2007) 42(3):285–288.]

DTT   DITHIOTHREITOL.

dual-fluorescence reporter/sensor plasmid   DFRS PLASMID.

dual-tropic strains (of HIV-1)   See HIV-1.

Duchenne muscular dystrophy   A genetic disorder characterized by the absence (or abnormality) of *dystrophin*, a protein found in normal muscle. (See also table in the entry GENETIC DISEASE.)

(See also NONSENSE-ASSOCIATED DISEASE.)

dUTP poisoning   In PCR: an inhibitory effect on certain types of DNA polymerase which results from deamination of dCTP to dUTP [Proc Natl Acad Sci USA (2002) 99:596–601]. Some commercial enzymes (for example *PfuUltra*™ DNA polymerase; Stratagene, La Jolla CA) are designed to overcome dUTP poisoning.

(See also ARCHAEMAXX.)

Dyggve–Melchior–Clausen syndrome   A syndrome, involving e.g. skeletal abnormalities, associated with mutation in the *DYM* gene (location 18q12–q21.1).

Dynabeads®   Microscopic spheres of precise size that contain a mixture of iron oxides (δFe_2O_3 and Fe_3O_4) encased within a thin polymer shell, giving the spheres SUPERPARAMAGNETIC properties. Dynabeads of 2.8 μm diameter are referred to as

Dynabeads M-280, those of 4.5 μm diameter are referred to as Dynabeads M-450. The surface of the polymer shell can be modified so as to exhibit any of a wide range of ligands, the choice of ligand being determined by the particular use for which the beads are required.

Dynabeads® (Dynal) have at least three main types of use:
• separation of a specific component from a mixture of similar components;
• isolation of a given component from a crude preparation;
• provision of a solid-phase support.

Separation (*biomagnetic separation*) may involve various types of target, including macromolecules (e.g. nucleic acid species and fragments), viruses and specific types or subtypes of cell. For example, mRNA spccies can be separated (and isolated) from a sample of total RNA by using Dynabeads Oligo (dT)$_{25}$ – Dynabeads coated with (covalently attached) 25-nucleotide-long chains of deoxythymidines. These ligands bind the oligo (dA) tails of mRNA molecules; retention of the bead–mRNA complexes, by means of a magnetic field, permits washing etc. and removal of unwanted components. If required, subsequently, the mRNA molecules can be eluted from the beads by incubation in a suitable buffer solution.

Separation of a particular type of blood cell from other cells in e.g. whole blood can be achieved by means of a BIOTIN-linked antibody (specific to the target cell) bound to streptavidin-coated Dynabeads. (This procedure is called *immuno-magnetic separation*.) After washing, the bound, magnetically retained cells can be lysed (while still attached to the Dynabeads), and mRNA can be recovered from the supernatant with Dynabeads Oligo d(T)$_{25}$.

The isolation of PCR-ready high-molecular-weight genomic DNA from a crude preparation, or e.g. whole blood, can be achieved e.g. by Dynabeads DNA DIRECT™. The DNA, released by cell lysis, is adsorbed to Dynabeads coated with an appropriate ligand; magnetic separation of the beads is followed by a series of washings. One advantage of this procedure is that the washing stages may assist in eliminating inhibitors of PCR.

The solid-phase characteristics of Dynabeads have been exploited e.g. for DNA sequencing by primer walking; for gene assembly; and for hybridization reactions.

The advantages of a solid-phase support include the ability to re-use a DNA template (e.g. for sequencing) several times.

Dynabeads: examples of use
Uses include e.g. purification of mRNA from total RNA with Dynabeads Oligo d(T)$_{25}$ [Plant Cell (2006) 18:1750–1765]; separation of T lymphocytes (T cells) from peripheral blood mononuclear cells of cancer patients [J Clin Invest (2006) 116(7):1946–1954]; selection of specific immunoglobulins from sera by Dynabeads coated with PROTEIN A and Dynabeads coated with PROTEIN G [Infect Immun (2005) 73(9): 5685–5696]; mRNA isolation from bovine peripheral blood mononuclear cells [BMC Immunol (2006) 7:10]; isolation of a streptavidin–tRNA fusion with BIOTIN-coated Dynabeads [Nucleic Acids Res (2006) 34(5):e44]; separation of B cells and T cells by using Pan B Dynabeads and Pan T Dynabeads, respectively [Proc Natl Acad Sci USA (2006) 103(13):4819–4824].

dynamic allele-specific hybridization (DASH) A method used for scoring SNPs and other short polymorphisms in single-stranded samples of the DNA under test. The single-stranded samples are commonly created by PCR amplification using one BIOTINylated primer; the strand formed by extension of this primer is immobilized on a streptavidin-coated surface to form the target sequence.

Essentially, a probe – with known complementarity to one possible version of the target sequence – is hybridized to the target sequence, and the probe–target duplex is monitored for denaturation (with increasing temperature) to determine the temperature at which denaturation occurs at a maximum rate; the different temperature maxima obtained in this approach indicate differences in relative stability, and the data are used to reveal the nature of the target sequences being examined.

DASH has been used e.g. in the analysis of polymorphisms in the paraoxonase gene [BMC Med Genet (2006) 7:28].

E

E L-Glutamic acid (alternative to Glu).

E. coli See ESCHERICHIA COLI.

EAF plasmid See PATHOGENICITY ISLAND.

EBER Epstein–Barr virus (EBV)-associated RNA: either of the two small (~170-nucleotide) RNA molecules (EBER-1 and EBER-2) expressed at high levels in cells latently infected with EBV; these molecules provide target sequences for the detection of EBV infection.

In latently infected B lymphocytes (B cells), EBERs inhibit α-interferon-induced apoptosis – and thus appear to promote viral persistence in these cells. It has been thought that such inhibition of apoptosis is due to the influence of EBERs on the role of dsRNA-dependent protein kinase PKR; however, the direct inhibition of PKR by EBERs now appears to be unlikely [J Virol (2005) 79(23):14562–14569].

(See also EPSTEIN–BARR VIRUS.)

Eberwine technique A technique used for amplifying RNA from a mixed population of mRNA molecules. Essentially, all the mRNAs are reverse transcribed with a poly(T) primer whose 5′ end includes a promoter sequence for the phage T7 RNA polymerase; following synthesis of the second strand, the now-functional T7 promoter is used for transcribing anti-sense copies of the mRNA.

EBNA-1 See EPSTEIN–BARR VIRUS.

EBV EPSTEIN–BARR VIRUS.

EBV-associated RNA See EBER.

Ecl18kI A type IIP RESTRICTION ENDONUCLEASE (recognition sequence: ↓CCNGG). [Mechanism of specificity: EMBO J (2006) 25:2219–2229.]

EcoKI A type I RESTRICTION ENDONUCLEASE which cleaves at random sites. The recognition sequence AA^{m}C(6N)GTGC (in which adenine is methylated at N-6) is not cleaved by EcoKI.

(See also HSD GENES.)

EcoKMcrA *Syn.* McrA (see entry MCRA GENE).

EcoKMcrBC *Syn.* McrBC (see entry MCRBC).

EcoRII-C See CPNPG SITES.

EcoR124I A type IC RESTRICTION ENDONUCLEASE which has random cleavage sites. [Mechanism of translocation: EMBO J (2006) 25:2230–2239.]

Ecotilling A method used for detecting SNPs (and other polymorphisms) (cf. TILLING). The principle of the method is outlined below.

Genomic DNA under test is initially mixed with a sample of the corresponding wild-type/reference DNA. With labeled gene-specific PCR primers, a target sequence of 1–1.5 kb is then amplified from the mixture of DNA. Denaturation of the products by heat is followed by cooling and then annealing of single-stranded products.

If the target sequence in *genomic* DNA contains an SNP, or a point mutation, then – during the annealing stage – some single-stranded amplicons copied from genomic DNA will hybridize with single-stranded wild-type amplicons (copied from the wild-type/reference DNA). The resulting (hetero-duplex) DNA amplicons (each containing a single-base-pair mismatch) are then exposed to a SINGLE-STRAND-SPECIFIC NUCLEASE which nicks at the site of the mismatch. The two parts of the nicked strand (on either side of the nick) can then be examined e.g. by gel electrophoresis to determine the site of the nick and, hence, the location of the SNP or point mutation.

[Example of use (discovery of rare human nucleotide polymorphisms): Nucleic Acids Res (2006) 34(13):e99.]

editing (1) See PROOF READING.

(2) See RNA EDITING.

editosome A complex involved in RNA EDITING. For example, in trypanosomatids the editosome may include proteins with functions such as: endonuclease, helicase, terminal uridylyl transferase, exouridylylase and ligase.

efavirenz A NON-NUCLEOSIDE REVERSE TRANSCRIPTASE INHIBITOR.

EFC ENZYME FRAGMENT COMPLEMENTATION.

eGFP *Syn.* EGFP.

EGFP (or eGFP) Enhanced GREEN FLUORESCENT PROTEIN: a mutant form of GFP which produces a higher level of fluorescence compared to the wild-type GFP. [Examples of use: J Virol (2004) 78(22):12333–12343; Appl Environ Microbiol (2005) 71(8):4856–4861; BioTechniques (2006) 40(1):91–100.]

EGFR family See EPIDERMAL GROWTH FACTOR RECEPTOR FAMILY.

EGS (1) External guide sequence: see SNRNAS.

(2) Ethyleneglycol-bis(succinimidyl succinate): see the entry CHROMATIN IMMUNOPRECIPITATION.

EGTA The chelating agent ethyleneglycol-bis(β-aminoethyl-ether)-*N,N,N′,N′*-tetra-acetic acid.

EGTA complexes various types of cation – including Ca^{2+}, Mg^{2+} and Zn^{2+}. Ca^{2+} is complexed much more strongly than Mg^{2+}.

eIF4E Part of the eukaryotic translation initiation complex that recognizes the CAP region of mRNA.

EK-Away™ resin An agarose-based product from Invitrogen (Carlsbad CA) which is designed for removing enterokinase (such as EKMax™) from reactions involving the cleavage of fusion proteins by this enzyme; the product contains soybean trypsin inhibitor, which has a high affinity for enterokinase.

EKMax™ An ENTEROKINASE (from Invitrogen, Carlsbad CA) which is reported to cleave proteins after the lysine residue in the sequence Asp-Asp-Asp-Asp-Lys.

(See also EK-AWAY RESIN.)

electroblotting A form of BLOTTING, faster than the method based on capillary action (i.e. SOUTHERN BLOTTING), in which nucleic acid fragments or proteins are transferred from gel to matrix by means of an electrical potential difference ('electric field') between gel and matrix.

electrocompetent cells See ELECTROPORATION.

electrophoresis Any method which is used e.g. for separating charged fragments, particles or molecules, in a heterogeneous population, by exploiting their different rates of movement produced by an electrical potential gradient in a liquid-based medium.

(cf. ISOTACHOPHORESIS.)

Electrophoresis is used e.g. for identification/quantitation of nucleic acid fragments, proteins etc., determination of the molecular weight of proteins, preparation of fingerprints (e.g. in typing procedures), and confirmation of specific amplicons in nucleic-acid-amplification techniques such as NASBA and PCR.

GEL ELECTROPHORESIS is widely used in nucleic acid technology.

electrophoretic mobility-shift assay See EMSA.

electroporation A method for inserting nucleic acid into cells by exposing a mixture of cells and nucleic acid to an electric field for a fraction of a second (or for several seconds); field strengths of up to ~16 kV/cm have been used (although field strengths are often lower than this). Electroporation has been used e.g. in bacterial, yeast, plant and mammalian cells.

[Example of protocol: PLoS Biology (2006) 4(10):e309.]

Specialized 'electrocompetent' cells, i.e. cells selected to be particularly suitable for electroporation, as indicated by their successful uptake and expression of DNA, are available from various commercial sources, for example, ElectroTen-Blue™ from Stratagene (La Jolla CA).

An electroporation protocol was reported to improve the expression of transgenes *after* microinjection of DNA into zebrafish muscle [BMC Biotechnol (2005) 5:29].

A procedure with >20% transfection efficiency in mammalian neurons has been reported in a 96-well electroporation format [BioTechniques (2006) 41(5):619–624].

Electroporation of *single* cells can be achieved with the use of a micromanipulator, a microscope and microelectrodes. One advantage, when dealing with adherent cells, is that contact with the electrode can create increased tension in the cell membrane – an effect that decreases the level of voltage required for electroporation. Difficulties associated with e.g. manual control of electrodes are addressed in an automated form of single-cell electroporation [BioTechniques (2006) 41 (4):399–402].

electrospray ionization See ESI.

ElectroTenBlue® See COMPETENT CELLS.

elementary body (EB) The infectious form of the organism in the development cycle of CHLAMYDIA (q.v.).

ELISA Enzyme-linked immunosorbent assay: a highly sensitive method for detecting specific antigens or antibodies. For example, to detect a given immobilized antigen, one can use antibodies (specific to the antigen) which are conjugated to a reporter system (e.g. the enzyme ALKALINE PHOSPHATASE). If the given antigen is present in the test sample it should bind antibodies and, hence, become labeled with the reporter system. With an alkaline phosphatase reporter, addition of a colorigenic (color-generating) substrate yields an amplified signal which can be used for assaying the antigen.

(See also ELISPOT and EMEA.)

ELISPOT Enzyme-linked immunospot: an assay, based on the ELISA principle, that is used e.g. for the detection of specific molecules or cells.

In one example, a sample of blood is assayed specifically to quantitate those T lymphocytes (T cells) which respond to the tuberculosis-associated antigen ESAT-6 by secreting the cytokine γ-interferon (gamma interferon). In the assay, cells in a given sample are first allowed to settle on the floor of the well. Then, on addition of ESAT-6, ESAT-6-specific cells in the sample react by secreting the cytokine – which is in high concentration in the immediate vicinity of each secreting cell. The cytokine is detected by adding a conjugate that consists of: (i) a molecule that binds to γ-interferon, linked to (ii) an exzyme capable of a colorigenic reaction with an appropriate (added) substrate. After adding the substrate, and incubating, the presence of ESAT-6-specific T cells is indicated by a visible spot of color at the location of each secreting T cell.

The principle of the ELISPOT assay has been used in a variety of contexts, for example: to screen dominant peptides recognized by CD8+ T cells in mice and in humans infected with *Trypanosoma cruzi* [PLoS Pathogens (2006) 2(8):e77], and for the characterization of T cell responses to immediate early antigens in humans with genital herpes [Virol J (2006) 3:54].

Elk-1 A protein which behaves as a transcription factor when activated appropriately (see also PATHDETECT SYSTEMS).

This protein also occurs in extranuclear locations and was reported to be associated with the mitochondrial permeability transition pore complex [Proc Natl Acad Sci USA (2006) 103 (13):5155–5160].

elongation arrest See PCR CLAMPING.

Elongator complex A complex of proteins, including histone acetyltransferases (HATs), associated with elongation during transcription mediated by RNA polymerase II.

(See also WOBBLE HYPOTHESIS.)

EMBL European Molecular Biology Laboratory. A source of nucleotide sequence data (EMBL-Bank) is available at: www.ebi.ac.uk/embl.html

EMBL-Bank See EMBL.

embryonic stem cells (ES cells) See STEM CELL.

EMCV Encephalomyocarditis virus.

(See also IRES.)

EMEA Exonuclease-mediated ELISA-like assay: a probe-based method used for detecting the binding of transcription factors to DNA.

The method involves dsDNA probes, immobilized at one end, which include a distal binding site for a given transcription factor and a proximal (internal) site labeled (in one strand) with DIGOXIGENIN. The plate with the immobilized probes is incubated with a sample of nuclear extract in order to permit the binding of the given transcription factor, if it is present. The whole is then exposed to the exonucleolytic activity of EXONUCLEASE III.

If the given transcription factor is present, and has bound to a probe, then exonuclease III will not be able to degrade that strand of the (dsDNA) probe which contains the digoxigenin label – because its activity will be blocked at the site of the bound transcription factor. As a consequence, the (internal) digoxigenin label will remain intact, and this label can be detected (as in the basic ELISA approach) by using an anti-digoxigenin antibody that is conjugated to an enzyme such as ALKALINE PHOSPHATASE; adding the enzyme's (colorigenic) substrate then permits *quantitative* estimation of the given transcription factor in the sample – as the signal's intensity is proportional to the quantity of transcription factor present.

If there are no copies of the given transcription factor in the sample then the dsDNA probes will not be protected from the activity of exonuclease III; in this case the digoxigenin label will be lost during strand degradation – leading to an absence of signal in the ELISA phase.

This method was used to assay the nuclear factor NF-κB [BioTechniques (2006) 41(1):79–90].

emission filter In fluorescence microscopy: a *bandpass* filter (see EXCITATION FILTER) with two primary functions: (i) to transmit radiation corresponding to the emission spectra of the fluorophore(s) in the sample, and (ii) to block radiation of other wavelengths.

EMRSA Epidemic MRSA.

EMSA Electrophoretic mobility-shift assay: a technique which has been used to investigate interactions between proteins (e.g. those found in cell lysates) and particular sequences of nucleotides in dsDNA. In one basic approach, differentially labeled fragments of DNA (containing different target sequences) are incubated with a lysate in order to permit DNA–protein binding. On subsequent electrophoresis, any protein-bound fragment of DNA will exhibit a lower electrophoretic mobility (i.e. it will move more slowly through the gel than unbound fragments) and can be identified, isolated and then examined.

[Use of EMSA in studies on the regulation of expression of histone deacetylase 4: Mol Biol Cell (2006) 17(2):585–597.]

A two-dimensional EMSA procedure has been used for mapping target sites of DNA-binding proteins along a 563-kb region of the human genome [BioTechniques (2006) 41(1): 91–96].

Enbrel® See BIOPHARMACEUTICAL (table).

End-It™ DNA end-repair kit A product (Epicentre) that includes enzymes T4 DNA polymerase and T4 polynucleotide kinase which convert PCR-derived amplicons with 3′ adenosine overhangs (see EXTENDASE ACTIVITY) to blunt-ended fragments; in this reaction, the 3′ adenosine overhangs are cleaved and the 5′ termini are phosphorylated, leaving the amplicons ready for blunt-ended ligation to a suitable type of vector.

[Uses (e.g.): Genetics (2006) 173(2):1007–1021; Nucleic Acids Res (2006) 34(12):e84; Infect Immun (2006) 74(1): 449–460.]

(See also POLISHING.)

end labeling Addition of a label to the 3′ or 5′ end of a strand of nucleic acid.

3′ labeling may be achieved e.g. by adding labeled nucleotide(s) to the 3′-OH group with the enzyme terminal deoxynucleotidyl transferase.

5′ labeling may be achieved e.g. by cleaving 5′-phosphate (with alkaline phosphatase) and replacing it with a labeled phosphate using (ATP-dependent) polynucleotide kinase.

end probe See CHROMOSOME WALKING.

endA **gene** See ESCHERICHIA COLI (table).

endogenote See MEROZYGOTE.

endogenous retroviral sequence The genome of a retrovirus (a DNA copy) integrated in a (eukaryotic) genome; retroviral genomes are common in eukaryotic genomes.

endogenous retrovirus Any complete or defective retroviral *provirus*, i.e. retroviral sequence, integrated in the host cell's genome. Endogenous retroviruses are widely distributed in the genomes of vertebrates, including humans. Some can be activated (e.g. by exposure to radiation or to chemicals such as 5-bromo-2-deoxyuridine) and may then form infectious or non-infectious virions.

endonuclease Any enzyme which can cleave internal phosphodiester bonds in a molecule of nucleic acid.

(See also SINGLE-STRAND-SPECIFIC NUCLEASE.)

endonuclease CEL I A SINGLE-STRAND-SPECIFIC NUCLEASE.

endonuclease P_1 A SINGLE-STRAND-SPECIFIC NUCLEASE.

endonuclease S_1 (endonuclease S1, nuclease S1, S1 nuclease) An endonuclease, first obtained from the fungus *Aspergillus oryzae*, which specifically degrades ssDNA and ssRNA. The enzyme is one of a range of nucleases in the SINGLE-STRAND-SPECIFIC NUCLEASE group. Endonuclease S_1 is used e.g. to remove 5′ single-stranded DNA in the preparation of NESTED DELETIONS.

Endonuclease S_1 differs from e.g. the mung bean nuclease in having the ability to cleave the DNA strand opposite a nick in a DNA duplex.

(See also RIBONUCLEASE PROTECTION ASSAY.)

endoribonuclease See RIBONUCLEASE.

endotoxin The term commonly used specifically to refer to a macromolecular complex (a PYROGEN) present in the normal cell envelope of Gram-negative bacteria (such as *Escherichia coli*): see LIPOPOLYSACCHARIDE.

enhancer (in chemiluminescence systems) See CHEMILUMINESCENCE ENHANCER.

enhancer (transcriptional) A *cis*-acting element that promotes transcription of certain genes; enhancers occur upstream or downstream of their promoters, within and outside genes, and may function independently of their orientation or distance from the promoter (cf. UAS). Some enhancers can function in a range of different cells; some are cell-specific. enhancer activity apparently depends on *trans*-acting proteins.

In yeast, DNA LOOPING was reported between an enhancer and a promoter – suggesting that apposition of these two elements is involved in transcriptional enhancement, at least in this case [Nucleic Acids Res (2005) 33(12):3743–3750].

enhancer (translational) Any sequence which is associated with the enhancement of translation (see e.g. DOWNSTREAM BOX).

The adenine-rich sequences that are found downstream of the start codon in many *Escherichia coli* mRNAs appear to influence the level of gene expression. One study, using site-directed mutagenesis, assessed the contribution made by the adenine-rich motifs to *in vivo* gene expression and to *in vitro* binding of mRNAs to ribosomes; the results suggested that these adenine-rich motifs may assist gene expression e.g. by facilitating mRNA–ribosome binding [J Bacteriol (2007) 189 (2):501–510].

(See also IRES.)

enoxacin See QUINOLONE ANTIBIOTICS.

enterobacteria A general (non-taxonomic) term that may refer to bacteria associated with the gut (i.e. intestine) but which often refers specifically to bacteria belonging to the family Enterobacteriaceae. All the bacteria in this family are Gram-negative, rod-shaped, non-spore-forming organisms that are facultatively anaerobic; they may adopt a fermentative or an oxidative metabolism according to conditions. The organisms usually grow well on simple (basal) media such as NUTRIENT AGAR. The family Enterobacteriaceae includes the following genera: *Erwinia*, *Escherichia*, *Klebsiella*, *Proteus*, *Salmonella*, *Serratia*, *Shigella* and *Yersinia*.

(See also ESCHERICHIA COLI and SALMONELLA.)

enterokinase (*syn.* enteropeptidase) A serine proteinase which is used e.g. for cleaving the components of fusion proteins; in at least some cases is reported to cleave proteins/peptides between the residues of lysine and isoleucine. EKMax™ (an enzyme from Invitrogen (Carlsbad, CA) is reported to cleave after the lysine residue in the sequence Asp-Asp-Asp-Asp-Lys.

(cf. THROMBIN; see also AFFINITY PROTEIN EXPRESSION AND PURIFICATION.)

enteropathogenic *Escherichia coli* See EPEC.

enteropeptidase *Syn.* ENTEROKINASE.

entry clone See e.g. GATEWAY SITE-SPECIFIC RECOMBINATION SYSTEM.

entry vector In the GATEWAY SITE-SPECIFIC RECOMBINATION SYSTEM: an initial vector (containing *att* sites) into which the gene, or sequence of interest, can be inserted e.g. by the use of restriction enzymes and ligase. After cloning in the entry vector, the gene/sequence can be transferred to a *destination vector* (see entry GATEWAY SITE-SPECIFIC RECOMBINATION SYSTEM (table) for examples of destination vectors) by site-specific recombination.

enucleation (in animal cloning) See SCNT.

env See RETROVIRUSES.

enzyme I (PTS) See PTS.

enzyme II (PTS) See PTS.

enzyme fragment complementation (EFC) A rapid technique for detecting specific recombinant proteins, either in purified form or from whole-cell lysates; unlike immunoblotting (a Western blot probed with labeled antibodies), this procedure does not require the use of antibodies.

The principle of EFC is related to α-complementation (see α-PEPTIDE). Essentially, a protein of interest is expressed as a fusion protein which includes the α-peptide as fusion partner. Such a fusion protein (present e.g. on a nitrocellulose filter) can complement the defective form of β-galactosidase, yielding a positive signal with e.g. a chemiluminescent substrate that is activated by the enzyme [BioTechniques (2006) 40(3): 381–383].

enzyme-linked immunosorbent assay See ELISA.

enzyme-linked immunospot See ELISPOT.

EPEC Enteropathogenic *Escherichia coli*: strains of food- and/ or water-borne pathogenic *E. coli* that are responsible e.g. for diarrhea-related infant mortality in developing countries. The characteristic lesions on the intestinal epithelium result from products encoded by the LEE PATHOGENICITY ISLAND.

[Molecular evolution of EPEC (an analysis by multilocus sequence typing): J Bacteriol (2007) 189(2):342–350.]

epidermal growth factor receptor family (the EGFR family; ERBB receptors) A family of membrane-spanning proteins characterized by (i) an extracellular ligand-binding domain, (ii) a transmembrane region, and (iii) a cytoplasmic (intracellular) domain associated with TYROSINE KINASE activity.

The family includes:

EGFR (HER1) (gene: c-*erbB1*, also called *ERBB1*)

HER2 (gene: c-*erbB2*, also called *ERBB2*)

HER3 (gene: c-*erbB3*, also called *ERBB3*)

HER4 (gene: c-*erbB4*, also called *ERBB4*)

Of these receptors, EGFR (170 kDa) and HER2 (185 kDa) have known roles in certain cancers. The ligand (activator) of EGFR is the epidermal growth factor (EGF); HER2 appears to have no known natural ligand. In cancer cells, these receptors may show gene amplification and/or overexpression. For example, overexpression of HER2 occurs in various tumors, including ~30% of breast carcinomas; overexpression is generally associated with apoor prognosis. Gene amplification and overexpression of EGFR (but not of HER2) have been reported in metaplastic breast carcinomas [Breast Cancer Res (2005) 7(6):R1028–R1035].

Types of anticancer therapy include e.g. agents that inhibit the ligand-binding domain or the tyrosine kinase activity of EGFR, and monoclonal antibodies (mAbs) against HER2. Herceptin® (= trastuzumab) is a humanized mAb that binds to HER2; it has been used therapeutically e.g. for those breast cancers in which this receptor is overexpressed or in which gene amplification has occurred.

epigenetics The study of certain (heritable) factors – other than nucleotide sequence – which influence gene expression. One factor is the pattern of methylation of bases in DNA. Methylation can influence gene expression e.g. by affecting transcription; for example, the methylation of specific bases may block access by transcription initiation factors (in a simple, mechanical way) and/or may promote recruitment of specific repressor protein(s). The inappropriate methylation of certain genes can give rise to specific diseases, such as cancer.

(See also GENETIC IMPRINTING.)

[DNA methylation patterns and epigenetic memory: Genes Dev (2002) 16(1):6–21.]

The Human Epigenome Project is looking at methylation over the entire human genome.

Methylation is an epigenetic factor in both eukaryotic and prokaryotic organisms.

(See also POLYCOMB-GROUP GENES.)

epigenotyping A term that has been used to refer, generally, to any method for assaying the methylation status of DNA – in particular the methylation of specific CPG ISLANDS in a given genome.

episome (1) Any PLASMID which is able to exist autonomously (extrachromosomally) in a cell – but which can also integrate into the cell's chromosome.

(2) *Syn.* PLASMID.

epitope tagging Addition of a specific peptide tag to a protein – e.g. by fusing the gene encoding the protein to a sequence encoding the peptide; the tag may be added to the C-terminal or the N-terminal of the protein. (See e.g. PESC VECTORS.)

Tagging may be carried out e.g. to facilitate the detection or recovery of the expressed protein. Detection or recovery of the given protein may be achieved e.g. by using monoclonal antibodies specific for the tagged region. One advantage of this approach is that the same tag can be used in different experiments with different proteins – thereby avoiding the need to generate a specific antibody for each of the proteins.

Various tags (both *ad hoc* and commercial) are used. One example is the FLAG® sequence (DYKDDDDK). This tag has been used e.g. in various studies on prion proteins [Mol Cell Biol (2006) 26(7):2697–2715; Mol Biol Cell (2006) 17 (8):3356–3368].

Detection of certain tagged proteins from an *in vivo* source may be problematic owing to low-level expression of such proteins. One approach to improving the signal-to-noise ratio has been to insert a sequence encoding *tandem* copies of the epitope into the genome to form a fusion that specifies both the target protein and the tandem epitope; this was carried out by using LAMBDA (λ) RED RECOMBINATION (for insertion of the sequence), and the resulting tagged proteins (transcription factors of *Escherichia coli*) were detected by Western blot analysis and CHROMATIN IMMUNOPRECIPITATION (the latter method to check that tagging had not negated the proteins' (DNA-binding) function) [BioTechniques (2006) 40(1):67–72].

Epstein–Barr virus (EBV) A ubiquitous human herpesvirus associated e.g. with various types of malignancy (including nasopharyngeal carcinoma); it is also found in some breast cancers in which it is reported to confer resistance to the drug paclitaxel and to promote overexpression of a gene encoding multidrug resistance [J Virol (2006) 80(2):845–853].

The EBV genome is linear dsDNA. Structurally, the virion resembles other herpesviruses. EBV infects various types of human cell, including B lymphocytes (B cells) and epithelial cells; the B cell membrane molecule CD21 is the receptor for EBV. In proliferating B cells the EBV genome occurs intranuclearly as a circular extrachromosomal molecule with an origin of replication, *oriP*. A virus-encoded protein, EBNA-1, binds to *oriP* and may be necessary for persistence of the viral genome within the cell's nucleus; EBNA-1 is detectable within several hours of infection by EBV.

(See also MINICHROMOSOME (sense 1).)

EBV infection is commonly latent, with a life-long carrier state. In latently infected cells, EBV expresses a range of microRNAs (miRNAs); the level of expression of a given miRNA depends e.g. on the particular stage of latency [PLoS Pathogens (2006) 2(3):e23]. (See also EBER.) [Control of latency: J Virol (2007) 81(12):6389–6401.]

Activation of viral replication in latently infected B cells can be induced by certain types of chemical (see ZEBRA).

erb (*ERB*) An ONCOGENE first detected in the avian erythroblastosis virus. v-*erb* comprises two contiguous genes: v-*erb*-A and v-*erb*-B; the cellular homologs (c-*erbA*, c-*erbB*) are not contiguous e.g. in the chicken genome.

The c-*erbA* protein lacks tyrosine kinase activity.

The c-*erbB* protein has TYROSINE KINASE activity.

The cell-transforming (i.e. oncogenic) agent of the virus is apparently a fusion protein containing the v-*erb*-B product.

ERBB receptors See EPIDERMAL GROWTH FACTOR RECEPTOR FAMILY.

ERIC sequence (enterobacterial repetitive intergenic consensus sequence) A highly conserved, repetitive element found in the genomes of e.g. enteric bacteria such as *Escherichia coli*; each contains a PALINDROMIC SEQUENCE. ERIC sequences have been exploited in TYPING (see REP-PCR).

erlotinib An anticancer agent which inhibits oncogenic (EGF receptor) tyrosine kinase activity.

(cf. IMATINIB.)

error-prone DNA polymerases See Y FAMILY.

ERV sequence ENDOGENOUS RETROVIRAL SEQUENCE.

ES cells Embryonic stem cells: see STEM CELL.

ESAT-6 A 6-kDa protein secreted by the bacterial pathogen *Mycobacterium tuberculosis* and by the species *M. bovis* and *M. africanum*; ESAT is an acronym for: *e*arly *s*ecreted *a*ntigenic *t*arget. Earlier it was reported that the operon encoding ESAT-6 also encodes a low-molecular-weight protein which was designated CFP-10.

The specificity of ESAT-6 for members of the so-called *M. tuberculosis* complex has been used for tracing contacts in epidemiological studies of human tuberculosis. When used in a skin test for tuberculosis in bovines, ESAT-6 was found to be more specific than PPD (purified protein derivative) [Vet Rec (2000) 146:659–665].

[Use of ESAT-6 in studies on latent tuberculosis in healthcare workers: PLoS Med (2007) 4(2):e55.]

(See also ELISPOT.)

Escherichia coli A much-studied, well-characterized species of Gram-negative, rod-shaped bacteria (of the family Enterobacteriaceae) that is found e.g. in the mammalian gut. *E. coli*

ESCHERICHIA COLI: genetic markers associated with some of the frequently used and commercial strains of *Escherichia coli*[a]

Genetic marker	Notes
Amp[r]	Resistant to the antibiotic ampicillin
Cam[r]	Resistant to the antibiotic chloramphenicol
dcm	See entry DCM GENE
endA	*endA* strains (inactivated endonuclease I) have been used e.g. to improve the quality/yield of cloned plasmid DNA
endA[+]	*endA*[+] strains have been used e.g. to reduce the level of contamination by double-stranded DNA when producing ssDNA
F′	Indicates the presence of an F PLASMID – which permits infection of an *Escherichia coli* host cell by phage M13 and related phages; these phages adsorb to specific plasmid-encoded pili (see PILUS) and do not infect cells which lack such pili. Infection by M13 and related phages is used e.g. for the production of ssDNA copies of a given sequence
galK	Inability to use galactose
gyrA	*gyrA* encodes a subunit of gyrase (a type II topoisomerase); mutation in *gyrA* can result in resistance to the antibiotic nalidixic acid
hsd	See entry HSD GENES
hsdR17(r_K^-, m_K^+)	Restriction-negative and modification-positive for this specific restriction–modification system
lacI[q]	High-level production of the *lac* operon repressor protein (LacI) which regulates activity of the *lac* promoter. This permits tight control of expression of proteins when transcription is regulated via the *lac* operator system
*lacZ*ΔM15	Deletion of part of the *lacZ* gene (encoding the enzyme β-galactosidase); this deletion is requird e.g. in strains used for 'blue–white screening' (see entry PBLUESCRIPT)
leuB	Requires leucine for growth in minimal media
Δ*lon*	The Lon protease degrades abnormal proteins in the heat-shock response (and is also functional in the SOS system in *E. coli*). Engineered (i.e. 'abnormal') fusion proteins and heterologous proteins are less susceptible to degradation in Δ*lon* host cells, and Δ*lon* strains are used e.g. in studies on fusion products and the overproduction of heterologous proteins (see also *rpoH*, below)
mcrA	See entry MCRA GENE. Some commercially available strains contain an inactivated *mrcA* gene. Such strains are used e.g. when cloning methylated DNA from eukaryotic sources
mcrBC	See entry MCRBC. Comments are similar to those for *mcrA* (above)
metB	Requires methionine for growth in minimal media
mrr	See entry MRR GENE. Strains with an inactivated *mrr* gene are used e.g. when cloning DNA containing methyladenine residues
ompT	See entry OMPT GENE. Cells lacking a functional OmpT protease are used e.g. for the display of heterologous (i.e. 'foreign') proteins at the cell surface; the heterologous gene, fused to one part of an autotransporter, is expressed as a cell-surface fusion protein in an *ompT*[−] strain
proAB	Requires proline for growth in minimal media
recA	*recA* mutants are used to inhibit homologous recombination (e.g. to prevent recombination between copies of a given plasmid present in the same cell). If required, a temporary *recA* facility can be provided on a SUICIDE VECTOR (q.v.) *(continued)*

Genetic marker	Notes
relA	The *relA* gene encodes the ribosome-associated enzyme pyrophosphotransferase (*stringent factor*). When activated by an uncharged tRNA at the A site, this enzyme catalyzes the synthesis of ppGpp; this results in inhibition of protein and RNA synthesis (*stringent response*). A null mutation in *relA* produces a so-called *relaxed* phenotype in which e.g. RNA synthesis can continue under conditions that would otherwise trigger the stringent response
rne131	See entry BL21 STAR.
rpoH	The *rpoH* gene encodes a sigma factor (σ^{32}) involved in activation of the heat-shock regulon – which includes the synthesis of Lon protease (see Δ*lon*, above). Intracellular accumulation of abnormal/heterologous proteins triggers the heat-shock response; *rpoH* mutants, deficient in the Lon protease, have been found to give increased yields during overproduction studies
rpsL	*rpsL* mutants used in recombinant studies are resistant to the antibiotic streptomycin (see RPSL GENE)
slyD	A *slyD* mutant is used to prepare a lysate for use in a commercial CELL-FREE PROTEIN SYNTHESIS system that employs a LUMIO tag in the fusion product; the *absence* of the SlyD protein in the lysate improves the signal-to-background ratio
supE/supF	Genes involved in suppression of amber mutations
Tet^r	Resistance to the antibiotic tetracycline
thi-1	Strains with this mutation need vitamin B_1 (thiamine) for growth in minimal medium
Tn5	A transposon that encodes e.g. resistance to kanamycin
Tn*10*	A transposon that encodes e.g. resistance to tetracyclines
tonA	Mutation in the *tonA* gene prevents infection by certain phages (e.g. phages T1, T5 and φ80) – for which the TonA protein acts as a cell-surface receptor
tonB	*tonB* mutants are resistant to various colicins
traD	In F$^+$ cells: *traD* mutations can inhibit conjugative transfer of the F plasmid

[a]An inactivated, mutant form of a gene may be written as e.g. *lon*, *lon*$^-$ or Δ*lon*.

is often used in DNA-based technology; it grows rapidly at ~37°C and can be cultured (grown) on/in inexpensive media such as NUTRIENT AGAR. (See also e.g. MACCONKEY'S AGAR and TERRIFIC BROTH.)

Certain strains of *E. coli* are well-characterized pathogens: see e.g. EPEC.

The *E. coli* genome is ~5×10^6 base pairs. [Genome of *E. coli* (sequence): Science (1997) 277:1453–1474; genome of *E. coli* strain O157:H7: Nature (2001) 409:529–533 – with an erratum: Nature 410:240.]

The GC% of the genomic DNA is ~50.5

Strains of *E. coli* frequently contain plasmids (see e.g. the F PLASMID)

(See also *E. coli* strain JM109.)

Genetic markers found in a number of strains of *E. coli* are listed in the table.

E. coli in recombinant protein production

The use of *E. coli* for producing heterologous proteins has a number of advantages, such as:
- Well-characterized genetics and metabolism.
- Easily cultured on inexpensive media.
- High-level expression of recombinant proteins is achievable with appropriately designed systems. In some cases, the recombinant protein can form >25% of the cell's total protein.
- *E. coli* cells are readily transfected by electroporation and other procedures.

However, this organism is also associated with certain disadvantages:
- Lack of ability to carry out post-translational modification (such as glycosylation) which is necessary for the biological activity of many recombinant proteins. (Despite this, *E. coli* has been used for the production of some (normally glycosylated) proteins: see e.g. Neupogen® in BIOPHARMACEUTICAL (table).)
- The recombinant protein may accumulate *intra*cellularly; this complicates the downstream processing as it is necessary

then to isolate the recombinant protein from the producing cells and to separate the required protein from the other (cell-associated) proteins.

● Part of the normal structure of the *E. coli* cell (and of other Gram-negative bacteria) is the so-called *outer membrane* – a permeability barrier that includes *lipopolysaccharide* (LPS). LPS, also called endotoxin, is a complex macromolecule that is harmful to humans (e.g. it behaves as a pyrogen) and its removal from any product is essential. Removal of LPS from recombinant products may be achieved by chromatographic fractionation. The presence of LPS in a product can be detected e.g. by the LAL TEST.

ESI Electrospray ionization: a technique used in mass spectrometry e.g. to study the kinetics of reactions by continuous monitoring.

Unlike the procedure in MALDI (q.v.), analytes are initially present in the *liquid* phase; the analyte-containing liquid is sprayed from an electrically charged capillary – forming fine droplets which quickly evaporate. As in MALDI, there is a detector system such as the time-of-flight (TOF) analyzer.

EST EXPRESSED SEQUENCE TAG.

etanercept See BIOPHARMACEUTICAL (Enbrel® in the table).

EtBr ETHIDIUM BROMIDE.

ethidium bromide (EtBr) 5-ethyl-3,8-diamino-6-phenylphenanthridinium bromide: an INTERCALATING AGENT used e.g. as a fluorophore for staining nucleic acids in electrophoresis strips; when bound to dsDNA, fluorescence occurs at ~605 nm (red) on appropriate excitation. Ethidium bromide is generally excluded from living cells, being unable to penetrate the cell membrane.

(See also DNA STAINING and PROPIDIUM IODIDE.)

Ethidium bromide is also used for separating ccc dsDNA from linear or nicked molecules of dsDNA by isopyknic ultracentrifugation. This procedure depends on the ability of the linear or nicked molecules to bind more molecules of ethidium bromide when compared to ccc dsDNA molecules; because the binding of ethidium bromide *decreases* the buoyant density of a molecule, those molecules which bind more ethidium bromide will separate in an upper (i.e. less dense) band during ultracentrifugation.

ethidium monoazide A fluorescent phenanthridinium intercalating dye reported to be excluded by the cell membrane in living cells. The dye can be covalently photo-crosslinked to DNA in dead cells.

ethyleneglycol-bis(β-aminoethylether)-*N,N,N′,N′*-tetraacetic acid See EGTA.

ethyleneglycol-bis(succinimidyl succinate) See CHROMATIN IMMUNOPRECIPITATION.

eukaryote Any animal, plant or microorganism in which the cellular structure includes a membrane-bounded nucleus and in which mitosis and/or meiosis precedes cell division.

(cf. PROKARYOTE.)

euploid (1) Refers to a cell or organism in which the number of chromosomes is the same as that characteristic of the species, i.e. a cell/organism containing the *normal* number of chromo-

somes.

(cf. HETEROPLOID.)

(2) Having a complement of chromosomes in which all the chromosomes are present in the same number of copies, e.g. one copy of each chromosome or two copies of each chromosome etc.

ex vivo **mode** (in gene therapy) See GENE THERAPY.

exBiFC *Extended* BIMOLECULAR FLUORESCENCE COMPLEMENTATION.

Exchanger™ system A range of expression vectors (Stratagene, La Jolla CA) which can be used e.g. for cloning in *Escherichia coli* (by using the ColEl origin of replication and selection on an ampicillin-containing medium) and protein expression in eukaryotic (including mammalian) cells (using a CMV promoter sequence and the SV40 polyadenylation signal). In this system, the required selectable marker can be introduced (*in vitro*) by site-specific recombination in which a linearized drug-resistance module is added by Cre-mediated recombination between *loxP* sites (CRE-LOXP SYSTEM); each module encodes resistance to hygromycin, neomycin or puromycin. In this way, the gene of interest can be located in each of several different vectors, with different selectable markers, without the need to move the gene itself.

In each vector the multiple cloning site (MCS, polylinker) is bracketed by T3 and T7 promoters, in opposite orientation. The vectors contain a FLAG or c-*myc* sequence that provides an EPITOPE TAGGING facility.

A phage f1 origin of replication in the vectors permits the recovery of ssDNA, if required.

excimer See e.g. BINARY PROBE.

excipient Any component of a BIOPHARMACEUTICAL which has the primary function of *stabilizing* the product, i.e. helping to prevent any change in the chemical/molecular structure of the active constituent(s).

Excipients often used in protein-based biopharmaceuticals include e.g. serum albumin, certain sugars (glucose, maltose etc.), amino acids (e.g. glycine, threonine), glycerol, sorbitol and polyethylene glycol (PEG).

excision repair Any of various DNA REPAIR processes in which the damaged/abnormal region of a strand of DNA is removed and replaced by the activity of a DNA polymerase; see e.g. BASE EXCISION REPAIR, MISMATCH REPAIR and UVRABC-MEDIATED REPAIR.

excitation filter (fluorescence microscopy) A bandpass filter (i.e. one which transmits radiation only within a given band of wavelengths) which has two main functions: (i) to transmit radiation corresponding to the excitation wavelength(s) of the *specific* fluorophore(s) in the sample, thus minimizing nonspecific fluorescence, and (ii) to block radiation of any other wavelengths.

(cf. EMISSION FILTER; see also DICHROIC BEAMSPLITTER.)

Exo⁻ Klenow Fragment A recombinant form of Klenow fragment (see DNA POLYMERASE I), marketed by Ambion (Austin TX), which lacks the 3′-to′-5′ exonuclease activity, i.e. it has only DNA polymerase activity.

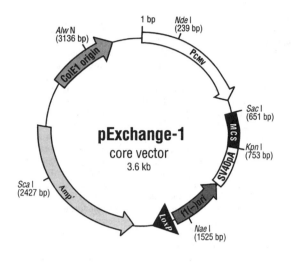

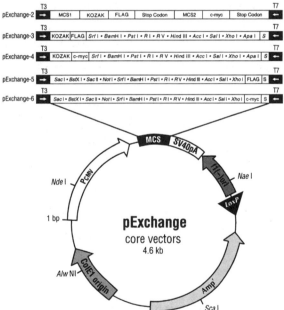

Exchanger™ SYSTEM VECTORS These vectors permit the *in vitro* insertion of a given antibiotic-resistance module by site-specific recombination at the *loxP* site. The vector below shows the expanded MCS (polylinker) in each of a range of vectors. See the entry for details of the system. (See also separate entries for FLAG and KOZAK SEQUENCE.)

Courtesy of Stratagene, La Jolla CA, USA.

exogenote　See MEROZYGOTE.

exon　See SPLIT GENE and SPLICING.

exon amplification　PCR-based amplification using, as template, cDNA copies of the spliced RNA produced during EXON TRAPPING. This approach may be used e.g. to recover exon(s) derived from the sample DNA.

exon-prediction program　Computer software that is designed to detect exons within sequences of nucleotides from cloned DNA, the object being to detect the presence of gene(s).

exon skipping　See ALTERNATIVE SPLICING.

exon trapping　A method used e.g. for demonstrating/detecting the presence of exon(s) – with functional splice sites – within a given fragment of sample DNA. Essentially, the fragment is inserted into a construct (a *minigene*) which already contains known exon and intron sequences; when the minigene (which is part of a plasmid) is transcribed *in vivo*, exons in the minigene may be spliced to any exon(s) that may be present in the fragment. If cDNA copies of the spliced transcript are then amplified by PCR, the length and composition of the amplicons can indicate whether the transcript contains only minigene exons or includes exon(s) from the sample fragment. If required, specific amplified exon(s) can then be recovered by the use of appropriate PCR primers.

In one scheme for exon trapping, the minigene forms part of a 6-kb plasmid shuttle vector which includes an origin of replication and an ampicillin-resistance gene for replication (and selection) in *Escherichia coli*. For replication and RNA splicing in suitable mammalian cells, one terminal region of the minigene consists of an origin of replication and promoter region from simian virus 40 (SV40), while the other terminal region consists of the SV40 polyadenylation signal (encoding the 3′ end of the transcript). The sequence between these two regions consists of two exons that are separated by an intron; the intron includes a multiple cloning site (i.e. POLYLINKER) into which the sample DNA fragment is inserted. Following transcription of the minigene in COS cells (recombinant cells prepared from a monkey cell line), several types of splicing pattern may be detected by amplifying cDNA copies of the transcripts. In the absence of (functional) exon(s) in the DNA sample fragment, the two exons in the minigene are spliced together (forming a sequence of known length). However, a functional exon present in the fragment may be spliced to the minigene's exons; in this case, primers that are complementary to sequences in the minigene's exons can be used to produce amplicons that indicate the composition of these transcripts.

This general approach – using minigenes in an expression system – has also been valuable for investigating the effect on splicing of mutations or SNPs and for studying the overall regulation of pre-mRNA splicing, including ALTERNATIVE SPLICING (which includes various tissue-specific forms of splicing). A recently proposed minigene plasmid vector may be useful e.g. for (i) assessing the effect of disease-associated mutations on the splicing of relevant gene(s); (ii) identifying *cis*-acting elements that are involved in normal regulation of

splicing; and (iii) examining the effects of specific regulatory factors and regions on alternative splicing [BioTechniques (2006) 41(2):177–181].

exonic splicing enhancer　See SPLICING.

exonic splicing silencer　See SPLICING.

exonuclease　Any enzyme which cleaves terminal nucleotides from a nucleic acid molecule.

The lambda exonuclease acts preferentially 5′-to-3′ on a 5′-phosphorylated strand of blunt-ended dsDNA. This enzyme is therefore useful e.g. for preparing single-stranded products (e.g. for SSCP ANALYSIS) from PCR amplicons. To prepare ssDNA products, PCR is carried out with *one* of the primers having a 5′-terminal phosphate – so that *one* strand of the amplicon will be susceptible to digestion by the lambda exonuclease.

(See also subsequent entries.)

exonuclease III　An enzyme (product of the *Escherichia coli* gene *xthA*) which degrades blunt-ended dsDNA (or dsDNA with 5′ overhangs) from the 3′ end of each strand, leaving the 5′ end intact and producing 5′-phosphomononucleotides; the enzyme, which does not degrade 3′ single-stranded overhangs, has been used e.g. for preparing NESTED DELETIONS in cloned DNA.

The enzyme also has activity similar to that of RNASE H and it can function as an AP endonuclease in the BASE EXCISION REPAIR process.

(See also EMEA.)

exonuclease VII　An enzyme (product of the *Escherichia coli* gene *xseA*) which degrades the ssDNA of 3′ and 5′ overhangs but does not degrade dsDNA.

exonuclease-mediated ELISA-like assay　See EMEA.

5′-exonuclease PCR　*Syn.* 5′-NUCLEASE PCR.

exoribonuclease　See RIBONUCLEASE.

exosome　(1) In eukaryotic cells: a multi-protein complex containing 3′-to-5′ exoribonucleases involved e.g. in degrading aberrant pre-mRNA, processing snRNAs and mediating the maturation of 5.8S rRNA; the RNA-binding protein MPP6 in HEp-2 cells is apparently needed for the latter role [Nucleic Acids Res (2005) 33(21):6795–6804].

(2) The term has also been used to refer to a DNA fragment that may replicate, and be expressed, when taken up by a cell but which may not be integrated in the host's DNA.

expanded gold standard　See GOLD STANDARD.

exponential silencing　Downregulation of promoters of specific bacterial gene(s) associated with rapid growth in a rich medium [EMBO J (2001) 20:1–11].

exportins　See KARYOPHERINS.

expressed sequence tag (EST)　A recorded sequence of nucleotides (often ~200–400 nt), derived e.g. from a cDNA library, which is kept in a database as a record of the expression of an unknown gene from a particular type of cell under given conditions.

A given EST, with a sequence of interest, may be located in a database by computer sequence-matching programs.

A pair of primers, specific for a given EST, can be designed and then used in a PCR assay of a large, cloned random fragment of genomic DNA; if this assay yields products that correspond to the given EST (i.e. if the fragment contains a homologous sequence), then the relevant sequence within the random fragment of DNA is referred to as a *sequence-tagged site* (STS).

Given an assortment of large, cloned random fragments of genomic DNA (collectively, covering a large region of the genome), each of these fragments can be assayed for STSs corresponding to a large number of different ESTs. If, as a result of all these assays, various STSs are located in each of the random fragments, this permits alignment of fragments with overlapping sequences; thus, for example, if fragment A has STSs X and Y, and fragment B has STSs Y and Z, then fragments A and B probably overlap at Y ('probably' because the Y STS may be a sequence that occurs more than once in the genome).

Analysis of 10000 ESTs, derived from a cDNA library, has been used to increase understanding of the immune system in the cynomolgus monkey (*Macaca fascicularis*) and – given the similarities between the genome of *M. fascicularis* and the human genome – may also prove to be useful for revising annotations of relevant genes in the human genome [BMC Genomics (2006) 7:82].

[Assembly of approximately 185000 ESTs from the cotton plant (*Gossypium*): Genome Res (2006) 16(3):441–450.]

expression bacmid   See BAC-TO-BAC.

expression platform   See RIBOSWITCH.

expression site (of trypanosomes)   See VSG.

expression vector   A VECTOR which encodes functions for the transcription/translation of a gene (or other sequence) carried by the vector (or subsequently inserted into the vector).

An expression vector may include: (i) an appropriate origin of replication; (ii) a marker gene (e.g. an antibiotic-resistance gene); (iii) one or more promoters (allowing e.g. transcription of the insert in either direction); (iv) a segment corresponding to the Shine–Dalgarno sequence in the transcript (for translation in bacteria); (v) a POLYLINKER (allowing flexibility when inserting target DNA); (vi) a transcription terminator (to avoid unwanted readthrough); (vii) an appropriate control system for initiating transcription of the insert.

Target DNA may be initially cloned by replication in the expression vector. Transcription can be initiated, as needed, e.g. via a *lac* operator (see LAC OPERON) located upstream of the coding sequence and controlled by the LacI repressor protein; in this case, repression can be lifted (i.e. transcription initiated) by adding IPTG.

Cloning and expression can be carried out as separate processes, in different organisms, in a SHUTTLE VECTOR.

Expression of a gene carried by an expression vector may be regulated by a chromosomally located control system (see e.g. CASCADE EXPRESSION SYSTEM) – or by a control system located on the vector itself.

The use of an EPITOPE TAGGING system may facilitate the detection/isolation of proteins.

(See also PESC VECTORS.)

The EXCHANGER SYSTEM of expression vectors is useful e.g. for epitope tagging of proteins and also for changing the selectable marker in a vector (by site-specific recombination) without the need to re-locate the insert/gene of interest.

Some expression vectors include a sequence that encodes a fusion partner for the gene of interest in order e.g. to increase the solubility of the target protein – the fusion product being more soluble than the target protein: see e.g. CHAMPION PET SUMO VECTOR.

Engineering gene expression in trypanosomes – a class of eukaryotic microorganisms – is associated with an additional problem. Apparently, trypanosomes generally do not regulate expression of their protein-encoding genes by controlling the initiation of transcription. Consequently, for studies on gene expression with an inducible transcription system in these organisms there is a requirement to construct such a system from exogenous sources. For *Trypanosoma cruzi* (the causal agent of Chagas' disease in Central and South America), a stable tetracycline-inducible expression vector (pTcINDEX), containing a multiple cloning site (MCS), was designed to integrate into the genome at a specific, transcriptionally silent location, thus avoiding some of the problems of integration within an endogenously transcribed site. [pTcINDEX: BMC Biotechnol (2006) 6:32.]

(See also the table of destination vectors in entry GATEWAY SITE-SPECIFIC RECOMBINATION SYSTEM.)

Expressway™ Plus expression system   A system (Invitrogen, Carlsbad CA) for *in vitro* protein synthesis (see CELL-FREE PROTEIN SYNTHESIS).

ExSite™ site-directed mutagenesis kit   A kit (Stratagene, La Jolla CA) used for PCR-based SITE-DIRECTED MUTAGENESIS in which deletions, insertions or point mutations can be introduced into almost any double-stranded plasmid, eliminating the need for e.g. phage M13-based vectors.

Essentially, the type of mutation produced depends on the design of the primers. A point mutation can be introduced by using primers with a single-base substitution. A deletion can be produced by primers which bind at sites separated by the sequence to be deleted. An insertion can be introduced by the use of primers with a 5′ extension.

Following PCR, the reaction mixture includes the following molecules: original template DNA (which had been methylated *in vivo*); linear, newly synthesized (unmethylated) DNA; and linear, hybrid DNA which consists of parental and newly synthesized strands. The reaction mixture is then subjected to restriction enzyme DpnI (see table in the entry RESTRICTION ENDONUCLEASE for details). Blunt-ended ligation of newly synthesized DNA is then carried out with T4 DNA ligase – this providing circular, mutagenized molecules suitable for transformation of *Escherichia coli*.

ExSite™ has been used e.g. to replace a GTC codon with a GAG codon [J Bacteriol (2006) 188(7):2604–2613], and to introduce mutations into the *hmuR* gene (encoding a hemin receptor) in a periodontitis-associated Gram-negative pathogen, *Porphyromonas gingivalis* [Infect Immun (2006) 74(2): 1222–1232].

extein See INTEIN.

extendase activity (template-independent polymerase activity) During PCR: the addition of an extra residue of an adenosine nucleotide to the 3′ end of the product strand (i.e. beyond the final, template-determined 3′ nucleotide) when synthesis is mediated e.g. by TAQ DNA POLYMERASE. Single-nucleotide (adenosine) 3′ overhangs can be exploited e.g. in facilitating insertion of the amplicons into certain types of vector which have terminal single-nucleotide thymidine overhangs – see e.g. TOPOISOMERASE I CLONING and CHAMPION PET SUMO VECTOR. (See also TOPO TA CLONING KIT.)

The expression of extendase activity is strongest when the last (template-determined) residue at the 3′ end of the product strand is a pyrimidine; if required, extendase activity can be promoted by including a purine (rather than a pyrimidine) in the relevant position in the template. If the last residue at the 3′ end of the product strand is a purine, extendase activity is less efficient.

If blunt-ended products are required from PCR, amplicons with the 3′ overhang can be subjected to exonuclease action: see POLISHING.

(See also END-IT DNA END-REPAIR KIT.)

extended BiFC See BIMOLECULAR FLUORESCENCE COMPLEMENTATION.

external guide sequence See SNRNAS.

extrachromosomal genes *Syn.* CYTOPLASMIC GENES.

extrachromosomal inheritance *Syn.* CYTOPLASMIC INHERITANCE.

extranuclear genes *Syn.* CYTOPLASMIC GENES.

EYFP *Enhanced* YELLOW FLUORESCENT PROTEIN (q.v.).

F

F L-Phenylalanine (alternative to Phe).

F⁻ recipient See F PLASMID.

F⁺ donor See F PLASMID.

F factor See F PLASMID.

F-like pili See PILUS.

F plasmid (formerly F factor) A specific, IncFI, conjugative, low-copy-number plasmid (~95 kb) found e.g. in *Escherichia coli*; the F plasmid can exist either as an extrachromosomal replicon or integrated in the host chromosome – and is able to mediate CONJUGATION in either location.

Cells containing the free, circular plasmid are conjugative *donor* cells (F⁺ cells); potential *recipient* cells (F⁻ cells) lack the plasmid. The F⁺ cells express (plasmid-encoded) donor functions (e.g. a PILUS) and are *derepressed* for conjugation – meaning that all, or nearly all, cells in an F⁺ population can function as donors (see FINOP SYSTEM); hence, in a mixed population of F⁺ and F⁻ cells, most or all F⁻ cells receive an F plasmid (through conjugation) and are converted to F⁺ cells.

Chromosomal integration of the F plasmid gives rise to an *Hfr donor* (Hfr means high frequency of recombination); Hfr donors transfer chromosomal (as well as plasmid) DNA to F⁻ recipients, the amount of DNA transferred increasing with increased length of uninterrupted mating. (The F plasmid in an Hfr cell is said to *mobilize* the chromosome for transfer.) (See also INTERRUPTED MATING.)

An F plasmid may excise from the chromosome aberrantly to form an F′ plasmid (see PRIME PLASMID).

A protein, SopA, involved in the partitioning of plasmids to daughter cells during cell division, was reported to polymerize into filaments, *in vitro*; these filaments elongated at a rate similar to the rate of plasmid separation *in vivo* [Proc Natl Acad Sci USA (2005) 102(49):17658–17663].

Transcription from the P_Y promoter of the *tra* (transfer) operon of the F plasmid was reported to be repressed by the host's H-NS protein [J Bacteriol (2006) 188(2):507–514]. (See also CCD MECHANISM and PIF.)

F′ plasmid See F PLASMID and PRIME PLASMID.

f1 phage See PHAGE F1.

Fab fragment (of an antibody) See ZENON ANTIBODY-LABELING REAGENTS.

Fabry disease An X-linked disease involving a deficiency in activity of the enzyme α-galactosidase A. Various manifestations are reported, including e.g. vascular-type skin lesions and cardiac symptoms; the cause of death is reported to be usually renal failure.

A recombinant enzyme, Fabrazyme®, is used for treatment (see entry BIOPHARMACEUTICAL (table)).

facile (of procedures) Able to be carried out easily – i.e. with no specific or unspecified difficulties.

FACS FLUORESCENCE-ACTIVATED CELL SORTER.

factor VIIa A factor involved in the blood-clotting mechanism (see NovoSeven® in entry BIOPHARMACEUTICAL (table)).

factor VIII A factor involved in the blood-clotting mech-

anism – see 'hemophilia' in the table in entry GENETIC DISEASE, and see also KOGENATE.

factor IX A factor involved in the blood-clotting mechanism – see CHRISTMAS FACTOR, and see also 'hemophilia' in entry GENETIC DISEASE (table).

factor essential for methicillin resistance (*fem*) See MRSA.

FAM 6-Carboxyfluorescein: a fluorescent reporter dye with an emission maximum at 525 nm and an excitation maximum at 493 nm.

farnesol A sesquiterpene alcohol reported to act as a QUORUM SENSING molecule in *Candida albicans* [autoregulation and quorum sensing in fungi: Eukaryotic Cell (2006) 5(4):613–619].

Farnesol and the antibiotic gentamicin were reported to act synergistically against the bacterium *Staphylococcus aureus* [Antimicrob Agents Chemother (2006) 50(4):1463–1469].

FBS Fetal bovine serum.

Fc portion (of an antibody) See ZENON ANTIBODY-LABELING REAGENTS.

fd phage See PHAGE FD.

feature The exact location (on a coated glass surface) where a given DNA probe is synthesized during the preparation of a GeneChip® (Affymetrix) MICROARRAY; a feature is ~5 μm in size.

feeder cells Cells which may be included in cultures of STEM CELLS in order to promote growth of the latter. For mouse ES cells in culture the engineered expression of Bcl-2 has been reported to override the requirement for feeder cells [Proc Natl Acad Sci USA (2005) 102(9):3312–3317].

feline immunodeficiency virus See LENTIVIRINAE.

feline syncytial virus See SPUMAVIRINAE.

***fem* genes** See MRSA.

female-specific phage Any of certain phages (e.g. T7, W31) whose replication is inhibited in cells containing particular plasmids; for example, production of intermediate and late phage proteins of T7 is inhibited in cells of *Escherichia coli* containing the F PLASMID.

Note that cells containing conjugative plasmids are said to be 'male' cells; cells lacking these plasmids are 'female' cells.

In *Pseudomonas aeruginosa*, the DNA of phages F116 and G101 is degraded by RESTRICTION ENDONUCLEASE activity in cells containing plasmid pMG7.

(See also PIF.)

femto- In SI (Système International) units: a prefix meaning 10^{-15}.

For a list of prefixes see the 'Ready reference' section at the front of the dictionary.

FEN1 (FEN-1) See FLAP ENDONUCLEASE.

Fenton reaction The reaction in which ferrous iron is oxidized to ferric iron by hydrogen peroxide with the production of hydroxyl radical (·OH):

$$Fe(II) + H_2O_2 \rightarrow Fe(III) + \cdot OH + OH^-$$

A Fenton reaction at the endoplasmic reticulum is reported to influence the expression of hypoxia-inducible genes [Proc Natl Acad Sci USA (2004) 101(12):4302–4307].

The highly reactive hydroxyl radical, produced in a Fenton reaction, can be employed to obtain fine resolution in FOOT-PRINTING studies [Nucleic Acids Res (2006) 34(6):e48].

In vivo footprinting (in frozen cells) has been achieved with a brief exposure to a synchrotron X-ray beam that produces hydroxyl radical footprints similar to those obtained *in vitro* using the Fenton reaction [Nucleic Acids Res (2006) 34(8): e64].

fermentation   (1) In an industrial/commercial context: any process involving the large-scale culture (i.e. growth) of micro-organisms, regardless of whether metabolism is fermentative or respiratory (oxidative). This use of the term 'fermentation' is in sharp distinction to that given in meaning (2), below.
(2) (*energy metab.*) A specific energy-converting process in which a substrate is metabolized without the involvement of an external electron acceptor, oxidation and reduction within the process being balanced. ATP is characteristically produced by substrate-level phosphorylation.

(cf. RESPIRATION.)

fes (*FES*)   An ONCOGENE in strains of feline sarcoma virus. The v-*fes* product has TYROSINE KINASE activity.

FHA   The filamentous hemagglutinin produced by the (Gram-negative) bacterium *Bordetella pertussis*.

(See also INTEGRINS.)

FhuA protein   See TONA GENE.

field inversion electrophoresis   See PFGE.

filament pyrolyser   See PYROLYSIS.

filamentous hemagglutinin (FHA)   In *Bordetella pertussis*: a cell-surface ligand which binds the $\alpha_M\beta_2$ INTEGRIN.

filgrastim   See Neupogen® in BIOPHARMACEUTICAL (table).

fimbria (*bacteriol.*)   A term often regarded (illogically) as a synonym of PILUS (q.v.). Fimbriae are thin, proteinaceous filaments which project from the surface of certain types of cell and which have roles e.g. in cell–cell adhesion, cell–substrate adhesion and (in some cases) in a type of motility referred to as 'twitching motility'.

fingerprint (DNA)   A pattern formed by a number of bands of stained (or labeled) fragments of DNA, of different sizes, that are present within a gel medium (generally following electro-phoresis of a restriction-digested sample) or, subsequent to a blotting procedure, on a nitrocellulose (or other) membrane; the nature of any given fingerprint will depend on the particular sample of DNA which is being examined and on the method used to produce the fingerprint.

Fingerprints are generated by various TYPING procedures (which often produce strain-specific fingerprints).

FinOP system   A regulatory system, involving plasmid genes *finO* and *finP*, which controls conjugative transfer in most F-like plasmids. The products of *finO* and *finP* jointly inhibit the expression of *traJ*, a gene in the 'transfer operon' which has a key role in the initiation of conjugative transfer.

The product of *finP* is a molecule of ANTISENSE RNA which binds to the *traJ* transcript. The product of *finO*, a poly-peptide referred to as an 'RNA chaperone', stabilizes the activity of the antisense RNA. With a fully active FinOP system in operation the transfer system remains repressed and conjugation remains inhibited.

The F PLASMID is (constitutively) derepressed for transfer, i.e. it is permanently conjugation-competent. Earlier, it had been thought that this was due to the absence of a *finO* locus in this plasmid. Later it was shown that *finO* is present but is inactivated by an insertion sequence, IS*3*, which disrupts the coding sequence of the gene. As a consequence, FinO is not available to act jointly with the *finP* product.

first strand (of cDNA)   The strand of DNA synthesized on an mRNA molecule by reverse transcriptase. If only a few types of mRNA are being targeted then gene-specific primers may be used. If many, or all, mRNAs are being targeted (e.g. for a microarray experiment) then oligo(dT) primers may be used; these primers bind to the 3′ poly(A) tails that are commonly present on eukaryotic mRNAs. Another possibility is the use of random primers (e.g. random hexamers); in one study it was found that the use of random pentadecamer (i.e. 15-mer) primers resulted in an improved range and yield of cDNAs compared with the use of random hexamers [BioTechniques (2006) 40(5):649–657].

mRNA is removed from the RNA/DNA hybrid – e.g. by RNASE H or by alkaline hydrolysis – and the *second strand* of DNA is synthesized, making ds cDNA.

In the Gubler–Hoffmann procedure, the hybrid RNA/DNA structure is treated by *controlled* enzymic action – leaving short sequences of RNA; DNA polymerase I (an enzyme with 5′-to-3′ exonuclease activity) is then used to synthesize the second strand. Hence, the second strand is produced without the use of an exogenous primer.

[Example of the Gubler–Hoffmann method: BioTechniques (2005) 38(3):451–458.]

(See also entry CDNA.)

FISH   Fluorescence *in situ* hybridization: a particular form of *in situ* hybridization (ISH) in which the label is a fluorophore. In one approach, BIOTINylated probes, bound to their target, are detected by a STREPTAVIDIN-conjugated fluorophore.

In an alternative approach, the probe itself incorporates a fluorophore (for example, ChromaTide™: see entry PROBE LABELING).

Increased sensitivity may be achieved by using TYRAMIDE SIGNAL AMPLIFICATION.

FLAG®   A peptide (sequence: DYKDDDDK) used for tagging proteins by creating protein–peptide fusions; a protein tagged with this sequence can be detected/recovered by monoclonal antibodies specific for the tagged region of the protein.

[Uses of FLAG® (examples): Mol Biol Cell (2006) 17(8): 3356–3368; Mol Cell Biol (2006) 26(7):2697–2715.]

flap (in lagging strand synthesis)   See OKAZAKI FRAGMENT.

flap endonuclease 1 (FEN1; FEN-1)   A structure-specific endo-nuclease involved e.g. in DNA replication (see OKAZAKI FRAGMENT). FEN1 was also reported to exhibit a gap endonuclease function which may have a part to play e.g. in the resolution of stalled replication forks [mode of FEN1 activity with gap substrates: Nucleic Acids Res (2006) 34(6):1772–1784].

FLASH® chemiluminescent gene mapping kit   A kit (Stratagene, La Jolla CA) designed for high-resolution restriction mapping.

Essentially, the gene (or fragment) – flanked by T3 and T7 promoter sites – is initially cloned in a vector. The gene is then excised from the vector, still flanked by the T3 and T7 sites. (Excision occurs at two NotI recognition sites; the NotI sites are used because they are the recognition sites of a 'rare-cutting' enzyme – an enzyme which is unlikely to interfere with the activity of the particular enzyme whose target sites are being mapped.)

The excised gene is exposed to partial digestion with the given RESTRICTION ENDONUCLEASE whose target sites are to be mapped.

The fragments produced by the restriction enzyme are subjected to electrophoresis in an agarose gel, and the bands of fragments are transferred to a hybridization membrane.

Bands of fragments on the membrane are probed with a T3 sequence that is conjugated to ALKALINE PHOSPHATASE. The hybridization membrane is then incubated with a chemiluminescent substrate (see CHEMILUMINESCENCE), and the light signal from the target–probe complex is detected within 30 minutes on radiographic film.

The position of each band in the resulting ladder reflects the distance between one end of the gene (i.e. the T3 site) and one of the cutting sites of the given restriction enzyme. The bands in the ladder therefore indicate the various cutting sites of the given enzyme within the gene.

By replicating the procedure with an alkaline phosphatase-conjugated T7 probe, a *complementary* set of bands are seen – each band reflecting the distance between one end of the gene (i.e. the T7 end in this case) and one of the cutting sites of the restriction enzyme. Hence, the second determination (with the T7 probe) serves to confirm the results obtained in the first determination.

flood plate   A PLATE whose surface has been flooded with a (concentrated) liquid suspension of a given organism (usually a suspension of bacteria) and excess liquid removed e.g. with a sterile Pasteur pipet.

A ('dried') flood plate is used e.g. in PHAGE TYPING.

floral dip method   A method first used for the transfection of *Arabidopsis thaliana* with *Agrobacterium tumefaciens*, which involves dipping developing floral tissues (including floral buds) into a solution containing 5% sucrose, 500 μL/l of the surfactant Silwet L-77 and cells of *A. tumefaciens*. [See also Methods Mol Biol (2005) 286:91–102, (2005) 286:103–110.] [Use of method in transcriptional profiling of the *Arabidopsis* embryo: Plant Physiol (2007) 143(2):924–940.]

*flox*ed **DNA**   A segment of DNA flanked, on both sides, by a *loxP* site (see CRE–LOXP SYSTEM).

Flp (FLP)   A site-specific recombinase (encoded by the two-micron plasmid) first isolated from the yeast *Saccharomyces*; Flp is a member of the integrase family of recombinases, and a tyrosine residue is found at the active site which mediates phosphodiester bond cleavage.

Within *S. cerevisiae* Flp catalyzes the inversion of a section of the plasmid flanked by a pair of (inverted) recognition sequences.

In recombinant DNA technology, Flp is used e.g. for the excision of specific sequences *in vivo*. The enzyme is active in both eukaryotes (e.g. *Drosophila*) and bacteria (including *Escherichia coli*). The enzyme can excise a sequence that is flanked, at both ends, with a so-called *Flp recognition target* (FRT) sequence – both FRTs being in the same orientation; the excised fragment is in the form of a circular molecule.

A plasmid containing one FRT site can be inserted, by the action of the Flp recombinase, into another replicon that also contains a copy of the FRT site.

[Example of use of the Flp recombinase: BioTechniques (2006) 40(1):67–72.]

[Modular and excisable molecular switch for the induction of gene expression by the Flp recombinase: BioTechniques (2006) 41(6):711–713.]

(See also the vector pEF5/FRT/V5-DEST™ in the table for entry GATEWAY SITE-SPECIFIC RECOMBINATION SYSTEM.)

Certain peptides which inhibit Flp have been reported from studies on the HOLLIDAY JUNCTION (q.v.).

(See also CRE–LOXP SYSTEM.)

Flp-In™ cell lines   Cell lines from Invitrogen (Carlsbad CA) in which the target site (FRT) of the Flp recombinase (see FLP) has been inserted stably into a transcriptionally active region of the genome. These cells are designed to be co-transfected with an FRT-containing Flp-In™ expression vector, carrying the gene of interest, and a plasmid (pOG44) encoding the Flp recombinase; within these cells, targeted integration of the expression vector occurs at the same location in each cell – promoting uniform levels of expression of the given gene of interest.

Flp-In™ cells have been prepared from various types of parental cell, including BHK, CHO, Jurkat and 293. In some of these cells a CMV promoter works well, but in others (e.g. BHK) expression from a CMV promoter is reported to be downregulated; in the latter cells, Flp-In™ vectors with the EF-1α promoter are recommended.

(See also vector pEF5/FRT/V5-DEST™ in GATEWAY SITE-SPECIFIC RECOMBINATION SYSTEM (table).)

fluctuation test   A classic, early (1943) test, devised by Luria and Delbrück, for examining the way in which populations of bacteria respond to changes in the environment.

Two hypotheses co-existed at the time: (i) genetic change is induced by environmental influences (i.e. an adaptive mechanism), and (ii) genetic change occurs spontaneously (that is, independently of environmental influences) – cells in which such changes have occurred being selected (and proliferating) if conditions become suitable.

Essentially the (statistics-based) test measured the variance between numbers of phage-resistant (mutant) cells in each of a set of individual, separate liquid cultures of phage-sensitive bacteria; this was compared with the variance in numbers of phage-resistant mutants in each of a number of samples taken from a single (bulk) liquid culture. (The numbers of phage-resistant mutants were ascertained by plating aliquots from the cultures on separate plates and then exposing the plates to virulent phage.)

The high variance (wide fluctuation) in numbers of mutants from the separate cultures indicated that the (phage-resistant) mutant cells had arisen spontaneously – at different times in different cultures – i.e. that the appearance of mutants was unrelated to exposure of the bacteria to phage.

(See also NEWCOMBE EXPERIMENT.)

fluorescence (*in vivo*) See IN VIVO FLUORESCENCE.

fluorescence-activated cell sorter (FACS) An instrument used for flow cytometry in which individual, fluorophore-labeled cells are counted by recording the fluorescence they emit, on excitation, when passing through a narrow aperture.

fluorescence *in situ* hybridization See FISH.

fluorescence resonance energy transfer See FRET.

fluoroquinolones See QUINOLONE ANTIBIOTICS.

FluoroTrans® PVDF membranes See PVDF.

5-FOA See YEAST TWO-HYBRID SYSTEM.

foamy viruses Viruses of the subfamily SPUMAVIRINAE.

footprinting A technique that is used to determine the location (i.e. sequence) at which a given ligand (e.g. a DNA-binding protein) binds to DNA.

Note. An *entirely unrelated* technique is known as GENETIC FOOTPRINTING.

This account refers specifically to *in vitro* footprinting – see also the entry for IN VIVO FOOTPRINTING.

Initially, two identical populations of end-labeled sample fragments of DNA are prepared, and the particular ligand is allowed to bind to fragments in one of the populations. Each of the populations is then subjected to either enzymatic or chemical cleavage under conditions in which each fragment is (ideally) cut at only one of a large number of possible sites. In each population of fragments, the result is a collection of subfragments, present in a range of different lengths, that are produced by cleavage at different sites.

In the population of ligand-bound fragments, cleavage will not have occurred at those cleavage sites which had been shielded from the enzyme (or chemical agent) by the bound ligand; this population will therefore lack a certain range of subfragments that are present in the other population. The *absence* of certain subfragments in the ligand-bound population will be seen as a *gap* when the two populations of subfragments are compared by gel electrophoresis; this gap is the ligand's *footprint*, and its position in the gel (in relation to the bands of subfragments) indicates the ligand's binding site on the DNA.

In one approach, cleavage of fragments is carried out by the enzyme DNase I. This tends to produce a large and clear footprint because DNase I is a large protein that will not cut the DNA at sites close to a large DNA-bound ligand (such as a DNA-binding protein).

Resolution can be improved (i.e. the footprint can be better defined) by using a small chemical agent to cleave the DNA. One such agent is hydroxyl radical (·OH) which brings about sequence-independent cleavage of DNA: any phosphodiester bond which is unprotected by the bound ligand is susceptible to cleavage. Footprinting with the hydroxyl radical can be achieved by means of the FENTON REACTION [Nucleic Acids Res (2006) 34(6):e48]. Footprinting with hydroxyl radical in frozed cells (i.e. *in vivo*) can be achieved by using a brief pulse of X-radiation from a synchrotron – which can generate hydroxyl radical footprints similar to those generated *in vitro* by the Fenton reaction [Nucleic Acids Res (2006) 34(8):e64].

forced cloning (directional cloning) Any procedure designed to ensure that target DNA is inserted into a vector molecule in a definite, known orientation; insertion in this way is required e.g. when the target DNA is subsequently to be transcribed from a promoter sequence within the vector.

forensic applications (of DNA-based technology) DNA-based technology can offer a range of possibilities for assisting with investigations. Moreover, given that DNA may survive for long periods of time, particularly in the right kind of tissue under appropriate conditions, current methods can sometimes resolve crimes that have remained unsolved for many years.

DNA-based identification

DNA is naturally important in the context of identification – including the identification of those killed in natural disasters such as earthquakes, floods and tsunamis as well as victims (or perpetrators) of crime; moreover, this technology also has a role e.g. in cases involving paternity issues.

Each investigation starts with one or more samples that are sources of DNA. The quality and quantity of DNA available from a given sample can vary enormously according to (i) the type of sample, (ii) the conditions under which the sample existed prior to collection, and (iii) the time for which it was exposed to those conditions.

Positive, unambiguous analysis of DNA requires a sample of at least a certain minimum quantity – e.g. of the order of nanograms – which has not been degraded to an extent that precludes its use. Fortunately, modern methods permit truly minute quantities of DNA to be characterized, and a number of commercial methods (e.g. CHARGESWITCH TECHNOLOGY) can efficiently recover the DNA from various types of crude sample. Even poor quality/damaged DNA may still be of use if it is susceptible to PCR amplification by the Y FAMILY of DNA polymerases [Nucleic Acids Res (2006) 34 (4):1102–1111].

Degraded DNA in small amounts is reported to be susceptible to isothermal whole-genome amplification with primers optimized, bioinformatically, for coverage of the human genome. Degraded DNA, pre-amplified by this procedure, was reported to be satisfactory for STR-based genotyping [DNA Res (2006) 13(2):77–88].

A system for *quantifying* the level of damage in a sample of

DNA has been devised in a *zoological* context and may be useful for forensic investigations involving domestic animals or wildlife [Frontiers Zool (2006) 3:11].

Both nuclear DNA and MITOCHONDRIAL DNA are of value for identification purposes. In general, analysis of nuclear (as opposed to mitochondrial) DNA is frequently the preferred option because nuclear DNA has a potentially greater power to discriminate between individuals. Samples of mtDNA may be unsatisfactory in certain cases, e.g. in that they can fail to distinguish between individuals of the same maternal line. Nevertheless, in the USA there is an extensive database of mtDNA – known as the mtDNA Popstats Population Database – containing over 5000 mtDNA profiles; this database is intended primarily for law-based and academic use. A given mtDNA profile in the database is described in relation to the (revised) standard 'Cambridge Reference Sequence'. Ongoing scrutiny continues to reduce errors in this database, which is considered to be a reliable resource for forensic case analysis [Forensic Sci Comm (2005) 7(10)].

A potential problem with the use of mtDNA targets is the existence of so-called 'mitochondrial pseudogenes': mtDNA-like sequences which occur in nuclear (chromosomal) DNA. Thus, unless appropriate precautions are taken, these nuclear sequences could be co-amplified by PCR when attempting *specifically* to amplify particular mtDNA targets. The importance of such potential contamination may be underestimated if it is assumed that the high copy number of mtDNA genes, compared with nuclear pseudogenes, may mask the effect of these nuclear targets: some pseudogenes are represented at *multiple* sites in nuclear DNA. Some 46 fragments of nuclear DNA – covering all of the human mitochondrial DNA – have been sequenced [BMC Genomics (2006) 7:185].

Voluntary samples of DNA are obtainable e.g. by BUCCAL CELL SAMPLING or from blood etc. Other sources of DNA include hairs, teeth and cells from the skin.

(See also DNA ISOLATION.)

Teeth as a source of DNA

Given adverse conditions, the remains of dead individuals, including isolated body parts, may be poor sources of DNA. However, the more-durable hard tissues, such as teeth, can be a valuable source; moreover, compared with other types of sample, hard-tissue samples may be easier to free from contamination by extraneous DNA.

Hair as a source of DNA

Hair can be useful as a source of DNA, and is particularly valuable when the origin of a given sample is a major factor in an investigation. Prior to DNA analysis, it is important to carry out a thorough macroscopic and microscopic examination of the hair sample because (particularly with a very small sample) the portion used for DNA analysis will no longer be available for physical characterization.

A hair in the active phase of growth is likely to provide a good source of both nuclear and mitochondrial DNA from cells in the root and sheath regions. However, hairs at the end of the growth cycle – lacking follicular components, and shed from the body – are likely to be poor/inadequate sources of nuclear DNA, although they may be adequate for the analysis of mitochondrial DNA.

[Guidelines for the forensic examination of human hair (including a glossary of descriptive terms): Forensic Sci Comm (2005) 7(2).]

Types of investigation used for identification purposes

Given adequate samples, human and non-human DNA can be readily distinguished (if necessary).

Identification can involve e.g. the analysis of genomic *short tandem repeats* (see STR) – an approach used in CODIS (q.v.). Male-specific STRs (i.e. those found on the Y chromosome) may be useful for investigations in sex-based cases.

The gender of a subject may be ascertained e.g. by a PCR-based assay of sequences from alleles of the amelogenin gene on the X and Y chromosomes: see DNA SEX DETERMINATION ASSAY. (See also BARR BODY.)

Results that exclude suspect(s) can be as valuable as those which incriminate.

The area of DNA sampling and identification has important ethical aspects. [Balancing crime detection, human rights and privacy (UK National DNA Database): EMBO Rep (2006) 7 (Special Issue):S26–S30.]

Disasters with mass fatalities

In exceptional events, e.g. major earthquakes and tsunamis, the problem of identification may be exacerbated by an overwhelming number of victims and, in many cases, by the lack of adequate technical facilities. Moreover – in any situation – dental, fingerprint and DNA-based data can be useful only if comparative data (e.g. in a database) are also available.

In the South Asian tsunami of December, 2004, an international collaborative effort assisted with the identification of victims. At the TTVI (Thai Tsunami Victim Identification) center, some 2010 victims had been identified 7 months post-tsunami. Of these victims, 1.3% had been identified on the basis of DNA analyses – as compared with 61% by dental records and 19% from fingerprints (some of the victims were identified by a combination of methods). In this scenario it has been considered that DNA-based identification should be reserved for those cases in which attempts at identification by other methods have been unsuccessful (instead of being used as a first-line approach).

[Management of mass fatality following the South Asian tsunami of 2004: PLoS Medicine (2006) 3(6):e195.]

Microbial forensics

Microbial forensics is a multi-disciplinary field of endeavor created in response to the ongoing threat of attack, on populations and/or individuals, by terrorists/criminals using pathogenic microorganisms or their toxins. A high-profile example of such attacks was the letter containing spores of *Bacillus anthracis* (causal agent of anthrax) sent to a member of the US government in 2001. A specialized laboratory facility, the National Bioforensics Analysis Center (NBFAC), was set up to examine and analyze relevant material.

[Sample collection, handling and preservation for an effective program of microbial forensics: Appl Environ Microbiol (2006) 72(10):6431–6438.]

Guidance is available for those physicians who believe that a given patient is a victim of bioterrorism (or other type(s) of biocrime). [Biocrimes, microbial forensics and the physician: PLoS Medicine (2005) 2(12):e337.]

The role of DNA-based technology in this field could be seen as central to tasks such as the identification of pathogens and determination of their source(s). Ideally, methods should be available to characterize a given isolate of a pathogen and to link it indisputably to a specific origin. However, this was not possible in the case of letter-borne spores of *B. anthracis*; in this case, TYPING based on the analysis of tandem repeats in DNA pointed to a laboratory source – but could not offer information that was more specific regarding the origin of the strain. A paper summarizing the requirements of the nascent field of microbial forensics [Appl Environ Microbiol (2005) 71(5):2209–2213] referred to a more informative and highly sophisticated (but not yet realized) typing system that could exploit our expanding knowledge of genome plasticity and bioinformatics. A future system for comparing genomic sequence data (suitable for detecting differences among isolates of a pathogen) was seen in terms of an approach that could accomodate genomic variation due to recombinational events and also possible genome-wide patterns of mutation.

Reliance on selected sequences of nucleotides for identification purposes can be problematic – as was shown e.g. by the finding of genes of *B. anthracis* virulence plasmid pXO2 in plasmids from other species of *Bacillus* [J Clin Microbiol (2006) 44(7):2367–2377]. Precision-based identification and comparison of isolates by whole-genome sequencing would require the availability of techniques that are faster and less expensive than those in current use; moreover, even with the development of such techniques, maximum use of the sequencing data is possible only if accessible databases on the pathogens, and related species, are in place.

Typing of *B. anthracis* on the basis of single-nucleotide repeats (see SNR) has been reported to permit differentiation of isolates with extremely low levels of genetic diversity – i.e. very closely related strains – even when such isolates could not be distinguished by other methods of typing [J Clin Microbiol (2006) 44(3):777–783].

Any typing procedure involving copying specific sequences of genomic DNA is likely to be facilitated by techniques that accelerate amplification – such as an ultra-fast form of PCR [Nucleic Acids Res (2006) 34:e77].

B. anthracis is, of course, only one of a number of possible microorganisms that can be considered in this context. Other, more common, types of pathogen, including those associated with natural outbreaks of disease, are also candidates. Less dramatic, covert events caused by this kind of pathogen may be correspondingly more difficult to detect against the background of routine, natural outbreaks.

It was suggested [Appl Environ Microbiol (2005) 71(5):2209–2213] that nucleic-acid-based techniques are unlikely

to be able to pinpoint the unique source of a given isolate of a pathogen (a requirement e.g. for tracing perpetrators of bioterrorism). This pointed to the need for chemical and physical analyses to supplement nucleic-acid-based methods in order to supply additional information; in particular, it was thought that the (chemical) composition of microbial cells might be able to reveal more information about their origin if more information were available on the way in which the chemical nature of miroorganisms reflects the type of environment in which they were grown.

Plant pathogen forensics
Bioterrorism directed at agricultural targets has the potential for creating widespread nutritional and economic damage as well as political instability. The diffuse nature of agriculture, and the (relatively) lower level of sophistication needed to target this area, makes this a particularly difficult problem to tackle. Moreover, the majority of plant pathogens are species of fungi which are, in general, technically less amenable than bacteria to laboratory investigation. Additionally, plant pathogens are generally harmless to humans, so that any would-be bioterrorist in the agricultural sphere is exposed to minimal risk. The total prevention of an attack on agricultural targets has been assessed to be impossible by the Banbury Microbial Forensics Group, so that vigilence and an effective response to any incident remain the optimal approach.

Information, technology and resources currently available in the agricultural sphere have been assessed for potential use in plant pathogen forensics [Microbiol Mol Biol Rev (2006) 70(2):450–471].

formamide (H.C=O.NH$_2$)   A denaturing agent which lowers T_m in the THERMAL MELTING PROFILE of dsDNA.

forward mutation   Any mutation that gives rise to a mutant phenotype, commonly by inactivating or modifying a gene.

forward primer   A PRIMER that binds to a *non-coding* strand (see CODING STRAND).

The fragment shown below identifies a forward primer as a sequence of nucleotides – in heavy type – within the coding strand. As an *isolated* oligonucleotide, this eight-mer primer, 5′-GCTATGCT-3′, would bind to the underlined sequence in the non-coding strand:

5′-**GCTATGCT**CTGCC/......./GGGACT<u>CGGCACGA</u>-3′
    (*coding strand*)

3′-<u>CGATACGA</u>GACGG/......./CCCTGA**GCCGTGCT**-5′
    (*non-coding strand*)

Consequently, when extended, this primer would give rise to a sequence identical to the coding strand.

A *reverse primer* binds to the coding strand. In the fragment shown, a reverse primer is identified (in heavy type) as a sequence of nucleotides within the non-coding strand. As an *isolated* oligonuleotide, 5′-TCGTGCCG-3′ would bind to the underlined sequence in the coding strand.

fosmid   A COSMID based on the F PLASMID; intracellularly, it occurs as a low-copy-number vector.

FPET Formalin-fixed paraffin-embedded tissue.

Fpg protein *Syn.* MutM: see 8-OXOG.

fps (*FPS*) An ONCOGENE in strains of avian sarcoma virus. The v-*fps* product has TYROSINE KINASE activity.

fragile X disease A hereditary disease characterized by mental retardation; the defect, on the X chromosome, arises through instability of MICROSATELLITE DNA.

(See also GENETIC DISEASE (table).)

frame-shift mutation (phase-shift mutation) Any mutation in which the addition or deletion of nucleotide(s) results in an out-of-phase message (altered reading frame) in the sequence downstream of the mutation. A frame-shift mutation may be induced e.g. by INTERCALATING AGENTS.

(cf. FRAMESHIFTING.)

frameshifting (ribosomal frameshifting; programed ribosomal frameshifting; translational frameshifting) A mechanism in which the precise product of translation is determined by an induced (programed) movement of the ribosome at a specific site in the mRNA: either a movement of one nucleotide upstream (i.e. in the 5′ direction) or one nucleotide downstream (in the 3′ direction) – translation continuing in the new −1 or +1 reading frame, respectively.

The ribosome's movement is induced by signals which are incorporated within the nucleotide sequence of the mRNA. In general, two kinds of signal have been reported. First, a so-called *slippery sequence*, downstream of the initiator codon, which contains groups of repeated nucleotides. Second, a so-called *stimulator sequence* – a short distance downstream of the slippery sequence – which appears to be often in the form of an RNA pseudoknot. It appears that, in at least some cases, frameshifting can occur through the influence of the slippery sequence alone, i.e. without assistance from a stimulator.

Frameshifting has been reported in relation to genes from viruses, bacteria, insects and animals. One of the functions of frameshifting is apparently to confer on a given coding sequence the ability to yield more than one type of product.

Studies on the translation of the 3a protein from the SARS (severe acute respiratory syndrome) virus have indicated that heptauridine and octouridine stretches in the mRNA are the sole signals needed for frameshifting in this instance [Nucleic Acids Res (2006) 34(4):1250–1260].

framycetin See AMINOGLYCOSIDE ANTIBIOTICS.

FRET (fluorescence resonance energy transfer) A phenomenon in which energy (that would otherwise be dissipated as fluorescence) is transferred from one molecule or moiety (donor) to another, *closely adjacent* molecule or moiety (acceptor) by a mechanism that does not involve emission of a photon; the energy received by the acceptor molecule or moiety is typically converted to fluorescence, but in some cases is absorbed (*quenched*) without the production of fluorescence.

(Compare BRET; see also IFRET.)

FRET can be exhibited between two regions on the same molecule, one region acting as the donor and the other as the acceptor. One example is the CCF2 substrate (which includes both coumarin and fluorescein moieties): see pcDNA™6.2/ GeneBLAzer™-DEST vector in the table in GATEWAY SITE-SPECIFIC RECOMBINATION SYSTEM.

In general, FRET requires that donor and acceptor molecules be separated by no more than ~100 Å; the separation in experimental protocols is often e.g. 30–70 Å. The donor and acceptor dipoles must also be orientated correctly for effective transmission of energy between the molecules.

In a TAQMAN PROBE (q.v.), energy received by the donor is quenched by the acceptor molecule that is bound adjacently on the oligonucleotide. When the probe is degraded (by the exonuclease activity of the DNA polymerase), the donor and acceptor molecules are separated; the donor molecule (i.e. reporter dye) can therefore exhibit fluorescence because its energy is no longer quenched.

The probes used in the LightCycler™ instrument involve a different arrangement (see REAL-TIME PCR). Fluorescence from the reporter dye (at a wavelength of 640 nm) is detected only if both halves of the probe bind correctly to the target sequence. When this happens, FRET-based excitation of the reporter dye, LightCycler™ Red 640 (present on one half of the probe) occurs by transfer of energy from the fluorescein molecule (on the other half of the probe) because, under these conditions, the donor and acceptor molecules are within the correct distance of one another for effective energy transfer.

In some donor–acceptor pairs the acceptor molecule is a non-fluorescent quencher such as DABCYL or one of the QSY dyes. The QSY dyes are derivatives of diarylrhodamine; their absorption spectra are largely insensitive to a wide range of pH values. The absorption maxima of QSY dyes include e.g. ~660 nm (QSY 21) and ~472 nm (QSY 35). Non-fluorescent acceptors are particularly useful in that they avoid the background fluorescence produced by non-specific excitation of fluorescent acceptor molecules.

The FRET principle has been used in a wide variety of studies involving e.g. detection of hybridization of nucleic acid molecules, the intracellular localization and distribution of specific molecules, the conformation of proteins, enzyme–substrate interaction etc. Note that, in all of these studies, the object is to determine whether or not the donor and acceptor molecules are located sufficiently close to one another in the experimental material to permit FRET-based interaction.

Examples of FRET-based studies include: determination of cell-cycle-dependent localization of proteins in the bacterium *Bacillus subtilis* [EMBO J (2002) 21:3108–3118]; studies on interactions between enzyme and substrate [Proc Natl Acad Sci USA (2002) 99:6603–6606]; studies on quadruplex and Watson–Crick DNA equilibrium [Nucleic Acids Res (2005) 33(21):6723–6732]; the detection of SNPs [BioTechniques (2006) 40(3):323–329]; studies on DNA bending [Proc Natl Acad Sci USA (2006) 103(49):18515–18520]; and studies on homodimer formation of the enzyme signal peptide peptidase [Mol Neurodegener (2006) 1:16].

(See also DARK QUENCHING.)

FRT The recognition site of the FLP recombinase (q.v.).

ftsZ **gene**   In *Escherichia coli*: a gene encoding the FtsZ protein, molecules of which form the Z RING.

fucosidosis   An autosomal recessive disease involving a defective lysosomal enzyme, α-fucosidase, and the accumulation of glycoproteins.

(See also GENETIC DISEASE (table).)

furocoumarins   See PSORALENS.

fusidic acid   A steroidal antibiotic, synthesized by various fungi (e.g. some species of *Acremonium* and *Cylindrocarpon*), that is active against a range of Gram-positive bacteria, including staphylococci; it inhibits protein synthesis by preventing the dissociation of the elongation factor EF-G from the ribosome following translocation.

Resistance to fusidic acid (in e.g. *Staphylococcus aureus*) can arise through mutations that affect EF-G. Such mutations in *S. aureus* are associated with a marked decrease in the biologic fitness of the bacterial cells – e.g. reduced growth in comparison to wild-type strains; this effect is reported to be compensated for by another mutation (designated S416F) in the gene for EF-G [Antimicrob Agents Chemother (2005) 49: 1426–1431].

fusion protein   (1) In some viruses (e.g. paramyxoviruses such as the Sendai virus): a protein that promotes fusion between the virus envelope and the membrane of target cells; these proteins can also promote fusion between host cells. (Another example is the GP64 protein of baculoviruses: see BACULO-VIRIDAE.)

(See also VP22.)

(2) In recombinant DNA technology/genetic engineering: a protein consisting of amino acid residues specified by coding sequences from two different proteins – i.e. a hybrid protein. Fusion proteins can be prepared by the techniques of GENE FUSION.

(See also ENZYME FRAGMENT COMPLEMENTATION.)

fusogen   See CELL FUSION.

G

G Glycine (alternative to Gly).

G-less cassette Essentially, a DNA template which, on transcription, yields RNA that contains no guanosine residues. G-less cassettes are used in *in vitro* transcription assays e.g. for studying transcriptional initiation; in such assays, unwanted transcripts (which contain guanosine residues) are eliminated by treatment of the reaction mixture with RNASE T1.

G loop A loop of unpaired ssDNA in the G region of phage Mu observed when DNA from an induced lysogenic population of the phage is first denatured and then re-annealed; a G loop reflects a local region of non-homology caused by inversion of the G region in the lysogenic population.

G-quadruplex See QUADRUPLEX DNA.

G-quartet A square, planar group of four guanine molecules held together by hydrogen bonds. A stack of G-quartets, with their planes parallel, forms the core of QUADRUPLEX DNA – in which each of four strands of DNA is associated with the N9 position of the aligned guanine molecules that form one corner of the stack of quartets.

Note that some authors [Nucleic Acids Res (2006) 34(Database issue):D119–D124] have used G-quartet as synonymous with G-quadruplex (quadruplex DNA); these authors refer to a G-quartet as a G-tetrad.

G-tetrad See G-QUARTET.

G418 sulfate An antibiotic, related to gentamicin (see AMINOGLYCOSIDE ANTIBIOTIC), active against prokaryotic, yeast, plant and mammalian cells; cell expressing the gene for an aminoglycoside phosphotransferase – such as a neomycin-resistance gene – exhibit resistance to G418 sulfate.

[Uses (examples): PLoS ONE (2007) 2(3):e269; PLoS Biol (2007) 5(3):e64.]

(See also HYGROMYCIN B.)

gag See RETROVIRUSES.

GAL4 A eukaryotic transcription activator. In yeast (*Saccharomyces cerevisiae*), GAL4 is involved in the utilization of galactose; in this role it binds to the corresponding upstream activator sequence (UAS).

(See also PATHDETECT SYSTEMS.)

Galacton™ See CHEMILUMINESCENCE.

β-galactosidase An enzyme (EC 3.2.1.23), encoded by the *lacZ* gene in *Escherichia coli*, which cleaves lactose to glucose and galactose.

(See also LAC OPERON and ONPG.)

The gene for β-galactosidase is widely used as a REPORTER GENE; it is used in various indicator systems such as BLACK–WHITE SCREENING, blue–white screening (see PBLUESCRIPT) and ENZYME FRAGMENT COMPLEMENTATION.

(See also CHEMILUMINESCENCE, α-PEPTIDE, Q TAG and X-GAL.)

gamete A type of cell involved in sexual reproduction – e.g. an egg or a sperm.

γδ (gamma delta) *Syn.* IS1000.

ganciclovir A nucleoside analog which inhibits DNA synthesis after it has been phosphorylated intracellularly.

gap (1) (in dsDNA) A single-stranded region produced by loss of one or more nucleotides. (cf. NICK; see also AP SITE.)

(2) Following SHOTGUN SEQUENCING of a genome (or other large molecule of DNA): a region for which no cloned fragments are available.

gapped vector A linear VECTOR molecule prepared e.g. by introducing a double-strand break in a ccc DNA vector [see e.g. Proc Natl Acad Sci USA (2005) 102(18):6413–6418].

Gateway® site-specific recombination system Various types of product (Invitrogen, Carlsbad CA) which can be used e.g. to move a given sequence into, or between, vector molecules for expression or directional cloning, and which are based on a site-specific recombination system of PHAGE LAMBDA that involves the ATT SITES.

Thus, e.g. a segment flanked by *att*P sites can be replaced by a segment flanked by *att*B sites. During this process, the inserted sequence becomes flanked by hybrid (*att*B–*att*P) sites referred to as *att*L sites; the displaced segment is also flanked by hybrid sites (referred to as *att*R sites). This procedure is mediated by BP CLONASE.

Similarly, a segment flanked by *att*R sites can be replaced with one flanked by *att*L sites; this results in reconstitution of the *att*B and *att*P sites (*att*B sites then flanking one of the segments, and *att*P sites flanking the other). This procedure is mediated by LR CLONASE.

Entry clones and destination vectors
Entry into the Gateway® system (for cloning, expression) can be achieved e.g. via PCR. Thus, the sequence of interest can be amplified with primers whose 5′ ends incorporate an *att*B sequence. The amplicons can be inserted (*in vitro*) e.g. into a pDONR™ vector to form a so-called *entry clone*; by inserting into a pDONR™ vector, an amplicon displaces the *ccdB* gene (see CCD MECHANISM) that is flanked by *att*P sites (thus permitting subsequent recovery of recombinants). The vectors are inserted (e.g. by transformation) into *Escherichia coli*; following growth, cells containing recombinant vectors are selected on a medium containing kanamycin or Zeocin™ (pDONR™ vectors contain either a kanamycin-resistance or a ZEOCIN-resistance gene).

The sequence of interest, within the entry clone, can then be transferred to any of a range of *destination vectors* (see accompanying table) in order to carry out a particular task.

Also available are so-called *entry vectors* (containing *att* sites) which include a polylinker for the insertion of a DNA sequence with restriction enzymes and ligase; the resulting entry clone can then be used to create an expression clone by transferring the sequence to a given destination vector.

(See also MULTISITE GATEWAY TECHNOLOGY and TOPOISOMERASE I CLONING.)

gatifloxacin See QUINOLONE ANTIBIOTICS.

GC-profile See ISOCHORE.

GC type See BASE RATIO.

Gateway® DESTINATION VECTORS: examples of some of the wide range of vectors to which a gene or fragment of interest can be transferred from a Gateway® entry clone. Every destination vector contains *att*R sites which can be used for recombination with any sequence that is flanked by *att*L sites[a]

Vector	Size	Properties/notes
Cell-free protein expression systems		
pEXP3-DEST	4.6 kb	T7 promoter and terminator for high-level expression. N-terminal SIX-HISTIDINE TAG and LUMIO tag to assist purification and detection; cleavage site for efficient removal of tags. (See also entry CELL-FREE PROTEIN SYNTHESIS.)
pEXP4-DEST	4.4 kb	T7 promoter and terminator for high-level expression. C-terminal SIX-HISTIDINE TAG and LUMIO tag for purification and detection
Expression of proteins in Escherichia coli		
Champion™ pET104-DEST	7.6 kb	T7 promoter and terminator for strong expression of recombinant proteins. Transcription regulation via a LacO operator. N-terminal BIOEASE tag permitting IN VIVO BIOTINYLATION of fusion proteins
pBAD-DEST49	6.2 kb	*araBAD* promoter providing tight regulation of expression of toxic proteins. Improved solubility of protein product provided by N-terminal thioredoxin fusion partner. SIX-HISTIDINE TAG to facilitate detection/purification of product
Expression of proteins in Saccharomyces cerevisiae		
pYES-DEST52	7.8 kb	High-level expression of protein product provided by the *GAL1* promoter. Detection and purification of the product facilitated by a C-terminal SIX-HISTIDINE TAG
Expression of proteins in insect cells		
BaculoDirect™		Insertion of gene/fragment of interest generates a recombinant baculovirus genome. Any non-recombinant vectors are negatively selected by expression of the thymidine kinase gene in the presence of ganciclovir. The *lacZ* gene (excised during insertion of the gene/fragment) permits checking of viral stock purity. C-terminal or N-terminal SIX-HISTIDINE TAG for purification. One version of the vector includes a MELITTIN secretion signal to promote secretion of the expressed protein
pMT-DEST48	5.3 kb	Designed for expression in *Drosophila* S2 cells. Transcription from a metallothionein promoter can be induced e.g. with copper sulfate or with cadmium chloride. SIX-HISTIDINE TAG for purification
Expression of proteins (and shRNAs) in mammalian cells		
pAd/CMV/V5-DEST™	36.7 kb	The plasmid includes a replication-deficient part of the adenovirus genome (lacking sequences in the E1 and E3 regions). A population of the recombinant molecules, consisting of the gene of interest integrated in the plasmid, is linearized (by restriction enzyme PacI), leaving the ITRs (inverted terminal repeats) of the viral genome as the flanking sequences. This construct is used to transfect specialized cells (cell line 293A) within which replication-incompetent (but infectious) virus particles are produced; these particles can be used to infect *target* cells and, hence, to deliver the gene of interest. The CMV promoter provides a high level of expression
pBLOCK-iT™3-DEST	5.9 kb	A vector designed for long-term expression of shRNAs (see entry SHORT HAIRPIN RNA). Expression may be made either constitutive or inducible, depending on the type of entry vector used. Geneticin®-selectable (neomycin-resistance gene)
pBLOCK-iT™6-DEST	5.5 kb	Similar to pBLOCK-iT™3-DEST but smaller, and blasticidin-selectable
pcDNA™6/BioEase™-DEST	7.0 kb	High-level expression from the CMV promoter. Blasticidin-selectable. The BIOEASE tag facilitates purification of *in vivo* biotinylated recombinant proteins; the fusion tag can be excised via an adjacent enterokinase cleavage site

(*continued*)

Vector	Size	Properties/notes
pcDNA™6.2/GeneBLAzer™-DEST		A fusion vector in which the gene of interest is fused (in N- or C-terminal orientation) to a mammalian-optimized β-lactamase gene (*bla*) which acts as a reporter gene. Reporter activity depends on the FRET (q.v.) principle. Cells are permeated with a FRET substrate (CCF2) – the molecule of which incorporates two fluorophores: coumarin and fluorescein. Cells in which *bla* is *not* expressed emit green light (520 nm) on excitation (409 nm) due to FRET-based interaction between coumarin and fluorescein. If *bla* is expressed, CCF2 is cleaved; excitation (at 409 nm) then causes simple (non-FRET-based) fluorescence from the coumarin moiety: blue light at 447 nm. The CMV promoter provides high-level expression of the fusion protein. Blasticidin-selectable. A related vector includes the option of topo cloning (see TOPOISOMERASE I CLONING) as well as the facility of a Gateway® destination vector; it also contains a CMV promoter and is blasticidin-selectable
pcDNA™6.2/nLumio™-DEST™	6.8 kb	High-level constitutive expression provided by the CMV promoter. The LUMIO tag facilitates detection and/or localization of the protein of interest either *in vivo* (in living cells) or *in vitro*
pEF5/FRT/V5-DEST™	7.5 kb	For inserting a gene of interest into cells of an FLP-IN CELL LINE. EF-1α promoter for use in those parental cells (e.g. BHK) in which the CMV promoter is not optimal. Bovine growth hormone (BGH) polyadenylation signal and transcription termination to promote stability of transcript. Hygromycin-resistance gene for selection of recombinant vectors
pLenti6/V5-DEST™	8.7 kb	A lentiviral expression vector incorporating the 5′-LTR and 3′-LTR sequences for insertion into the target cell's genome. The vector, carrying the gene of interest, is co-transfected into a producer cell line (293FT) together with plasmids encoding (i) the lentiviral packaging proteins, and (ii) the VSV-G envelope protein (the latter protein confers on a viral particle the ability to infect a broad range of types of mammalian cell). The recombinant (replication-incompetent) lentiviral particles, produced in the 293FT cells, can be used to infect *target* cells, within which the gene of interest is expressed. The CMV promoter normally provides high-level expression. The pLenti6/UbC/V5-DEST™ vector contains the (human) ubiquitin C (UbC) promoter (instead of CMV) for efficient expression when CMV is inappropriate. A blasticidin-resistance gene is incorporated for selection of stable cell lines
pT-REx™-DEST31	7.5 kb	Strong, tetracycline-regulated CMV promoter, two copies of the $TetO_2$ operator being downstream of the promoter. Geneticin®-selectable. SIX-HISTIDINE TAG to facilitate purification
pVAX™200-DEST		A small vector designed specifically for use in the development of DNA VACCINES. In order to minimize the possibility of integration into the chromosome, the plasmid includes only the minimal amount of eukaryotic DNA necessary for expression. The polylinker permits insertion of DNA from PCR-generated fragments etc. as well as from Gateway® entry clones

[a]Descriptions of products are derived from data provided by courtesy of Invitrogen Corporation, Carlsbad CA, USA.

GC% (GC value; %GC; mol% G + C etc.)   Of *bacterial* DNA: the ratio (G + C)/(A + T + G + C) in which A, T, G and C are the relative molar amounts of adenine, thymine, guanine and cytosine residues, respectively, in the DNA of a given organism; the ratio is expressed as a percentage. (cf. BASE RATIO.)

The value of GC% depends on genus and species. It is one of the criteria used in taxonomy, although similarity in GC%, in itself, is not an indicator of taxonomic affinity. In bacteria, GC% values range from ~25 to ~75; for example, the GC% of *Staphylococcus aureus* is ~33, and that of *Mycobacterium tuberculosis* is ~66.

GC% is useful as a descriptor e.g. for chromosomal DNA, for specific sequences of nucleotides in chromosomal DNA, and for plasmid DNA etc. In some pathogenic bacteria the genome includes certain sequences of nucleotides (so-called *pathogenicity islands*) in which the GC% differs from that of

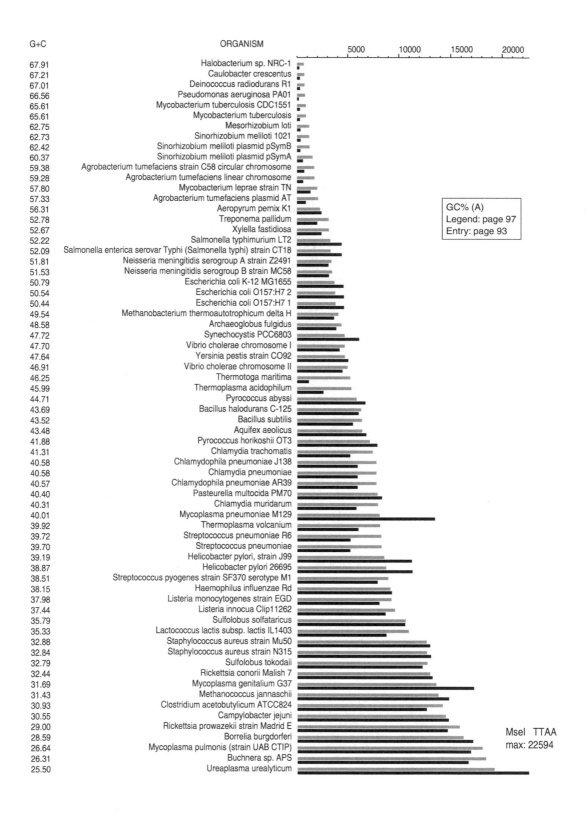

G+C	ORGANISM		
		5000 10000 15000 20000	

67.91 Halobacterium sp. NRC-1
67.21 Caulobacter crescentus
67.01 Deinococcus radiodurans R1
66.56 Pseudomonas aeruginosa PA01
65.61 Mycobacterium tuberculosis CDC1551
65.61 Mycobacterium tuberculosis
62.75 Mesorhizobium loti
62.73 Sinorhizobium meliloti 1021
62.42 Sinorhizobium meliloti plasmid pSymB
60.37 Sinorhizobium meliloti plasmid pSymA
59.38 Agrobacterium tumefaciens strain C58 circular chromosome
59.28 Agrobacterium tumefaciens linear chromosome
57.80 Mycobacterium leprae strain TN
57.33 Agrobacterium tumefaciens plasmid AT
56.31 Aeropyrum pernix K1
52.78 Treponema pallidum
52.67 Xylella fastidiosa
52.22 Salmonella typhimurium LT2
52.09 Salmonella enterica serovar Typhi (Salmonella typhi) strain CT18
51.81 Neisseria meningitidis serogroup A strain Z2491
51.53 Neisseria meningitidis serogroup B strain MC58
50.79 Escherichia coli K-12 MG1655
50.54 Escherichia coli O157:H7 2
50.44 Escherichia coli O157:H7 1
49.54 Methanobacterium thermoautotrophicum delta H
48.58 Archaeoglobus fulgidus
47.72 Synechocystis PCC6803
47.70 Vibrio cholerae chromosome I
47.64 Yersinia pestis strain CO92
46.91 Vibrio cholerae chromosome II
46.25 Thermotoga maritima
45.99 Thermoplasma acidophilum
44.71 Pyrococcus abyssi
43.69 Bacillus halodurans C-125
43.52 Bacillus subtilis
43.48 Aquifex aeolicus
41.88 Pyrococcus horikoshii OT3
41.31 Chlamydia trachomatis
40.58 Chlamydophila pneumoniae J138
40.58 Chlamydia pneumoniae
40.57 Chlamydophila pneumoniae AR39
40.40 Pasteurella multocida PM70
40.31 Chlamydia muridarum
40.01 Mycoplasma pneumoniae M129
39.92 Thermoplasma volcanium
39.72 Streptococcus pneumoniae R6
39.70 Streptococcus pneumoniae
39.19 Helicobacter pylori, strain J99
38.87 Helicobacter pylori 26695
38.51 Streptococcus pyogenes strain SF370 serotype M1
38.15 Haemophilus influenzae Rd
37.98 Listeria monocytogenes strain EGD
37.44 Listeria innocua Clip11262
35.79 Sulfolobus solfataricus
35.33 Lactococcus lactis subsp. lactis IL1403
32.88 Staphylococcus aureus strain Mu50
32.84 Staphylococcus aureus strain N315
32.79 Sulfolobus tokodaii
32.44 Rickettsia conorii Malish 7
31.69 Mycoplasma genitalium G37
31.43 Methanococcus jannaschii
30.93 Clostridium acetobutylicum ATCC824
30.55 Campylobacter jejuni
29.00 Rickettsia prowazekii strain Madrid E
28.59 Borrelia burgdorferi
26.64 Mycoplasma pulmonis (strain UAB CTIP)
26.31 Buchnera sp. APS
25.50 Ureaplasma urealyticum

GC% (A)
Legend: page 97
Entry: page 93

Msel TTAA
max: 22594

G+C	ORGANISM	
		50 100 150 200 250 300 350

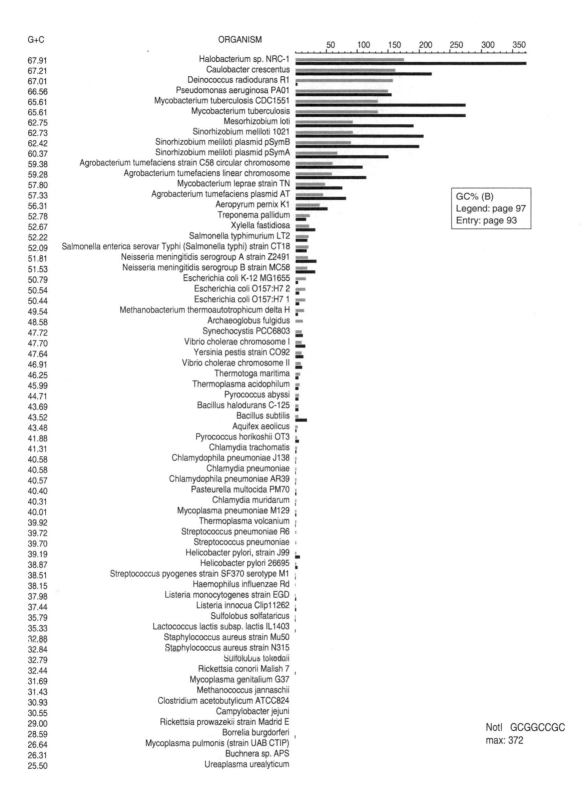

G+C	ORGANISM
67.91	Halobacterium sp. NRC-1
67.21	Caulobacter crescentus
67.01	Deinococcus radiodurans R1
66.56	Pseudomonas aeruginosa PA01
65.61	Mycobacterium tuberculosis CDC1551
65.61	Mycobacterium tuberculosis
62.75	Mesorhizobium loti
62.73	Sinorhizobium meliloti 1021
62.42	Sinorhizobium meliloti plasmid pSymB
60.37	Sinorhizobium meliloti plasmid pSymA
59.38	Agrobacterium tumefaciens strain C58 circular chromosome
59.28	Agrobacterium tumefaciens linear chromosome
57.80	Mycobacterium leprae strain TN
57.33	Agrobacterium tumefaciens plasmid AT
56.31	Aeropyrum pernix K1
52.78	Treponema pallidum
52.67	Xylella fastidiosa
52.22	Salmonella typhimurium LT2
52.09	Salmonella enterica serovar Typhi (Salmonella typhi) strain CT18
51.81	Neisseria meningitidis serogroup A strain Z2491
51.53	Neisseria meningitidis serogroup B strain MC58
50.79	Escherichia coli K-12 MG1655
50.54	Escherichia coli O157:H7 2
50.44	Escherichia coli O157:H7 1
49.54	Methanobacterium thermoautotrophicum delta H
48.58	Archaeoglobus fulgidus
47.72	Synechocystis PCC6803
47.70	Vibrio cholerae chromosome I
47.64	Yersinia pestis strain CO92
46.91	Vibrio cholerae chromosome II
46.25	Thermotoga maritima
45.99	Thermoplasma acidophilum
44.71	Pyrococcus abyssi
43.69	Bacillus halodurans C-125
43.52	Bacillus subtilis
43.48	Aquifex aeolicus
41.88	Pyrococcus horikoshii OT3
41.31	Chlamydia trachomatis
40.58	Chlamydophila pneumoniae J138
40.58	Chlamydia pneumoniae
40.57	Chlamydophila pneumoniae AR39
40.40	Pasteurella multocida PM70
40.31	Chlamydia muridarum
40.01	Mycoplasma pneumoniae M129
39.92	Thermoplasma volcanium
39.72	Streptococcus pneumoniae R6
39.70	Streptococcus pneumoniae
39.19	Helicobacter pylori, strain J99
38.87	Helicobacter pylori 26695
38.51	Streptococcus pyogenes strain SF370 serotype M1
38.15	Haemophilus influenzae Rd
37.98	Listeria monocytogenes strain EGD
37.44	Listeria innocua Clip11262
35.79	Sulfolobus solfataricus
35.33	Lactococcus lactis subsp. lactis IL1403
32.88	Staphylococcus aureus strain Mu50
32.84	Staphylococcus aureus strain N315
32.79	Sulfolobus tokodaii
32.44	Rickettsia conorii Malish 7
31.69	Mycoplasma genitalium G37
31.43	Methanococcus jannaschii
30.93	Clostridium acetobutylicum ATCC824
30.55	Campylobacter jejuni
29.00	Rickettsia prowazekii strain Madrid E
28.59	Borrelia burgdorferi
26.64	Mycoplasma pulmonis (strain UAB CTIP)
26.31	Buchnera sp. APS
25.50	Ureaplasma urealyticum

GC% (B)
Legend: page 97
Entry: page 93

NotI GCGGCCGC
max: 372

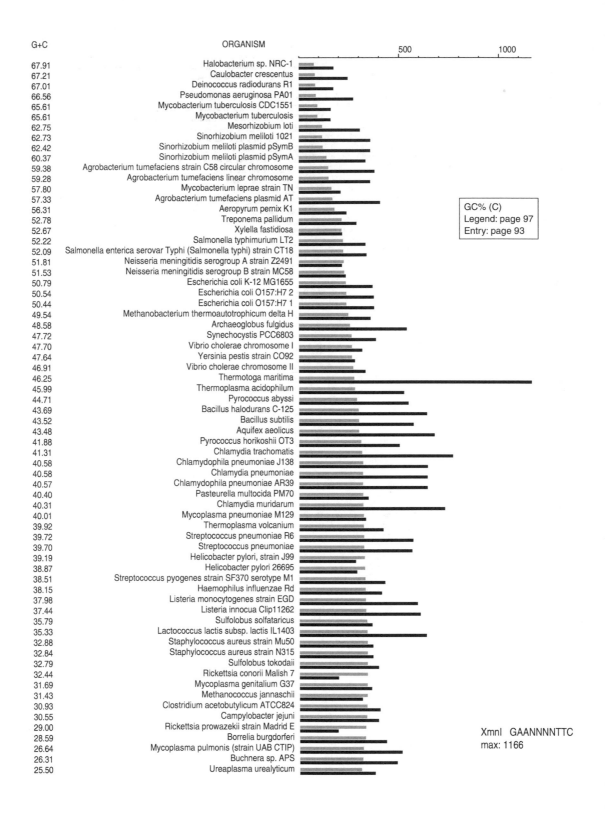

G+C	ORGANISM		500	1000
67.91	Halobacterium sp. NRC-1			
67.21	Caulobacter crescentus			
67.01	Deinococcus radiodurans R1			
66.56	Pseudomonas aeruginosa PA01			
65.61	Mycobacterium tuberculosis CDC1551			
65.61	Mycobacterium tuberculosis			
62.75	Mesorhizobium loti			
62.73	Sinorhizobium meliloti 1021			
62.42	Sinorhizobium meliloti plasmid pSymB			
60.37	Sinorhizobium meliloti plasmid pSymA			
59.38	Agrobacterium tumefaciens strain C58 circular chromosome			
59.28	Agrobacterium tumefaciens linear chromosome			
57.80	Mycobacterium leprae strain TN			
57.33	Agrobacterium tumefaciens plasmid AT			
56.31	Aeropyrum pernix K1			
52.78	Treponema pallidum			
52.67	Xylella fastidiosa			
52.22	Salmonella typhimurium LT2			
52.09	Salmonella enterica serovar Typhi (Salmonella typhi) strain CT18			
51.81	Neisseria meningitidis serogroup A strain Z2491			
51.53	Neisseria meningitidis serogroup B strain MC58			
50.79	Escherichia coli K-12 MG1655			
50.54	Escherichia coli O157:H7 2			
50.44	Escherichia coli O157:H7 1			
49.54	Methanobacterium thermoautotrophicum delta H			
48.58	Archaeoglobus fulgidus			
47.72	Synechocystis PCC6803			
47.70	Vibrio cholerae chromosome I			
47.64	Yersinia pestis strain CO92			
46.91	Vibrio cholerae chromosome II			
46.25	Thermotoga maritima			
45.99	Thermoplasma acidophilum			
44.71	Pyrococcus abyssi			
43.69	Bacillus halodurans C-125			
43.52	Bacillus subtilis			
43.48	Aquifex aeolicus			
41.88	Pyrococcus horikoshii OT3			
41.31	Chlamydia trachomatis			
40.58	Chlamydophila pneumoniae J138			
40.58	Chlamydia pneumoniae			
40.57	Chlamydophila pneumoniae AR39			
40.40	Pasteurella multocida PM70			
40.31	Chlamydia muridarum			
40.01	Mycoplasma pneumoniae M129			
39.92	Thermoplasma volcanium			
39.72	Streptococcus pneumoniae R6			
39.70	Streptococcus pneumoniae			
39.19	Helicobacter pylori, strain J99			
38.87	Helicobacter pylori 26695			
38.51	Streptococcus pyogenes strain SF370 serotype M1			
38.15	Haemophilus influenzae Rd			
37.98	Listeria monocytogenes strain EGD			
37.44	Listeria innocua Clip11262			
35.79	Sulfolobus solfataricus			
35.33	Lactococcus lactis subsp. lactis IL1403			
32.88	Staphylococcus aureus strain Mu50			
32.84	Staphylococcus aureus strain N315			
32.79	Sulfolobus tokodaii			
32.44	Rickettsia conorii Malish 7			
31.69	Mycoplasma genitalium G37			
31.43	Methanococcus jannaschii			
30.93	Clostridium acetobutylicum ATCC824			
30.55	Campylobacter jejuni			
29.00	Rickettsia prowazekii strain Madrid E			
28.59	Borrelia burgdorferi			
26.64	Mycoplasma pulmonis (strain UAB CTIP)			
26.31	Buchnera sp. APS			
25.50	Ureaplasma urealyticum			

GC% (C)
Legend: page 97
Entry: page 93

XmnI GAANNNNTTC
max: 1166

the remainder of the chromosomal DNA; this has been taken to indicate that such sequences of nucleotides were imported into the genome from an extracellular source.

A knowledge of the GC% of an organism's DNA may be useful for assessing the susceptibility of the DNA to a given RESTRICTION ENDONUCLEASE. For example, the restriction enzyme NotI (recognition site GC↓GGCCGC) lacks cutting sites in the genomic DNA of *Staphylococcus aureus* but has more than 250 cutting sites in *Mycobacterium tuberculosis*. Charts which show the cutting frequency of various types of restriction endonuclease in the genomic DNA of a range of bacteria and archaeans can be found on the Internet (see entry REBASE for details of access); some examples of these charts are shown in the figure. The choice of restriction enzyme is important e.g. in RFLP ANALYSIS.

An indirect indication of the GC% of a given sample of DNA may be obtained from its 'melting point' (see THERMAL MELTING PROFILE) owing to the linear relationship between T_m and GC% (a high T_m correlating with a high GC%). It is also possible to assess GC% by ultracentrifugation in a CsCl density gradient.

In any determination of genomic GC%, the presence of a plasmid (especially a high-copy-number plasmid) may affect the observed value because the GC% of the plasmid may not be similar to that of the chromosomal DNA. When isolating chromosomal DNA it is therefore necessary to use a method that discriminates against extrachromosomal DNA.

GC% in eukaryotic/mammalian DNA

G + C content is also used to describe regions in eukaryotic/mammalian DNA. For example, human genomic DNA can be divided into >3000 regions called *isochores*, each isochore characterized by a uniform or near-uniform G + C content; the isochores in human genomic DNA fall into five groups on the basis of their G + C values. [Isochore mapping of the human genome: Genome Res (2006) 16(4):536–541.]

The DNA of CPG ISLANDS is typically characterized by a value higher than ~60%. This high value of G + C content is associated with susceptibility to certain types of 'rare-cutting' RESTRICTION ENDONUCLEASE; for example, more than 85% of the recognition sites of the restriction endonuclease NotI in the human genome are found in CpG islands.

G-CSF Granulocyte colony-stimulating factor – see e.g. entry

GEL ELECTROPHORESIS: examples of concentrations of agarose and acrylamide in gels used for separating nucleic acid fragments of different sizes (from various sources)

Nucleic acid fragment (linear dsDNA, in bp)	Agarose gel (% agarose)	Polyacrylamide gel (% acrylamide)
20000–100000	0.3	
1000–30000	0.5	
800–12000	0.7	
500–10000	1.0	
400–7000	1.2	
200–3000	1.5	
100–1000		3.5
50–2000	2.0	
60–400		8.0
50–200		12.0
10–500	4.0	
5–100		20.0

BIOPHARMACEUTICAL (table).

gefitinib An anticancer agent which inhibits oncogenic (EGF receptor) TYROSINE KINASE activity.
(cf. IMATINIB.)

gel electrophoresis A form of ELECTROPHORESIS used e.g. for separating fragments of nucleic acid, of different sizes and/or conformations, in a gel medium. (cf. ISOTACHOPHORESIS.)

Following electrophoresis, the separated fragments may be stained *in situ* (i.e. in the gel), extracted from the gel (for ongoing study), or transferred to another medium (see e.g. SOUTHERN BLOTTING). In some cases, fragments are labeled (e.g. with a fluorophore) before electrophoresis; in such cases the label is read from the bands of fragments that develop in the gel during electrophoresis.

In methods such as NASBA and PCR, gel electrophoresis is

GC% (*opposite*) The effect of GC% on the cutting frequencies of three restriction endonucleases in the genomic DNA of various bacteria and archaeans.

The organisms are arranged in order of the GC% of their genomic DNA – the highest value (67.91) at the top, the lowest (25.5) at the bottom.

For a given organism, the solid black bar represents the observed number of recognition sites (see scale at top of chart) in the genomic DNA of that organism. The adjacent gray bar represents the expected number of cutting sites.

(A) Restriction endonuclease MseI. Cutting site: T↓TAA
(B) Restriction endonuclease NotI. Cutting site: GC↓GGCCGC
(C) Restriction endonuclease XmnI. Cutting site: GAANN↓NNTTC

Charts supplied by, and reproduced by courtesy of, Dr Janos Posfai and Tamas Vincze, New England Biolabs, Ipswich MA, USA.

used e.g. to check that amplicons of the expected length are produced in the reaction. To facilitate measurement of length, use can be made of a 'DNA ladder'; this consists of a set of DNA fragments, in a range of known sizes, which undergo electrophoresis in a lane parallel to the lane(s) in which test sample(s) are being examined. Following electrophoresis, the size of the fragment in a given 'experimental' band is assessed by comparison with those bands in the DNA ladder that have migrated at a similar rate.

For nucleic acids, the matrix used in gel electrophoresis is commonly AGAROSE or POLYACRYLAMIDE; agarose is used for separating large fragments, while polyacrylamide is used for the smaller fragments (see table).

(See also NOVEX GELS.)

gel shift assay *Syn.* EMSA.

geldanamycin A benzoquinoid compound, produced by strains of *Streptomyces*, that inhibits heat-shock protein 90 (Hsp90) and which was reported to inhibit the expression of c-*myc* in murine lymphoblastoma cells.

gellan gum A bacterial product (a linear polymer containing residues of glucose, rhamnose and glucuronic acid) that has been recommended as a gelling agent for bacterial growth media used in the context of PCR (agar inhibits PCR) [J Med Microbiol (2001) 50:108–109].

Purified gellan gum is available commercially (Gelrite®; Kelco, San Diego CA).

Gelrite® See GELLAN GUM.

gemifloxacin See QUINOLONE ANTIBIOTICS.

GenBank A major DATABASE forming part of the INTERNATIONAL NUCLEOTIDE SEQUENCE DATABASE COLLABORATION.

(See also gene ACCESSION NUMBER.)

gender determination assay See DNA SEX DETERMINATION ASSAY.

gene A specific sequence of nucleotides in DNA (in cells and certain viruses), or in RNA (in other viruses), that encodes a given polypeptide or an RNA molecule with a biosynthetic or control function.

(See also ALLELE.)

gene cassette See CASSETTE.

gene cloning See CLONING.

gene conversion Conversion of one allele into another. Gene conversion can occur e.g. following hybridization between one strand from each of a pair of non-identical alleles; during the repair of this heteroduplex (in which *one* of the strands is used as template) the sequence of one strand is converted to a sequence which is complementary to that of the other.

(See also MATING TYPE.)

gene-delivery system Any system used for inserting gene(s) (or other fragments of DNA) into target cell(s) – often with the object of expression within those cells.

There are various types of gene-delivery vehicle – such as e.g. plasmids, cosmids and viruses (including animal viruses, phages, phagemid particles); these generally involve circular molecules of nucleic acid into which target DNA is inserted

prior to TRANSFECTION (sense 1). (Compare LAMBDA (λ) RED RECOMBINATION and BIGEASY LINEAR CLONING SYSTEM.) (See also SPINOCULATION.)

Viral vectors (in which the target DNA is incorporated in a recombinant or modified viral genome) internalize this DNA when they infect cells. Commercial gene-delivery systems include e.g. the AAV HELPER-FREE SYSTEM, the ADEASY XL ADENOVIRAL VECTOR SYSTEM and the VIRAPORT RETROVIRAL GENE EXPRESSION SYSTEM.

Plasmids, and other molecules of naked nucleic acid which contain target DNA, are often inserted into cells by transformation or by ELECTROPORATION.

Other modes of gene delivery include LIPOFECTION, MAGNETOFECTION and MICROINJECTION. (See also PEI.)

(See also GENE GUN.)

gene expression profile The pattern of *expression* (i.e. active, non-active, level of activity) of the genes in a given tissue, cell or organism at a particular time under given conditions.

gene-for-gene concept (*plant pathol.*) An early concept – relating to interactions between plants and plant pathogens – in which e.g. a specific *avirulence gene* in a given pathogen interacts with the corresponding *resistance gene* in one or more strains of the host species. Such interaction enables the host strain(s) to give a defensive response (*hypersensitivity reaction*) and hence exhibit resistance to the given pathogen.

Interaction between the products of avirulence and resistance genes was reported e.g. in rice plants challenged with the pathogen which causes rice blast disease, *Magnaporthe grisea* (*Pyricularia oryzae*) [EMBO J (2000) 19:4004–4014].

gene fusion In recombinant DNA technology/genetic engineering: any process in which sequences of nucleotides from two distinct genes are joined together, with their reading frames in phase, so that transcription from a single promoter region produces an mRNA transcript that encodes a hybrid *fusion protein*; the fusion protein may or may not have biological activity – or functionality may be limited to particular part(s) of the protein.

Gene fusion may be carried out in various ways – e.g. by deleting a sequence of nucleotides between two contiguous genes so as to provide a single, continuous coding sequence controlled via the first (upstream) gene. More generally, it can be achieved e.g. by using a plasmid vector to insert a given gene, in frame, with a *partner* gene; such a procedure may be carried out *in vitro* or *in vivo*.

Fusions of the type described above are sometimes referred to as *translational fusions* because they give rise to a fusion protein whose synthesis requires both transcription and translation signals from the upstream fusion partner. By contrast, a *transcriptional fusion* is one in which, through engineering, the genes of interest are subjected to a common mode of regulation; in this case the genes themselves are not fused, and no fusion protein is formed.

Uses of gene fusion

● To facilitate detection/isolation of a specific gene product. If a gene product is difficult to detect (or to assay), the gene may be fused with a partner gene (= *carrier gene*) encoding a readily detectable product. The partner gene might encode, for example, glutathione *S*-transferase (GST) – in which case the fusion protein (with a GST *affinity tail*) can be isolated by using AFFINITY CHROMATOGRAPHY with glutathione in the stationary phase. A target protein from a thermophilic organism might be isolated e.g. by fusion with a temperature-stable lectin-based affinity tail [BioTechniques (2006) 41(3):327–332].

(See also FLAG and PESC VECTORS.)

● To determine the intracellular location of a given protein using a reporter system such as GFP (GREEN FLUORESCENT PROTEIN) as a fusion partner. Fusion with GFP permits the (intracellular) target protein to be detected by fluorescence microscopy. In one early study, the gene for FtsZ protein (see Z RING) was fused to that of GFP, enabling a remarkable photographic image of the Z ring of *Escherichia coli* to be obtained [Proc Natl Acad Sci USA (1996) 93:12998–13003].

The use of GFP (or other fluorescent protein partners such as MONOMERIC RED FLUORESCENT PROTEIN) places limitations on this technique in terms of excitation/emission wavelengths. In an alternative approach, a fusion protein consists of the protein of interest fused with O^6-alkylguanine-DNA alkyltransferase (AGT). The advantage here is that AGT can be labeled *in vivo*, i.e. within living cells, by any of a range of fluorophores (derivatives of O^6-benzylguanine) – of which many are cell-permeable; thus, an AGT fusion protein which is expressed intracellularly can be labeled by incubating the cells in a medium that contains one of the cell-permeable fluorophores. (O^6-benzylguanine derivatives that are not cell-permeable may be internalized by microinjection.) Labeling of AGT fusion proteins with an O^6-benzylguanine derivative involves a covalent bond. The AGT approach permits flexibility because the O^6-benzylguanine derivatives are available with a wide range of emission spectra (from 472 nm to 673 nm) [BioTechniques (2006) 41(2):167–175].

AGT is a normal (eukaryotic) DNA repair enzyme which transfers alkyl groups from a guanine residue to a cysteine residue on the enzyme (thereby inactivating the enzyme). The (unwanted) labeling of *endogenous* molecules of AGT within the cells under test has been regarded as a disadvantage of the AGT technique, although such labeling apparently does not occur to any significant degree in at least some mammalian cell lines. Moreover, use can be made of a mutant form of AGT (^{M}AGT); this mutant form of AGT can be labeled in the presence of N^9-cyclopentyl-O^6-(4-bromo-thenyl)guanine – a compound which blocks labeling of wild-type AGT. Another advantage of ^{M}AGT is that its affinity for alkylated DNA is lower than that of the wild-type protein; thus, it is less likely (than the wild-type AGT) to be inactivated by functioning as a repair enzyme.

● To increase the solubility of a target protein: see, for example, CHAMPION PET SUMO VECTOR.

● To obtain a gene product which is normally not highly expressed. The relevant (target) gene may be fused downstream

of a highly expressed gene in an expression vector; given an appropriate choice, the partner gene may contribute increased solubility/stability to the fusion product.

● To modify the mobility of the target protein. For example, the fusion partner VP22 confers on a target protein the ability to translocate from a given mammalian cell to an adjacent cell in a cell culture (see VOYAGER VECTORS).

● To engineer the secretion of a given protein that normally remains intracellular. Fusion with a gene whose product is normally secreted may enable secretion of the target protein as part of the fusion product.

● To study the regulation of gene expression. For example, if there are problems in monitoring the expression of a given gene (perhaps due to difficulty in assaying the gene product), it may be possible to monitor activity of the gene's *promoter* (rather than the whole gene). For this purpose, a promoterless *reporter gene* (encoding a readily detectable product) can be fused downstream of the target gene's promoter; the promoter's activity can then be monitored via the product of the reporter gene. Examples of reporter genes include those encoding GFP, galactokinase and chloramphenicol acetyltransferase. Expression of the *lacZ* gene (encoding β-galactosidase) in a *lacZ* fusion product can be monitored on media containing X-GAL.

The use of reporter genes in this way generally works well. However, an early report [J Bacteriol (1994) 176:2128–2132] indicated that certain reporter genes are able to influence the activity of certain promoters; this serves as a useful reminder that unpredictable interactions between components may take place in recombinant DNA systems.

● To detect/identify specific organisms. In a novel approach, GFP was fused to the coat protein of a strain-specific phage and used for the rapid detection of the pathogenic bacterium *Escherichia coli* strain O157:H7 [Appl Environ Microbiol (2004) 70:527–534].

● See also ENZYME FRAGMENT COMPLEMENTATION.

Cleavage of fusion proteins

It may be possible to obtain a separate product from each of the two fusion genes by cleavage of the fusion protein. Given an appropriate and accessible sequence of amino acids at the junction region, cleavage may be achieved by a site-specific protease (see e.g. GST in GENE FUSION VECTOR).

(See also CHAMPION PET SUMO VECTOR and TEV protease in the entry TEV.)

Cleavage may also be carried out with chemical agents, e.g. hydroxylamine (which cleaves between adjacent residues of glycine and asparagine) or cyanogen bromide (which cleaves at methionine residues); the problems with chemical cleavage include unwanted modification (by the agent) and cleavage at sites *within* the target protein.

gene fusion vector An EXPRESSION VECTOR that includes a sequence encoding a *partner gene* – such as glutathione *S*-transferase (GST); the sequence from a target gene is inserted in the correct reading frame, adjacent to the partner gene, and both genes are jointly transcribed and translated as a single product (a so-called *fusion protein*). The fusion protein may be cleavable to separate products; for example, a GST partner has a recognition site for a site-specific protease close to the fusion boundary.

gene gun A device used e.g. for the intraepidermal inoculation of a DNA VACCINE. The DNA is coated onto μm-scale gold particles which are internalized via a pressure-based system. [Example of use (in mice): Infect Immun (2005) 73(5):2974–2985.]

gene knock-out *Syn.* KNOCK-OUT MUTATION.

gene product (gp) The (final) product formed by the expression of a given gene: either a protein (formed via the mRNA intermediate) or an RNA molecule which is not translated – e.g. a molecule of rRNA or tRNA.

Specific gene products, i.e. products formed by the expression of specific genes, may be designated e.g. as gp32, gp120 etc., the numbers reflecting particular genes in a given organism.

gene shuffling See DNA SHUFFLING.

gene silencing A term applied to any (natural or *in vitro*) process that tends to block gene expression (see, for example, EXPONENTIAL SILENCING, MICRORNA, MORPHOLINO ANTISENSE OLIGOMER, PTGS, RIBOSWITCH, RNA INTERFERENCE).

(See also transcriptional gene silencing in the entry SIRNA.)

In many eukaryotes (including plants), methylation of DNA sequences may promote the recruitment of specific binding proteins which – either by themselves or as part of a complex – recruit other agents (such as histone deacetylases), resulting in a localized region of repressed chromatin.

DNA methylation is involved in gene silencing in various contexts, including e.g. imprinting, differentiation and tumor development

(See also DEMETHYLATION.)

gene targeting A procedure used to produce precise *in vivo* changes in genomic DNA at predetermined sites. Typically, this has been achieved by transfecting cells with a vector, e.g. a plasmid, containing an insert (and a selectable marker) that is flanked by sequences homologous to the targeted genomic DNA; replacement of a given sequence of genomic DNA by the insert relies on the (relatively rare) occurrence of homologous recombination.

Gene targeting can be used e.g. to inactivate a specific gene (a so-called knock-out mutation) or to modify the expression of a given gene e.g. by replacing part(s) of the gene's coding sequence. In the context of therapy, gene targeting may be used to attempt to correct a mis-functioning gene.

The efficiency of gene targeting has been improved by the development of certain phage-encoded recombinase systems (see e.g. RECOMBINEERING).

(cf. GENE TRAPPING; see also TARGETED TRAPPING.)

(See also FLP-IN CELL LINES.)

gene therapy Any form of therapy that involves genetic modification of (particular) cells with the object of correcting a genetic disorder or of treating certain types of infectious disease. Public awareness of gene therapy focuses primarily on the treatment of inherited disorders (such as CYSTIC FIBROSIS and ADENOSINE DEAMINASE DEFICIENCY) but much work has also been carried out on infectious diseases, such as those caused by hepatitis, influenza and human immunodeficiency viruses and by *Mycobacterium tuberculosis*.

Two basic approaches in gene therapy are: (i) the *ex vivo* mode, in which cells are removed from the body, genetically modified *in vitro*, and then returned to the body; (ii) the *in vivo* mode, in which genetic modification is carried out *in situ*, the modifying agent being internalized.

Inherited disease involving a single malfunctioning gene may be remediable by installing the normal (i.e. functional, wild-type) gene in order to counteract the specific deficiency. For example, successful therapy for ADENOSINE DEAMINASE DEFICIENCY has been achieved by inserting the normal gene into STEM CELLS; in this case, adenosine deaminase is formed in the T cells derived from those stem cells. Stem cells suitable for gene therapy have been isolated e.g. by exploiting the CD34$^+$ marker in IMMUNOMAGNETIC ENRICHMENT techniques. Following *in vitro* modification, the target stem cells are isolated by appropriate selective procedures; selection that is *not* based on drug-resistance can be achieved e.g. with reporter genes encoding different fluorophores (i.e. fluorophores with different emission spectra) instead of drug-resistance genes, the target cells being detected and separated by FACS (fluorescence-activated cell sorter) [Proc Natl Acad Sci USA (2005) 102(45):16357–16361].

Vectors in gene therapy

Vectors (i.e. vehicles used for inserting genetic material into cells) include certain types of virus which have been made replication-deficient and from which pathogenic potential has been eliminated. A gene which is to be inserted into cells (a *transgene*) is incorporated into the viral genome and enters a cell during viral infection of that cell.

Viral vectors include certain lentiviruses (a class of RETROVIRUSES), adenoviruses and adeno-associated viruses (the so-called AAVs); these viruses can infect both dividing and non-dividing cells.

AAVs are able to carry small sequences (inserts), while the adenoviruses can carry larger sequences.

(See also ADEASY XL ADENOVIRAL VECTOR SYSTEM.)

AAVs have been used e.g. for introducing genes into mice, by intracranial inoculation, for studying GM2 gangliosidoses [Proc Natl Acad Sci USA (2006) 103 (27):10373–10378].

Some viral vectors infect many types of cell. This can be a disadvantage because, to deliver a transgene to a *specific* type of cell, it may be necessary to administer the vector in high doses in order to allow for wastage (i.e. the take-up by other types of cell); the use of high doses of the given vector may increase the risk of adverse reactions. For other viral vectors the range of host cells may be too narrow. In either case, the problem may be solved by PSEUDOTYPING (q.v.).

Virus-mediated transfer of genes into cells can be enhanced by certain peptides and also by certain types of polycationic compound. From *in vitro* studies on the effect of peptides and polycationic agents on the transfer of genes from lentiviral and adenoviral vectors into human tumor cells, it was concluded that protamine sulfate may be the most suitable agent for clinical use [BioTechniques (2006) 40(5):573–576].

Strains of the Gram-positive bacterium *Lactococcus lactis* were reported to be able to deliver DNA into mammalian epithelial cells [Appl Environ Microbiol (2006) 72(11):7091–7097], suggesting a possible use in this context. (So far, the use of bacteria as gene delivery vectors has been considered less frequently than viral vectors.)

Certain modified phages (see BACTERIOPHAGE) have been reported to act as vectors for gene delivery to mammalian cells, and a similar role has been reported for PHAGEMID *particles*. To fulfill this role, the coat proteins of phages or phagemid particles are modified to display certain targeting ligands which can facilitate uptake by eukaryotic cells. In the case of phagemid particles, coat proteins can be encoded by the helper phage so that more of the phagemid's sequence can be used for the gene of interest; phagemid particles with a specific ligand have been prepared by using a coat-modified strain of phage M13 as helper phage [BioTechniques (2005) 39(4):493–497]. For phage or phagemid vectors, low levels of transgene expression in the recipient cells may reflect e.g. factors such as the need to convert ssDNA to dsDNA and the translocation of nucleic acid into the nucleus.

In cystic fibrosis, gene therapy is aimed at epithelial cells of the respiratory tract. So far, benefit has been achieved for only a limited period of time. Because extended benefit needs repeated dosing, this tends to exclude the use of viral vectors because repeat dosing with viral vectors can compromise the treatment as a result of a developing immune response to the vector. In this context, a novel, non-primate (caprine) adeno-associated virus (see AAVS) may be useful because it shows high resistance to neutralization by human antibodies and has a marked tropism for (murine) lung tissue [J Virol (2005) 79: 15238–15245].

For cystic fibrosis, attention has been focused on increasing the effectiveness of liposome-mediated delivery of the transgene, e.g. by facilitating transgene internalization, and escape from the endosome, as well as import into the nucleus [see e.g. Bioch J (2005) 387(1):1–15].

Gene therapy against infectious diseases

With infectious diseases, the possibilities for intervention by gene therapy are greater owing to the nature of infection and the diversity of infectious agents. Some approaches/ideas:

● Antisense oligonucleotides which bind to the pathogen's mRNAs, blocking transcription (see e.g. VITRAVENE).

● Suicide genes whose expression – leading to cell death – occurs only in infected cells.

● RIBOZYMES targeting specific sequence(s) in an infected cell. A single vector may encode many different ribozymes. The ribozyme's double requirement for correct binding and cleavage sites offers good specificity. The catalytic activity allows ongoing destruction of targets. To be useful, though, a ribozyme must be stabilized against intracellular degradation

by RNase. Useful results were reported in a simian immuno-deficiency virus (SIV) model using an anti-SIV *pol* ribozyme [J Gen Virol (2004) 85:1489–1496].

[Catalytic nucleic acid enzymes for study and development of therapies in the central nervous system: Gene Ther Mol Biol (2005) 9A:89–106.]

● RNA INTERFERENCE (q.v.) *in vitro* can inhibit replication of e.g. HIV-1 and the viruses that cause hepatitis, influenza and poliomyelitis. Moreover, siRNA-mediated downregulation of a cell's co-receptor for HIV can block *infection* of cells by HIV.

Synthetic siRNAs can be introduced into mammalian cells directly by the use of appropriate systems for internalization; alternatively, expression cassettes encoding siRNAs for intracellular expression can be transfected by an appropriate gene transfer vector.

(See also SHORT HAIRPIN RNA.)

A novel form of delivery of siRNA to mammalian cells has been carried out with an siRNA conjugated to an aptamer via a streptavidin bridge (the aptamer having been previously demonstrated to bind to prostate tumor cells); the conjugate (i.e. siRNA + aptamer) was internalized within 30 minutes of addition to the cells, and the siRNA was found to produce an efficient inhibition of gene expression [Nucleic Acids Res (2006) 34(10):e73].

Problems with RNAi in gene therapy

(a) Mutation in the target sequences can permit escape from RNAi, a consequence of the high-level specificity of RNAi cutting [e.g. escape of HIV-1 from RNAi: J Virol (2004) 78: 2601–2605]. One study indicated that RNAi can be effective against highly conserved sequences but was inhibited when mutations occur in the central, target-cleavage region [Blood (2005) 106(3):818–826].

[Computational design of RNAi strategies that resist escape of HIV: J Virol (2005) 79(3):1645–1654.]

(b) Non-specific ('off-target') modification of gene expression can occur, especially under high-dose conditions.

(c) There is a need for a highly efficient delivery system to avoid a residue of unprotected cells – in which target viruses can replicate and mutate to RNAi-insensitivity.

● Intrabodies (= single-chain antibodies): molecules, encoded by engineered antibody genes, which *remain intracellular* and which have antigen-binding properties.

[The *de novo* production of intracellular antibody libraries: Nucleic Acids Res (2003) 31(5):e23.]

An intrabody without disulfide bonds was found to perform better during *in vitro* studies on (non-infectious) Huntington's disease [Proc Natl Acad Sci USA (2005) 101 (51):17616–17621].

An intrabody has been used against vIL-6, a form of IL-6 (interleukin-6) encoded by human herpesvirus-8 (HHV-8) and associated with pathogenesis in certain types of disease, e.g. Kaposi's sarcoma [J Virol (2006) 80(17):8510–8520].

● Transdominant negative proteins (TNPs): modified, inhibitory forms of a pathogen's normal (regulatory or structural) proteins; TNPs may block activity of wild-type proteins e.g. by forming inactive complexes or by competing for specific binding sites.

Negative immune reactions against cells containing TNPs must be avoided.

A transdominant negative version of the human immunodeficiency virus-1 (HIV-1) regulatory REV PROTEIN (which e.g. mediates the export of certain viral transcripts from the nucleus) was found to inhibit replication of HIV-1 *in vitro*.

● DNA VACCINES have shown promise in animal models. In some early studies a DNA vaccine encoding the 65-kDa heat-shock protein of *Mycobacterium tuberculosis* (Hsp65) was able to act therapeutically as well as prophylactically in mice; a plasmid encoding interleukin-12 (IL-12) gave even better results.

DNA vaccines are being developed against e.g. papillomavirus type 16 (a virus associated with human cervical cancer) [J Virol (2004) 78(16):8468–8476]; the protozoa *Leishmania donovani* [Infect Immun (2005) 73(2):812–819] and *Plasmodium falciparum* [Infect Immun (2004) 72(1):253–259]; and *Mycobacterium tuberculosis* [Infect Immun (2005) 73 (9):5666–5674].

Genetic immunization (in animals) by intravenous delivery of antibody-specifying plasmid DNA was described as an efficient method for inducing antigen-specific antibodies in laboratory animals [BioTechniques (2006) 40(2):199–208].

gene transfer agent   See CAPSDUCTION.

gene-trap vector   See GENE TRAPPING.

gene trapping   A procedure which is used e.g. for introducing random insertional mutations into *cultured* mouse embryonic stem cells (ES cells); the inserts used for mutagenesis include a selectable marker or reporter which also acts as a 'tag' (i.e. a known sequence of nucleotides) so that a disrupted gene can be readily identified and investigated.

ES cells which have been genetically modified in this way can be injected into an (isolated) blastocyst which is then re-implanted in a mouse and allowed to develop. This procedure is therefore a valuable method for studying gene function, including studies on genetic modification of the germ line.

The insertional mutations are introduced by transfecting ES cells with a *gene-trap vector* that integrates randomly in the genome. Two common types of vector are described.

One type of gene-trap vector (used in 'promoter trapping') contains a promoter-less selectable sequence which is flanked on one side by an upstream splice acceptor sequence and on the other side by a polyadenylation signal; expression of the vector depends on chance integration into a host gene, the host gene supplying a promoter function. Transcription of the integrated vector produces an mRNA in which the poly(A) tail is transcribed from the vector's sequence. Note that genes which are transcriptionally silent in the target cell will fail to express the vector.

The second type of gene-trap vector contains a promoter-competent selectable sequence which lacks a polyadenylation signal but which includes a downstream splice donor site; the downstream splice donor site allows exploitation of the host's polyadenylation signal.

mRNA formed by transcription of either type of integrated vector can be used to determine the site of integration of the vector.

(See also TARGETED TRAPPING and GENE TARGETING.)

GeneChip®   See MICROARRAY.

GeneMorph™ PCR mutagenesis kit   A product (Stratagene, La Jolla CA) designed to generate random mutations during PCR-based amplification; the product includes an error-prone DNA polymerase (Mutazyme™) that is reported to generate from one to seven mutant bases per kilobase in a given PCR reaction.

Examples of use of GeneMorph: generation of temperature-sensitive mutants [Mol Biol Cell (2006) 17(4):1768–1778]; studies on the transcriptional regulator Mga of *Streptococcus pyogenes* [J Bacteriol (2006) 188(3):863–873].

(See also MUTAGENESIS.)

generalized transduction   See TRANSDUCTION.

GeneTailor™ site-directed mutagenesis system   A system (Invitrogen, Carlsbad CA) used for introducing specific point mutations, deletions, or insertions of up to 21 nucleotides in length. DNA of up to 8 kb, from any bacterial source, can be mutagenized.

(See also SITE-DIRECTED MUTAGENESIS.)

Initially, methylation of the (circular) molecule of DNA is carried out with a DNA methylase and *S*-adenosylmethionine as methyl donor.

A point mutation can be introduced by synthesizing copies of the DNA with a pair of primers which bind to overlapping sites, one of the primers incorporating the required mutation. Progeny strands anneal to form (nicked) circular molecules which are inserted into an appropriate strain of *Escherichia coli*, by transformation, for replication; the *mcrBC*⁺ strain of *E. coli* digests the (methylated) parental DNA (see the entry MCRBC).

The GeneTailor™ system has been used e.g. in studies on the fatty-acid-binding protein aP2 [Proc Natl Acad Sci USA (2006) 103(18):6970–6975] and in studies on HIV-1 [J Virol (2006) 80(7):3617–3623].

genetic code   The form of the information which enables a sequence of nucleotides in DNA (or, in some viruses, RNA) to direct the synthesis of a polypeptide – such direction usually involving the relay of information to an intermediate effector molecule: *messenger RNA* (mRNA); consecutive triplets of nucleotides in the mRNA (see CODON) encode consecutive AMINO ACID residues in the polypeptide, while certain of the codons (see the table) specify the termination of synthesis.

(In certain viruses with a *positive*-sense ssRNA genome the genomic RNA itself is translated into polyproteins – without the need for relaying information to an intermediate effector molecule.)

(Compare synthesis of oligopeptides by NON-RIBOSOMAL PEPTIDE SYNTHETASE.)

In that a given amino acid may be specified by more than

GENETIC CODE[a-e]

First base in codon (5' end)	Second base in codon				Third base in codon (3' end)
	U	C	A	G	
U	Phe	Ser	Tyr	Cys	U
	Phe	Ser	Tyr	Cys	C
	Leu	Ser	*ochre*	*opal*	A
	Leu	Ser	*amber*	Trp	G
C	Leu	Pro	His	Arg	U
	Leu	Pro	His	Arg	C
	Leu	Pro	Gln	Arg	A
	Leu	Pro	Gln	Arg	G
A	Ile	Thr	Asn	Ser	U
	Ile	Thr	Asn	Ser	C
	Ile	Thr	Lys	Arg	A
	Met	Thr	Lys	Arg	G
G	Val	Ala	Asp	Gly	U
	Val	Ala	Asp	Gly	C
	Val	Ala	Glu	Gly	A
	Val	Ala	Glu	Gly	G

[a]A = adenine; C = cytosine; G = guanine; U = uracil.
[b]Amino acid symbols are explained in the entry AMINO ACID (table).
[c]Codons are conventionally written in the 5'-to-3' direction.
[d]The *ochre*, *opal* and *amber* codons are normally stop signals.
[e]See text for some variations in the code.

one codon (see e.g. Leu in the table), the genetic code is said to be *degenerate*.

A given amino acid may be specified preferentially by a certain codon in one species but by another codon in different species. (See also CODON BIAS.)

Although widely applicable, the code shown in the table – often called the 'universal' genetic code – is not invariable. In the mitochondria of at least some plants, animals and fungi the codon UGA specifies tryptophan (rather than acting as a stop codon), while codons UAA and UAG specify glutamine in ciliate macronuclei.

Among the arthropods, AGG is reported to specify serine in certain species and either lysine or arginine in others – with some species not using the codon at all [PLoS Biol (2006) 4(5):e127; PLoS Biol (2006) 4(5):e175].

genetic counseling Advice given to e.g. parents regarding the possibility/probability of genetically based problems in their existing or future offspring, or, in general, to others regarding their susceptibility to particular genetically based problem(s).

genetic disease A term generally used to refer specifically to a *heritable* disease or disorder, i.e. one which is determined by an individual's genotype.

Some examples of genetic diseases are listed in the table.
(See also ONLINE MENDELIAN INHERITANCE IN MAN.)

genetic disorder *Syn.* GENETIC DISEASE.

genetic engineering The manipulation of genetic material – DNA and/or RNA – with the object of bringing about any desired change or innovation, either *in vitro* or *in vivo*, as carried out during the study, or modification for any purpose, of genes or genetic systems.

Genetic engineering therefore includes, for example, those *in vitro* techniques involved in the study of genes and their regulation; various techniques used in GENE THERAPY; and the creation of novel strains of existing microorganisms for medical or industrial use.

genetic footprinting A technique that can be used to examine gene function – e.g. to determine whether the expression of specific genes is required for growth under given conditions; the method is used in eukaryotic and prokaryotic microorganisms, including *Saccharomyces cerevisiae* and various Gram-negative bacteria.

Note. This technique is completely unrelated to the method, used for studying DNA–protein interactions, that is referred to as FOOTPRINTING.

Genetic footprinting involves three basic stages. One of the formats for genetic footprinting in bacteria is as follows. The first step involves random, transposon-mediated mutagenesis of a population of bacteria. This may be carried out e.g. by (i) transposon mutagenesis of DNA fragments *in vitro* followed by insertion of the mutagenized fragments into cells by transformation, or (ii) use of the transposome approach (see TN5-TYPE TRANSPOSITION) in which mutagenesis occurs *in vivo*. (The latter approach has certain advantages which include the possibility of limiting insertions to one per cell, by using an appropriate transposome–cell ratio, and the lack of a requirement for preparing a special transposon-delivery vector.) An aliquot of the (mutagenized) population is set aside for subsequent analysis; it is labeled T0 (for time zero).

The remainder of the mutagenized population is then grown for many generations under conditions in which further transposition is inhibited.

Finally, genomic DNA from (i) T0 cells, and (ii) cells from the cultured, mutagenized population is isolated, and nucleotide sequences from specific genes are determined, e.g. by a PCR-based approach.

If, under the given conditions of growth, a specific gene is essential for cell viability, then transposon insertions in that gene should be easily detectable in cells of the T0 population but not in cells of the cultured population.

[Example of genetic footprinting in the bacterial pathogen *Pseudomonas aeruginosa* strain PA14: Proc Natl Acad Sci USA (2006) 103(8):2833–2838.]

genetic immunization See GENE THERAPY (DNA vaccine).

genetic imprinting (genomic imprinting) The phenomenon in

Adenosine deaminase deficiency	An autosomal recessive disorder, involving abnormal susceptibility to infectious diseases, caused by deficiency of a functional adenosine deaminase (EC 3.5.4.4) encoded by gene *ADA* (20q13.11); deficiency in this enzyme inhibits normal development of T lymphocytes so that the patient's immune system is inefficient
Angelman syndrome	A condition characterized by mental impairment, defective balance, abnormal behavior, and severe speech defects. At least four genetic mechanisms are believed to be capable of causing Angelman syndrome. Most cases appear to result from a deletion at 15q11.2–q13, a small number result from imprinting defects, and some are reported to be due to mutation in the gene for ubiquitin protein ligase E3A
Axenfeld–Rieger syndrome	An autosomal dominant disorder affecting eyes and certain systemic features. Associated with mutation in the *PITX2* gene (encoding a transcription factor). In some cases the syndrome is reported to involve aberrant splicing of pre-mRNA
Bardet–Biedl syndrome	A genetically heterogeneous disorder, involving at least 11 chromosomes, characterized by e.g. renal and retinal abnormalities
Bernard–Soulier syndrome	A rare autosomal recessive condition involving a tendency to abnormal/excessive bleeding. Relevant mutations are found on chromosomes 3, 17 and 22, affecting proteins which form the subunits of a receptor for von Willebrand factor. See entry BERNARD–SOULIER SYNDROME. See also Hemophilia and Wiskott–Aldrich syndrome, below, for further examples of abnormal/excessive bleeding disorders
Charcot–Marie–Tooth disease	Any of a group of heterogeneous inherited neuropathies that include demyelinating and axonal types; autosomal dominant, autosomal recessive and X-linked forms of the disease are recognized (see entry CHARCOT–MARIE–TOOTH DISEASE)
Citrullinemia	Deficiency in arginosuccinate synthetase, with accumulation of citrulline and ammonia in the plasma and damage to the nervous system. The *classic* (type I) form involves mutation in gene *ASS* (9q34) which encodes arginosuccinate synthetase The *adult-onset* (type II) form is caused by mutation in gene *SLC25A13* (7q21.3) encoding *citrin*; this leads to a deficiency of the enzyme arginosuccinate synthetase
Cockayne syndrome	Poor development, photosensitivity and (generally) failure to survive beyond early adulthood. Forms A and B, resulting from mutation in genes (encoding DNA-repair proteins) at locations 5q12 (*CSA*) and 10q11 (*CSB*)
Cystic fibrosis	Commonly: abnormal secretion in the respiratory tract, with risk of infection, associated with a defective gene for the cystic fibrosis transmembrane conductance regulator (CFTR) protein (7q31.2)
Down's syndrome	Mental impairment and characteristic facial features. It is associated with trisomy (chromosome 21)
Duchenne muscular dystrophy	Muscular abnormality due to absence or abnormality of the (normal) muscle protein dystrophin, encoded by gene *DMD* (Xp21.2)
Dyggve–Melchior–Clausen syndrome	A condition, involving e.g. skeletal abnormalities, associated with mutation in the *DYM* gene (18q12–q21.1)
Emphysema (one type)	Deficiency of the protease inhibitor α-1-antitrypsin (gene location 14q32.1). Deficiency in this protein is also associated with cirrhosis
Fabry disease	An X-linked condition involving deficiency in the activity of α-galactosidase A (gene location Xq22). The range of manifestations apparently include e.g. vascular-type skin lesions and cardiac symptoms; renal failure is reported to be a common cause of death Fabrazyme® is used for treating this condition (see the table in the entry BIOPHARMACEUTICAL) *(continued)*

Fragile X disease	An X-linked disorder, characterized e.g. by mental impairment, associated with instability of MICROSATELLITE DNA (the CGG triplet) near the promoter of the *FMR1* gene, which results in gene silencing
Fucosidosis	An autosomal recessive disease involving a defective lysosomal enzyme, α-L-fucosidase (gene *FUCA1*, location 1p34) and the consequent accumulation of glycoproteins
Glanzmann's thrombasthenia	An autosomal recessive disease characterized by a deficiency in platelet agglutination; it is associated with abnormalities in the $\alpha_{IIb}\beta_3$ INTEGRIN
Glycogen storage disorder	Dysfunctional glycogen metabolism. Various types. Type I disease is characterized by a deficiency of the enzyme glucose 6-phosphatase (EC 3.1.3.9) (gene location 17q21); infants exhibit e.g. severe hypoglycemia and an enlarged liver
Hemophilia	Defective blood-clotting mechanism characterized e.g. by a tendency to hemorrhage, easy bruising etc. There is more than one type of hemophilia. *Hemophilia A* is an X-LINKED DISORDER resulting from a deficiency in the activity of clotting factor VIII; the genetic lesion is at Xq28. *Hemophilia B*, also an X-LINKED DISORDER, results from a deficiency in the activity of factor IX (the Christmas factor); the genetic lesion is at Xq27.1–q27.2. The term hemophilia has also been used to include the hemorrhagic condition von Willebrand disease – typically an autosomal dominant disorder associated with chromosomal location 12p13.3. See also Bernard–Soulier syndrome, above, and Wiskott–Aldrich syndrome, below, for some other examples of abnormal/excessive bleeding disorders. Various recombinant products are available for the therapeutic treatment of these disorders: see, for example, Kogenate® and NovoSeven® in the table in BIOPHARMACEUTICAL
Huntington's disease	An autosomal dominant disorder that involves chorea (i.e. involuntary movements) and progressive dementia; it is caused by expansion of MICROSATELLITE DNA (the CAG triplet) associated with a gene on chromosome 4
Hurler's syndrome	See Mucopolysaccharidosis type IH
Hyper-IgM syndrome	Immunodeficiency, with normal or elevated levels of IgM but a deficiency in IgG and other isotypes; patients with hyper-IgM syndrome are highly vulnerable to bacterial infections. There is an X-linked form and an autosomal recessive form. The *X-linked* form (HIGM1) is associated with mutation in the *CD40L* gene (affecting T cell–B cell interaction) The *autosomal recessive* form (HIGM2) may be due to mutation in the *CD40* gene or to a deficiency in the enzyme activation-induced cytidine deaminase (which may be involved in RNA editing)
ICF syndrome	Immunodeficiency, centromere instability and facial abnormality syndrome. A rare syndrome possibly caused by dysregulation of genomic methylation due to mutation in the *DNMT3B* gene (20q11.2)
Lesch–Nyhan syndrome	An X-linked syndrome, with e.g. neurologic and metabolic abnormalities, associated with mutation in the *HPRT* gene (Xq26–q27.2)
Leukocyte adhesion deficiency	An autosomal recessive disorder characterized by a low resistance to certain infectious diseases. Leukocytes are deficient in the β_2 INTEGRIN component of cell-surface adhesion molecules (involved in binding to pathogens)
Mucopolysaccharidosis type IH	An autosomal recessive disease (also called Hurler's syndrome) affecting various organs, including the heart. It results from mutation in the *IDUA* gene (encoding the lysosomal enzyme α-L-iduronidase). (*continued*)

Niemann–Pick disease	Mental retardation. Several types. Types A and B associated with lysosomal accumulation of sphingomyelin in the tissues due to deficiency in the enzyme sphingomyelin phosphodiesterase
Peutz–Jeghers syndrome	An autosomal dominant condition with intestinal hamartomatous polyposis, pigmentation in the oro-facial region, and an increased risk of gastrointestinal malignancy. Mutation in the coding region of a serine-threonine kinase gene, *STK11/LKB1* (chromosomal locus 19p13.3), appears to be present in most of the cases
Phenylketonuria	An autosomal recessive disease with e.g. mental retardation. Phenylpyruvate is found in the urine, and phenylalanine is found in blood and other tissues; the disorder is caused by inadequacy of the enzyme phenylalanine 4-mono-oxygenase (EC 1.14.16.1) (gene location: 12q24.1)
Prader–Willi syndrome	Obesity, mental retardation etc. Error in genetic imprinting. In at least some cases it may result from a deficiency of paternal copies of certain genes, including the gene (*SNRPN*) encoding small nuclear ribonucleoprotein polypeptide N (chromosomal location: 15q12)
Rett syndrome	Neurodevelopmental disorder. Commonly: mutation in the *MECP2* gene (encoding a methyl-CpG-binding protein); the condition apparently can also result from mutation in gene *CDKL5* (which encodes a cyclin-dependent kinase)
Sandhoff disease	A condition related to Tay–Sachs disease (see below) but involving the β-subunit of hexosaminidase A
SCID	Severe combined immunodeficiency: a group of diverse diseases involving the failure of T lymphocytes to develop normally. One of these diseases is adenosine deaminase deficiency (see above). Another is an X-linked disorder involving a defective γc subunit in a cell-surface cytokine receptor which (e.g.) inhibits normal development of T cells; this disorder is called XSCID or SCIDX1
Severe combined immunodeficiency	See SCID, above
Sickle-cell anemia	Anemia, involving the β-chain of hemoglobin (see the entry SICKLE-CELL ANEMIA)
Smith–Lemli–Opitz syndrome	An autosomal recessive disorder, involving mental retardation, reported to involve defective cholesterol metabolism owing to mutation in the *DHCR7* gene (encoding 3β-hydroxysterol-Δ7 reductase)
Tay–Sachs disease	An autosomal recessive condition resulting from mutation in the gene for the α-subunit of hexosaminidase A (EC 3.2.1.52) located at 15q23–q24, a lysosomal enzyme required for the breakdown of gangliosides. This neurodegenerative disease is commonly seen early in life: infants show poor development, with mental impairment and blindness, and the condition is often fatal within the first few years of life. See also Sandhoff disease, above
Thalassemia	Anemia, resulting from a disorder involving the α-chain or β-chain of hemoglobin
von Willebrand disease	See Hemophilia, above, and Wiskott–Aldrich syndrome, below
Wiskott–Aldrich syndrome	An X-LINKED DISORDER: thrombocytopenia (and defective blood clotting), eczema, and a susceptibility to recurrent infection (see entry WISKOTT–ALDRICH SYNDROME). See also Hemophilia, above

which particular genes are methylated, at specific loci, as a marker of their origin – i.e. from the male or female parent; only *one* allele of an imprinted gene (from the male or female parent) is expressed under given circumstances.

Errors in imprinting may cause serious disorders – e.g. the Prader–Willi syndrome (which is characterized by obesity, mental retardation and hypogonadism).

Imprinting is an epigenetic phenomenon, that is, it directs a heritable phenotype that is not dependent on the sequence of nucleotides in the given genes. It occurs during the formation of germ cells and persists in somatic cells.

genetic screening Any procedure used for detecting/selecting individual cells or organisms with specific genetic characteristic(s) from among a population of those cells or organisms.

In a clinical context: test(s) carried out on patients in order to detect the risk of possible or probable genotype-based disorders in the patients themselves or in their offspring.

genetically modified food (GM food) Any food (such as GM soya) which has been produced after specific and intentional alteration of the genome of a given type of plant or animal.

The construction of a GM organism is not necessarily the accelerated production of an organism that could be obtained by a naturally occurring process. This is because it is possible to modify genomes with sequence(s) of nucleotides designed on a computer – sequences that do not necessarily reflect any that occur, have ever occured, or may ever occur, in nature.

Geneticin® A commercial brand of G418 SULFATE (Invitrogen, Carlsbad CA).

genistein 4′,5,7-Trihydroxyisoflavone: a strong inhibitor of the tyrosine kinases; it acts as a competitive inhibitor of ATP at the binding site.

(cf. TYRPHOSTIN.)

(See also TYROSINE KINASE.)

genome (1) The genetic content of a cell or virus – in terms of either (a) the information (coding) content or (b) the physical content of nucleic acid (i.e. a cell's DNA or the DNA or RNA of a virus).

In this sense, DNA in mitochondria (including kinetoplast DNA) and chloroplasts forms part of the genome.

In bacteria, which often contain plasmids, *genome* is sometimes used specifically to refer to *chromosomal* DNA; this use of the term may be justified in that plasmids are often dispensable to the cell, and in that cells of a given species may contain different assortments of (dissimilar) plasmids (which would indicate a 'variable genome' for the species). However, 'genome' is also used to include bacterial plasmids, particularly when cells of a given species commonly contain a stable complement of plasmid(s) – or the plasmid(s) have a particular relevance to the organism's biological activity or pathogenicity; the term has been used in this way e.g. for *Bacillus anthracis* [J Bacteriol (2000) 182(10):2928–2936], for *Pseudomonas syringae* pv. tomato [Proc Natl Acad Sci USA (2003) 100(18):10181–10186] for *Rhizobium leguminosarum* [Genome Biol (2006) 7(4):R34] and for *Rhodococcus* RHA1 [Proc Natl Acad Sci USA (2006) 103:15582–15587].

(2) The *haploid* set of genes or chromosomes in a cell.

(3) The complete set of *different* genes in an organism.

(4) The term 'genome' has even been used in the context of *viroids* (i.e. non-coding, single-stranded molecules of RNA that infect plants) [BMC Microbiol (2006) 6:24].

Genome Deletion Project (for *Saccharomyces cerevisiae*) A project that systematically replaced each open reading frame (ORF) in the genome of the yeast *Saccharomyces cerevisiae* with a kanamycin-resistance cassette – creating a collection of strains in which a different ORF has been replaced in each strain. This collection of (GDP) strains provides a comprehensive source of knock-outs for *S. cerevisiae*, facilitating studies on gene function.

In addition to their intended application, these strains can also be used e.g. to copy any desired *S. cerevisiae* promoter; a copy of this promoter can then be inserted into a strain of interest and used for controlling the expression of a given gene. For this purpose, one first identifies the particular GDP strain in which the desired promoter is flanked by a kanamycin knock-out immediately on its 5′ side. This promoter, together with its contiguous kanamycin cassette, is amplified by PCR, using primers having 5′ extensions homologous to sites of insertion in the strain of interest. The PCR products can then be inserted into the genome of the given strain by homologous recombination, replacing the existing promoter [Method: BioTechniques (2006) 40:728–734.]

genome walking *Syn.* CHROMOSOME WALKING.

genomic cloning See CLONING.

genomic imprinting *Syn.* GENETIC IMPRINTING.

genomic island In a bacterial genome: a discrete region of the chromosome, acquired from an exogenous source, that differs in GC% (and codon usage) from the rest of the chromosome and is often located near tRNA genes; genomic islands are typically flanked by direct repeat sequences and may include any of various genes as well as mobile genetic elements.

Recombination may result in fragmentation of a genomic island with re-location of part(s) of the island to different regions of the chromosome.

Genomic islands are reported to be generated, for example, at the sites of insertion of transposon Tn7 [J Bacteriol (2007) 189(5):2170–2173].

A 54-kb genomic island in the (Gram-negative) bacterium *Leptospira interrogans* serovar Lai (containing 103 predicted coding sequences) is reported to excise from the chromosome and to exist as a (replicative) plasmid [Infect Immun (2007) 75(2):677–683].

genomic library See LIBRARY.

genomic masking See PHENOTYPIC MIXING.

genospecies Any group of (microbial) strains between which genetic exchange can occur.

genotoxin Any agent that damages nucleic acid. [Detection of genotoxic compounds: Appl Environ Microbiol (2005) 71(5): 2338–2346.]

GenoType MTBDR See LINE PROBE ASSAY.

gentamicin An AMINOGLYCOSIDE ANTIBIOTIC used e.g. as a

selective agent for bacteria containing a vector which carries a gentamicin-resistance gene.

germ line cells Cells whose development leads to the formation of gametes (reproductive cells).

GFP See GREEN FLUORESCENT PROTEIN.

GFP reactivation technique An approach designed to facilitate (drug-mediated) analysis of DNA methylation (see entry DEMETHYLATION); the protocol published in BioTechniques [(2006) 41(4):461–466] uses the methylation-inhibitory drug 5-aza-2′-deoxycytidine, but this approach may also be useful for studying the effects of some other chromatin-modifying drugs (such as TRICHOSTATIN A).

The method improves our ability to identify genes that have been activated by drug treatment – such activation resulting from the removal of methylation-induced repression. In this method, cells in which drug-induced activation has occurred are selected by using a reporter gene whose activation, by the drug, indicates 'global' drug-induced de-repression of genes in these cells.

This method uses transgenic female mice with an X-linked reporter gene for GREEN FLUORESCENT PROTEIN (GFP). The relevant transgene in this method is the one present on the *inactivated* X chromosome.

The GFP reactivation technique involves several stages of screening of a population of cells isolated from the transgenic mouse. The final stage of screening isolates those cells in the population which exhibit drug-induced activation of the GFP reporter gene present on the *inactive* X chromosome. All the screening is carried out with a FLUORESCENCE-ACTIVATED CELL SORTER (FACS).

Cells from the animal were first sorted by flow cytometry to select for those containing an inactive, *non*-expressed gene for GFP (see X-INACTIVATION). After treatment with 5-aza-2′-deoxycytidine this population of cells was again sorted by flow cytometry to separate those cells containing active GFP from those containing inactive GFP – i.e. separating cells in which the reporter gene had been activated by the drug from those in which no activation had occurred.

Subsequent MICROARRAY-based gene expression profiling on the three populations of cells – i.e. (i) the GFP-inactive untreated cells, (ii) GFP-inactive drug-treated cells and (iii) GFP-active drug-treated cells – indicated the potential of this method for identifying genes that were activated by global demethylation as a result of drug treatment.

giant chromosome See POLYTENIZATION.

Gigapack® Any of a range of products (Stratagene, La Jolla CA) used for packaging certain types of lambda-based vector molecules ('packaging' referring to the process in which each (DNA) vector molecule is enclosed in phage components to form an infective phage particle). Gigapack® products are used e.g. with the LAMBDA FIX II VECTOR.

GISA Strains of MRSA with decreased susceptibility to glycopeptide antibiotics (e.g. vancomycin), the abbreviation referring to 'glycopeptide intermediately susceptible S. aureus'.

Glanzmann's thrombasthenia An autosomal recessive disease that is characterized by a deficiency in platelet agglutination and linked to abnormalities of the $\alpha_{IIb}\beta_3$ INTEGRIN.

[Review of Glanzmann's thrombasthenia: Orphanet J Rare Dis (2006) 1:10.]

glargine See INSULIN GLARGINE.

Glucuron™ See CHEMILUMINESCENCE.

glucose effect See CATABOLITE REPRESSION.

glutathione *S*-transferase See GENE FUSION (uses).

glycogen storage disorder Any of various human diseases that involve dysfunctional glycogen metabolism.

The type I disease is characterized by deficiency of glucose 6-phosphatase in the liver. In infants it involves severe hypoglycemia and an enlarged liver containing abnormally high levels of glycogen.

The type VIII form of glycogen storage disorder, which is generally less severe, is characterized by inadequate levels of the enzyme phosphorylase kinase.

(See also GENETIC DISEASE (table).)

glycosylation (of recombinant proteins) Post-translational modification of recombinant proteins, carried out in cells capable of adding glycosyl residue(s) to the appropriate amino acid residue(s). In many cases such glycosylation is an essential requirement for normal activity of the recombinant protein.

Some types of cell (e.g. bacteria) do not normally carry out the patterns of glycosylation that are found in mammalian proteins; however, bacteria have been used for the production of certain mammalian proteins (e.g. interleukin-2) in which a lack of post-translational glycosylation apparently does not significantly affect biological activity.

(See also Neupogen® in the entry BIOPHARMACEUTICAL (table).)

GM food GENETICALLY MODIFIED FOOD.

GM2 gangliosidoses Certain GENETIC DISEASES in which non-degraded gangliosides accumulate in lysosomes.

One example of such diseases is TAY–SACHS DISEASE.

goi Gene of interest.

gold standard Any well-established and trusted procedure (e.g. a particular form of test) regarded by workers in the field as being superior (in e.g. sensitivity/specificity/reliability) when compared to other (alternative or proposed) methods. In the diagnosis of infectious diseases a *combined* or *expanded* gold standard is generally taken to mean both culture *and* nucleic-acid-based methods.

Goldberg–Hogness box See CORE PROMOTER.

gp (1) GENE PRODUCT.

(2) A *glycoprotein* gene product encoded by retroviruses.

gp41 (in HIV-1) See HIV-1.

***gp64* gene** (in baculoviruses) See BACULOVIRIDAE.

gp120 A major envelope glycoprotein of the HIV-1 virion.

(See also DC-SIGN.)

Grace's medium A liquid medium used for the culture of (i.e. growth of) insect cells. Grace's medium includes a number of inorganic salts, sugars (fructose, D-glucose and sucrose) and a variety of amino acids.

(See also BACULOVIRUS EXPRESSION SYSTEMS.)

granulin A protein, encoded by GRANULOSIS VIRUSES, which forms the matrix of the intracellular *occlusion bodies* of these viruses: see BACULOVIRIDAE for details.

(cf. POLYHEDRIN.)

granulocyte See PMN.

granulosis viruses (GVs) A category of baculoviruses that are distinguished from NUCLEAR POLYHEDROSIS VIRUSES (q.v.) e.g. on the basis of characteristics of their occlusion bodies: see BACULOVIRIDAE.

Unlike the NPVs, granulosis viruses appear to be confined to lepidopteran hosts.

Viruses in this group include e.g. a pathogen of the cabbage looper (*Trichoplusia ni*) (TnGV), a pathogen of the codling moth (*Cydia pomonella*) (CpGV), and viruses isolated from a variety of other lepidopterans.

granzymes Agents, released e.g. by $CD8^+$ T cells, which are lethal for target cells. Granzyme A brings about single-strand damage to DNA and causes caspase-independent cell death; it was reported to target a protein (Ku70) involved in the repair of *double*-stranded breaks in DNA [EMBO Rep (2006) 7(4):431–437].

GRAS Acronym for 'generally regarded as safe'.

gratuitous inducer (of an operon) Any compound which acts as an inducer of an operon but which has no metabolic role in the cell (see e.g. IPTG).

gray A unit of the amount of radiation absorbed: 1 joule/kg. Symbol: Gy.

(cf. RAD.)

green fluorescent protein (GFP) A naturally fluorescent protein found e.g. in the jellyfish *Aequorea*; on irradiation with blue light ($\lambda = \sim395$ nm) GFP emits green light ($\lambda = 508$ nm).

The GFP gene is widely used as a partner in GENE FUSION, and has been used e.g. for tracking viral proteins [J Virol (2004) 78:8002–8014] and virions [J Virol (2005) 79:11776–11787]. (See also EGFP, GFP REACTIVATION TECHNIQUE and REPORTER GENE.)

The GFP from *Aequorea* has been associated with a certain level of toxicity in mammalian cells in which it is expressed. GFP from *Renilla reniformis* (see HRGFP) has been used as a less-toxic alternative.

For fluorescence microscopy of GFP, the usual (expensive, inconvenient) mercury arc lamp may be substituted with a light-emitting diode (LED) which appears to give comparable results [BioTechniques (2005) 38:204–206].

(See also IN VIVO FLUORESCENCE and MONOMERIC RED FLUORESENT PROTEIN.)

grepafloxacin See QUINOLONE ANTIBIOTICS.

grooves (in the DNA helix) In B-DNA, the *minor groove* is the helical groove between the two base-paired strands (see also BOXTO), while the *major groove* is the helical groove that runs between the overall turns of the double helix.

Grunstein–Hogness procedure See COLONY HYBRIDIZATION.

GT...AG rule (GU...AG rule) A rule stating that the 5′ and 3′ ends of an intron (i.e. the donor splice site and acceptor splice site, respectively) have the dinucleotide sequences GT and AG respectively; the rule apparently applies in most (but not all) cases.

GTA Gene transfer agent: see CAPSDUCTION.

GTP Guanosine 5′-triphosphate.

GU...AG rule *Syn.* GT...AG RULE.

guanidine salts Agents that inhibit certain viruses (e.g. polioviruses) by inhibiting viral RNA synthesis. Resistant mutants develop readily.

guanosine A riboNUCLEOSIDE.

guanosine nucleotide exchange factor (guanyl nucleotide exchange factor) See e.g. CYTOTRAP TWO-HYBRID SYSTEM.

Gubler–Hoffmann technique See FIRST STRAND.

guide sequence (external guide sequence) See SNRNAS.

Guthrie card A card used for collecting and storing specimens of blood. Blood is spotted onto each of several circular areas and then allowed to dry. The card includes an area on which details of the patient etc. can be written.

GVs GRANULOSIS VIRUSES.

GW678248 A potent benzophenone NON-NUCLEOSIDE REVERSE TRANSCRIPTASE INHIBITOR; the prodrug GW695634 is being developed for the treatment of HIV-1 infection [Antimicrob Agents Chemother (2005) 49(10):4046–4051].

GW695634 See GW678248.

gyrase See TOPOISOMERASE.

H

H (1) A specific indicator of ambiguity in the recognition site of a RESTRICTION ENDONUCLEASE or in another nucleic acid sequence; for example, in GDGCH↓C (enzyme SduI) the 'H' indicates A or C or T. (In RNA 'H' indicates A or C or U.) In the example, 'D' is A or G or T.

(2) L-Histidine (alternative to His).

H-DNA See TRIPLEX DNA.

H′-DNA See TRIPLEX DNA.

H-ras See RAS.

H strand (of dsDNA) The 'heavy' strand: that strand found in the lower band when a given sample of denatured DNA is subjected to density gradient centrifugation; the other strand is the 'light' (L) strand.

The designation 'heavy' may also refer to a strand of DNA labeled with a heavy isotope.

H1 histone See HISTONE.

H2A, H2B histones See HISTONE.

H3, H4 histones See HISTONE.

H37rv The reference strain of MYCOBACTERIUM TUBERCULOSIS.

Ha-ras See RAS.

HAART Highly active antiretroviral therapy, i.e. chemotherapy used in the treatment of AIDS which involves a *combination* of various types of antiretroviral agent, including e.g. a NONNUCLEOSIDE REVERSE TRANSCRIPTASE INHIBITOR, a NUCLEOSIDE REVERSE TRANSCRIPTASE INHIBITOR and a PROTEASE INHIBITOR.

Such a regime should theoretically block all replication of HIV. However, low-level viremia can occur and may be due e.g. to (i) replication in long-lived HIV-infected cells, and (ii) selection of new drug-resistant mutants of the virus [J Virol (2005) 79(15):9625–9634].

hadacidin ($CHO.NOH.CH_2.CO_2H$) A compound which acts as a structural analog of L-aspartic acid, inhibiting the enzyme adenylosuccinate synthetase and inhibiting the biosynthesis of adenine-containing nucleotides.

Hadacidin has antimicrobial and antitumor activity.

(See also AZASERINE and DON.)

haemophilia See HEMOPHILIA.

Haemophilus A genus of Gram-negative bacteria that occur as parasites (e.g. on mucous membranes) and opportunist pathogens in man and other animals. The cells are coccoid, small rods (e.g. ~0.4–1.5 μm) or filaments, according e.g. to growth conditions. Growth requires rich media (e.g. *chocolate agar* i.e. heat-treated blood agar), X FACTOR and/or the V FACTOR (according to species).

The GC% of genomic DNA in species of *Haemophilus* is within the range 37–44.

The type species is *H. influenzae*.

hairpin See e.g. PALINDROMIC SEQUENCE.

halocins BACTERIOCINS produced by certain species of the domain Archaea.

hammerhead ribozyme A type of *trans*-acting RIBOZYME that is found naturally in certain types of VIROID and which has been subjected to extensive experimentation and engineering.

Essentially, the hammerhead ribozyme consists of a single, folded (structured) strand of RNA with a central, catalytic component that is flanked by two recognition sequences. The recognition sequences base-pair with a complementary target sequence that has a central triplet such as GUC – or a similar variant triplet with a central U; cleavage of the target sequence occurs at the 3′ end of this central triplet.

handcuffing A proposed mechanism for inhibition of replication in plasmids that contain ITERONS: a replication-control protein, bound to iterons, couples the origins of replication of two plasmids and, in this way, blocks initiation of replication.

In plasmid R6K, handcuffing appears to involve dimers of the plasmid-encoded π protein [J Bacteriol (2005) 187(11): 3779–3785].

A mechanism such as handcuffing appears to contribute to replication control in the iteron-containing plasmid P1 [Proc Natl Acad Sci USA (2005) 102(8):2856–2861].

haploid See PLOIDY.

haploinsufficiency An effect in which a loss of function in one of a pair of alleles causes a change in phenotype – the nature of which depends on gene and conditions.

haplotype A term which is used in various (distinct) ways by different authors. The meanings of 'haplotype' include:

(1) The specific sequence of alleles in a given chromosome, part of a chromosome, or another, specified region of DNA; in human DNA such a sequence may be either maternal or paternal in origin.

(2) The sequence of alleles encoding the major histocompatibility complex (MHC): components of the immune system that include cell-surface antigens on leukocytes and various other types of cell. In humans, these alleles are designated HLA (human leukocyte antigen); they occur on chromosome 6.

(3) The complete complement of MHC *antigens* encoded by genes derived from *a given* parent (i.e. of either maternal or paternal origin).

Hardy–Weinberg equilibrium In a given, large population, if the frequency of the alleles A and a be represented by p and q ($q = 1 - p$), respectively, then, in general, the expected ratio of the genotypes AA, Aa and aa is given by $p^2:2pq:q^2$.

HAT Histone acetyltransferase: see ACETYLATION.

(See also WOBBLE HYPOTHESIS.)

HAT medium See HYBRIDOMA.

HCV pseudoparticle See PSEUDOPARTICLE.

HDA HELICASE-DEPENDENT AMPLIFICATION.

HDAC Histone deacetylase: see ACETYLATION.

(See also TRICHOSTATIN A.)

headful mechanism See e.g. PHAGE T4.

headloop suppression PCR A form of PCR used for selectively suppressing the amplification of one or more related sequences without affecting amplification of the (required) target sequence; it is reported to be particularly useful when a rare target sequence occurs among a large number of copies of a closely related, but unwanted, sequence.

Each primer has a 5′ tag (the 'head') which can bind to an internal region of the *unwanted* sequence. After extension of a primer, the head can loop over and hybridize with the complementary region in an unwanted sequence, thereby forming a hairpin-type structure which is not readily amplifiable. The head does not hybridize with the (required) target sequence because there is no complementary region; accordingly, the required sequence is amplified normally.

Headloop suppression PCR has been used with BISULFITE-treated DNA for the (selective) amplification of sequences containing methylated cytosines (the amplification of non-methylated sequences being suppressed). [Method: Nucleic Acids Res (2005) 33(14):e127.]

heated-lid cycler See THERMOCYCLER.

heavy strand (of dsDNA) See H STRAND.

helicase (DNA helicase; unwinding protein) A type of protein which can separate (unwind) the strands of a DNA duplex, in an ATP-dependent fashion.

Escherichia coli helicases include the Rep protein (*rep* gene product); helicase II (= UvrD protein), involved e.g. in DNA repair; and the DnaB protein (*dnaB* gene product), a hexameric ring of which is involved in chromosomal replication [J Mol Biol (2002) 321(5):839–849].

The F plasmid's helicase I (encoded by gene *traI*) may be used to nick the plasmid's *oriT* site and unwind plasmid DNA during bacterial conjugation.

Some phages use the host cell's helicase – while others, e.g. T4 (the *dda* gene product) and T7 (gp4), encode their own helicases.

A thermostable helicase (from *Thermoanaerobacter tengcongensis*) is used in HELICASE-DEPENDENT AMPLIFICATION.

Some enzymes which are referred to as 'helicases' may not be able to unwind DNA. For example, the type IC restriction endonuclease EcoR124I, which has ATP-dependent translocation, is reported to be able to move along a DNA molecule even when there are interstrand cross-links (preventing strand separation); translocation in this enzyme appears to depend primarily on contact with the sugar–phosphate backbone and bases in the 3′–5′ strand – although contact with the 5′–3′ strand appears to be important for stabilizing the enzyme's motor on the DNA [EMBO J (2006) 25:2230–2239].

helicase I A HELICASE encoded by the F PLASMID (gene *traI*).

helicase II *Syn.* UvrD (see UVRABC-MEDIATED REPAIR).

helicase-dependent amplification (HDA) An isothermal DNA AMPLIFICATION method in which the need for temperature cycling is avoided by the use of a helicase (which separates the strands of dsDNA to reveal target sequence(s)). [Original description of method: EMBO Reports (2004) 5(8):795–800.]

More recently, both specificity and performance of HDA were improved by carrying out the process at higher temperatures (60–65°). To do this, use was made of a thermostable helicase derived from *Thermoanaerobacter tengcongensis* [J

Biol Chem (2005) 280(32):28952–28958].

Helicobacter pylori A species of Gram-negative bacteria; the cells are typically curved or spiral rods up to ~3 μm in length. This organism is catalase-positive, oxidase-positive and also (strongly) urease-positive.

H. pylori is associated e.g. with gastric disease in man – but the organism is apparently present in the stomach (without symptoms) in a significant part of the human population.

The (circular) genome of *H. pylori* is ~1.6 kb.

The GC% of the genomic DNA is ~39.

helix (double) See B-DNA.

helix–coil transition (of dsDNA) Transition from an ordered helical conformation to a 'random coil'; this generally refers to MELTING.

(See also THERMAL MELTING PROFILE.)

helix-destabilizing protein *Syn.* SINGLE-STRAND BINDING PROTEIN.

helix-turn-helix A structural feature in certain DNA-binding proteins: two helical regions linked by a β-turn.

helper phage Any phage (e.g. M13K07) which, on infecting a cell, can promote replication of a vector (e.g. a PHAGEMID) which contains a phage f1 (or similar) origin of replication – leading to encapsidation of single-stranded copies of vector DNA in phage particles. Such *single-strand rescue* has been used e.g. to prepare samples of DNA for sequencing.

(See also PILUS.)

hemiphosphorothioate site See e.g. SDA.

hemophilia Any of several distinct types of disorder involving a failure of the normal blood-clotting (coagulation) process: see GENETIC DISEASE (table).

Recombinant proteins are used for treatment/prophylaxis (see e.g. NovoSeven® in the table in BIOPHARMACEUTICAL).

hemorrhagiparous thrombocytic dystrophy *Syn.* BERNARD–SOULIER SYNDROME.

HEPA filter See SAFETY CABINET (class I).

hepatitis C virus pseudoparticle See PSEUDOPARTICLE.

HER2 See EPIDERMAL GROWTH FACTOR RECEPTOR FAMILY; see also NEU.

Herceptin® See HER2 in entry EPIDERMAL GROWTH FACTOR RECEPTOR FAMILY.

heteroauxin (auxin) See AUXINS.

heteroduplex (1) Any double-stranded nucleic acid in which each of the strands is derived from a different parent duplex (the strands may or may not be fully complementary).

(See also HOMOLOGOUS RECOMBINATION.)

(2) Any double-stranded nucleic acid in which the strands are not complementary.

heterogeneous nuclear RNA (hnRNA) Within a (eukaryotic) nucleus: various types of RNA that include pre-mRNA and the RNA components of ribonucleoproteins.

heterogeneous test A nucleic-acid-amplification test in which the amplified product is transferred from the reaction mixture (e.g. to a gel) for detection/quantitation.

(cf. HOMOGENEOUS TEST.)

heterogenote See MEROZYGOTE.

heterologous From a source other than the organism, or entity, under consideration. For example, expression of a protein-encoding mammalian gene in a bacterium would involve the synthesis of a heterologous protein in the bacterial cell.

heteromerous See MACRONUCLEUS.

heteroplasmy Refers to the condition in which both wild-type and mutant copies of given mitochondrial gene(s) coexist in the same cell. (cf. HOMOPLASMY.)

The ratio of mutant to wild-type copies of mtDNA appears to be a major factor in determining the development or otherwise of clinical disease; this ratio can vary between different tissues in the body. mtDNA recombination has been reported from studies on skeletal muscle in heteroplasmic individuals [Nature Genet (2005) 37(8):873–877]. [Heteroplasmy in *Caenorhabditis elegans*: BMC Genet (2007) 8:8.]

heteroploid (1) Refers to any cell or organism in which the number of chromosomes is different from that characteristic of the species. (cf. EUPLOID, sense 1.)

(See also ANEUPLOID.)

(2) Refers to a cell or organism which has a complement of chromosomes other than the haploid or diploid number.

heterosome (heterochromosome; also sex chromosome) A sex-linked chromosome – e.g. the human X or Y chromsome.

(cf. AUTOSOME.)

heterothallism (*fungal genetics*) The need for two (different) thalli in the process of sexual reproduction.

Morphological heterothallism (*dioecism*) refers to the need for separate male and female thalli.

Physiological heterothallism involves compatibility of the sexual partners which is based on MATING TYPE (q.v.).

heterozygous See ALLELE.

hexadimethrine bromide See POLYBRENE.

hexidium iodide A fluorescent phenanthridinium dye which binds to DNA; the cell membrane in mammalian cells, and in Gram-*positive* bacteria, is permeable to hexidium iodide.

(See also DNA STAINING and LIVE BACLIGHT BACTERIAL GRAM STAIN KIT.)

Hfr donor See F PLASMID.

Hi-Res Melting™ A system for DNA melting analysis (Idaho Technology Inc., Salt Lake City UT) in which the methodology used permits an increased amount of information to be obtained; the LightScanner® instrument is employed in this procedure.

(See also HRM.)

high frequency of recombination donor See F PLASMID.

high-mobility group proteins (HMG proteins) See HMG BOX.

high-resolution melt See HRM.

high-stringency conditions See e.g. PROBE and STRINGENCY

(See also PCR.)

highly active antiretroviral therapy See HAART.

HIGM1, HIGM2 See HYPER-IGM SYNDROME.

Himar1 **transposon** See MARINER FAMILY.

HimarFT **transposon** See MARINER FAMILY.

hirudin A potent anticoagulant found in the leech, *Hirudo medicinalis*; it binds to, and inhibits, thrombin.

A recombinant form of hirudin, which is used therapeutically, is produced in the yeast *Saccharomyces cerevisiae* – see Refludan® in the entry BIOPHARMACEUTICAL (table).

his **operon** See OPERON.

histidine kinase A kinase in which the active site includes a histidine residue. Histidine kinases are involved e.g. in TWO-COMPONENT REGULATORY SYSTEMS.

histidine operon See OPERON.

(See also AMES TEST.)

histone A type of small, basic protein present in CHROMATIN; there are three main groups: H1 (lysine-rich); H2A and H2B (slightly lysine-rich); H3 and H4 (arginine-rich).

Constitutive, non-allelic, histone *variants*, which can differ in different species, can alter both structure and dynamics of chromatin. Unlike other histones, these are formed throughout the cell cycle and they may affect e.g. DNA transcription, replication and repair [Genes Dev (2005) 19(3):295–316].

Genome-wide plotting of the yeast variant histone H2A.Z indicated global localization to *inactive* genes and a role in nucleosome positioning [PLoS Biol (2005) 3(12):e384].

histone acetyltransferase See ACETYLATION.

histone deacetylase See ACETYLATION and TRICHOSTATIN A.

HIV-1 Human immunodeficiency virus-1: a virus of subfamily LENTIVIRINAE (family Retroviridae – see RETROVIRUSES for general information); infection with HIV-1 can lead to AIDS.

HIV-1 was linked to AIDS in 1983. Later, another (distinct but related) retrovirus was associated with AIDS patients in West Africa; this virus was designated HIV-2.

The HIV-1 virion is approx. 100 nm in diameter (see entry RETROVIRUSES for basic structure and genome).

Interaction with (susceptible) cells occurs via the envelope glycoprotein gp120, which is located at the distal (outermost) end of a trans-envelope protein, gp41. The main high-affinity binding site for gp120 is cell-surface antigen CD4 (found e.g. on 'helper' T lymphocytes). However, the entry of HIV-1 into cells apparently depends not only on gp120–CD4 binding but also on the presence of particular cell-surface receptors for chemokines (e.g. CXCR4 and CCR5); thus, CXCR4 appears to be required for entry of T-cell-tropic strains of the virus, while CCR5 is needed for entry of M-tropic strains of HIV-1 (M-tropic strains being those able to infect cells of both the T lymphoid and macrophage/monocyte lineages). Some ('dual-tropic') strains of HIV-1 can use both of these receptors. The various strains of HIV-1 have been categorized as X4, R5 or R5X4 strains on the basis of their use of these receptors.

Following reverse transcription of viral RNA (see RETRO-VIRUSES) the dsDNA provirus is circularized before integration into the host's chromosome. Integration involves the viral integrase (encoded by the *pol* region).

HIV-2 See HIV-1.

HLA Human leukocyte antigen (see HAPLOTYPE).

HMG box The DNA-binding region of the small, non-histone *high-mobility group proteins* of eukaryotes; it consists of a region of ~80 amino acid residues. Like the LrpC protein in the (prokaryote) *Bacillus subtilis* [Nucleic Acids Res (2006)

34(1):120–129], HMG proteins apparently bind to HOLLIDAY JUNCTIONS.

HMG proteins High-mobility group proteins: see HMG BOX.

hMUTYH See 8-OXOG.

hnRNA HETEROGENEOUS NUCLEAR RNA.

H-NS protein A small, multi-functional prokaryotic protein associated e.g. with condensation of DNA into the compact NUCLEOID [Nucleic Acids Res (2000) 28:3504–3510]. It also appears to be needed for synthesis of the transposase of IS*1* (insertion sequence 1) [J Bacteriol (2004) 186:2091–2098] and for the (temperature-dependent) repression of P fimbriae in *Escherichia coli* – as well as the transcriptional regulation (often repression) of various other genes. [Regulation of the sigma factor RpoS (by H-NS): J Bacteriol (2006) 188(19): 7022–7025.] H-NS also appears to repress transcription from the P_Y promoter of the transfer (*tra*) operon of the F plasmid [J Bacteriol (2006) 188(2):507–514].

Homologs of H-NS occur in many Gram-negative bacteria, and although sequence homology may be rather low, these homologs appear to have analogous DNA-binding properties [J Bacteriol (2005) 187(5):1845–1848].

(cf. HU PROTEIN.)

HO endonuclease See MATING TYPE.

Hogness box See CORE PROMOTER.

Holliday junction (Holliday structure) A conformation formed by two DNA duplexes as an essential intermediate in the process of homologous recombination (which occurs e.g. during meiosis). In the Holliday junction, one strand in one of the duplexes becomes covalently linked to (i.e. continuous with) a strand in the other duplex and the strand in the other duplex becomes continuous with the strand in the first duplex; two duplexes are therefore held together by two single-stranded regions of DNA. So-called *branch migration* of the Holliday junction leads to the formation of stretches of heteroduplex DNA – duplex DNA containing one strand from each of the participating duplexes. Resolution of a Holliday junction (i.e. restoration of two separate duplexes) involves introduction of a nick in each of the strands by a junction-resolving enzyme, followed by ligation – thus completing the recombinational event.

Holliday junctions are also formed during site-specific recombination mediated by the phage lambda-encoded integrase (Int) protein (involved in integration of the phage genome into the bacterial chromosome) – as well as in other instances of site-specific recombination mediated by tyrosine recombinases.

Resolution of Holliday junctions in homologous recombination is clearly important for the integrity of the genome, and resolution of these structures in site-specific recombination mediated by tyrosine recombinases is also important because this kind of recombinational event is involved e.g. in certain kinds of regulation of gene expression.

Resolution of Holliday junctions can be inhibited by certain peptides (e.g. WRWYCR) which bind to these structures and antagonize junction-processing enzymes; these peptides are also reported to be inhibitory for certain other recombinases, including the Cre protein (see CRE–LOXP SYSTEM) and the Flp protein (see FLP). These peptide inhibitors are likely to be valuable in studies on relevant recombination processes [Proc Natl Acad Sci USA (2005) 102(19):6867–6872].

(See also HMG BOX.)

Holliday structure *Syn.* HOLLIDAY JUNCTION.

homeobox A conserved, 180-bp sequence found within HOX GENES.

homeotic gene Any gene which is associated with the identity of a given part of an organism.

(See also HOMEOBOX, HOX GENE and POLYCOMB-GROUP GENES.)

homing endonuclease Any of a range of highly site-specific endonucleases found in some mobile genetic elements.

(See also INTRON HOMING and INTEIN.)

[The directed evolution of homing endonucleases: Nucleic Acids Res (2005) 33(18):e154.]

homodiaphoromixis See SECONDARY HOMOTHALLISM.

homodimixis See SECONDARY HOMOTHALLISM.

homogeneous test Any nucleic-acid-amplification test which is carried out entirely in a single, closed vessel.

(cf. HETEROGENEOUS TEST.)

homogenote See MEROZYGOTE.

homoheteromixis *Syn.* SECONDARY HOMOTHALLISM.

homoiomerous See MACRONUCLEUS.

homologous (1) Refers to the similarity or 'relatedness' of given samples of nucleic acid in terms of nucleotide sequences; if samples of nucleic acid have *identical* sequences then they are said to be 100% homologous.

(2) Refers to the *corresponding* sequence(s) of nucleotides in nucleic acids from different sources, i.e. sequences encoding similar functions – although not necessarily identical in terms of nucleotide sequence.

(3) Refers to the two chromosomes that form each pair (so-called 'homologous pair') in meiosis.

homologous recombination A type of RECOMBINATION which requires an extensive region of sequence homology between the two participating duplexes. Homologous recombination is involved in events as diverse as CROSSING OVER in meiosis and certain modes of DNA repair in bacteria.

A feature of homologous recombination is the development of a so-called *nucleoprotein filament*: a structure consisting of the free 3′ end of a strand of DNA coated with monomers of a protein which has the ability to promote the juxtaposition (*synapsis*) of homologous sequences of DNA; this leads to the formation of a hybrid duplex (*heteroduplex*) between the strand in the nucleoprotein filament and a homologous strand in the target duplex. In bacteria, the DNA strand within the nucleoprotein filament is coated with RECA protein; in other types of cell the DNA strand may be coated with e.g. RADA or RAD51.

In *Escherichia coli*, the development of the nucleoprotein filament may be initiated by the RecBCD system or the RecF system – or by a hybrid system consisting of elements from both of these 'recombination machines'.

RecBCD is a large multisubunit protein which exhibits both helicase and nuclease functions; it also has a synaptogenic function. RecBCD appears to be involved e.g. in the repair of double-stranded breaks.

The RecF system, involving a number of separate proteins, appears to be responsible e.g. for the repair of single-stranded gaps in circular molecules.

Following synapsis, and the formation of a heteroduplex, the process of homologous recombination proceeds to the development of an intermediate structure called a HOLLIDAY JUNCTION (q.v.) which is subsequently resolved to complete the process of recombination.

(Enzymes that mediate resolution of the Holliday junction can be inhibited by certain peptides which may be useful for experimentation in this area: see HOLLIDAY JUNCTION.)

In *Escherichia coli* homologous recombination is facilitated in certain regions of the chromosome. Thus, recombination is enhanced up to 10-fold in regions containing a so-called chi (χ) site:

$$5'\text{-GCTGGTGG-}3'$$

with which RecBCD has been found to interact. Chi sites are commonly found at or near the 3′ terminus in a nucleoprotein filament.

(See also INTEIN.)

homology (1) In general usage: similarity or relatedness. Thus, e.g. the phrase 'homologous chromosomes' refers to those chromosomes, in a given nucleus, which contain a similar or identical sequence of genes (although not necessarily alleles). When comparing fragments or molecules of nucleic acid, the sequences of nucleotides are often described as exhibiting a certain percentage homology (e.g. 'the sequences are 80% homologous') – meaning that, in this case, 80% of the nucleotides in one sample are the same as those, in corresponding positions, in the other sample(s).

(2) In some cases the term is given a meaning which is not equivalent to the general concept of 'level of similarity'. This meaning refers specifically to the relatedness of two or more sequences which have evolved, divergently, from a common ancestral sequence.

homology arm One of the two terminal sequences that bracket a given fragment of DNA which is designed to be inserted, by recombination, into a given target molecule that contains the corresponding sequences.

Homology arms can be quite short; for example, arms of 36–50 nucleotides in length are used in the protocol referred to in LAMBDA (λ) RED RECOMBINATION.

homomixis *Syn.* HOMOTHALLISM.

homoplasmy Refers to the (normal) condition in which there is a single mitochondrial genotype in a given cell.

(cf. HETEROPLASMY.)

homopolymer tailing See TAILING.

homothallism (homomixis) (*fungal genetics*) Self-fertility – in which there is no barrier to the fusion of gametes etc. from the same individual; MATING TYPES are not involved.

(cf. SECONDARY HOMOTHALLISM and HETEROTHALLISM.)

homozygous See ALLELE.

Hoogsteen base-pairing Base-pairing in which the pattern of hydrogen bonding differs from that in Watson–Crick base-pairing. In Hoogsteen base-pairing the C–G pair involves only two hydrogen bonds: (i) cytosine N-4 to guanine O-6, and (ii) (protonated) cytosine N-3 to guanine N-7. (Cytosine is protonated at pH <5.) T–A pairing involves O-4 and N-3 of thymine and the N-6 and N-7, respectively, of adenine.

Hoogsteen base-pairing is found e.g. in TRIPLEX DNA.

horizontal transmission (of genes) The transmission of genes from one individual to another, contemporary, individual. An example is the transmission of genes from one bacterium to another by the process of CONJUGATION.

(cf. VERTICAL TRANSMISSION.)

horseradish peroxidase (HRP) A hemin-containing peroxidase used e.g. for enzyme-amplified immunodetection procedures (immunoperoxidase assays) in which an antibody-conjugated peroxidase is used to locate a specific antigen e.g. on cells or tissues. HRP produces a brown precipitate with the substrate 3,3′-diaminobenzidine tetrahydrochloride dihydrate (DAB).

This peroxidase is also used e.g. in the TYRAMIDE SIGNAL AMPLIFICATION procedure and in an assay for pyrophosphate (PIPER PYROPHOSPHATE ASSAY KIT).

(See also ZENON ANTIBODY-LABELING REAGENTS.)

hot-start PCR A form of PCR in which cycling does not begin until the temperature of the mixture is, for the first time, sufficient to inhibit the non-specific binding of primers; the object is to avoid mispriming, i.e. the binding of primers to sequences other than their fully complementary binding sites. The avoidance (or minimization) of mispriming promotes specificity of the assay and reduces the background against which the actual target is to be detected. This approach may also enhance sensitivity by minimizing wastage of potential on the formation of non-specific products. Various types of procedure have been used for the hot-start approach.

One commercial system uses a modified form of the DNA polymerase that is inactive when added to the reaction mixture; activation of the enzyme occurs at the initial stage of denaturation when a temperature of ~95° is reached.

In another system the polymerase is inactivated by its own antibody. Inactivation is lost as the temperature rises for the initial stage of denaturation.

(See also PLATINUM TAQ DNA POLYMERASE.)

Yet another method involves the use of a physical barrier of wax (AmpliWax™, Applied Biosystems) which – initially – separates some of the components of the mixture from others (above and below the layer of wax). Cycling begins once the wax has melted (75–80°C).

[Some examples of the use of AmpliWax™: Appl Environ Microbiol (2005) 71(12):8335–8345; Virol J (2005) 2:41.]

(See also PRIMER SEQUESTRATION.)

housekeeping gene (constitutive gene, or reference gene) Any gene that is expressed constitutively in a given type of active/ functional cell, such expression being essential for the cell's normal activity.

Examples of housekeeping genes include any of those that encode species of rRNA.

HOX gene (*Hox* gene)   A generic designation for a HOMEOTIC GENE (which contains a HOMEOBOX).

(See also POLYCOMB-GROUP GENES.)

HPr kinase   See CATABOLITE REPRESSION.

HPr protein   See PTS.

hprK gene   See CATABOLITE REPRESSION.

HPRT deficiency   *Syn.* LESCH–NYHAN SYNDROME.

hrGFP   Humanized *Renilla* GFP: a HUMANIZED, recombinant form of GREEN FLUORESCENT PROTEIN from the invertebrate *Renilla reniformis* which is used (in mammalian cells) as a less-toxic alternative to the GFP from *Aequorea victoria*.

hrGFP is available commercially (Stratagene, La Jolla CA).

Examples of use: studies on intercell mitochondrial transfer [Proc Natl Acad Sci USA (2006) 103(5):1283–1288] and the activation of nuclear receptor FXR [Proc Natl Acad Sci USA (2006) 103(4):1006–1011].

(See also PATHDETECT SYSTEMS.)

HRM™   High-resolution melt: DNA melting analysis (Corbett Life Science) in which the methodology employed permits an increased amount of information to be obtained; the Rotor-Gene™ 6000 instrument is a real-time rotary analyzer used for this procedure.

(See also HIGH-RES MELTING.)

HRP   HORSERADISH PEROXIDASE.

hsd genes   In *Escherichia coli*: genes encoding the functions of a type I RESTRICTION ENDONUCLEASE (such as EcoKI).

Gene *hsdR* is required for restriction activity; it is transcribed from the promoter P_{RES}.

Genes *hsdM* and *hsdS* are both transcribed from promoter P_{MOD}.

Gene *hsdM* is required for the modification function.

Gene *hsdS* is the specificity determinant for both *hsdR* and *hsdM*. A null mutation in *hsdS* abolishes both restriction and modification activities.

(See also ESCHERICHIA COLI (table).)

hSos   A human guanosine nucleotide exchange factor involved e.g. in the CYTOTRAP TWO-HYBRID SYSTEM.

hTERT   Human telomerase reverse transcriptase.

(See also TELOMERASE.)

htpR gene   *Syn. rpoH* gene: see ESCHERICHIA COLI (table).

HTS assay   High-throughput screening assay.

Hu protein   One of a number of RNA-binding proteins which induce neuronal differentiation and which are associated (as targets) with human autoimmune disease.

Studies in mice suggested that the HuD protein is involved at multiple points in the development of neurones [Proc Natl Acad Sci USA (2005) 102(12):4625–4630].

Note. There is a possibility of confusion with the HU protein: see next entry.

HU protein   In various bacteria: a small NUCLEOID-associated DNA-binding protein which may contribute to compaction of the nucleoid and which is reported to have roles in chromosomal replication and site-specific recombination in *Escherichia coli*. Other roles may include e.g. regulating expression of gene *rpoS* (which encodes a sigma factor) [Mol Microbiol (2001) 39:1069–1079].

The binding of *Helicobacter pylori* HU protein is reported to differ from that of the *E. coli* protein in that e.g. it does not exhibit a strong preference for DNA with mismatches [Biochem J (2004) 383 (2):343–351].

In vitro, the HU protein is reported to dictate the morphology of the DNA condensates formed by crowding agents and polyamines – favoring a shift from toroidal to rod-like forms [Nucleic Acids Res (2007) 35(3):951–961].

Human Epigenome Project   See EPIGENETICS.

human foamy viruses   See SPUMAVIRINAE.

human immunodeficiency virus   See HIV-1.

human insulin *crb*   Recombinant human insulin (see INSULINS) which is synthesized as two separate chains (A and B) within bacterial cells. When isolated from the cells, the two chains are incubated under suitable conditions in order to promote the development of interchain disulfide bonds.

(cf. HUMAN INSULIN PRB.)

human insulin *prb*   Recombinant human insulin (see INSULINS) which is synthesized in bacteria as a single molecule (i.e. the precursor form, *proinsulin*). When isolated from the cells, the proinsulin is processed (cut) enzymatically to form the A and B chains – which are then incubated under suitable conditions for the development of interchain disulfide bonds.

(cf. HUMAN INSULIN CRB.)

humanized   (of a non-human gene)   Engineered in order to be expressed more readily in human cells – e.g. by changing certain codon(s) in order to avoid problems associated with CODON BIAS.

(See also HRGFP.)

Huntington's disease   A hereditary disorder, characterized by chorea and progressive dementia, which is associated with a gene on chromosome 4. The disorder involves expansion of MICROSATELLITE DNA.

Hurler's syndrome   *Syn.* MUCOPOLYSACCHARIDOSIS TYPE IH.

HvrBase++   A database which includes details of hypervariable regions in the mitochondrial DNA (mtDNA) from a range of primate species, including humans. The source also includes details of 1376 complete mitochondrial sequences as well as sequences from autosomal and X chromosomes [HvrBase++: Nucleic Acids Res (2006) 34(Database issue):D700–D704].

hybrid-arrested translation   A technique used in the identification of a protein encoded by a given cDNA. Essentially, mRNAs from the particular cell are translated *in vitro* in the presence of cloned (single-stranded) copies of the particular cDNA. The mRNAs which fail to hybridize with this cDNA yield proteins that incorporate a labeled amino acid; mRNA complementary to the cDNA will hybridize with it and will not be translated. Translation is repeated without cDNAs; the mRNA previously blocked by hybridization to the cDNA can now be translated. The protein of interest is the *extra* protein produced in the second translation, and it can be identified by comparison of the two sets of proteins – e.g. by gel electrophoresis.

hybridization-based sequencing   A method for sequencing a DNA fragment (e.g. 100 nt in length) by finding a set of short oligonucleotides which hybridize to the fragment in an overlapping pattern, and which – collectively – cover the whole fragment. This set of oligonucleotides is then arranged, by computer, into an order that reflects the complete sequence of the sample fragment.

In practice, the short oligonucleotides are present in an array of probes on a solid support (chip), the array covering all possible combinations of nucleotides in a probe of given length; for example, an 8-nt probe has 4^8 (65536) possible combinations of nucleotides, and this number of probes is present on the chip. The chip is exposed to labeled copies of the unknown sequence, and the particular set of probes to which they hybridize (under very stringent conditions) is determined and used in the computer analysis.

(See also DNA SEQUENCING and SHOM.)

hybridization protection assay   See ACCUPROBE.

hybridoma   The product (and progeny) of CELL FUSION (q.v.) between a tumor cell and a non-tumor cell; the purpose of making a hybridoma is to obtain a cell in which some/all of the properties of the non-tumor cell are exhibited on a long-term basis due to ongoing replication specified by the tumor cell.

A hybridoma formed by the fusion of a B lymphocyte (a B cell) and a myeloma cell is a source of *monoclonal antibodies*.

During the preparation of a hybridoma the efficiency of cell fusion may be low – e.g. 1 in 10^4. Moreover, it is necessary to prevent overgrowth of the tumor cells during incubation/culture of fusogen-treated cells. Therefore, use is made of (mutant) tumor cells which are blocked in *one* of two normal pathways for nucleotide synthesis; these mutant cells lack the *ancillary* pathway and are therefore unable to use exogenous thymidine or hypoxanthine. Consequently, *non*-fused tumor cells can be suppressed by the use of an incubation medium (HAT medium) that contains *aminopterin* (which blocks the *main* pathway of nucleotide synthesis) together with hypoxanthine and thymidine. In HAT medium, the fused (hybrid-

oma) cells are able to grow by using the ancillary pathway of the non-mutant partner cells.

hydroxyl radical (·OH)   See e.g. FENTON REACTION.

hydroxylamine (as a mutagen)   *In vitro*, this agent (NH_2OH) reacts primarily with cytosine residues in DNA, particularly in ssDNA, where it replaces the amino group with a hydroxyamino group (NHOH); adenine also reacts with the agent, but much more slowly. Bases modified in this way tend to undergo mispairing during the next round of DNA replication – leading e.g. to GC→AT mutations.

(See also NITROUS ACID.)

hygromycin B   An AMINOGLYCOSIDE ANTIBIOTIC that is active against plant and mammalian cells. It is used as a selective agent for cells stably transfected with (and expressing) a gene encoding resistance to hygromycin B (such as the *hyg* gene of *Escherichia coli*).

[Examples of use of hygromycin B (for selection): PLoS Biology (2006) 4(10):e309; Proc Natl Acad Sci USA (2006) 103(30):11346–11351.]

(See also G418 SULFATE.)

hyperauxiny   See AUXINS.

hyper-IgM syndrome (HIGM)   A rare immunodeficiency that is characterized by a high level of vulnerability to bacterial infections, normal or elevated levels of IgM, a lack of IgG and other isotypes, and lymph node hyperplasia.

The X-linked form of the syndrome (HIGM1) has been attributed to mutation in the *CD40L* gene. CD40L is a cell-surface molecule on T lymphocytes (T cells) which interacts with CD40 on B cells; interaction promotes the development of B cells in processes such as *class switching* (in which IgG and other isotypes are produced by the B cells as part of the normal antibody response).

The autosomal recessive form of the syndrome (HIGM2) may result from mutation in the *CD40* gene or a deficiency in the enzyme *activation-induced cytidine deaminase* (AID), an enzyme found in germinal center B cells. AID is essential for the processes of affinity maturation and class switching in B cells, and its activity may involve RNA EDITING.

hyphenated dyad symmetry   See PALINDROMIC SEQUENCE.

hypoxanthine   The product formed by oxidative deamination of adenine.

hypoxanthine guanine phosphoribosyltransferase deficiency   *Syn.* LESCH–NYHAN SYNDROME.

I

I L-Isoleucine (alternative to Ile).

I-like pili See PILUS.

IAA Indole 3-acetic acid. (See also AUXINS.)

IAN Indole 3-acetonitrile. (See also AUXINS.)

IAN-PCR Inverse affinity nested PCR: see METAGENOME.

ICF syndrome Immunodeficiency, centromere instability and facial abnormality syndrome: a (human) autosomal recessive disorder caused by mutation in *DNMT3B*, the gene encoding DNA methyltransferase 3B. The normal methylation of cytosine residues in the satellite DNA in certain loci is almost completely lacking in patients with ICF syndrome. This syndrome is characterized by low levels of the serum immunoglobulins, and many of the patients contract fatal infectious disease before reaching adulthood.

(See also GENETIC DISEASE (table).)

icosahedron A geometric figure bounded by 20 plane faces, all of which are equilateral triangles of the same size. Icosahedral symmetry (also called 5-3-2 symmetry) is a characteristic of the CAPSID of some viruses, including some phages.

identifier DNA Essentially, DNA synthesized with a unique (totally specific) sequence and used to identify a particular object; the DNA is immobilized on a 'tag' which is secured to the object. A tagged object can be rapidly identified e.g. by using sequence-specific molecular beacon probes.

idiogram A systematized, diagrammatic representation of a KARYOTYPE; a photographic version may be referred to as a *karyogram*.

idling In DNA replication: ongoing enzymic activity in which the conversion of dNTP to dNMP does not result in any *net* synthesis or degradation of DNA; it involves the addition and removal of nucleotides at a 3′ terminus.

Idling by DNA polymerase δ (delta) has been implicated in a mechanism for the maturation of OKAZAKI FRAGMENTS in lagging strand synthesis [see Genes Dev (2004) 18(22):2764–2773].

iduronidase See MUCOPOLYSACCHARIDOSIS TYPE IH.

ie-1 gene See BACULOVIRIDAE.

iFRET (induced FRET) A modified form of FRET designed as an improved fluorescence system for DNA melting analyses [original description: Genome Res (2002) 12(9):1401–1407]. The system involves a conventional FRET acceptor, bound to the DNA, and a donor consisting of a dsDNA-binding intercalating dye (such as SYBR GREEN I); in this arrangement, a positive signal is generated in a duplex setting and is lost on strand separation.

IGR Intergenic region.

IHF INTEGRATION HOST FACTOR.

IκB See NF-κB.

imatinib An agent which inhibits oncogenic TYROSINE KINASE activity (encoded e.g. by *bcr–abl* or *kit*); an anticancer agent. (cf. ERLOTINIB.) Mutant target molecules can inhibit binding of the drug.

[Inhibition of drug-resistant mutants: Proc Natl Acad Sci USA (2005) 102(31):11011–11016.]

immuno-PCR A PCR-based method used for the ultrasensitive detection of antigens. Monoclonal antibodies, specific to the antigen of interest, are immobilized on microtiter plate wells and exposed to the sample under test. Molecules of specific antigen, if present within the sample, are captured by the monoclonal antibodies. Any bound molecules of antigen are subsequently detected by homologous antibodies which are conjugated – via a STREPTAVIDIN–protein A chimera – to a biotinylated DNA fragment. Amplification of a segment of the DNA by PCR, and analysis of the PCR products by gel electrophoresis, provides a highly sensitive indication of the presence of the specific antigen.

More recently, the method has been simplified by using a recombinant phage that has a surface-displayed *single chain variable fragment* (scFv) which binds to the specific antigen; when the phage has bound to the antigen, the phage DNA is exposed, by lysis of the phage particle, and this DNA serves as a template for the PCR reaction. [Phage display-mediated immuno-PCR: Nucleic Acids Res (2006) 34(8):e62.]

immunoblotting (Western blot analysis) A form of BLOTTING in which a Western blot (see WESTERN BLOTTING) is exposed to specific, labeled *antibodies* in order to detect/identify particular proteins by antibody–protein binding.

Multiplex detection of proteins on a Western blot requires the use of a range of different labels; difficulties involved in using multiple types of fluorescent dye may be overcome by the use of QUANTUM DOT PROBES.

Recombinant proteins may be detected or identified by an antibody-independent procedure called ENZYME FRAGMENT COMPLEMENTATION.

immunodeficiency, centromere instability, facial abnormality syndrome See ICF SYNDROME.

immunomagnetic enrichment Any procedure, involving e.g. the use of antibody-coated superparamagnetic beads (such as DYNABEADS), for isolating a given type of cell or molecule, which binds to the antibody, from a mixture of cells or molecules. Beads are added to the mixture and are allowed to bind ('capture') the cells or molecules of appropriate specificity; the beads, with their adsorbed cells or molecules, are retained by a magnetic field while other components of the mixture are removed by washing.

In an alternative approach, antibodies are bound indirectly to the beads (rather than being bound directly).

(See also GENE THERAPY.)

immunomagnetic separation (IMS) See e.g. DYNABEADS.

immunoperoxidase assay See HORSERADISH PEROXIDASE.

importins See KARYOPHERINS.

IMS Immunomagnetic separation: see e.g. DYNABEADS.

in silico By computer.

in situ hybridization See ISH.

in situ solid-phase DNA amplification See SOLID-PHASE PCR.

in vitro protein synthesis See CELL-FREE PROTEIN SYNTHESIS.

in vitro **transcription–translation** See CELL-FREE PROTEIN
SYNTHESIS.

in vitro **transposition** See TN5-TYPE TRANSPOSITION.

in vivo **bioluminescence** (engineered) BIOLUMINESCENCE produced in LUCIFERASE-expressing (genetically engineered)
living cells/animals following the provision of luciferin. In
one experiment, tumor cells that constitutively expressed luciferase were implanted in the forebrain and flank region of
mice and allowed to develop into tumors. Subsequently, luciferin was injected intraperitoneally. (Intraperitoneal or intravenous injection of luciferin apparently permits the molecule
to penetrate cell membranes and to cross the blood–brain
barrier – allowing the detection of luciferase throughout the
animal's soft tissues.) In this experiment it was found that the
intensity of bioluminescence varied with time after injection
of luciferin, peak emission being recorded ~20 minutes after
injection and subsequently decaying slowly [BioTechniques
(2003) 34(6):1184–1188].

in vivo **biotinylation** (engineered) BIOTINylation of a specified
protein within living cells engineered by the action of the enzyme *protein–biotin ligase* on a target protein which has been
genetically modified to exhibit a biotin-binding tag: a *biotin
ligase recognition peptide* (BLRP). The protein–biotin ligase
may be an endogenous enzyme but is usually one expressed
from an imported plasmid-borne gene – usually the *birA* gene
encoding the protein–biotin ligase of *Escherichia coli*. Thus,
when a recombinant (i.e. BLRP-tagged) target protein is co-
expressed in a cell with the *Escherichia coli* BirA ligase,
BirA mediates the attachment of biotin to the BLRP tag. This
procedure has been carried out e.g. in mammalian cells as
well as in the cells of bacteria and the yeast *Saccharomyces
cerevisiae*.

(See also BIOEASE.)

The BLRP tags used for engineering biotinylation *in vivo*
are much shorter than the biotin-binding sequences present
on naturally biotinylated proteins. The natural tags are long
(>50 amino acid residues), and were these to be used in the
preparation of a recombinant (tagged) protein they may affect
the protein's properties. Moreover, these (natural) tags can be
recognized by endogenous biotin ligases, making it difficult
to regulate the biotinylation of a specific target protein. For
these reasons, shorter, artificial tags have been prepared by
carrying out multiple rounds of screening of peptide libraries
for those peptides which exhibit optimal biotinylation by the
BirA biotin ligase. The resulting tags, of e.g. ~23 amino acid
residues, have an efficacy in biotinylation comparable to that
of the natural tags.

Biotinylation of a specified protein *in vivo* has been used,
for example, to facilitate subsequent detection, recovery and
purification of the target protein from the cell lysate. This is
often achieved by using STREPTAVIDIN-coated DYNABEADS;
this procedure (in which the target protein is securely held by
the Dynabeads) permits efficient washing and purification.

In general, the *in vivo* biotinylation of proteins is likely to
be valuable as an affinity purification method in the field of
proteomics.

Biotinylation of transcription factors *in vivo* has been found
to facilitate studies involving chromatin immunoprecipitation
– in which the DNA-binding characteristics of a particular
protein are investigated by cross-linking proteins to DNA and
then isolating the required protein by an appropriate selective procedure.

[Examples of *in vivo* biotinylation using BirA: J Biol Chem
(2006) 281(7):3899–3908; Proc Natl Acad Sci USA (2006)
103(16):6172–6177; Nucleic Acids Res (2006) 34(4):e33.]

in vivo **expression technology** See IVET.

in vivo **fluorescence** Fluorescence produced in live, genetically
engineered cells/animals.

One factor which has facilitated *in vivo* fluorescence is the
availability of modified forms of the GREEN FLUORESCENT
PROTEIN with altered absorbance/emission characteristics. In
comparison to wild-type GFP (major absorbance at ~395 nm,
minor absorbance at ~475 nm), some genetically modified
forms of this protein have enhanced absorbance at 475 nm,
permitting excitation solely with blue light; the significance
of this is that excitation can be achieved in the absence of
ULTRAVIOLET RADIATION (thus avoiding a factor which is
potentially harmful to the cells/animals under investigation).
In one development, live transgenic mice expressing a fusion
protein (GFP fused to the tau microtubule-binding protein)
were seen as fluorescent animals when placed under radiation
from five blue LEDs (light-emitting diodes) [BioTechniques
(2003) 34(3):474–476].

Increased flexibility in the use of *in vivo* fluorescence has
been achieved by the development of O^6-alkylguanine-DNA
alkyltransferase (AGT) as a fusion partner: see GENE FUSION.

(See also LUMIO.)

As mentioned above, one of the problems which can affect
fluorescence imaging of living cells is the phototoxicity that
results from exposure to ultraviolet radiation used to excite
many types of fluorophore. One approach to protecting cells
from phototoxicity is the use of stroboscopically controlled
excitation; thus, the use of 1 ms pulses of radiation enabled
sharp images to be obtained of a rapidly moving flagellum –
and also reduced the level of phototoxicity, as indicated by
extended viability/activity of the cells used in the experiment
[BioTechniques (2006) 41(2):191–197].

A similar approach to problems of phototoxicity has been
employed for the fluorescent imaging of mouse and bovine
preimplantation embryos: the use of a spinning-disk confocal
microscope; embryos examined in this way were reported to
maintain full developmenal potential [BioTechniques (2006)
41(6):741–750].

Dual-fluorescence reporter/sensor plasmids have been used
to study the dynamics of microRNA formation in living cells
of zebrafish and mouse [BioTechniques (2006) 41(6):727–
732].

in vivo **footprinting** A form of FOOTPRINTING in which cells
are treated with a reagent that penetrates the nucleus, causing
e.g. modification of chromosomal DNA at a number of sites;

any given sequence of nucleotides in the DNA will be resistant to such modification if it is protected from the reagent by a closely bound protein. When extracted from the cell, the modified DNA is cleaved, at the sites of modified bases, into a number of fragments; the fragments are then analyzed and compared with control preparations. Analysis may be carried out by subjecting the fragments to LIGATION-MEDIATED PCR.

When the final experimental and control preparations are compared by gel electrophoresis, the *absence* of particular bands of fragments in the experimental preparation indicates that DNA-binding protein(s) have protected the corresponding cleavage sites in the DNA.

in vivo **mode** (in gene therapy)   See GENE THERAPY.

in vivo **protein analysis**   See e.g. TEV.

Inc groups (among plasmids)   See PLASMID (Compatibility: Inc groups).

IncFI group   See PLASMID (Compatibility: Inc groups).

IncFII group   See PLASMID (Compatibility: Inc groups).

inclusion (inclusion body)   In *Chlamydia* infections: an intracellular population of elementary bodies: see CHLAMYDIA.

inclusion bodies (*DNA technol.*)   See OVEREXPRESSION.

IncN group   See PLASMID (Compatibility: Inc groups).

incompatibility groups (among plasmids)   See PLASMID (Compatibility: Inc groups).

IncP group   See PLASMID (Compatibility: Inc groups).

IncX group   See PLASMID (Compatibility: Inc groups).

indel   An insertion–deletion polymorphism.

indinavir   See PROTEASE INHIBITORS.

indirect suppression   See SUPPRESSOR MUTATION.

induced FRET   See IFRET.

inducer exclusion   See CATABOLITE REPRESSION.

induction (of a lysogen)   See LYSOGENY.

INH   Isonicotinic acid hydrazide: see ISONIAZID.

INN   International non-proprietary name. (rINN may be used to mean recommended international non-proprietary name.)

INNO-LiPA Mycobacteria®   A PCR-based PROBE system from Innogenetics (Ghent, Belgium) which is used for identifying medically important mycobacteria (cf. ACCUPROBE). Amplification of spacers in the 16S–23S rRNA genes of the test strains (by PCR) is followed by reverse hybridization of the products to a range of membrane-bound probes [see J Clin Microbiol (2001) 39:3222–3227 and J Clin Microbiol (2004) 42:3083–3088].

INNO-LiPA Rif TB   See LINE PROBE ASSAY.

inorganic pyrophosphate (PP_i)   See PYROPHOSPHATE.

inosine   A ribonucleoside.

INSDC   INTERNATIONAL NUCLEOTIDE SEQUENCE DATABASE COLLABORATION.

insect-cell-based expression systems   Those systems used for the expression of recombinant proteins in either cultures of insect cells or in live insects: see BACULOVIRUS EXPRESSION SYSTEMS and DES.

insertion sequence (IS; IS element)   A type of TRANSPOSABLE ELEMENT (q.v.) which encodes only those functions that are necessary for transposition. (cf. TRANSPOSON.) The structural gene(s) of an insertion sequence are bracketed by a pair of INVERTED REPEAT sequences; usually, these inverted repeats form the terminal parts of an insertion sequence, but in some IS elements (e.g. members of the IS1111 FAMILY) the inverted repeats are *sub*terminal.

A specific insertion sequence is commonly designated by 'IS' followed by an *italic* number (e.g. IS*1*, IS2 etc.); in some cases the designation of an IS element includes an indication of the source organism – e.g. ISHP608 (q.v.), which is present in the Gram-negative bacterial pathogen *Helicobacter pylori*.

Insertion sequences exist in their own right, and they also form the terminal parts of class I (composite) transposons.

Insertion sequences commonly transpose by a cut-and-paste mechanism (see figure in entry TRANSPOSABLE ELEMENT) – but some transpose in the replicative mode (see e.g. IS1071) and some (see TRANSPOSABLE ELEMENT for details) transpose with the formation of a circular intermediate.

In bacteria, the chromosomal REP sequences have been reported to be common targets for insertion sequences [BMC Genomics (2006) 7:62].

Transposition frequency varies with insertion sequence and with the physiological state of the host cell. In general, the frequency of transposition ranges from ~10^{-9} to ~10^{-5} per IS per cell division.

The presence of an insertion sequence may be indicated e.g. by the effects of its insertion. For example, the presence of IS*3* in the *finO* gene of the F plasmid inactivates the *finO* gene and results in the ability of this plasmid to behave as a constitutively derepressed conjugative plasmid.

Some insertion sequences are used as markers for detecting or typing particular bacteria – e.g. IS*900* has been used as a specific marker for *Mycobacterium paratuberculosis*. IS6110 is regarded as specific for the *Mycobacterium tuberculosis* complex; different strains contain different numbers of copies of IS*6110* – e.g. the genome of the reference strain of *M. tuberculosis* (H37rv) contains 16 copies, while some strains apparently lack the sequence. Strains of *M. bovis* generally contain a single copy.

[Diversity of insertion sequences in the Archaea: Microbiol Mol Biol Rev (2007) 71(1):121–157.]

(See also entries for some individual insertion sequences under 'IS'.)

insertion vector   A CLONING VECTOR into which target DNA can be inserted, at *one* restriction site, without the need to remove non-essential DNA

(cf. REPLACEMENT VECTOR.)

insertional targeting vector   See VECTOR.

insulator   See CHROMATIN INSULATOR.

insulin aspart   The (non-commercial) name for a genetically engineered short-acting form of human insulin: see INSULINS.

insulin glargine   The (non-commercial) name for a genetically engineered long-acting form of human insulin in which the C-terminal residue in the A chain is replaced with a glycine residue and the B chain has two additional arginine residues. The recombinant protein is produced in *Escherichia coli*.

(See also INSULINS.)

[Use of insulin glargine for studying streptozotocin-induced diabetic mice: Cardiovasc Diabetol (2007) 6:6.]

insulins (recombinant) Any of various forms of insulin, some short-acting and some long-acting, which are produced by recombinant DNA techniques in a range of commercial organizations; some of these engineered insulins are synthesized in *Escherichia coli* and others are synthesized in the yeast *Saccharomyces cerevisiae*.

The native (human) insulin molecule consists of two polypeptide chains, A and B, of 21 and 30 amino acid residues, respectively, that are held together by two disulfide bridges. Even small changes in this molecule can cause significant changes in biological activity. For example, replacement of the proline residue at position B28 by an aspartic acid residue gives rise to a short-acting insulin (insulin aspart – compare INSULIN GLARGINE).

(See also HUMAN INSULIN CRB and HUMAN INSULIN PRB.)

Porcine insulin differs from human insulin by only a single amino acid residue, and it has little immunogenicity in man; it can be converted enzymically/chemically to a form which has the same composition as human insulin.

Bovine insulin differs from human insulin by three amino acid residues, and it does trigger an immunological response in humans.

int **gene** (phage λ) See PHAGE LAMBDA.

integrase See RECOMBINASE.

integration host factor (IHF) In *Escherichia coli*: a multifunctional, heterodimeric protein with contributory roles that include e.g. expression of the F plasmid, on–off switching of type I fimbriae, promotion of sigma factor specificity, and integration of the phage λ genome into the host cell chromosome.

integrin Any of a specific category of cell adhesion molecules which form part of the cytoplasmic membrane in many types of eukaryotic (including mammalian) cell and which have roles in various aspects of physiology. The integrin molecule is a heterodimer consisting of α and β protein subunits linked non-covalently. There are many types of α subunit but only relatively few types of β subunit; the particular combination of α and β subunits in any given integrin determines its distribution and biological properties.

The β_1 integrins, which occur e.g. in epithelial cells, have important roles in cell–cell and cell–matrix interactions; the matrix components to which these integrins bind include e.g. collagen, fibronectin and laminin. As well as the maintenance of tissue structure such binding is also involved in generation of signals that influence a range of cell functions, including aspects of the cell cycle.

Integrins of the β_1 group may also act as receptors for the specific adhesins of invasive pathogenic bacteria.

The β_2 integrins can be expressed by leukocytes and may also serve as receptors for bacterial adhesins. Many integrins bind, via their α subunit, to ligands containing the RGD motif (arginine–glycine–aspartic acid motif); this motif is mimicked by the FHA (i.e. filamentous hemagglutinin) of the Gram-negative bacterial pathogen *Bordetella pertussis* – binding between FHA and the $\alpha_M\beta_2$ integrin (= Mac-1) on an activated macrophage facilitating uptake by the macrophage [see also Infect Immun (2005) 73(11):7317–7323].

Inadequate expression of β_2 integrins by leukocytes results in the failure of these cells to respond normally in the process of inflammation (= *leukocyte adhesion deficiency*, LAD); those with this condition are more susceptible than others to infectious diseases.

A β_3 integrin ($\alpha_{IIb}\beta_3$), found e.g. on blood platelets, binds to ligands which include fibrinogen, von Willebrand factor and fibronectin; deficiency of this integrin leads to defective platelet agglutination (GLANZMANN'S THROMBASTHENIA).

A given integrin may be denoted by *two* CD numbers, one number referring to the α subunit, the other to the β subunit; for example, LFA-1 (leukocyte function-associated antigen-1) is CD11a/CD18, and the Mac-1 integrin is CD11b/CD18.

integron A segment of DNA containing (i) a gene encoding a recombinase (integrase) and (ii) site(s) (att) for the insertion or excision of one or more gene cassettes – such insertion or excision being mediated by the integrase.

Resistance integrons characteristically contain genes that encode resistance to antibiotics and/or to disinfectants. These integrons are found in bacterial chromosomes and also in plasmids and transposons. They have been divided into three classes on the basis of e.g. structure and distribution; resistance integrons of class 2 are associated with transposons of the Tn7 family and are found in Gram-negative species.

Super-integrons are species-specific elements which may contain up to ~100 gene cassettes that encode a variety of functions; they are chromosomal elements.

intein In some proteins: an *internal* sequence of amino acids which is able to catalyze its own excision (self-splicing) and to join the flanking regions (*exteins*) to form a functional protein; a branched polypeptide (having two N terminals and one C terminal) is formed as an intermediate product in the splicing process.

At least some excised inteins exhibit the properties of a site-specific endonuclease (*homing endonuclease*). Such an intein can (in e.g. the *VMA1* gene of *Saccharomyces cerevisiae*) mediate insertion of an intein-encoding sequence into an intein-less copy of the gene; the latter is cleaved (at the site normally occupied by an intein) and an intein sequence that is copied from the intein-containing allele is inserted. The ability of an intein to mediate the insertion of its own coding sequence into an intein-less copy of the gene is called *intein homing*.

(See also INTRON HOMING.)

The sequence-specific characteristic of the homing endonucleases – which are also called *meganucleases* – has been exploited e.g. in promoting homologous recombination in the vicinity of their specific target sequences. It was suggested that these enzymes might be useful for inserting transgenes at specific (rather than random) locations in the context of gene therapy. However, given the limited repertoire of naturally occurring homing endonucleases, it would probably be difficult to find an enzyme that could promote the insertion of a particular, chosen transgene; for this reason, a combinatorial approach has been used to create artificial homing endonucleases that cleave specific, chosen sequences [Nucleic Acids Res (2006) Nov 27 doi: 10.1093/nar/gkl720].

First discovered in the yeast *VMA1* gene, inteins also occur e.g. in the bacterium *Mycobacterium tuberculosis* (*recA* gene [Nucleic Acids Res (2003) 31(14):4184–4191]), the archaean *Thermococcus litoralis* (DNA polymerase gene) and in some algal viruses (DNA polymerase gene [Appl Environ Microbiol (2005) 71(7):3599–3607]); they have also been reported in the alga *Chlamydomonas reinhardtii* [BMC Biol (2006) 4: 38].

intein homing See INTEIN.

intercalating agents Molecules that contain a planar chromophore which can insert (intercalate) between adjacent base pairs in double-stranded nucleic acids; a *bifunctional intercalating agent* has two planar chromophores per molecule. The effects of intercalation may include e.g. local unwinding of the duplex.

In linear dsDNA, intercalation results in an increase in viscosity and a reduction in the sedimentation coefficient. In ccc dsDNA intercalation results e.g. in a local increase in pitch and changes in the viscosity of the DNA solution – and in the sedimentation coefficient of the DNA. Nicked circular (or linear) molecules of DNA can bind more molecules of an intercalating agent than can an equivalent ccc dsDNA molecule (see also ETHIDIUM BROMIDE).

When one molecule of an intercalating agent inserts at a given site it inhibits the insertion of another molecule in the adjacent two or three base pairs (the *neighbor exclusion principle*).

Intercalation *in vivo* can inhibit transcription and replication and may also induce mutations. Lower concentrations of e.g. some acridines, or of ethidium bromide, may selectively block replication of small bacterial plasmids (see CURING).

Intercalating agents include ACTINOMYCIN D, anthracyclines, ETHIDIUM BROMIDE, PSORALENS, QUINOXALINE ANTIBIOTICS and tilorone.

intergenic repeat unit *Syn.* ERIC SEQUENCE.

intergenic spacer region (ISR) See RRN OPERON.

intergenic suppression See SUPPRESSOR MUTATION.

internal resolution site (IRS) See TN3.

internal ribosomal entry site See IRES.

International Nucleotide Sequence Database Collaboration A joint, collaborative project involving the DNA DataBank of Japan (DDBJ), European Molecular Biology Laboratory (EMBL) and GenBank (NCBI: National Center for Biotechnology Information).

interrupted gene *Syn.* SPLIT GENE.

interrupted mating A method once used to study the transfer of genes, from donor to recipient cell, during conjugation. At time zero, a population of (Hfr) donors is mixed with a population of recipients; samples are removed from the mating mixture at regular intervals and are plated in order to select recombinants. Donor genes are transferred to recipient cells sequentially (according to their positions on the chromosome) so that a given donor gene will appear in recombinants after a characteristic interval from time zero.

In *Escherichia coli* the entire chromosome may be transferred in ~100 minutes, although, as time progresses, there is an increasing chance of strand breakage.

Interrupted mating has been used for genetic mapping.

interstitial junction sequence See TRANSPOSABLE ELEMENT.

intervening sequence *Syn.* INTRON.

intrabody A genetically engineered form of an antibody which remains within the cell in which it is synthesized. Intrabodies have been used in studies on GENE THERAPY (q.v.).

intragenic suppression See SUPPRESSOR MUTATION.

intramer An (intracellular) APTAMER (sense 1) which has been transcribed within a cell.

[Example of use: Proc Natl Acad Sci USA (2004) 101(31): 11221–11226.]

intron (intervening sequence) A sequence that occurs between those regions (*exons*) in a SPLIT GENE (q.v.) which, collectively, make up the coding sequence of that gene; introns are found in the split genes of eukaryotes, archaeans, bacteria and viruses.

Normally, the expression of a given split gene requires (i) transcription followed by (ii) excision of those sequences that correspond to the introns – and ligation (i.e. joining together) of the exonic regions to form a continuous coding sequence (i.e. a *mature* mRNA).

In human pre-mRNA, the excision of introns occurs by a complex process involving a SPLICEOSOME (see SPLICING).

At least some of the introns in bacteria and bacteriophages are autocatalytic (i.e. self-splicing).

(See also INTRON HOMING.)

intron homing (in bacteria) The replicative spread of a given intron to an intron-less allele. For a group I intron, homing begins with a typically double-stranded cut in the intron-less allele made by a *homing endonuclease* (which is encoded by the intron). During repair, the intron is used as template, so that a copy of that intron is inserted into the intron-less gene.

(See also INTEIN.)

For a group II intron, an RNA copy of the intron complexes with an intron-encoded protein. This complex makes a double-stranded cut in the target site and inserts the strand of RNA; a cDNA copy is made and the RNA is replaced by DNA. This process has been termed *retrohoming* (because of the involvement of an RNA intermediate).

[Review of intron homing: J Bacteriol (2000) 182:5281–5289.]

intron retention See ALTERNATIVE SPLICING.

inv–spa genes See PATHOGENICITY ISLAND (*Salmonella*).

inverse affinity nested PCR (IAN-PCR) See METAGENOME.

inverse PCR A form of PCR which is used e.g. for amplifying the (unknown) DNA that *flanks* a known sequence (on both sides) in a circular molecule. Inverse PCR is useful e.g. for investigating the site of insertion of a transposon in a plasmid or a chromosome.

In inverse PCR the primers are complementary to the two terminal (end) regions of the known sequence. However, unlike the normal arrangement in PCR, when these primers are bound to their complementary sequences they are extended in *opposite* directions, i.e. outwards, into the unknown flanking sequence on each side.

If the known sequence (e.g. transposon) has inserted into a long molecule (e.g. a bacterial chromosome), the initial task is to cut the molecule (with a RESTRICTION ENDONUCLEASE) and obtain the known sequence, together with both flanking regions, on a small, linear restriction fragment. This fragment is then circularized through hybridization and ligation of the STICKY ENDS. (Circularization can be promoted by carrying out the ligation with low concentrations of the fragments; in this way, the sticky ends on a given fragment are more likely to hybridize with each other than with sticky ends on another fragment.)

The *circularized* fragments are amplified by PCR, using the primers as described above. The resulting amplicons contain parts of the known sequence, i.e. the primer-binding sites at each end, and also the unknown (original flanking sequences) which now form the main (continuous) central region of each amplicon. The amplicons can then be cloned and sequenced etc.

Other uses of inverse PCR include e.g. the preparation of deletion mutations (see e.g. SITE-DIRECTED MUTAGENESIS) and preparation of full-length cDNAs (see CAPFINDER).

inverted repeat (IR)   In a given, double-stranded molecule of nucleic acid, either of two sequences such as:

$$5'....CCATC..........GATGG.....3'$$
$$3'....GGTAG..........CTACC.....5'$$

i.e. sequences which are identical, with the same polarity, but opposite in orientation. The two sequences may or may not be contiguous. (cf. PALINDROMIC SEQUENCE.)

In single-stranded nucleic acids an IR is equivalent to one of the two strands in a double-stranded IR; such IRs can e.g. form hairpin structures.

Typically, a pair of inverted repeats form the two terminal sequences in each TRANSPOSON and INSERTION SEQUENCE, although in some transposable elements (see e.g. IS111) the inverted repeats are in *sub*terminal locations.

IPTG   Isopropyl-β-D-thiogalactoside: a synthetic inducer of the *lac* operon, i.e. it inhibits the repressor system of that operon. As IPTG is not a substrate for β-galactosidase it is referred to as a *gratuitous* inducer.

(See also ALLOLACTOSE.)

IR   INVERTED REPEAT.

IRES   Internal ribosomal entry site: a specific segment of RNA (first obtained from the encephalomyocarditis virus, EMCV) which, when present in mRNAs, promotes high-level, CAP-independent synthesis of proteins in mammalian cells (and in *in vitro* systems) in monocistronic and bicistronic vectors. (The designation IRES is also used to refer to segments from other organisms/cells which promote cap-independent translation in eukaryotes.)

Versions of the EMCV IRES, that differ in sequence, have been widely used in a range of studies. These versions do not behave in the same way (e.g. they can exhibit a requirement for different types of translation factor) and so may behave differently in different types of cell. Accordingly, the results reported in studies involving EMCV IRES should include precise details of the particular IRES sequence used. [Translational efficiency of EMCV IRES in bicistronic vectors: BioTechniques (2006) 41(3):283–292].

iRNA/DNA   See OKAZAKI FRAGMENT.

IRS   Internal resolution site: see TN3.

IS   INSERTION SEQUENCE.

IS element   *Syn.* INSERTION SEQUENCE.

IS1   A 768-bp INSERTION SEQUENCE present e.g. in some R plasmids (which encode antibiotic-resistance), in the chromosome of *Escherichia coli* K12, and in the genome of phage P1.

Target sites for IS1 appear to occur preferentially in AT-rich regions, and insertion may generate 9-bp or 8-bp target-site duplication.

IS5   A 1195-bp INSERTION SEQUENCE present in the chromosome of strains of *Escherichia coli* K12.

IS10 (IS10L, IS10R)   See TN10.

IS50 (IS50L, IS50R)   See TN5.

IS101   A 209-bp defective (gene-less) INSERTION SEQUENCE; transposition of IS101 depends on functions encoded by the insertion sequence IS1000. (The inverted repeat sequences of IS101 are similar, but not identical, to those of IS1000.)

IS911   An INSERTION SEQUENCE which forms a circular intermediate ('minicircle') between excision and insertion into the target sequence. During circularization (see TRANSPOSABLE ELEMENT) juxtaposition of the inverted repeats (separated by the intervening junction sequence) brings together a −35 box and a −10 box at an optimal distance to provide an efficient promoter.

IS1000 (γδ)   A 5.8-kb INSERTION SEQUENCE that has extensive homology with the DNA of transposon Tn3.

IS1071   A 3.2-kb INSERTION SEQUENCE, often associated with xenobiotic-degrading genes, in which the 110-bp terminal inverted repeats and the transposase gene are related to those of class II transposons. Transposition of IS1071 involves the formation of a cointegrate, and a 5-bp target-site duplication is produced at the site of insertion.

[Functional analysis of IS1071: Appl Environ Microbiol (2006) 72(1):291–297.]

IS1111   An atypical INSERTION SEQUENCE that is characterized by *sub*terminal inverted repeats, the absence of target-site duplication on transposition, and the formation of a circular intermediate between excision and insertion into the target site.

(See also ISEC11.)

IS6110 An insertion sequence apparently specific to members of the *Mycobacterium tuberculosis* complex – see INSERTION SEQUENCE for further details.

(See also W-BEIJING STRAIN.)

ISEc11 An INSERTION SEQUENCE, related to members of the IS1111 family, present in the chromosome (and the virulence plasmid pINV) in a strain of enteroinvasive *Escherichia coli* (EIEC) [J Bacteriol (2006) 188(13):4681–4689].

ISH *In situ* hybridization: a PROBE-based procedure for detecting a target sequence *in situ* (at a normal or aberrant location within cells or tissues or e.g. within an *in vitro* preparation of chromosomes). A probe used for ISH – or a conjugate which is subsequently bound to a hybridized probe – may exhibit any of various types of label. Radioactive labels were widely used in the early protocols; fluorescent labeling (see FISH) is currently popular.

ISH has various applications in the study of structure and function in the biological sciences. In medicine it can be used e.g. to detect certain pathogens in clinical samples by using probes that bind to pathogen-specific sequences; in certain cases (e.g. *Mycobacterium tuberculosis*) a pathogen may be detected by ISH significantly earlier than it could be detected by culture. (ISH may also be able to distinguish virulent from non-virulent strains of an organism by the use of probes for specific virulence factors.)

ISHp608 An INSERTION SEQUENCE, present in a plasmid in *Helicobacter pylori*, which excises as a circular element; the break in the parent molecule is resealed. Transposition is site-specific (5′-TTAC-3′) [EMBO J (2005) 24(18):3325–3338].

island rescue PCR A form of PCR which has been used e.g. for the amplification of CPG ISLAND sequences from inserts in artificial chromosomes (e.g. YACs). This approach relies on the presence, in the insert, of (i) an ALU SEQUENCE (Alu sequences are common in the human genome), and (ii) a GC-rich recognition site for a RESTRICTION ENDONUCLEASE such as BSSHII; GC-rich cleavage sites are commonly found to be associated with CpG islands.

Artificial chromosomes are cut with the restriction enzyme, and the linear fragments are ligated to *vectorette* linkers (see VECTORETTE PCR). PCR is then carried out with a primer specific for an Alu sequence and a vectorette-specific primer.

isochore In human genomic DNA: a long sequence of nucleotides (of the order of hundreds of kilobases in length) that is characterized by a uniform, or near-uniform, content of the bases guanine + cytosine (G + C); the G + C content differs among different isochores. Isochores can be classified in five groups according to their G + C content.

Isochore mapping of the human genome revealed ~3200 isochores (which cover the entire genome) [Genome Res (2006) 16(4):536–541].

A web-based tool (called GC-profile) has been devised for analyzing variation in G + C content in sequences of genomic DNA [GC-profile: Nucleic Acids Res (2006) 34(Web Server issue): W686–W691].

isoniazid (INH) Isonicotinic acid hydrazide: a synthetic antibiotic, used as an anti-tuberculosis drug, which is bactericidal for actively growing cells of e.g. *Mycobacterium tuberculosis* (and some other mycobacteria). The antibacterial function of isoniazid depends on its intracellular activation by a catalase (the *katG* gene product). The catalase-activated drug appears to inhibit synthesis of the essential cell-wall mycolic acid.

Resistance to isoniazid may result from mutation in any of several genes, including *katG* and *ahpC*.

(See also LINE PROBE ASSAY.)

isonicotinic acid hydrazide See ISONIAZID.

isopeptidase *Syn.* SUMO protease (see SUMOYLATION).

isopropyl-β-D-thiogalactoside See IPTG.

isopsoralen See AMPLICON INACTIVATION.

isoschizomer A RESTRICTION ENDONUCLEASE whose recognition site is identical to that of another restriction enzyme. In general, the restriction enzyme which is first shown to recognize a particular sequence is called the *prototype* (in relation to that sequence); a prototype may have many isoschizomers (which can occur in different species).

An isoschizomer whose *cutting* site (*within the recognition site*) differs from that of the prototype is referred to as a *neoschizomer*.

isotachophoresis (ITP) A form of ELECTROPHORESIS in which fragments of nucleic acid *of different sizes* can be focused into a single band, i.e. in this procedure the electrophoretic mobility of polynucleotides is independent of size. DNA has been isolated from biological fluids by ITP and then analyzed by PCR [BioTechniques (2005) 39(5):695–699]; the DNA in such fluids may contain specific mutant alleles associated with cancer, so that ITP may be useful for the diagnosis and monitoring of cancer.

isotopic labeling (of probes) See PROBE LABELING.

ISR Intergenic spacer region: see RRN OPERON.

iteron One of a series of tandemly repeated ('reiterated') sequences of nucleotides found e.g. in the origin of replication of certain types of PLASMID. [Example of use: Proc Natl Acad Sci USA (2005) 102(8):2856–2861.]

The term 'iteron' (singular) has also been used for a *series* of these sequences.

(See also HANDCUFFING.)

ITP ISOTACHOPHORESIS.

ITR Inverted terminal repeat – see e.g. ADENOVIRUS.

***iutA* gene** In *Escherichia coli*: the gene encoding an outer membrane protein that acts as a receptor for the siderophore aerobactin (and for a colicin: cloacin DF13).

IVET *In vivo* expression technology: a method used originally to detect those genes (in a pathogen) that are expressed only *during infection* of the host animal; genes expressed only during infection *may* be virulence genes, and their identification can be followed-up e.g. with animal tests using strains of the pathogen which have mutations in the relevant genes.

The principle of IVET is shown diagrammatically in the figure.

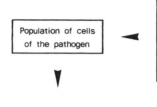

Population of cells of the pathogen

Population of small cccDNA molecules, constructed *in vitro*, *each* containing (in order of transcription):
(1) a random fragment of the pathogen's chromosome
(2) a *promoter-less* gene encoding chloramphenicol acetyl-transferase
(3) a *promoter-less* gene encoding β-galactosidase

Population of recombinant cells of the pathogen used to infect a test animal whose food has been supplemented with chlor-amphenicol

Recover the bacteria from test animal and plate on a medium containing Xgal; select white colonies

IVET (*in vivo* expression technology): a method used e.g. for detecting those genes (in a bacterial pathogen) which are expressed *only during infection of the host animal*. The figure shows, diagrammatically, one of several versions of IVET; other versions are described at the end of the legend.

Vector molecules (see *top, right*) are inserted, by transformation, into a population of cells of the pathogen. In each cell the (random) fragment of chromosome in the vector inserts into the corresponding part of the pathogen's chromosome by an insertion–duplication mechanism; thus, the genes that are present in the vector are inserted into a specific part of the chromosome. Because the vector molecules contain different fragments of the chromosome, they will insert into different chromosomal sites in different cells – forming a heterogeneous population of recombinant cells.

In some of the recombinant cells the vector's two promoter-less genes will have inserted 'in frame' with an upstream promoter; in such cells both of these genes are transcribed *if the promoter is active*.

The recombinant cells are used to infect a test animal whose food contains the antibiotic chloramphenicol. Under these conditions, a recombinant cell can grow if it produces chloramphenicol acetyltransferase (CAT), i.e. if the CAT gene (in the vector) is controlled by an active promoter in the cell's chromosome; thus, if the given recombinant cell *grows* in the test animal this indicates that its CAT gene is controlled by a promoter *which is active within the test animal*. The cells that produce CAT can form large populations which will greatly outnumber those cells which do not form CAT: a cell that does not produce CAT will be inhibited by the chloramphenicol present in the animal's food.

We need to know whether the promoter controlling a CAT gene is active *only* when the pathogen is infecting a test animal – or whether it is also active when the pathogen is cultured (e.g. on agar media). If it is active only in the test animal, this indicates that the gene *normally* controlled by that promoter is induced ('switched on') during infection; such a gene is of interest because of its possible association with virulence.

To resolve this question we need to study promoter activity further. The bacteria recovered from the test animal are plated on a medium lacking chloramphenicol but containing the agent Xgal; all the cells can grow on this medium. If the promoter regulating the vector's genes is active in culture, then β-galactosidase will be formed in the cell, giving rise to a *blue-green* colony; hence, such a colony indicates that activation of the given promoter does not occur *only* in the test animal. By contrast, a *white* colony (a *lac⁻* colony) indicates

The IVET principle is now exploited in different contexts. For example, the method was used to identify those genes of the plant pathogen *Erwinia amylovora* which are induced during infection of immature pear tissue [J Bacteriol (2005) 187(23):8088–8103], and has also been used to investigate *in vivo* gene expression in *Lactobacillus reuteri* during fermentation of sourdough [Appl Environ Microbiol (2005) 71(10): 5873–5878].

[IVET for exploring niche-specific gene expression: Microbiol Mol Biol Rev (2005) 69(2):217–261.]

IVET (*in vivo* expression technology): (*continued*) that β-galactosidase and CAT are formed *only* within the test animal (not in culture) – i.e. the relevant promoter is active only during infection of the animal. The gene which is normally controlled by this promoter can be identified, cloned and sequenced, and its role in virulence can be investigated.

A different version of IVET uses an *auxotrophic* population of the pathogen. These cells can (i) grow on agar media supplemented with the given growth requirement, but (ii) cannot grow within the test animal unless they contain the relevant – and functional – gene. Each vector molecule includes (in addition to the random fragment of chromosome) the genes encoding (i) the specific growth requirement and (ii) β galactosidase – both of these genes being promoter-less. The rationale is analogous to that given above.

In another version of IVET, each vector molecule includes (i) a tetracycline-resistance transposon and (ii) promoter-less genes encoding a transposase and β-galactosidase. If the relevant promoter is active in the test animal, transposase is synthesized and excises the transposon; the excised transposon does not replicate – leading to a clone of tetracycline-*sensitive* cells. Tetracycline-sensitive cells can be detected by replica plating using media which (i) lack, and (ii) contain tetracycline. The β-galactosidase has the same function as in other versions of the method.

Figure reproduced from *Bacteria in Biology, Biotechnology and Medicine*, 6th edition, Figure 11.3, pages 360–361, Paul Singleton (2004) John Wiley & Sons Ltd, UK [ISBN 0-470-09027-8] with permission from the publisher.

J

Jacob–Monod model An early model (~1960) for the system now known as an OPERON.

JAK kinase A member of the family of JANUS KINASES.

janiemycin A polypeptide with antibacterial activity; it inhibits transglycosylation during synthesis of the cell-wall polymer peptidoglycan.

Janus kinases A family of cell-membrane-associated tyrosine kinases – see e.g. SIGNAL TRANSDUCERS AND ACTIVATORS OF TRANSCRIPTION.

(See also TYROSINE KINASE.)

Java codon adaptation tool See CODON BIAS.

JC virus An icosahedral virus with a ccc dsDNA genome that belongs to the polyomavirus group. JC virus infects humans and other mammals; it can be oncogenic in newborn rodents, can transform certain types of cell in culture, and in immuno-compromised humans (e.g. AIDS patients) it can give rise e.g. to a fatal demyelinating condition known as progressive multifocal leukoencephalopathy (PML).

JC virus is similar to another human polyomavirus, the BK virus. Detection and differentiation of these two viruses (in cerebrospinal fluid, serum and urine) has been reported with a commercial hybridization assay [J Clin Microbiol (2006) 44(4):1305–1309].

JCat See CODON BIAS.

JM109 A strain of *Escherichia coli* used e.g. for cloning; it has mutations in various genes, including *endA*, *recA*, *relA* and *supE*, and is suitable for blue–white screening and for single-strand rescue.

juglone A compound, 5-hydroxy-1,4-naphthoquinone, found in leaves and roots of walnut (*Juglans*), with antibacterial and antifungal activity. [Transcription-blocking activity: Nucleic Acids Res (2001) 29:767–773; possible immunosuppressant activity: PLoS ONE (2007) 2(2):e226.]

jumping gene *Syn.* TRANSPOSABLE ELEMENT.

junction-resolving enzyme See HOLLIDAY JUNCTION.

K

K (1) A specific indicator of ambiguity in the recognition site of a RESTRICTION ENDONUCLEASE or in another nucleic acid sequence; for example, in CMG↓CKG (enzyme NspBII) the 'K' indicates G or T. (In RNA 'K' indicates G or U.) In this example, 'M' is A or C.

(2) L-Lysine (alternative to Lys).

K-*ras* See RAS.

Kaiso protein A protein that binds to DNA containing methyl-CpGs; the binding involves a characteristic zinc finger motif. The protein also binds to the sequence: CTGCNA.

Mice with a null mutation in the *Kaiso* gene were found to show resistance to intestinal cancer; this has suggested the possibility that Kaiso may be a potential target for therapeutic intervention [Mol Cell Biol (2006) 26(1):199 208].

The Kaiso-like proteins designated ZBTB4 and ZBTB38, unlike Kaiso, can bind to *single* methylated CpGs [Mol Cell Biol (2006) 26(1):169–181].

(See also MBD PROTEINS.)

kanamycin An AMINOGLYCOSIDE ANTIBIOTIC used e.g. as a selective agent for bacteria containing a vector which carries a kanamycin-resistance gene.

Kaposi's sarcoma A form of sarcoma found e.g. in immuno-suppressed patients, including those with AIDS. It has been associated with human herpesvirus 8 (HHV-8).

In vitro activation of latent HHV-8 was achieved by promoter demethylation using the reagent tetradecanoylphorbol acetate (TPA); a relationship was suggested between methylation status, transactivation, and the occurrence of HHV-8-mediated disease.

vIL-6, a form of interleukin-6 which is encoded by HHV-8, and which is apparently associated with pathogenesis, has been targeted by an intrabody [J Virol (2006) 80(17):8510–8520].

karyogram See IDIOGRAM.

karyolysis (*histopathol.*) Degradation of a eukaryotic nucleus with loss of affinity for basic dyes.

(cf. KARYORRHEXIS.)

karyomere See MACRONUCLEUS.

karyonide (*ciliate protozool.*) A clone of cells whose macronuclei are derived from the same parental macronucleus.

karyopherins In eukaryotic cells: agents involved in transport of proteins/nucleoprotein complexes between the nucleus and the cytoplasm; they include the *exportins* and the *importins*. Exportin 1 is also called CRM1.

karyoplast An isolated eukaryotic nucleus enclosed within a sac of cytoplasmic membrane that includes a small amount of cytoplasm.

karyorrhexis (*histopathol.*) The fragmentation of a eukaryotic nucleus.

(See also KARYOLYSIS and PYKNOSIS.)

karyosome A nucleolus-like body, or a nucleolus.

karyotic Refers to those cells which contain a nucleus: most of the cells of eukaryotes – but not e.g. erythrocytes (red blood cells).

karyotype A representation of (all) the chromsomes in the nucleus of a given type of eukaryotic cell, showing their size and morphology (usually) at metaphase.

(cf. IDIOGRAM.)

kasugamycin An AMINOGLYCOSIDE ANTIBIOTIC which has antibacterial activity mainly against Gram-positive species; it has also been used to control rice blast disease caused by the fungus *Pyricularia oryzae*.

(See also ANTIBIOTIC.)

katG **gene** See ISONIAZID and LINE PROBE ASSAY.

kb Kilobase, i.e. a length of 10^3 bases in a single-stranded (or sometimes double-stranded) nucleic acid. In double-stranded nucleic acids a length may be given in *base pairs* (bp) or in *kilobase-pairs* (kbp).

kbp Kilobase-pairs: see KB.

kDNA See KINETOPLAST.

kdpABC **operon** See TWO-COMPONENT REGULATORY SYSTEM.

Kemptide sequence The sequence of amino acid residues – leucine-arginine-arginine-alanine-serine-leucine-glycine (also written LRRASLG) – in a peptide tag which is used e.g. in a test system for the enzyme cAMP-dependent protein kinase A (PKA); the Kemptide sequence is phosphorylated by PKA.

The Kemptide sequence is also used as a tag that is suitable for *in vitro* labeling of recombinant proteins expressed in *E. coli*.

Kepivance® See BIOPHARMACEUTICAL (table).

Ki-*ras* See RAS.

Kid See PARD SYSTEM.

(See also R1 PLASMID.)

killer factor (in *Saccharomyces cerevisiae*) In 'killer' strains of *S. cerevisiae*: any of several secreted protein toxins encoded by a cytoplasmically inherited dsRNA element. Type 1 (or K1) killer strains form the K1 toxin – which binds initially to the cell wall of a sensitive cell and subsequently disrupts the cytoplasmic membrane.

(cf. KILLER PLASMIDS.)

killer plasmids (in yeasts) In some strains of *Kluyveromyces marxianus*: two linear, multicopy dsDNA plasmids (pG*l*1 and pG*l*2); cells containing these plasmids produce a glycoprotein toxin that kills (sensitive) strains of e.g. *Candida*, *Kluyveromyces* and *Saccharomyces*.

Killer plasmids can be transferred to other yeasts, e.g. by protoplast fusion; the recipients then exhibit the killer pheno-

type.

(cf. KILLER FACTOR.)

kilobase See KB.

Kineret® See BIOPHARMACEUTICAL (table).

kinetochore In eukaryotic chromosomes: either of the two multi-protein structures that assemble on both sides of the centromere at cell division; they are involved e.g. in attachment to the spindle and in regulating alignment of chromosomes prior to anaphase.

The outer part of a vertebrate's kinetochore includes microtubule-binding proteins (such as CENP-E), while the inner part includes e.g. CENP-A, -B, -C, -H and -I proteins, which keep their positions throughout the cell cycle.

A knock-out mutation of CENP-A was reported to result in misaggregation of the kinetochore [Mol Cell Biol (2005) 25 (10):3967–3981].

kinetoplast A complex network of catenated DNA molecules (kDNA) within the mitochondrion in protozoa of the order Kinetoplastida (e.g *Trypanosoma*). There are ~20–50 large circular molecules (*maxicircles*) and several thousand small circles (*minicircles*).

Maxicircles appear to be equivalent to mitochondrial DNA in other eukaryotes (encoding e.g. rRNA and proteins).

Minicircles encode most of the guide RNAs (gRNAs) that are involved in RNA EDITING [kDNA: Eukaryotic Cell (2002) 1:495–502].

The mitochondrion (including the kinetoplast) divides prior to cell division.

Division of the kinetoplast can be inhibited by certain intercalating agents, e.g. some phenanthridine derivatives such as ethidium bromide.

Kis See PARD SYSTEM.

kit (*KIT*) An ONCOGENE present in a strain of feline sarcoma virus. The c-*kit* product is a transmembrane protein with tyrosine kinase activity in the cytoplasmic region; it binds to, and enhances the activity of, *stem cell factor* (= kit ligand; mast cell growth factor; steel factor), an agent which can e.g. stimulate the proliferation of mast cells and regulate the growth/survival of hemopoietic precursors.

c-*kit* is strongly expressed in certain types of cancer.

kit ligand See KIT.

Kleinschmidt monolayer technique A method used for examining molecules of nucleic acid by electronmicroscopy. Nucleic acid is first coated with e.g. cytochrome *c* and it then forms extended (relaxed) molecules in a monolayer of denatured protein at an air–liquid interface; part of the monolayer is transferred to a grid, shadowed with heavy metal, and examined under the electronmicroscope.

Klenow fragment See DNA POLYMERASE I.

knockdown Refers to an organism in which one or more genes have been inactivated, or to the inactivated genes themselves.

knock-in mutation Any engineered change in nucleotide sequence that is designed to promote the expression of a given gene or genes – including gene(s) previously inactivated e.g. by a KNOCK-OUT MUTATION.

knock-out mutation Any engineered mutation that is designed to nullify the expression of a given gene or genes.

[Improved method for generating knock-out and knock-in mutations in cultured human cells: Nucleic Acids Res (2005) 33(18):e158.]

Kogenate® Recombinant human factor VIII (Bayer) which is used e.g. for therapy in cases of hemophilia A.

[Use (as a standard) for the *in vitro* assay of factor VIII: Biochem J (2006) 396(2):355–362.]

(See also table in the entry BIOPHARMACEUTICAL.)

Kornberg enzyme *Syn.* DNA POLYMERASE I.

Kozak sequence A sequence of nucleotides, flanking the init-iator codon, reported to optimize initiation of translation by eukaryotic ribosomes. In the original paper the sequence was reported as ACCATGG.

[Example of use: Clin Vaccine Immunol (2007) 14(1):28–35.]

The Kozak sequence is also used e.g. in some vectors of the EXCHANGER SYSTEM.

KpnI A type IIP RESTRICTION ENDONUCLEASE (see table in the entry).

KpnI family (of LINEs) See LINE.

KRAS proto-oncogene See QUADRUPLEX DNA.

Ku70 protein See GRANZYMES.

L

L L-Leucine (alternative to Leu).

L-complex The EDITOSOME in trypanosomatids.

L-SIGN *Syn.* CD209L.

L strand (of dsDNA) See H STRAND.

***lac* operon** (lactose operon) In e.g. *Escherichia coli* (and some other bacteria): an OPERON that encodes proteins involved in the transport (uptake) and use of β-galactosides (e.g. lactose); in *E. coli* this operon is located at ~8 minutes on the chromosome map.

The operon contains (i) three regulated genes: *lacZ*, *lacY* and *lacA*; (ii) a promoter (P), (iii) an operator (O) between the promoter and the first structural gene (*lacZ*), and (iv) the regulator gene (*lacI*) which is upstream of the promoter and which encodes a repressor. The *lacI* gene is transcribed constitutively, at a low rate, from an independent promoter.

The *lacZ* gene encodes β-galactosidase, an enzyme which cleaves lactose to glucose and galactose; this reaction also yields a minor product, ALLOLACTOSE, which is the *in vivo* inducer of the *lac* operon.

The *lacY* gene encodes β-galactoside permease, a protein involved in the transport of β-galactosides.

The *lacA* gene encodes thiogalactoside transacetylase, an enzyme which catalyzes the transfer of an acetyl group from acetyl-CoA to a β-galactoside. The *in vivo* function of the LacA protein in lactose metabolism is apparently unknown; one suggestion was that it might detoxify non-metabolizable sugars by acetylating them and facilitating their excretion.

In the absence of inducer, the regulator protein, LacI, binds to the operator and minimizes transcription of the operon by the RNA polymerase. A low level of transcription appears to occur in each cell under these conditions.

In the presence of lactose, the enzyme β-galactosidase converts some of the lactose to *allolactose*; allolactose acts as an inducer of the *lac* operon by binding to – and inactivating – LacI (the regulator protein). Once the regulator protein has been inactivated, the genes can be transcribed. The single mRNA transcript (i.e. a *polycistronic* transcript) includes an initiator codon and a stop codon for each of the genes. Note, however, that the *lac* operon is regulated not only by the LacI protein but also by CATABOLITE REPRESSION.

When the lactose has been used up, transcription of the operon is no longer needed; the inducer (allolactose) is not formed, and the (now active) regulator protein switches off the operon. The mRNA is degraded.

In recombinant DNA technology the *lac* operon can be switched on (induced), as required, by adding the compound isopropyl-β-D-thiogalactoside (IPTG) – which blocks the repressor protein. Unlike lactose, IPTG is a *gratuitous* inducer of the *lac* operon – i.e. although it induces the operon it is not metabolized by the cell. (This switching mechanism can be used when the expression of other genes is regulated via the *lac* operator sequence.)

Although this account describes the essential operation of the *lac* operon, the actual process is rather more complex. For example, the regulator protein can bind to more than one site: it also binds to sites designated O-2 and O-3, albeit with a lower affinity. During repression of the operon it appears that a tetramer of regulator protein binds at the main operator (O) and at O-2 (or O-3) – thus forming a loop of DNA – and that this may stabilize binding between the regulator and operator. Gene repression in the *lac* operon has been investigated in the context of DNA looping [PLoS ONE (2006) 1(1):e136].

As well as the main promoter (designated P1), the operon includes various overlapping promoter-like sequences. Some of these promoter-like sequences can be modified by a single base-pair substitution to yield a Lac$^+$ phenotype independent of the catabolite activator protein (CRP – see CATABOLITE REPRESSION).

Mutants with defective regulation of the lac operon Constitutive transcription of the operon occurs in those *lacI*$^-$ strains which fail to produce a repressor or which produce an inactive one.

The *lacI*^{s} mutants form a super-repressor which binds to the operator but which has little or no affinity for the inducer; as a result, the repressor binds to the operator even when an inducer is present – so that the operon is non-inducible.

In *lacO*^{c} (= *o*^{c}) mutants the operator has an altered affinity for the repressor; if the affinity is too low the *lac* genes are expressed constitutively.

Cells with a *lacI*^{q} gene produce higher-than-normal levels of repressor protein. This allele is included in some expression vectors in order to obtain 'tight' control of the expression of gene(s) that are regulated via a *lac* operator.

Lac plasmid LACTOSE PLASMID.

***lacI*^{q}** A mutant repressor gene of the *lac* operon associated with high-level production of repressor protein.

***lacI*^{s} mutant** See LAC OPERON.

***lacO*^{c} mutant** See LAC OPERON.

LacR An alternative designation of the LacI repressor/regulator protein of the *lac* operon.

β-lactam antibiotics A class of antibiotics in which the molecule is characterized by the 4-membered, nitrogen-containing β-lactam ring; all the antibiotics in this group kill or inhibit bacteria by targeting enzymes (so-called *penicillin-binding proteins*, PBPs) involved in the synthesis and maintenance of the cell wall polymer peptidoglycan.

A given β-lactam antibiotic may be more effective against Gram-positive species than against Gram-negative species, or vice versa; in general, a given β-lactam is ineffective against a number of bacterial species.

Bacterial resistance to these antibiotics commonly involves (i) the production of β-LACTAMASES and/or (ii) synthesis of a (*mecA*-encoded) PBP (designated PBP 2a, or PBP2′) which is resistant to a range of β-lactams. Resistance may also be due e.g. to reduced permeability of the cell envelope to particular antibiotic(s).

These antibiotics include CEPHALOSPORINS, carbapenems, CEPHAMYCINS, clavams, nocardicins and the penicillins (see PENICILLIN).

β-lactamases Enzymes, produced by certain bacteria, which inactivate susceptible β-LACTAM ANTIBIOTICS by cleaving the β-lactam ring at the C–N bond. Some β-lactam antibiotics are inherently resistant to some β-lactamases; in some cases the resistance of a given β-lactam antibiotic to specific β-lactamases may be attributed to particular structural features (such as the 7-α-methoxy group in cephamycins and the cysteamine side-chain of thienamycin).

The β-lactam antibiotic clavulanic acid (a clavam) has only weak antibacterial activity but it strongly inhibits a number of β-lactamases; it is used therapeutically e.g. in combination with certain β-lactamase-sensitive β-lactams that have greater antibacterial activity.

A β-lactamase gene (*bla*) is employed as a reporter gene in various commercial fusion vectors (GeneBLAzer™) that are marketed by Invitrogen: see pcDNA™6.2/GeneBLAzer™ in the entry GATEWAY SITE-SPECIFIC RECOMBINATION SYSTEM (table).

The detection of β-lactamases *in vitro* can be facilitated e.g. by the use of certain substrates which give a color reaction when they are cleaved by these enzymes – see e.g. NITROCEFIN and PADAC.

lacticin 3147 See LANTIBIOTIC.

lactose operon *Syn.* LAC OPERON.

lactose plasmid (Lac plasmid) In certain types of bacteria (e.g. some strains of lactococci): a plasmid that encodes the uptake and metabolism of lactose.

lacZ A gene encoding β-galactosidase (EC 3.2.1.23), an enzyme that hydrolyzes lactose to glucose and galactose; *lacZ* occurs in the LAC OPERON in *Escherichia coli* and in some other organisms.

lacZ **fusion** See GENE FUSION.

lacZΔM15 **mutation** See e.g. PBLUESCRIPT.

ladder (DNA ladder) See GEL ELECTROPHORESIS.

Laemmli electrophoresis See SDS–PAGE.

LAL test *Limulus* amebocyte lysate test: a procedure used for detecting or quantitating the pyrogen LIPOPOLYSACCHARIDE (LPS). [Example of use: Genet Vaccines Ther (2007) 5:2.] In DNA technology it is used for detecting LPS in recombinant products synthesized in Gram-negative bacteria.

The LAL test is based on the ability of LPS to bring about gelation of a lysate of amebocytes (blood cells) of the horseshoe crab (*Limulus polyphemus*). As little as 10^{-9} gram of LPS per milliliter can be detected in this way; the test is read within 1 hour, and the formation of a clot (i.e. a coagulated lysate) is recorded as a positive test (i.e. LPS present).

The capacity to cause gelation differs in different types of LPS.

Some substances other than LPS – including lipoteichoic acid and polynucleotides – are reported to cause gelation in this test.

As an alternative procedure, the product under test is introduced parenterally into three rabbits. The presence or absence of pyrogen in the product is subsequently inferred from the presence or absence of a specified rise in temperature in the animals. This test is useful for pyrogens in general (not only LPS). However, the test is precluded (in favor of the LAL test) if the product itself (apart from any contaminating LPS) has known pyrogenic properties.

lambda exonuclease See EXONUCLEASE.

lambda FIX® II vector A CLONING VECTOR (Stratagene, La Jolla CA), derived from PHAGE LAMBDA, used as a REPLACEMENT VECTOR after removal of a ~14-kb central region; it accomodates inserts of ~9–23 kb. [Use (e.g.) Proc Natl Acad Sci USA (2006) 103(15):5887–5892.]

The central region of the genome is removed by digestion with the RESTRICTION ENDONUCLEASE XhoI. This permits two terminal regions of the genome (20 kb, 9 kb), each with an outer *cos* sequence, to be subsequently ligated on either side of the gene or insert of interest. The vector–insert–vector construct can then be packaged (e.g. by a GIGAPACK product) to form an infective phage particle.

The initial digestion of the genome (with XhoI) produces 5′-TCGA overhangs on the 20-kb and 9-kb fragments. These overhangs are subjected to a *partial fill-in* procedure, with a DNA polymerase and the deoxyribonucleoside triphosphates dTTP and dCTP, to produce 5′-TC overhangs; this avoids subsequent self-ligation between the two vector fragments.

The sample DNA is digested with BamHI, MboI, BglII or Sau3AI and a partial fill-in carried out with dGTP and dATP, leaving 5′-GA overhangs; the inability of these fragments to anneal avoids the problem of subsequent ligation of multiple inserts to the vector ends.

Binding can now occur between the partially filled-in ends of the vector and the partially filled-in ends of the fragments.

Prior to ligation, the fragments of sample DNA, produced by restriction, can be size-fractionated in a sucrose gradient, allowing selection of fragments within a given range of sizes; this permits use to be made of those fragments which, when inserted into the cloning vector, will yield products of a size suitable for packaging.

The Lambda FIX® II vector includes T7 and T3 promoter sequences on either side of the cloning gap to permit transcription, if required.

The central region of the lambda genome (that is removed, and not used) contains the ATT SITE and also the genes for the LAMBDA (λ) RED RECOMBINATION system; the lack of these features in the vector discourages (unwanted) recombination between the insert-containing lambda FIX® II vector and the bacterial chromosome.

lambda phage See PHAGE LAMBDA.

lambda (λ) Red recombination Engineered recombination, in cells of *Escherichia coli* (or other bacteria), mediated by the Red recombinase function of PHAGE LAMBDA (genes γ, β and *exo* – encoding products Gam, Bet and Exo, respectively); the Red system permits *linear* fragments of DNA (generated e.g. by PCR) to be inserted into cells by transformation, or by electroporation, and then undergo recombination at *targeted* sites in the chromosome.

Linear fragments of DNA are usually degraded within *E. coli* by exonuclease activity. However, the Gam component of the Red system inhibits the (*recD*-encoded) exonuclease activity of the host cell's RecBCD recombination system.

The λ Red system can be used in either a plasmid-encoded or chromosome-encoded format.

This recombination system permits targeted replacement, inactivation or mutagenesis of genes, *in vivo*, using linear fragments of DNA. For example, PCR-derived products have been used to inactivate a range of genes in *E. coli* strain K-12 [Proc Natl Acad Sci USA (2000) 97(12):6640–6645]. Each targeted gene was first inactivated by replacement with an antibiotic-resistance gene (allowing selection of recombinant cells) and the antibiotic-resistance gene was then excised. In this experiment, the initial step involved amplification of the antibiotic-resistance gene by PCR. One of the primers carried a 5′ extension homologous to the terminal sequence of the gene *on one side of the target gene*; the other PCR primer carried a 5′ extension homologous to the terminal sequence of the gene on the other side of the target gene. Furthermore, the antibiotic-resistance gene being copied was bracketed by a pair of FRT (Flp-recognition target) sequences: sequences recognized by the site-specific recombinase FLP (q.v.).

Following transformation of cells with these PCR products, the two end sections of an amplicon undergo λ-Red-mediated recombination with the genes *flanking* the target gene – thus replacing the target gene with an antibiotic-resistance gene. Selection of recombinant cells is facilitated by their ability to grow in the presence of the given antibiotic encoded by the amplicon.

Finally, the antibiotic-resistance gene is removed by inserting a helper plasmid encoding the Flp recombinase – which excises the gene via the FRT sites.

In this protocol, the 5′ extensions on the PCR primers were only 36–50 nucleotides long, yet this allowed effective site-directed insertion. Moreover, while it is possible to transform *recD* mutants with linear fragments, this protocol can be carried out in wild-type cells.

A similar procedure was used to insert tagging sequences into specific chromosomal locations, enabling the production of protein–tag fusion products [BioTechniques (2006) 40(1):67–72].

A lambda (λ) Red recombination system has been used for inserting TEV protease cleavage sites into the *putA* gene of *Salmonella enterica* in order to carry out probing of protein structure/function *in vivo* [BioTechniques (2006) 41(6):721–724].

The efficiency of this system was reported to be improved by co-expressing the RecA protein with the Gam, Bet and Exo proteins [Mol Biotechnol (2006) 32:43–53].

[Preparation of an improved cassette, encoding resistance to gentamicin, for use in chromosomal gene replacement in *Escherichia coli* by the lambda Red recombination technique:

BioTechniques (2006) 41(3):261–264.]

lambdoid phages A category of phages whose genomes can undergo mutual recombination. The lambdoid phages, which have a similar *sequence* of genes (although they produce a number of genome-specific products), include e.g. phages λ, P22 and φ80.

lamivudine The (–) enantiomer of 2′-deoxy-3′-thiacytidine: an antiviral agent which is active against e.g. retroviruses (see NUCLEOSIDE REVERSE TRANSCRIPTASE INHIBITOR) and also some DNA viruses.

The drug has achieved seroclearance of HBsAg in patients chronically infected with hepatitis B virus [J Clin Microbiol (2004) 42(10):4882–4884].

A new resistance-conferring mutation has been reported in the hepatitis B virus [Antimicrob Agents Chemother (2005) 49:2618–2624].

landmark enzyme See RESTRICTION LANDMARK GENOMIC SCANNING.

lantibiotic Any of the (typically pore-forming) polycyclic BACTERIOCINS in which the molecule includes certain unusual residues – such as D-amino acids and the (sulfur-containing) amino acid lanthionine.

Lantibiotics are produced by Gram-positive bacteria (e.g. species of *Bacillus* and *Lactococcus*); they are active against other Gram-positive bacteria.

The food preservative *nisin* is one example of a lantibiotic.

Lacticin 3147 is a lantibiotic which consists of two peptide components – both being necessary for activity; each of the components requires modification by a separate enzyme.

Lantus® See BIOPHARMACEUTICAL (table).

lariat See SPLICING.

lawn plate A Petri dish containing an agar gel medium whose surface bears a continuous (confluent) growth of microorganisms (usually bacteria) of one species or strain.

LB broth A liquid medium used for the growth/maintenance of *Escherichia coli* and other bacteria. LB broth contains (grams per liter): tryptone 10, yeast extract 5, sodium chloride 5; pH 7.

LCR LIGASE CHAIN REACTION.

LCx® assays Diagnostic assays (Abbott Diagnostics), based on the LIGASE CHAIN REACTION, that are carried out on clinical samples for detecting certain types of pathogen (such as e.g. *Chlamydia trachomatis*).

leader peptide See 5′-UTR.

leader sequence (leader) (in mRNA) See 5′-UTR.

LEE (pathogenicity island) See PATHOGENICITY ISLAND (locus of enterocyte effacement).

***lef* genes** (in baculoviruses) Late expression factor genes: see BACULOVIRIDAE.

Lentivirinae A subfamily of viruses (within the family Retroviridae – see RETROVIRUSES) which replicate in, and kill, host cells; members of this group include the human immunodeficiency viruses (see HIV-1 and AIDS), feline immunodeficiency virus, visna virus (cause of a progressive, fatal meningoencephalitis in sheep) and the zwoegerziekte virus.

At least some lentiviruses – including e.g. HIV-1 and visna virus – can replicate in cell cultures.

Atypically, for retroviruses, lentiviruses infect non-dividing as well as dividing cells.

lentiviruses Viruses of the subfamily LENTIVIRINAE (q.v.).

lepirudin See Refludan® in BIOPHARMACEUTICAL (table).

Lesch–Nyhan syndrome (*syn.* HPRT deficiency) An X-linked syndrome, involving neurologic and metabolic abnormalities, associated with mutation in the gene encoding hypoxanthine guanine phosphoribosyltransferase (at chromosomal location Xq26–q27.2).

letA **gene** See CCD MECHANISM.

letB **gene** See CCD MECHANISM.

leucine-responsive regulator protein (Lrp) A homodimeric protein in *Escherichia coli* that contributes to the regulation of a range of genes and operons – commonly as an activator (but sometimes as a repressor) of transcription.

The activity of Lrp is inhibited by exogenous leucine.

[Lrp: J Biol Chem (2002) 277:40309–40323.]

Lrp and H-NS protein have been referred to as cooperative partners in the regulation of transcription of rRNA genes in *Escherichia coli* [Mol Microbiol (2005) 58(3):864–876].

leucine zipper In certain DNA-binding (and other) proteins: a (possibly helical) region in which leucine residues are repeated at every seventh residue in the chain.

leukemia inhibitory factor (LIF) A protein, encoded by gene *LIF* on (human) chromosome 22 (and produced by various types of cell), which is used e.g. in cultures of embryonic STEM CELLS; LIF promotes the pluripotent phenotype, i.e. it inhibits differentiation of ES cells.

leukocyte adhesion deficiency See GENETIC DISEASE (table).

levofloxacin See QUINOLONE ANTIBIOTICS.

LexA protease See SOS SYSTEM.

LFA-1 *Syn.* CD11a/CD18 (q.v.).

library (1) (genomic library) A set of DNA fragments (often in cloned form in vector molecules) which, collectively, may represent the entire genome of a given organism. This kind of library is prepared by isolating genomic DNA, cutting it into fragments with a restriction enzyme, inserting the pieces into vector molecules (e.g. plasmids) and then transforming cells with the recombinant plasmids; intracellular replication of the plasmids yields a clone of each fragment. (By contrast, a library prepared from a METAGENOME includes fragments from an unknown number of uncharacterized genomes.)

A library may be *screened* for a particular gene or sequence by various methods: see e.g. COLONY HYBRIDIZATION and RECACTIVE system.

(2) (cDNA library) A collection of cDNA molecules prepared from mRNAs obtained from a given type of cell under given conditions. This type of library reflects only the actively expressed genes of the given organism under the particular set of conditions (cf. genomic library).

(See also EXPRESSED SEQUENCE TAG.)

(3) A population of shRNAs (see SHORT HAIRPIN RNA), or other molecules, consisting of selected pieces of nucleic acid prepared by recombinant technology.

(4) (phage library) A population of phages, of a given type, in which different individuals have different coat proteins – the population as a whole exhibiting an extensive range of types of coat protein; this kind of population is prepared by *in vitro* mutagenization and is used in PHAGE DISPLAY technology.

(5) Any population of diverse synthetic molecules prepared for a given purpose or function.

LIF LEUKEMIA INHIBITORY FACTOR.

lif **gene** (in *Staphylococcus simulans*) A gene that encodes an enzyme which modifies the organism's peptidoglycan; such modification makes the organism resistant to the effects of its own BACTERIOCIN.

LIF **gene** (in humans) See LEUKEMIA INHIBITORY FACTOR.

ligase (early name: synthetase) Any enzyme of EC class 6 that forms a bond (C–O, C–S, C–N, C–C) using energy obtained from cleavage of a pyrophosphate bond (e.g. ATP → AMP). One example is DNA LIGASE. Another is protein–biotin ligase – see e.g. IN VIVO BIOTINYLATION.

(See also BINARY DEOXYRIBOZYME LIGASE.)

ligase chain reaction (LCR) A (probe-based) method for DNA AMPLIFICATION involving thermal cycling and the activity of a heat-stable DNA ligase. (Compare PCR.)

Essentially, in the basic scheme, sample dsDNA is initially heat-denatured to expose the target sequence (the *amplicon*) on one strand and a sequence complementary to the amplicon on the other strand. On lowering the temperature, two target-specific probes anneal, end-to-end, on the target sequence, the 3′ end of one probe being juxtaposed to the 5′ end of the other – i.e. the two probes jointly cover the precise sequence of the amplicon. With the probes bound to the amplicon, a heat-stable DNA LIGASE joins the two probes covalently.

Another two probes bind to the sequence *complementary* to the amplicon – on the other strand of the sample DNA – and are similarly ligated.

In this scheme, the 5′ juxtaposed nucleotide in one of the probes must be phosphorylated in order for ligation to occur.

Note that each pair of ligated probes forms a sequence to which another pair of probes can subsequently bind following a further phase of denaturation; hence, the quantity of product (i.e. ligated probe-pairs) rises exponentially with ongoing temperature cycling.

When probe–target hybridization occurs under sufficiently stringent conditions, the ability to amplify the target sequence argues for the presence of that specific sequence in the DNA sample; this is the basic principle underlying the use of the ligase chain reaction in diagnostic tests.

In the commercial form of the ligase chain reaction (LCx® assays; Abbott Diagnostics) the two target-hybridized probes are separated by a gap of one to several nucleotides (rather than being hybridized in a contiguous, end-to-end fashion); the gap between one pair of bound probes is staggered in relation to the gap between the other pair of bound probes. After the probes have bound to the target sequence a DNA polymerase fills in the gap and ligation then follows.

Detection of products

In LCx® assays the products of LCR (i.e. the pairs of ligated probes) are detected by a *microparticle enzyme immunoassay* (MEIA). For the purpose of this assay, the outer terminal of each probe (i.e. that end of the probe which is *not* ligated during cycling) carries a *hapten*: a molecule which binds to a specific antibody. The hapten on one probe of a pair differs from that on its partner probe (i.e. the probe to which it is ligated during cycling), i.e. the two haptens bind to different types of antibody.

After cycling, any probe pair which has been ligated will consist of a single strand bearing hapten 1 at one end and hapten 2 at the other end. The unligated probes carry only a single terminal hapten (hapten 1 or 2, depending on probe).

Ligated probe-pairs bind, via hapten 1, to microparticles (<1 μm in diameter) that are coated with antibodies specific to hapten 1. The microparticles are subsequently immobilized on a solid surface; note that these microparticles will have bound (i) ligated probe-pairs and (ii) any individual (non-ligated) probes which carry a terminal hapten 1.

To the immobilized microparticles is then added a conjugate consisting of the enzyme ALKALINE PHOSPHATASE (AP) linked to an antibody specific for hapten 2. This conjugate binds to hapten 2 on probe-pairs that are bound to the microparticles. On addition of the substrate for AP (MUP: 4-methylumbelliferyl phosphate), the MUP is cleaved by AP to a compound, 4-methylumbelliferone, which fluoresces under appropriate excitation. Monitoring of fluorescence provides quantitation of the LCR product. Note that *unligated* probes bearing hapten 2 are eliminated by washing during the assay; unligated probes bearing hapten 1 bind to the microparticles but, as they lack hapten 2, they do not bind conjugate and, hence, do not contribute to the measured fluorescence.

Anticontamination measures

As in other methods for *in vitro* DNA amplification (such as PCR), LCR can give false-positive results if extraneous DNA (e.g. from previous assays) contaminates the specimen and/or reagents. In general, anti-contamination measures include (i) use of anti-aerosol pipet tips, (ii) use of dedicated laboratory areas, and (iii) inactivation of products in the reaction vial (after the final reading) by automatic addition of a chelated metal complex and an oxidizing agent which jointly bring about almost total degradation of the DNA.

ligation (in DNA) The formation of a phosphodiester bond, mediated by a DNA LIGASE, between suitably juxtaposed 3′-OH and 5′-phosphate terminals.

ligation-mediated PCR (LMPCR) A procedure used e.g. for analyzing the products from an IN VIVO FOOTPRINTING assay – i.e. helping to define the locations at which proteins bind to DNA (e.g. in the promoter region of a given gene).

Essentially, the cleaved fragments of chromosomal DNA from a footprinting experiment are hybridized to copies of a gene-specific primer which binds to a site near the promoter sequence of the given gene; primer extension gives rise to a population of products of various sizes which reflect all the (accessible) cleavage sites in the promoter region of the gene. These products are blunt-ended at the 3′ end of the extended primer.

To these blunt-ended products are ligated double-stranded linkers. The linker-bound products are PCR-amplified with a second gene-specific primer and a primer that binds to the linker sequence. Finally, the PCR products are amplified with a third, end-labeled gene-specific primer. The final products are then examined by gel electrophoresis and compared with fragments produced by control experiments.

light strand (of dsDNA) See H STRAND.

LightCycler™ An apparatus (Roche) which is used for temperature cycling and monitoring in REAL-TIME PCR. Samples, each in a sealed capillary tube, are rapidly heated and cooled by a forced air current, permitting protocols to be completed in a short period of time.

Monitoring of progress in a PCR assay is carried out by means of a probe-based system. Essentially, when a BINARY PROBE binds to the target sequence on an amplicon (at the *annealing* stage) it fluoresces by a FRET-based mechanism. In the extension stage, DNA synthesis from the primer on the amplicon displaces (but does not degrade) both parts of the binary probe (cf. TAQMAN PROBE); fluorescence then stops, and the probes are free to take part (at the annealing stage) in the next temperature cycle.

The probe system can use e.g. fluorescein as a FRET donor and LightCycler Red 640 as the FRET acceptor; the latter compound fluoresces at 640 nm.

LightCycler™ Red 640 A fluorophore used in the LIGHT-CYCLER system: see REAL-TIME PCR.

LightScanner® See HI-RES MELTING.

LightUp® probe A commercial probe (LightUp Technologies, Huddinge, Sweden) used e.g. for monitoring amplification in REAL-TIME PCR. The probe consists of a PNA oligomer and an associated cyanine dye, thiazole orange, which is tethered to the oligomer; when the PNA binds to target DNA the ability of the dye to fluoresce is greatly increased.

[Examples of use: J Virol (2005) 79(3):1966–1969; J Clin Microbiol (2005) 43(8):4057–4063.]

limited enrichment method See AUXOTROPHIC MUTANT.

***Limulus* amebocyte lysate test** See LAL TEST.

LINE Long interspersed element: any one of a number of repetitive sequences, typically >1 kb long, which are found dispersed in at least some mammalian genomes (including the human genome); they are capable of retrotransposition. The human genome includes approximately 50000 copies of elements of the KpnI family.

(cf. SINE.)

line probe assay A PROBE-based assay used e.g. for detecting bacteria of the *Mycobacterium tuberculosis* complex and for simultaneously detecting mutations which confer resistance to specific antibiotic(s). One assay, the INNO-LiPA Rif TB (Innogenetics, Ghent, Belgium), detects mutations within a particular region of the pathogen's *rpoB* gene (which encodes the β-subunit of RNA polymerase), mutations that are usually responsible for resistance to rifampin (rifampicin) – a major anti-tuberculosis drug (see RIFAMYCINS). The assay involves a set of probes that are immobilized, in a line, on a membrane.

To detect the mutations, the 'resistance region' of the *rpoB* gene (in which these mutations commonly occur) is initially amplified by PCR in a reaction in which one of the primers is BIOTINylated. The resulting amplicons are denatured, and the single-stranded (biotinylated) products are exposed to the line of immobilized probes under stringent conditions.

Five probes (the S probes) consist of wild-type sequences which, collectively, cover the entire resistance region.

Another four probes (the R probes) cover sections of the resistance region associated with common mutations. Each of the four probes carries a specific mutation.

Any amplicons that bind to a given probe are subsequently detected by a STREPTAVIDIN–alkaline phosphatase conjugate which gives a purple coloration with an added reagent.

Coloration of all the S probes, with no staining of the R probes, indicates a wild-type strain (sensitive to rifampin).

Amplicons that contain one of the four specific mutations covered by the R probes will bind to the appropriate R probe; coloration of this probe will then indicate a particular mutant genotype.

There are opportunities in the assay for both false-positive and false-negative results.

False-positive results may derive from contamination with amplicons from a previous assay and/or from using a temperature below 62°C for the hybridization step. Also, a *silent mutation* may (falsely) indicate resistance by preventing hybridization of amplicons to relevant S probe(s).

False-negative results may arise if the temperature used for hybridization is too high (>62°C) or the concentration of the amplicons is too low. A false-negative result may also occur if a specimen contains a wild-type strain *and* a strain with a mutation that is not covered by the R probes; in this case the wild-type strain would cause coloration of all the S probes, indicating rifampin sensitivity, but the mutant strain would give no indication of its presence.

Another commercial line probe assay, GenoType MTBDR (Hain Lifescience, Nehren, Germany), detects resistance to both rifampin and ISONIAZID. Resistance to isoniazid is frequently due to mutation in the *katG* gene (often in codon 315), and this is reflected in the probes used in this assay.

Evaluation of the line probe assays referred to above found that both are useful for rapid screening, the GenoType assay having an advantage in being able to detect resistance to two antibiotics simultaneoulsy [J Clin Microbiol (2006) 44(2): 350–352].

linear cloning vector Any type of CLONING VECTOR which is either produced in a linear form or produced by linearization of a circular vector.

(See e.g. BIGEASY LINEAR CLONING SYSTEM.)

linearization Cleavage of a covalently closed circular molecule of nucleic acid to form a linear molecule.

linkage (of eukaryotic genes) The degree of association of two or more genes on the same chromosome; the shorter the distance between two genes (i.e. the closer the linkage) the more likely they are to be transmitted together to a daughter cell during cell division. Linkage can be estimated from the recombination frequency.

linker (*DNA technol.*) A short, synthetic, double-stranded fragment of DNA which is designed to be ligated (i.e. covalently joined) to one end of a given dsDNA molecule in order e.g. to facilitate manipulation of that molecule. For example, the sequence of nucleotides in a linker may include the recognition site of a particular RESTRICTION ENDONUCLEASE; thus when the (bound) linker is cleaved by the given restriction enzyme it can provide a desired STICKY END e.g. to facilitate insertion of the target molecule into a vector.

A (blunt-ended) linker may be joined to the target molecule by BLUNT-ENDED LIGATION.

Before using a particular linker it is necessary to ensure that the linker's restriction site does not occur also in the target DNA molecule itself; any cleavage sites within the target molecule may be methylated, prior to ligation, in order to protect such site(s) from the restriction enzyme.

A linker may also be ligated to a target molecule in order to provide a primer-binding site for amplification of the target sequence by PCR (see e.g. ANCHORED PCR).

Note. The term 'linker' is sometimes used for a *spacer arm*: a sequence used to link a reactive reagent to a particular position on a molecule; see e.g. BIOTIN for the meaning of spacer arm.

linker DNA (*in vivo*) See CHROMATIN.

linking number (α, *Lk*, topological winding number) In a given molecule of double-stranded cccDNA lying in a plane: the number of times one strand winds around the other.

Lipofectamine™ Any of several reagents (Invitrogen, Carlsbad CA) used for LIPOFECTION.

Lipofectamine™ 2000 is a cationic lipid reagent which is designed for high-efficiency transfection; it is reported to be suitable for nucleic acid delivery to a wide range of types of eukaryotic cell.

Lipofectamine™ 2000 CD transfection reagent is a chemically defined reagent which is 100% free of components of animal origin; it may be used e.g. in any protocol designed to ensure that the downstream product is free of animal-derived entities – such as prions or viruses.

lipofection Lipid-assisted insertion of nucleic acids into cells: one alternative to the use of a viral vector. In some procedures, a mixture of cationic and neutral lipids (in the correct proportions) form liposome complexes with nucleic acids and facilitate internalization. (cf. MAGNETOFECTION.)

Specific reagents are available commercially for particular types of application and/or particular types of cell. Thus, for example, Lipofectamine™ 2000 CD reagent is intended for use when there are concerns about the presence of animal-derived components (such as viruses) in the downstream product. Again, the 293fectin™ reagent has been optimized for transfection of FreeStyle™ 293-F cells.

Lipofection has been used e.g. in studies on the activation of T cells [J Clin Invest (2006) 116(10):2817–2826]; in GENE THERAPY for cystic fibrosis [Biochem J (2005) 387(1):1–15]; for studying mammalian mRNA synthesis [PLoS Biology (2006) 4(10):e309]; and for studies on the design of siRNAs [PLoS Genetics (2006) 2(9):e140].

A brief heat shock was reported to increase stable integration of lipofected DNA [BioTechniques (2005) 38(1):48–52].

(See also LIPOFECTAMINE.)

lipopolysaccharide (LPS)   A component of the outer membrane – the outermost layer of the cell envelope – in Gram-negative bacteria (such as *Escherichia coli*).

LPS is a macromolecule consisting of three linked regions: (i) lipid A, (ii) core oligosaccharide, and (iii) the O-specific chain; the O-specific chains in the outer membrane form the outermost part of the cell envelope, i.e. that part which is in direct contact with the environment. The (glycolipid) lipid A is associated with endotoxic properties.

LPS is a PYROGEN that must be removed from recombinant protein products synthesized in Gram-negative bacteria. This can be achieved by the chromatographic separation processes involved in downstream processing of the product.

(See also LPXC GENE.)

Listeria   A genus of Gram-positive, facultatively anaerobic bacteria; the organisms range from coccobacilli and rods (~0.5 μm in width to ~0.5–2 μm in length) to filaments. Most of the strains are catalase-positive. Oxidase-negative. Species occur e.g. in silage and decaying vegetation and also in some dairy products.

L. monocytogenes is a human pathogen which can cross the blood–brain barrier; it causes (sometimes fatal) disease which ranges from gastroenteritis to meningitis and abortion.

The GC% of genomic DNA in *L. monocytogenes* is 38.

LIVE *Bac*Light™ bacterial Gram stain kit   A commercial kit from Molecular Probes Inc. (Eugene OR) which is used for determining the Gram reaction of *living* bacteria by the use of a pair of DNA-staining fluorescent dyes: SYTO®9 (see SYTO DYES) and HEXIDIUM IODIDE. When treated with a mixture of these two dyes, Gram-positive bacteria are preferentially stained by the (orange-fluorescent) hexidium iodide – even though both dyes can penetrate the cell membrane. Gram-negative bacteria are stained by (green-fluorescent) SYTO®9 because hexidium iodide is excluded by the cell envelope in Gram-negative species.

live cell fluorescence   See the entries GENE FUSION and IN VIVO FLUORESCENCE.

LIVE/DEAD® *Bac*Light™ bacterial viability kit   A product (Molecular Probes Inc., Eugene OR) designed as a one-step staining technique for distinguishing between live and dead bacteria. The method is based on the use of two fluorescent dyes – SYTO®9 and propidium iodide – which stain the genomic DNA. SYTO®9 (green fluorescence) can enter both living and dead cells, but propidium iodide (red fluorescence)

can enter only cells with damaged/permeable cell membranes (a characteristic of dead cells). In this procedure, the living cells fluoresce green. In the dead cells, propidium iodide competes with SYTO®9 for binding sites on the DNA, and these cells fluoresce red. [Use of method in flow cytometry: Appl Environ Microbiol (2007) 73(10):3283–3290.]

Lk   LINKING NUMBER.

LMPCR   LIGATION-MEDIATED PCR.

LNA   See LOCKED NUCLEIC ACIDS.

locked nucleic acids (LNAs)   Nucleic acids, constructed *in vitro*, whose (modified) bases bind more strongly, and with greater specificity, to complementary bases [see: Tetrahedron (1998) 54:3607–3630].

Locked nucleic acids are used in PROBES [e.g. BioTechniques (2005) 38:29–32]. In genotyping, LNAs in (unlabeled) probes have been found to improve mismatch discrimination in melting analysis (T_m) studies [BioTechniques (2005) 39(5):644–650]. LNAs have been used to enhance activity of triplex-forming oligonucleotides [*purine*: J Biol Chem (2005) 280(20):20076–20085; *pyrimidine*: Nucleic Acids Res (2005) 33(13):4223–4234].

In some cases, the inclusion of LNAs in 2′-O-methyl oligonucleotides has been found to enhance stability of RNA/RNA duplexes (which may permit e.g. improved design for probes in Northern blot analysis) [Nucleic Acids Res (2005) 33(16): 5082–5093].

[Improvement of mismatch discrimination in LNA probes: Nucleic Acids Res (2006) 34(8):e60.]

[Position-dependent effects of LNA on DNA sequencing and PCR primers: Nucleic Acids Res (2006) 34(20):e142.]

locus of enterocyte effacement   See LEE pathogenicity island in the entry PATHOGENICITY ISLAND.

lon **gene** (in *Escherichia coli*)   A gene encoding the Lon heat-shock protein: an ATP-dependent protease.

In the SOS response to damaged DNA, Lon inactivates the SulA protein, thereby regulating the ability of SulA to block septation (see SOS SYSTEM).

Strains of *E. coli* with an inactivated *lon* gene are used e.g. in the production of fusion proteins (see ESCHERICHIA COLI (table), and see also 'The problem of proteolysis' in the entry OVEREXPRESSION).

long terminal repeat (LTR)   See RETROVIRUSES.

LongSAGE   See SAGE.

loop (*microbiol.*)   A simple instrument, used e.g. in bacteriology and mycology, for manipulating small quantities of liquid or solid material (e.g. during the inoculation of a medium); it consists of a metal rod (the handle) to which is attached, at one end, a piece of platinum or nickel-steel wire formed into a closed loop (~2–3 mm diam.) at the free end.

A loop (the wire portion) is flamed before and after use in order to sterilize it.

looping (in DNA)   The phenomenon in which separate sites in a DNA molecule are physically linked, via specific DNA-binding proteins, such that an intervening sequence of DNA forms a loop between the pair of sites. Looping occurs e.g.

when operator sequences are linked by regulatory proteins in the transcriptional control of certain genes/operons (e.g. in the LAC OPERON). (See also ENHANCER.) Gene repression in the *lac* operon was analyzed in the context of DNA looping [PLoS ONE (2006) 1(1):e136].

[DNA looping by restriction endonucleases: Nucleic Acids Res (2006) 34(10):2864–2877. Real-time observation of the DNA looping dynamics of the type IIE RESTRICTION ENDO-NUCLEASES NaeI and NarI: Nucleic Acids Res (2006) 34: 167–174.]

low-stringency conditions See e.g. PROBE and STRINGENCY.
(See also PCR.)

loxP See CRE–LOXP SYSTEM.

lpp **gene** (in *Escherichia coli*) A gene encoding the Braun lipoprotein, molecules of which link the outer membrane to the underlying layer of peptidoglycan in the cell envelope.

LPS LIPOPOLYSACCHARIDE.

lpxC **gene** (in *Escherichia coli*) A gene encoding deacetylase, a zinc-containing enzyme essential for the biosynthesis of lipid A in the outer membrane LIPOPOLYSACCHARIDE.

LR Clonase™ An enzyme that is used in the GATEWAY SITE-SPECIFIC RECOMBINATION SYSTEM; it can mediate *in vitro* exchange between a segment flanked by *att*L sites and one flanked by *att*R sites; both of the segments may be in circular molecules.

(cf. BP CLONASE.)

Lrp (in *Escherichia coli*) LEUCINE-RESPONSIVE REGULATOR PROTEIN.

LRRASLG The KEMPTIDE SEQUENCE (q.v.).

LTR (long terminal repeat) See RETROVIRUSES.

luciferase An oxidoreductase involved in the generation of light (BIOLUMINESCENCE) e.g. in certain species of bacteria, fungi and insects. The (ATP-dependent) luciferase of the firefly (*Photinus pyralis*) (EC 1.13.12.7) generates light when it oxidizes *luciferin*: 4,5-dihydro-2-(6-hydroxy-2-benzothiazolyl)-4-thiazolecarboxylic acid. In experimental systems, the intensity of the light generated can be monitored by means of (for example) a charge-coupled device camera.

Experimentation may be facilitated by the use of CAGED LUCIFERIN.

Luciferase is used in techniques for detecting and/or quantitating ATP (e.g. PYROSEQUENCING) and in reporter systems for studying e.g. promoter activity [Appl Environ Microbiol (2005) 71:1356–1363] and the efficacy of antisense oligomers [Antimicrob Agents Chemother (2005) 49:249–255].

(See also PATHDETECT and REPORTER GENE.)

Three luciferases, emitting green, orange and red light – with the same substrate – have been used for simultaneously monitoring expression levels in three genes [BioTechniques (2005) 38:891–894].

luciferin See BIOLUMINESCENCE and LUCIFERASE.

luciferin (caged) See CAGED LUCIFERIN.

Lumio™ A six-amino-acid-residue tag, encoded by some types of expression vector (Invitrogen, Carlsbad CA), which binds a fluorescent substrate, permitting e.g. fluorescence-based detection and localization of proteins in living mammalian cells (see e.g. pcDNA™6.2/nLumio™-DEST™ in the entry GATEWAY SITE-SPECIFIC RECOMBINATION SYSTEM (table)).

The Lumio™ tag also permits real-time detection of protein synthesis in a CELL-FREE PROTEIN SYNTHESIS system.
(See also IN VIVO FLUORESCENCE.)

lymphoid lineage Cells which include e.g. B lymphocytes (B cells), plasma cells (derived from B cells) and T lymphocytes (T cells).
(See also MYELOID LINEAGE.)

lysogen Any cell, or strain of bacteria, in which a BACTERIO-PHAGE genome has established a stable, non-lytic presence – as in LYSOGENY.

lysogenic bacteria See BACTERIOPHAGE and LYSOGENY.

lysogenic conversion (*syn.* phage conversion) See LYSOGENY.

lysogeny A stable, non-lytic relationship between a BACTERIO-PHAGE genome and a bacterial host cell in which no progeny virions are formed; in most cases (e.g. PHAGE LAMBDA) the phage genome (the *prophage*) is maintained by integration into the bacterial chromosome, but in some cases (e.g. PHAGE P1) the prophage persists as an extrachromosomal 'plasmid'. A cell containing a prophage is termed a *lysogen*; a lysogen continues to grow and divide, and replication of the prophage is coordinated with that of the host cell.

In some cases the prophage alters the phenotype of the host cell (a phenomenon termed *bacteriophage conversion*, *phage conversion* or *lysogenic conversion*). This may involve (i) the inactivation of host cell genes during integration of the prophage and/or (ii) expression of phage genes within the host cell. For example, integration of phage L54a into the chromosome of *Staphylococcus aureus* causes a loss of lipase activity. Phage conversion in some Gram-negative pathogens, e.g. species of *Salmonella* and *Shigella*, has been shown to alter cell-surface antigens; such modification of serotype has to be borne in mind when developing vaccine strains of these organisms. Phage conversion involving the expression of *phage* genes is responsible e.g. for toxin production in the causal agents of cholera (*Vibrio cholerae*) and diphtheria (*Corynebacterium diphtheriae*), and the shiga-like toxins of enterohemorrhagic strains of *Escherichia coli* (including O157:H7) are also encoded by a phage.

Commonly, the prophage retains a lytic potential, i.e. under certain conditions it is able to initiate the lytic cycle with the production of progeny virions and lysis of the host cell; in many cases this may occur spontaneously in a small number of cells in a lysogenic population. *Induction* of the lytic cycle in most or all cells in a lysogenic population may be achieved experimentally by certain agents – particularly by agents that damage DNA, e.g. ULTRAVIOLET RADIATION or MITOMYCIN C (both of which can trigger the SOS response in bacteria). In at least some cases, induction involves cleavage/inactivation of a phage-encoded repressor protein whose activity mediates the lysogenic state.

lysostaphin A BACTERIOCIN, produced by *Staphylococcus simulans*, which acts against strains of *Staphylococcus aureus* –

cleaving peptide bridges in the (cell wall) polymer peptido-glycan).

Lysostaphin has been used e.g. to isolate PROTEIN A.

lysozyme An enzyme (*N*-acetylmuramidase; EC 3.2.1.17) that hydrolyzes *N*-acetylmuramyl-(1→4)-β links in the bacterial cell-wall polymer peptidoglycan. The enzyme is found e.g. in saliva, tears and egg-white and is also found in macrophages. Lysozyme is used e.g. for the preparation of SPHEROPLASTS from Gram-positive cells.

lytic bacteriophage Any BACTERIOPHAGE which lyses the host bacterial cell.

M

M (1) A specific indicator of ambiguity in the recognition site of a RESTRICTION ENDONUCLEASE or in another sequence of nucleic acid; for example, in GT↓MKAC (restriction enzyme AccI) the 'M' indicates A or C. In the example, 'K' is T or G. (2) L-Methionine (alternative to Met).

M plasmid See MICROCIN.

M-tropic strains (of HIV-1) See HIV-1.

M13 phage See PHAGE M13.

M13K07 A HELPER PHAGE (q.v.).

mAbs MONOCLONAL ANTIBODIES.

Mac-1 See (β_2) INTEGRIN.

MacConkey's agar A selective, AGAR-based MEDIUM which contains peptone, lactose, sodium chloride, bile salts (e.g. sodium taurocholate) and the pH indicator neutral red. The bile salts inhibit non-enteric bacteria but permit the growth of enteric species such as *Escherichia coli* and *Salmonella typhi*.

Some species form acid from the fermentation of lactose and give rise to red colonies (the pH indicator, neutral red, is red below pH 6.8); these species include *E. coli* and some other members of the Enterobacteriaceae. The non-lactose-fermenting bacteria (for example, most strains of *Salmonella*) do not form acid and therefore give rise to colorless colonies.

macroarray A term used for a test system which is similar in principle to a MICROARRAY but which employs fewer – and often significantly longer – probes. Macroarrays have been used e.g. to analyze gene expression in the porcine immune system (probes: 200–650 nt) [Clin Diag Lab Immunol (2004) 11(4):691–698] and analyze transcription of simian varicella virus in tissue cultures (probes: 200–600 nt) [J Virol (2005) 79:5315–5325].

macronucleus (*ciliate protozool.*) The larger of the two types of ciliate nucleus (cf. MICRONUCLEUS); a cell may have more than one macronucleus, depending on species. Macronuclei (which contain a nucleolus) are usually polyploid, but are typically diploid in some ciliates – e.g. *Loxodes*; they encode the cell's somatic functions and usually disintegrate during conjugation, a replacement arising from the micronucleus.

A macronucleus is *heteromerous* if it is divided into two dissimilar *karyomeres* (parts): the *orthomere* and *paramere*. Most ciliate macronuclei are *homoiomerous*, i.e. they are not divided into karyomeres.

magnetic resonance imaging (for monitoring gene expression) See MRI.

magnetic separation See e.g. DYNABEADS.

magnetofection A process in which DNA – coated on super-paramagnetic nanoparticles – is introduced into cells (both *in vitro* and *in vivo*) by a strong magnetic field.

[Enhancement of the efficiency of non-viral gene delivery by application of a pulsed magnetic field: Nucleic Acids Res (2006) 34(5):e40.]

(See also LIPOFECTION.)

ᴹAGT See GENE FUSION.

major groove (in DNA) See GROOVES.

MALDI Matrix-assisted laser desorption/ionization: a method which is used e.g. for accurate determination of the relative masses of nucleic acid and protein molecules.

The analyte is initially embedded in a *matrix* which often consists of an aromatic carboxylic acid containing group(s) that can absorb laser radiation of wavelength approximately 340 nm. Pulses of laser, directed onto the embedded analyte, cause desorption (i.e. volatilization and ionization) of matrix material and of at least some analyte molecules. (Without the matrix, laser energy would be more likely to cause fragmentation of the analyte molecules.)

The ions (in gas phase) are initially accelerated with an electric field and then pass into a region of constant field at the end of which is a detector; the detector records the time taken by each species of ion to travel a specific distance, and a so-called time-of-flight (TOF) analyzer provides data based on the relationship between travel time and mass.

Analytes with low solubility may precipitate on the wall of the flight tube; such analytes may give better results when examined by ESI.

MALDI has been used e.g. to study acetylation by the p300 histone acetyltransferase [Biochem Biophys Res Commun (2005) 336(1):274–280] and has also found use e.g. in SNP genotyping [Nucleic Acids Res (2006) 34(3):e13].

MALDI–TOF See MALDI.

map unit (1) A CENTIMORGAN.

(2) Any unit which is able to indicate the locations of specific markers in a genome – e.g. the chromosome of *Escherichia coli* is divided into a number of *minutes* (used in interrupted mating experiments).

MAPH MULTIPLEX AMPLIFIABLE PROBE HYBRIDIZATION.

MAR2xT7 transposon See MARINER FAMILY.

mariner family A family of TRANSPOSONS that are widespread in animals, from humans and flatworms to arthropods; related transposons have been found in plants and fungi. The first transposon in the category to be isolated (*Mos1*) was obtained from a species of *Drosophila* (fruit-fly).

In appropriate constructs, certain *mariner* transposons, or their derivatives, can insert into the chromosomes of various species of bacteria.

This type of transposon has been widely used for insertional studies.

Characteristically, the *mariner* transposon inserts into TA-dinucleotide target sites with a cut-and-paste mechanism and with little or no requirement for host-specific factors.

The *mariner* transposon *Himar1* was used e.g. for insertional mutagenesis in *Leptospira interrogans* [J Bacteriol (2005) 187(9):3255–3258]. *mariner*-based transposons have been used e.g. for studies on *Bacillus subtilis* (transposon Tn*YLB-1*) [Appl Environ Microbiol (2006) 72(1):327–333], *Francisella tularensis* (transposon *HimarFT*) [Appl Environ Microbiol (2006) 72(3):1878–1885] and the PA14 strain of *Pseudomonas aeruginosa* (*MAR2xT7*) [Proc Natl Acad Sci

USA (2006) 103(8):2833–2838].

marker rescue The re-location of a given marker (e.g. a gene) from an inactivated (or defective) replicon to a functional replicon (through recombination) and, hence, acquisition of the capacity to be expressed or to replicate.

mast cell growth factor See KIT.

MAT See MATING TYPE.

maternal inheritance A type of CYTOPLASMIC INHERITANCE in which particular characteristics are inherited only from the female parent. For example, only the maternal mitochondrial genes can be inherited when paternal mitochondria are excluded from the zygote.

In the *poky mutant* of *Neurospora*, a (defective) gene that affects growth rate is transmitted from the female parent cell to sexually derived progeny.

mating type (*fungal genetics*) In general, any strain which can mate (i.e. interact sexually) only with a genetically distinct strain of the same species. Mating types have been studied particularly well e.g. in the yeast *Saccharomyces cerevisiae*.

The somatic (i.e. vegetative) cells of *S. cerevisiae* that give rise to gametes are haploid, and there are two mating types. Cells can mate only if they are of *different* mating types. The mating type of a given cell is determined by the particular allele which occupies the *MAT* (mating) locus: the *MAT*a allele or the *MAT*α allele; the *MAT*a allele is in the *MAT* locus in cells of the **a** mating type, while *MAT*α is in the *MAT* locus in cells of the α mating type.

All the cells (of both mating types) contain α-specific genes (which specify the α phenotype) *as well as* **a**-specific genes (which specify the **a** phenotype). These genes are controlled from the *MAT* locus: with *MAT*α in the *MAT* locus, α-specific genes are expressed and the cell exhibits the α phenotype; in cells of the **a** phenotype the *MAT* locus is occupied by *MAT*a.

*MAT*α encodes two products: the α1 and α2 proteins. The α1 protein is needed for the expression of α-specific genes; products of these genes include a pheromone, the α-*factor*. The α2 protein acts as a repressor of the **a**-specific genes.

*MAT*a encodes only a single product (the **a**1 protein) which appears not to be active in *vegetative* cells. With this allele in the *MAT* locus, the **a**-specific genes are expressed; products of the **a**-specific genes include a pheromone, the **a**-*factor*.

On mixing cells of **a** and α mating types, the pheromone of a given mating type promotes fusion with cells of the other mating type. The resulting (diploid) zygote, which has no mating potential, is designated **a**/α. Within the zygote, the α2 and **a**1 proteins (jointly) switch off both the α-specific and **a**-specific genes – and also switch off the so-called 'haploid-specific genes' which are normally expressed in cells of both mating types.

Isolates of *S. cerevisiae* often exhibit a spontaneous (and reversible) change from one mating type to another. Such switching involves replacement of the resident allele (in the *MAT* locus) by a *copy* of an allele of the other mating type. This mechanism depends on the presence of 'silent' copies of the *MAT*a and *MAT*α alleles that are kept transcriptionally

inactive by the structure of their chromatin. Switching involves a double-stranded cut in the *MAT* locus (by the HO endonuclease) and removal of the resident allele; this allele is replaced by an allele copied from the silent gene of the other mating type (*gene conversion*).

matrix-assisted laser desorption/ionization See MALDI.

Maxam–Gilbert method (of DNA sequencing) (*syn.* chemical cleavage method) A method of DNA SEQUENCING involving four separate reactions – in each of which an aliquot of end-labeled sample DNA is subjected to a chemical agent which cleaves at *one* of the four types of nucleotide; conditions are arranged so that, ideally, each fragment of the sample DNA in a given reaction is cleaved only once, i.e. at only one of the residues of the relevant nucleotide within the fragment.

As each of the fragments is labeled at one end, the products of a reaction include a number of end-labeled subfragments of various lengths – each subfragment extending from the labeled end to one of the positions at which cleavage has occurred, at the given nucleotide, within the fragment.

The reaction is repeated for each of the other three nucleotides – using an appropriate chemical cleavage agent in each case.

The four sets of subfragments (one from each reaction) are then subjected to gel electrophoresis in four separate lanes. As the subfragments are separated according to their lengths (i.e. according to the number of nucleotide residues in each), the position of a given band in the gel will indicate the identity of the nucleotide at a given location in the sample DNA; hence, the sequence of nucleotides in the fragment can be read directly from the gel.

A procedure analogous to the Maxam–Gilbert method, but using base-specific endoribonucleases (rather than chemical agents), has been employed for sequencing single-stranded RNA. Ribonucleases used: T_1 (Gp↓N), U2 (Ap↓N), Phy M (Ap↓N, Up↓N) and the enzyme from *Bacillus cereus* (Up↓N, Cp↓N).

maxicell A *recA*, *uvrA* mutant bacterial cell which has been subjected to ultraviolet radiation and in which the chromosomal DNA has been extensively damaged and degraded. Some of the small, multicopy plasmids within such cells may escape damage and may be able to direct the synthesis of proteins.

(cf. MINICELL.)

maxicircles (in trypanosomatids) See KINETOPLAST.

maxizyme An engineered, allosterically controllable, dimeric, Mg^{2+}-dependent NUCLEIC ACID ENZYME that is able to carry out cleavage of mRNA, *in vivo*, in a highly sequence-specific manner [original paper: Mol Cell (1998) 2(5):617–627].

A maxizyme has been used e.g. in studies on Alzheimer's disease [Gene Ther Mol Biol (2005) 9A:89–106].

(See also BINARY DEOXYRIBOZYME LIGASE.)

MBD proteins Methyl-CpG-binding domain proteins: a family of proteins that bind preferentially to a symmetrically methylated CpG motif in DNA.

These proteins can e.g. repress *in vitro* transcription.

(See also CPG ISLAND and KAISO PROTEIN.)

Mcc plasmid   See MICROCIN.

MCP   Methyl-accepting chemotaxis protein: a protein which acts as sensor in a TWO-COMPONENT REGULATORY SYSTEM that is involved in chemotaxis (i.e. movement in response to a chemical-gradient stimulus) in e.g. *Escherichia coli*.

mcrA **gene** (*syn. rglA*)   In *Escherichia coli*: a gene encoding a type IV RESTRICTION ENDONUCLEASE which is reported to cleave DNA e.g. at the sequence 5'-C^mCGG-3' (in which the *second* cytosine residue is methylated).

Inactivation of *mcrA* apparently permits greater efficiency when cloning DNA which is methylated in the above sequence.

(See also ESCHERICHIA COLI (table).)

mcrBC (*syn. rglB*)   In *Escherichia coli*: a sequence encoding a type IV RESTRICTION ENDONUCLEASE which is reported to cleave DNA at 5'-GC-3' loci in which the cytosine residue is methylated.

Inactivation of *mcrBC* apparently permits greater efficiency when cloning DNA that contains methylation in the above sequence.

An *mcrBC+* strain (i.e. one with an active form of this restriction system) is used in the GENETAILOR SITE-DIRECTED MUTAGENESIS SYSTEM.

Note. This sequence is also written *mcrCB*.

(See also ESCHERICHIA COLI (table).)

MCS (multiple cloning site)   *Syn.* POLYLINKER.

MDA   See MULTIPLE DISPLACEMENT AMPLIFICATION.

mecA **gene**   In strains of the Gram-positive bacterium *Staphylococcus aureus* (see MRSA): a gene that encodes a cell-wall-synthesizing enzyme (PBP 2a or PBP 2'; penicillin-binding protein 2a or 2') which is resistant to the antibiotic methicillin (and to other β-lactam antibiotics); this gene can confer high-level resistance to β-lactam antibiotics. [Evidence for *in vivo* transfer of *mecA* between staphylococci: Lancet (2001) 357: 1674–1675.]

The *mecA* gene occurs in the SCCMEC element (q.v.).

media   The plural of MEDIUM.

medium (microbiological)   Any solid (gel) or liquid preparation formulated specifically for the growth, maintenance (storage) or transportation of microorganisms (particularly bacteria or fungi).

Solid media are typically prepared with AGAR or with gelatin (cf. GELLAN GUM) and are usually dispensed into Petri dishes, glass screw-cap bottles or similar containers.

Liquid media are generally used in test tubes, screw-cap containers or flasks. *Any* medium must be sterile prior to use, and it must be inoculated and incubated with strict regard to avoidance of extraneous contamination.

(See also ASEPTIC TECHNIQUE and SAFETY CABINET.)

(Entries for specific types of medium: COMPLETE MEDIUM, MACCONKEY'S AGAR, NUTRIENT AGAR, SOC MEDIUM and TERRIFIC BROTH.)

meganuclease (*syn.* homing endonuclease)   See INTEIN.

megaprimer mutagenesis   A PCR-based technique for SITE-DIRECTED MUTAGENESIS involving e.g. a small primer, containing a mutant site, which binds to an *internal* site on one strand of target DNA. Extension of this primer to the 5' end of the template strand forms the *megaprimer*. Ongoing temperature cycling – with a conventional flanking primer to copy the *other* strand of the template – produces a large population of the megaprimer and *complementary* copies of the megaprimer sequence. The *complementary* copies are isolated, e.g. via gel electrophoresis, and are used as one of the two types of primer to copy the target DNA in a further round of PCR, leading to dsDNA amplicons containing the mutation.

[Examples of megaprimer mutagenesis: J Bacteriol (2006) 188:5055–5065; J Virol (2006) 80(16):7832–7843; Mol Cell Biol (2006) 26(18):6762–6771; Retrovirology (2007) 4:1.]

MEIA   Microparticle enzyme immunoassay: see LIGASE CHAIN REACTION.

melittin   A cationic, 26-amino acid, membrane-lytic peptide. If covalently bound to poly(ethyleneimine) (PEI), it forms complexes with DNA in which the DNA condenses into discrete particles (<100 nm diameter) which have enhanced entry into the cytoplasm during transfection; this approach also appears to promote entry of DNA into the nucleus (indicated by enhanced expression of transgenes) and may have potential as a non-viral gene-delivery system [see e.g. J Biol Chem (2001) 276:47550–47555].

A sequence encoding melittin is included in some versions of the BACULODIRECT vector in order to promote secretion of the expressed protein (see e.g. BaculoDirect™ vector in the table in GATEWAY SITE-SPECIFIC RECOMBINATION SYSTEM).

melting (of dsDNA)   Strand separation. Analysis of samples of DNA, based on their melting characteristics, can be carried out by using commercial systems such as HIGH-RES MELTING and HRM. (cf. TM-SHIFT PRIMERS.)

(See also HELIX–COIL TRANSITION and THERMAL MELTING PROFILE.)

membrane anchor sequence   See SIGNAL SEQUENCE.

2-mercaptoethanol (HO(CH$_2$)$_2$SH)   A reducing agent present e.g. as a constituent in buffers used for storing enzymes (e.g. many restriction endonucleases); it maintains sulfhydryl (SH) groups in the reduced state.

merodiploid   A partial diploid: a term used e.g. to refer to a (haploid) bacterial cell which has two copies of certain gene(s) – extra copies having been acquired e.g. by transformation.

merozygote   A prokaryote which has received exogenous DNA (e.g. by conjugation or transformation) and which, as a consequence, has become diploid in respect of certain allele(s). The recipient's genetic complement is the *endogenote*, while the imported DNA is termed the *exogenote*.

If the sequence in the exogenote is the same as that in the endogenote, the merozygote is a *homogenote*; if not identical, the merozygote is a *heterogenote*.

MessageAmp™ aRNA amplification kit   A commercial kit (Ambion, Austin TX) used for the high-level amplification of RNA (for example, for microarray gene expression profiling) when only limited quantities are available. Essentially, total (or poly(A)) RNA is used for FIRST STRAND synthesis of cDNA with an oligo(dT) primer which has a 5′ promoter sequence for T7 RNA polymerase. The hybrid RNA/DNA duplexes are treated with RNase H (fragmenting the RNA) and the RNA fragments are used as primers for synthesis of the second strand. Synthesis of the second strand provides a double-stranded template for the T7 polymerase and permits ongoing *in vitro* transcription to produce large amounts of antisense RNA (aRNA).

The aRNA product may be labeled during, or after, synthesis. For example, aminoallyl UTP may be incorporated at the time of synthesis; this allows a choice of the dye which is subsequently coupled to the reactive amino group. (The range of available amine-reactive fluorophores includes a number of the Alexa Fluor® dyes.)

[Uses (e.g.): Plant Physiol (2007) 143(2):924–940; PLoS Med (2007) 4(1):e23.]

meta operon (in the TOL plasmid)   See TOL PLASMID.

metacentric   Refers to a CHROMOSOME in which the CENTRO-MERE is located at, or close to, the center.

(cf. ACROCENTRIC.)

metagenome   The totality of genomes of all microflora found in nature, or in a given environmental location (e.g. 'groundwater metagenome'), including both cultured and uncultured species. [MEGAN: computer-based analysis of metagenomic data: Genome Res (2007) 17(3):377–386.]

The genomes of uncultured species are believed to form the major part of genetic information in the natural world and to constitute a rich source of information on e.g. novel products. Accordingly, various methods have been used for the *direct* screening of a metagenome with the object of isolating novel genes without prior isolation of the organisms from which the genes are derived.

One type of screening detects and amplifies target genes by means of probes or PCR primers based on known, *conserved* sequences of nucleotides.

A different approach starts with the preparation of a metagenomic library and uses it to screen for novel phenotypes in an *Escherichia coli* or other host species. (See also SIGEX.)

One difficulty in studies on a metagenome is the inefficient amplification of *rare* sequences, i.e. sequences that occur in samples in low-copy-number fragments. One approach to this problem is to use inverse affinity nested PCR (IAN-PCR) in which the initial step is a standard inverse PCR with one of the primers carrying an affinity tag (such as BIOTIN); the resulting PCR products are affinity purified (thus enriching the wanted product and removing background products) and are then subjected to a nested PCR. [BioTechniques (2006) 41(2):183–188].

methicillin   6-(2,6-dimethoxybenzamido) penicillanic acid: a semi-synthetic PENICILLIN which is resistant to cleavage by a range of β-lactamases. Bacterial resistance to methicillin can be due e.g. to penicillin-binding protein 2a (PBP 2a): see e.g. MRSA.

methicillin-resistant *Staphylococcus aureus*   See MRSA.

methoxyamine (as a mutagen)   An agent (NH_2OCH_3) with activity similar to that of HYDROXYLAMINE.

methyl-binding PCR   A method for detecting methylation of CpG sequences in genomic DNA. Essentially, genomic DNA in the test sample is fragmented by restriction endonucleases, and the fragment of interest (such as a CpG island associated with the promoter of a given gene) is allowed to bind to the (immobilized) molecules of recombinant protein that have a high affinity for methylated CpG sequences; in the tube containing the immobilized proteins (and the bound DNA fragments) PCR is carried out with gene-specific primers.

[Method: Nucleic Acids Res (2006) 34(11):e82.]

methyl-CpG-binding domain   See CPG ISLAND.

(See also MBD PROTEINS.)

***N*-methyl-*N*′-nitro-*N*-nitrosoguanidine**   See DNA REPAIR.

***N*-methyl-*N*-nitrosourea**   See DNA REPAIR.

3-methyladenine DNA glycosylase II   See DNA REPAIR.

methylation (of DNA)   The addition of a methyl group ($-CH_3$) to specific bases in DNA. For notes on the roles of methylation in prokaryotes and eukaryotes see entry DNA METHYL-TRANSFERASE. (Other relevant entries include: BISULFITE, CPG ISLAND, CPNPG SITES, EPIGENETICS, GENETIC IMPRINT-ING, METHYL-BINDING PCR, METHYLATION-SPECIFIC PCR, METHYLOME, REBASE, RESTRICTION ENDONUCLEASE and RESTRICTION LANDMARK GENOMIC SCANNING.)

Methylation-based gene silencing has been studied e.g. by methods that promote DEMETHYLATION (q.v.).

Methylation of specific bases may be achieved *in vitro* and *in vivo* by TAGM. More recently it was reported that targeted methylation had been achieved with mutant methyltransferases linked to zinc-finger arrays, the latter giving specificity; the pattern of methylation imparted to the DNA (*in vivo*) was transmitted through successive cell divisions [Nucleic Acids Res (2007) 35(3):740–754].

Methylation in specific alleles has been studied by ALLELE-SPECIFIC DNA METHYLATION ANALYSIS.

[Microarray-based DNA methylation profiles: technology and applications: Nucleic Acids Res (2006) 34:528–542.]

Detection of (5′-methylated) cytosine residues in genomic DNA was reported in a microarray-based protocol employing monoclonal antibodies [DNA Res (2006) 13(1):37–42].

PCR-based analysis of DNA methylation has been carried out with BISULFITE-treated – but initially non-desulfonated – DNA (SafeBis DNA) that is resistant to uracil-*N*-glycosylase (UNG), the enzyme used in a standard anti-contamination procedure; in this method, the desulfonation of SafeBis DNA occurs (in PCR) during an initial prolonged (30-minute) stage of denaturation at 95°C [Nucleic Acids Res (2007) 35(1):e4].

methylation (of RNA)   See e.g. CAP.

methylation-deficient cells   Mutants defective in methylation of DNA bases. For example, strain SCS110 of *Escherichia coli* (Stratagene, La Jolla CA) lacks *dam* (adenine methylase) and *dcm* (cytosine methylase) functions; strains such as this are useful e.g. for producing cloned DNA that can be cut by methylation-sensitive RESTRICTION ENDONUCLEASES (such as EcoRII and XbaI).

methylation-specific PCR (MSP)   A form of PCR which is used for monitoring the methylation status of CpG sites in DNA, i.e. for detecting changes in methylation at these sites.

Essentially, BISULFITE-treated genomic DNA is examined with different pairs of primers that can distinguish sites in the original (pre-treatment) sample which are methylated or non-methylated. The primers are designed to reflect the changes in sequence that result from treatment with bisulfite, i.e. the conversion of (non-methylated) cytosine to uracil.

A quantitative multiplex form of MSP has been developed [BioTechniques (2006) 40(2):210–219].

methylation-specific single-base extension (MSBE)   A method used for monitoring methylation at CpG sites in genomic DNA. Genomic DNA is initially treated with BISULFITE to convert *non*-methylated cytosine to uracil. Bisulfite-modified DNA is then amplified by PCR with primers that bind to the modified template.

A *specific* CpG that was *non*-methylated before treatment with bisulfite will, after PCR, exhibit a change from GC to AT. The presence of A (or T), in a particular strand, can be determined by using a primer whose 3′ end is extended by a T (or A) complementary to the base *at the given site*. This primer is extended, for a single base only, by using a labeled, chain-terminating dideoxyribonucleoside triphosphate; extension of the primer by ddT or ddA (signaled by the labeled products) indicates that the given CpG is non-methylated in the original sample of genomic DNA.

[Method: BioTechniques (2005) 38:354–358.]

***N,N′*-methylene-*bis*-acrylamide** (Bis)   A cross-linking agent which is used in the preparation of POLYACRYLAMIDE gels from ACRYLAMIDE.

In polyacrylamide gels used for the separation of fragments of nucleic acid by GEL ELECTROPHORESIS, the ratio of acrylamide to Bis is often ~19:1.

methylome   The totality of DNA methylation in a given cell, and its inherent content of information. It varies with time in the life of the cell.

methylotrophic fungi   Those fungi – e.g. species of the yeasts *Hansenula* and *Pichia* – which are able to carry out oxidative metabolism of C_1 compounds (such as methanol) with the assimilation of formaldehyde as a major source of carbon. An example is *Pichia pastoris*.

methyltransferase   See DNA METHYLTRANSFERASE.

***mfd* gene**   A gene (*mutation frequency decline*) which encodes the *transcription repair coupling factor* (TRCF): a protein which facilitates the release of a stalled RNA polymerase at a lesion on the DNA template.

While, as the name indicates, the Mfd protein is associated with a reduction in mutation frequency, a loss of Mfd has been reported to depress stationary-phase mutagenesis in the Gram-positive bacterium *Bacillus subtilis* [J Bacteriol (2006) 188(21):7512–7520].

microarray (DNA chip; chip)   Typically: thousands or millions of short, single-stranded DNA molecules, having diverse but known sequences, attached, at one end, to specific, known locations on the surface of a small piece of glass or silica etc.; acting as PROBES, the immobilized molecules have a range of uses (see below).

A microarray can also be constructed with PNA (see below). (cf. MACROARRAY.)

A microarray can be made in two ways. In one method, a mechanical device is used to attach the oligonucleotides to a prepared solid support – either non-covalently (as in earlier chips) or covalently (see e.g. ATMS, DENDRICHIP).

In the second method ('on-chip synthesis'), a high-speed robotic device is used for the *in situ* synthesis of probes at specific locations (see FEATURE) on the surface of the chip; each probe can be synthesized with any desired sequence of nucleotides. Synthesis of probes involves so-called *random access combinatorial chemistry* – for details see: http://www.affymetrix.com/technology/chemistry.affx

On-chip synthesis is used for manufacturing GeneChip® arrays (Affymetrix Inc.). In GeneChip® arrays the probes, in at least some cases, are 25 nucleotides in length. Probes in other microarrays reported in the literature have sizes ranging from ~10 to ~70 nucleotides; a certain minimum length is necessary for adequate specificity in probe–target binding.

Using a high-density microarray, a given labeled sequence of nucleotides may be identified by allowing it to bind to the probe which has a *complementary* sequence; the location of the probe, on the chip, indicates the probe's sequence – and, therefore, indicates the sequence of the target. (Hybridization must be carried out with an appropriate level of stringency.)

The use of *multiple copies* of each probe – at a given spot on the chip – increases the sensitivity of the test system and also allows a comparison to be made of populations of (differentially labeled) test samples (see later).

The opportunity for target–probe hybridization to occur is reported to be optimized (for accurate and reproducible data) by active mixing [BioTechniques (2005) 38:117–119].

Following hybridization, the intensity of a fluorescent label may depend on the position of the label in the target sequence [Nucleic Acids Res (2005) 33(19):e166].

Factors potentially disruptive to probe–target hybridization, and to the interpretation of signals, include the effects of the so-called 'dangling ends' – i.e. non-hybridized parts of target strands which project beyond the free ends of the probes; the dangling ends may affect binding between probes and their legitimate targets and may also bind to other strands in the reaction mixture – leading e.g. to cross-hybridization signals [Appl Environ Microbiol (2007) 73(2):380–389].

Microarrays are used (e.g.) to study gene expression under different conditions. In one method, two samples of mRNA – obtained from the same cells under different conditions – are each converted to (differentially labeled) cDNAs; these two, labeled populations are then simultaneously hybridized to an appropriate microarray. After hybridization, a comparison of the two labels at a given spot (i.e. cluster of identical probes) may indicate the relative level of expression of a given gene under each set of conditions; detection of only *one* label at a particular spot would suggest that the given gene is expressed under only one of the two sets of conditions examined. The labels used are often fluorescent dyes, e.g. dyes which fluoresce red and green; this is the so-called two-color strategy.

If there is only limited material for gene profiling it may be possible to address the problem by carrying out a preliminary amplification (see e.g. MESSAGEAMP ARNA AMPLIFICATION KIT).

Another use for the microarray is expression profiling of microRNAs (short, gene-regulatory RNAs). When hybridized to a microarray, labeled cDNA copies of microRNAs from a sample of tissue may indicate the pattern of expression of the microRNAs under given conditions. In one study, expression profiling revealed a particular spectrum of microRNAs under hypoxic conditions (in low concentrations of oxygen) [Mol Cell Biol (2007) 27(5):1859–1867].

A microarray-based assay for detecting 5′-methylated cytosine residues in genomic DNA (without BISULFITE treatment *or* DNA amplification) makes use of monoclonal antibodies (mAbs) which specifically recognize 5′-methylated cytosines in strands that are hybridized to oligonucleotide probes. This assay involves initial binding of the mAbs to the target (i.e. 5′-methylated) cytosine residues; this is followed by exposure of the array to a secondary antibody – a (dye-labeled) anti-immunoglobulin antibody that binds to mAbs and is detected by fluorescence of its (cyanine) dye. The design of probes in the microarray was guided by analysis of predicted promoter sequences for possible methylation sites. [Method: DNA Res (2006) 13(1):37–42.]

[Clinical applications of microarray-based diagnostic tests: BioTechniques (2005) 39(4):577–582. Microarrays in studies on DNA methylation profiles: Nucleic Acids Res (2006) 34: 528–542.]

Among microorganisms, microarrays have been used e.g. to identify *Mycobacterium* spp (and *simultaneously* to test for antibiotic resistance) [J Clin Microbiol (1999) 37:49–55], and also to investigate attenuation of virulence in *Pseudomonas aeruginosa* by a quorum sensing inhibitor (furanone) [EMBO J (2003) 22:3803–3815]. Other uses include the profiling of mutant strains of *Staphylococcus aureus* [J Bacteriol (2006) 188(2):687–693].

A microarray of 14283 probes was developed for sequence-independent identification of organisms from samples of their genomic DNA. Essentially, DNA from a given sample was digested with restriction enzymes, labeled, denatured, and then applied to the microarray. The patterns of hybridization of the restriction fragments from different species were able, reproducibly, to differentiate the test organisms on the basis of their species-dependent hybridization signatures [Nucleic Acids Res (2004) 37(4):654–660].

PNA-based microarray

A microarray consisting of PNA probes was used for detecting mutations in the gene for hepatocyte nuclear factor-1α that are responsible for one type of maturity-onset diabetes in the young. First, the relevant mutation-prone genomic region was amplified by PCR (using allele-specific primers), and the resulting amplicons were used as follows. Mutant nucleotides in these amplicons were detected by various primers, each *type* of primer having (i) a 5′ binding site for a *specific* PNA probe, and (ii) a 3′ end capable of SINGLE-BASE EXTENSION at *one particular type* of mutant nucleotide. SBE primers were extended by BIOTIN-labeled ddNTPs; when bound to PNA probes, the (extended) primers were detected by dye-linked STREPTAVIDIN. The binding of an extended primer to a *particular* PNA probe thus indicated one type of mutation present in the sample DNA [Nucleic Acids Res (2005) 33(2): e19].

Non-optimal probe–target binding

One problem with a microarray is that the binding of a range of target sequences to their complementary probes is carried out at one temperature, even though the various probe–target pairs may have a range of different T_m values (see THERMAL MELTING PROFILE); therefore, the operating temperature is likely to be optimal, or near-optimal, for some probe–target pairs but suboptimal for others. This temperature problem has been addressed with a ZIPCODE ARRAY.

microbial forensics See FORENSIC APPLICATIONS.

microbicidal (*adj.*)   Able to kill at least certain types of microorganism under given conditions.

(cf. MICROBISTATIC.)

microbiota See MICROFLORA.

microbistatic (*adj.*)   Able to arrest the growth of certain microorganisms under given conditions.

(cf. MICROBICIDAL.)

microcin Any of a range of low-molecular-weight, typically thermostable BACTERIOCINS produced by enterobacteria and active e.g. against related bacteria. Unlike COLICINS, the synthesis of microcins is not induced by conditions that trigger the SOS response. Microcins are usually synthesized in the stationary phase of growth, and rich media may depress their synthesis.

Microcins range in size from microcin A15 (a single, modified amino acid – apparently a derivative of methionine) to peptides of up to ~50 amino acid residues.

Microcin B7 inhibits DNA gyrase, and microcin C7 blocks protein synthesis. Microcin A15 inhibits the enzyme homoserine succinyltransferase in the pathway for methionine biosynthesis.

Microcin-encoding plasmids include both conjugative and non-conjugative types. These plasmids are called M plasmids or (preferably) Mcc plasmids.

microflora (*microbiol.*)   Collectively, the microorganisms that are normally associated with a given environment or niche; the term is sometimes abbreviated to 'flora'.

Some authors have used the term 'microbiota', in place of microflora, with the apparent aim of excluding the 'plant-like' connotation. However, 'microflora' is a long-established and widely accepted term which is generally understood to have the meaning given above.

microinjection   Direct injection of nucleic acid into a cell – a purely physical alternative to chemically assisted or vector-assisted methods of internalizing nucleic acid. Microinjection was chosen as the preferred method e.g. in a study on the fate of internalized DNA within cytoplasm and nucleus; methods such as LIPOFECTION were regarded (by the authors) as unsuitable for this particular type of study because they result in the deposition of large amounts of DNA at the *surface* of the cell [Nucleic Acids Res (2005) 33(19):6296–6307].

In a more general sense, the term includes any procedure involving injection of a microorganism – such as the transfer of parasitic bacteria from one vector organism to another [as used in: Appl Environ Microbiol (2005) 71:3199–3204].

micron (μ)   A trivial name for the micrometer (10^{-6} m).

micronucleus (*ciliate protozool.*)   The smaller of two types of ciliate nuclei (cf. MACRONUCLEUS); each cell may contain one, two or more micronuclei, depending on species. Micronuclei are usually diploid; they lack a nucleolus and appear to be involved mainly in recombination and the development of new macronuclei.

microparticle enzyme immunoassay   See entry LIGASE CHAIN REACTION.

microRNAs (miRNAs)   Small, genomically encoded molecules of RNA, typically ~21–22 nucleotides in length, whose roles (where known) appear to be regulatory; thus, miRNAs bind to particular target transcripts and appear generally to inhibit translation (one form of GENE SILENCING). This is one of the phenomena known as post-transcriptional gene silencing – see PTGS.

A given miRNA may target more than one transcript (and may target many transcripts).

An miRNA often binds to the 3′-UTR region of an mRNA, although hybridization usually appears to involve an inexact matching of sequences. It appears that, in humans, miRNAs bind preferentially to AT-rich 3′-UTRs [Proc Natl Acad Sci USA (2005) 102(43):15557–15562].

Some miRNAs in plants are reported to be almost perfectly matched to their (known) target sequences; however, only a limited number of these miRNAs have been characterized to date. Plant miRNAs have been quantitated by real-time PCR from total polyadenylated RNA [BioTechniques (2005) 39 (4):519–525]. [Artificial miRNA-mediated antiviral activity in plants: J Virol (2007) 81(12):6690–6699.]

In eukaryotic cells, the *maturation* of miRNAs involves the activity of several enzymes. An initial stage of processing by the so-called Drosha enzyme occurs intranuclearly, and the product is exported to the cytoplasm in a process mediated by an exportin. In the cytoplasm, a further stage of processing is carried out by the DICER enzyme – which is also functional in processing siRNAs in RNA INTERFERENCE.

Many miRNAs have been identified but not all have known function(s). At least some appear to have major roles in the differentiation and/or development of cells. In *Drosophila*, cardiac differentiation is influenced by miRNA1 [Proc Natl

Acad Sci USA (2005) 102(52):18986–18991], and miRNAs seem to occur in diverse spatial patterns in the embryo [Proc Natl Acad Sci USA (2005) 102(50):18017–18022]. Maternal miRNAs are reported to be essential for mouse zygotic development [Genes Dev (2007) 21:644–648].

Expression profiling of miRNAs has been carried out with a microarray, and the identification of miRNA functions has been studied by combining expression profiling with target prediction [Nucleic Acids Res (2006) 34(5):1646–1652]. One study, involving expression profiling, found that a particular spectrum of miRNAs is associated with hypoxic conditions (conditions of low levels of oxygen); it was pointed out that many of the miRNAs expressed under these conditions are also overexpressed in various human tumors [Mol Cell Biol (2007) 27(5):1859–1867].

The Epstein–Barr virus is reported to express a number of miRNAs in latently infected B cells. The level of expression of a given miRNA depends on factors such as the type of cell and the stage of latency [PLoS Pathogens (2006) 2(3):e23].

The formation of miRNAs in (living) cells of zebrafish and mouse was investigated by dual-fluorescence reporter/sensor plasmids [BioTechniques (2006) 41(6):727–732].

Synthetic molecules, termed ANTAGOMIRS, have been used for *in vivo* silencing of endogenous miRNAs in mice.

Details of miRNAs may be obtained at miRNAMap: mirnamap.mbc.nctu.edu.tw

MicroSAGE   See SAGE.

microsatellite DNA   In various genomes (including e.g. human, fungal, bacterial): regions of DNA that consist of multiple tandem repeats of *short* sequences of nucleotides; *short* has been interpreted (by different authors) as e.g. <6 bp, 2–10 bp.

Microsatellite sequences vary in length (i.e. in number of repeated subunits), even in closely related subjects, and are useful e.g. as genetic markers and in forensic profiling.

A given microsatellite sequence may exhibit *expansion* (i.e. increase in the *number* of tandemly repeated units) or *contraction* (involving deletion of nucleotides). Variation in the number of repeated units may arise e.g. by SLIPPED-STRAND MISPAIRING; microsatellite DNA is found in both coding and non-coding sequences of certain genes, and such instability may give rise to disorders such as HUNTINGTON'S DISEASE, myotonic dystrophy and FRAGILE X DISEASE. (An analogous event causes PHASE VARIATION in the *opa* genes of *Neisseria gonorrhoeae*.) [Advances in mechanisms of genetic instability related to hereditary neurological diseases: Nucleic Acids Res (2005) 33(12):3785–3798.]

(See also REPEAT-EXPANSION DETECTION.)

[The synthesis of disease-linked repeats to study instability: BioTechniques (2005) 38(2):247–253.]

[Novel technique for identifying microsatellite markers in genomic DNA: BioTechniques (2007) 42(4):479–486.]

Mimic™ Sf9 insect cells   A cell line, derived from SF9 CELLS and marketed by Invitrogen (Carlsbad CA), in which the cells have been genetically engineered to enable them to express various mammalian glycosyltransferases – thereby permitting production of recombinant proteins which are more similar to those produced in mammalian systems.

minicell (1) The product of an abnormal cell division process in certain mutant rod-shaped bacteria (such as *Escherichia coli*); it consists of the polar part (end) of a cell lacking a chromosome. Minicells cannot grow. Nevertheless, they contain the machinery for transcription and translation and have been of use in genetic studies.

The minicell phenotype can be obtained experimentally e.g. with engineered *minC* mutations (which affect the position of the septum during the process of bacterial cell division) [e.g. J Bacteriol (2005) 187(8):2846–2857].

(cf. MAXICELL.)

(2) (minicell; MiniCell; Minicell etc.) A device (also called a French press) used for disrupting cells – for example, for preparing whole-cell lysates.

minichromosome (1) The intracellular form of the genome of certain DNA viruses (in animals and plants); the circular viral genome complexes with histones to form a structure similar to that of the host's histone-associated DNA. Minichromosomes formed by simian virus 40 (SV40) each contain about 25 *nucleosomes* (see entry CHROMATIN). Minichromosomes are also formed e.g. by the cauliflower mosaic virus and the Epstein–Barr virus.

(2) In *Tetrahymena thermophila*: a stage in the development of the macronuclear rRNA-encoding sequence following its excision from the micronucleus [Nucleic Acids Res (2006) 34(2):620–634].

(3) A plasmid in which the sole origin of replication is one derived from a bacterial host.

minichromosome maintenance protein 1 See ARS.

minicircles See KINETOPLAST.

minigene An *in vitro* construct (commonly part of a plasmid vector) which contains certain features of a typical eukaryotic gene such as a promoter/polyadenylation region, exonic and intronic sequences, and a polylinker (multiple cloning site) at which a fragment of sample DNA can be inserted.

Minigenes are used in EXON TRAPPING.

minimal medium See AUXOTROPHIC MUTANT.

minor groove (in DNA) See GROOVES.

minus strand (of a gene) See CODING STRAND.

MIP genotyping See MOLECULAR INVERSION PROBE GENOTYPING.

miRNAs See MICRORNAS.

MIRU Mycobacterial interspersed repetitive unit.

(See also W-BEIJING STRAIN.)

mismatch extension (of a primer) The inefficient extension of a primer with a 3′ terminal mismatched base. The nature of the mismatch influences the readiness with which extension can occur; a G/T mismatch is reported to be one of the least inhibitory mismatches.

mismatch repair (MMR) A system involved in the response to (i) mismatched nucleotides, incorporated during replication of DNA, and (ii) (in e.g. humans) DNA damage (as well as mismatched nucleotides – see below).

Mismatched nucleotides which escape proofreading by the DNA polymerase can be corrected by a mismatch repair system that operates in both prokaryotes and eukaryotes.

MMR in Escherichia coli

In *Escherichia coli*, the incorporation of a mismatched nucleotide during DNA replication can be detected by the MutS protein. (Using a direct, electrochemical method, MutS was found to interact with a mismatch more strongly than with a normally base-paired site [Nucleic Acids Res (2006) 34(10): e75].) During interaction between MutS and a mismatch, a hydrogen bond is formed between a glutamate residue in MutS and the mismatched base; this interaction promotes the triggering of downstream events [EMBO J (2006) 25(2):409–419].

Detection of a mismatch by MutS is followed by activation of an endonuclease, MutH, which cleaves the new daughter strand (identified by its initial state of undermethylation) at an unmethylated GATC (Dam) site; the cleavage site may be some distance from the mismatch, and co-ordination between the mismatch and cleavage sites seems to involve the MutL protein. [Identification of a site of interaction between MutH and the C-terminal of MutL: Nucleic Acids Res (2006) 34 (10):3169–3180.] (In that Dam sites are involved in MMR in *E. coli*, this system has been referred to as *Dam-directed mismatch repair*, DDMR, in this organism.)

After strand cleavage by MutH, the sequence of nucleotides between the cleavage site and a site on the other side of the lesion is removed (apparently in a process involving helicase II) and replaced by a sequence that is newly synthesized on the template.

A strain defective in MMR is associated with a mutator phenotype.

Interestingly, *dam* mutants of *E. coli* (i.e. cells unable to carry out Dam methylation of their DNA) are killed by an MMR-related mechanism on treatment with the base analog 2-aminopurine (which forms pairs with thymine and cytosine that trigger MMR); in these cells the DNA suffers double-strand breakage, the chromosomal DNA then being totally degraded, leaving DNA-free cells [J Bacteriol (2006) 188(1): 339–342].

The role of MutS in humans

In humans, MutS has an *additional* role: it is involved in the initiation of cell death following damage to DNA; a defect in this role can promote carcinogenesis. In the presence of DNA damage the role of MutS differs from its role in the context of mismatched nucleotides; the mechanism by which DNA damage is recognized has been studied with MutS homologs [Nucleic Acids Res (2006) 34(8):2173–2185].

mis-sense mutation Any mutation in which a codon specifying a given amino acid is changed to one which specifies a different amino acid.

mis-sense suppressor See SUPPRESSOR MUTATION.

mitochondrial DNA (mtDNA) DNA associated with the mitochondrion (as opposed to the nucleus). Human mtDNA (~16 kbp) derives from the female parent [diversity of mtDNA in humans: Nucleic Acids Res (2007) 35(9):3039–3045].

(See also NUMTS.)

Details of the mitochodrial DNA have been reported from various other species: e.g. the complete sequence of mtDNA in zebrafish (*Danio rerio*) (~16.6 kbp) [Genome Res (2001) 11(11):1958–1967] and in the teleost fish *Scleropages formosus* (Osteoglossidae) (~16.6 kbp) [BMC Genomics (2006) 7:242].

mtDNA is examined e.g. in studies on population genetics and in certain FORENSIC APPLICATIONS of DNA technology.

Information on mtDNA (e.g.): a US government database (the mtDNA Popstats Population Database) and HVRBASE++. [Enhanced MITOMAP with global mtDNA mutational phylogeny: Nucleic Acids Res (2007) 35(Database issue): D823–D828.]

(See also CYBRID and HETEROPLASMY.)

mitochondrial pseudogenes See NUMTS.

(See also FORENSIC APPLICATIONS.)

mitomycin C An antibiotic, produced by *Streptomyces* spp, in which the molecule includes both a quinone group and an aziridine ring. *In vivo* activity depends on intracellular reduction to a hydroquinone derivative that e.g. forms covalent cross-links between the strands of dsDNA.

Mitomycin C has been used e.g. for inducing a lysogenic population (see LYSOGENY) and for CURING plasmids.

MLPA See MULTIPLEX LIGATION-DEPENDENT PROBE AMPLIFICATION.

MLST (multilocus sequence typing) A method of TYPING, used for various (commonly) pathogenic microorganisms, which is designed to allow the long-term and global tracking of (e.g.) antibiotic-resistant and virulent strains – with dissemination of information on the Internet.

In this approach, strains of a given pathogen are characterized/classified according to nucleotide sequences in *specific* alleles, this type of categorization generally being regarded as stable for long periods of time.

Originally used for typing bacterial pathogens, MLST has also been used e.g. for the fungal pathogen *Candida albicans* [Eukaryotic Cell (2007) 6:1041–1052].

Uses of MLST (e.g.): analysis of uropathogenic strains of *Escherichia coli* (UPEC): [J Clin Microbiol (2005) 43:5860–5864]; studies on typable and non-typable strains of *Streptococcus pneumoniae* (the pneumococcus) [J Bacteriol (2005) 187(17):6223–6230; Microbiology (2006) 152:367–376].

MLST typing of the bacterium *Wolbachia pipientis* [Appl Environ Microbiol (2006) 72(11):7098–7110]: see database at http://pubmlst.org/wolbachia/

MLST has also been used to study the population genetic structure of strains of (non-pathogenic) nodulating rhizobia [J Bacteriol (2006) 188(15):5570–5577].

[MLST network: Nucleic Acids Res (2005) 33(Web Server issue):W728–W733.]

[Molecular evolution of enteropathogenic strains of *E. coli* (EPEC) (clonal analysis by MLST): J Bacteriol (2007) 189 (2):342–350.]

MLVA Multiple loci VNTR analysis (in which VNTR means 'variable number of tandem repeats'): a method used e.g. for TYPING bacteria in which strains are compared on the basis of loci containing tandemly repeated sequences; strains may differ in the number of tandem repeats at a given locus, and in the number of such loci. Relevant sequences are copied by PCR and the amplicons from each strain can be compared by gel electrophoresis.

[Selection of tandem repeat loci for typing *Streptococcus pneumoniae*: BMC Microbiol (2005) 5:66.]

[MLVA used in the molecular characterization of *Coxiella burnetii*: BMC Microbiol (2006) 6:38.]

[MLVA used for the subtyping of *Neisseria meningitidis*: BMC Microbiol (2006) 6:44.]

Strains of *Bacillus anthracis* that were indistinguishable by routine MLVA procedures have been differentiated by means of single-nucleotide repeats (SNRs) [J Clin Microbiol (2006) 44(3):777–782].

MMF Mycophenolate mofetil: a prodrug which is conveted to the active agent MYCOPHENOLIC ACID.

MMLV reverse transcriptase Moloney murine leukemia virus reverse transcriptase (see e.g. FIRST STRAND).

MMR (1) MISMATCH REPAIR.

(2) Measles–mumps–rubella (vaccine).

MMS Methylmethane sulfonate: an alkylating agent which can e.g. methylate guanine residues in DNA.

MNNG *N*-methyl-*N*′-nitro-*N*-nitrosoguanidine (see entry DNA REPAIR).

MNU *N*-methyl-*N*-nitrosourea (see entry DNA REPAIR).

mobile genetic element Any nucleic acid sequence which can re-locate to a different site, or insert a copy of itself at a new location; such elements occur e.g. in chromosomes, plasmids and viral genomes.

Examples of mobile genetic elements: insertion sequences, introns, retrotransposons, transposons (including conjugative transposons).

(See also TRANSPOSABLE ELEMENT.)

mobilization (of chromosomes) See e.g. CONJUGATION and F PLASMID.

modification methylase A trivial name for any enzyme that methylates particular bases in DNA.

modulator protein See TN21.

MOI MULTIPLICITY OF INFECTION.

molecular beacon probe A PROBE which consists of a single-stranded linear oligonucleotide in which the complementary *ends* hybridize, forming a stem–loop structure. The sequence in the loop is complementary to the target sequence. Within the stem, one of the strands carries a fluorescent dye and the other contains a quencher of fluorescence.

The *unbound* probe is non-fluorescent.

If the loop region binds to a target sequence, the two ends of the probe separate and the quencher ceases to be effective – so that the dye fluoresces.

These probes were reported to have greater *specificity* than other probes of equivalent length [Proc Natl Acad Sci USA

(1999) 96:6171–6176]. They are used for real-time monitoring of nucleic acid amplification, and have also been used for detecting specific nucleic acids in solution by flow cytometry [Nucleic Acids Res (2005) 33(2):e13].

A novel molecular beacon probe has been developed by the use of the *intrinsically* fluorescent nucleotides 2-aminopurine and pyrrolo-dC [Nucleic Acids Res (2006) 34(6):e50].

(See also REAL-TIME PCR.)

molecular cloning See CLONING.

molecular epidemiology Epidemiology involving nucleic-acid-based TYPING of isolates of a given pathogen.

molecular inversion probe genotyping (MIP genotyping) A technique capable (e.g.) of multiplexed SNP GENOTYPING of more than 10000 targeted loci.

The molecular inversion probe (MIP) technique is based on the use of a type of linear, oligonucleotide probe whose *end-sequences* are complementary to two *adjacent* genomic sequences that are separated by only a single nucleotide; that is, when bound to the target, the probe is circularized except for a one-nucleotide gap. For a given probe, this one-nucleotide gap corresponds to the exact location of one of the SNPs that are being assayed. In any given assay, thousands of different oligonucleotide probes are used, each type of probe being highly specific for one of the SNPs being scored.

The one-nucleotide gap in each (bound) probe is filled in (by polymerase/ligase activity) during one of four separate reactions – each reaction involving *one* of the four types of dNTP.

The probes are released from genomic DNA, and the fully (covalently) circularized probes are amplified by PCR. All of the probes (regardless of specificity) contain identical primer-binding sites for PCR – so that a universal primer pair can amplify all the circularized probes.

In addition to primer-binding sites, each probe includes a unique 'tag' sequence *which indicates its target specificity*, i.e. a given tag corresponds to a specific SNP.

The (labeled) PCR products are treated with restriction enzymes, in order to release the tag sequences, and the tags are then detected by an array of probes that are complementary to the tag sequences.

The system of unique tag sequences, described above, has been termed *barcoding*. (Compare ZIPCODE ARRAY.) The large number (thousands) of unique sequence tags used in a given assay are designed to have minimal similarity, and tag design also aims to avoid problems associated with secondary structures. Furthermore, the tags are designed so that the overall range of melting temperatures is narrow.

[Multiplexed molecular inversion probe genotyping: Genome Res (2005) 15:269–275.]

molecular zipper A construct used in a method for the *in vitro* isothermal amplification of DNA.

The sequence of nucleotides to be copied is initially present as an ssDNA circle. A forward primer binds to the circle and is extended by the ROLLING CIRCLE mechanism, producing a long strand of DNA consisting of many tandem repeats of the target sequence.

Multiple molecular zippers bind to the ssDNA multimer. Each molecular zipper consists of a 48-nt 'positive' strand of DNA (labeled with a quencher of fluorescence at the 5′ end) hybridized (at the 5′ end) to a 25-nt 'negative' strand of DNA labeled with a fluorophore at its 3′ end; the 23-nt (single-stranded) 3′ terminal region of the positive strand acts as a reverse primer and binds to the ssDNA target multimer.

The 3′ ends of the (bound) molecular zippers are extended by DNA polymerases, and this results in the displacement of other (bound and extended) *downstream* molecular zippers – creating multiple free copies of the extended zippers to which *forward* primers can bind. Extension of a forward primer displaces the negative strand from a zipper, thus releasing the fluorophore from the quenching effect of the positive strand. Ongoing amplification thus gives rise to an increasing level of fluorescence as there is an ongoing increase in the number of displaced negative strands (with active, i.e. non-quenched, fluorophores).

[Method: Nucleic Acids Res (2006) 34(11):e81.]

Moloney murine leukemia virus reverse transcriptase See e.g. FIRST STRAND.

monoclonal antibodies (mAbs) Any population of antibodies derived from a *specific clone* of B lymphocytes (B cells); all the antibodies obtained from a given clone of B cells recognize the same antigenic determinant(s).

Monoclonal antibodies can be obtained from a HYBRIDOMA and are used e.g. for the study and identification of specific macromolecules.

monomeric red fluorescent protein (mRFP1) A monomeric derivative of DsRed – a naturally tetrameric red fluorescent protein derived from the coral *Discosoma* [Proc Natl Acad Sci USA (2002) 99(12):7877–7882]. Excitation and emission wavelengths for mRFP1 are 584 and 607 nm, respectively.

(cf. GREEN FLUORESCENT PROTEIN and YELLOW FLUORESCENT PROTEIN.)

(See also DFRS PLASMID.)

mononucleotide repeat *Syn.* single-nucleotide repeat: see SNR.

monosomic See CHROMOSOME ABERRATION.

Morgan A unit of length on a (eukaryotic) chromosome: the length within which, on average, one cross-over occurs in each meiosis.

morpholino antisense oligomer Any of a range of synthetic, non-ionic, oligonucleotide analogs in which the pyrimidine and purine bases are carried on a backbone of morpholine residues linked by phosphorodiamidate bonds (morpholine = tetrahydro-1,4-oxazine). The oligomers are typically 10–20 morpholine residues in length; they are resistant to nucleases and are used e.g. for GENE SILENCING.

Phosphorodiamidate morpholino oligomers (PMOs) can bind to mRNAs by Watson–Crick base-pairing and block translation; the duplex is resistant to RNase H. These oligomers have been used e.g. for studying antiviral activity [J Virol (2007) 81(11):5637–5648].

[Antisense PMOs: (the effects of length and target position

on gene-specific inhibition): Antimicrob Agents Chemother (2005) 49(1):249–255.]

Mos1 See MARINER FAMILY.

moxifloxacin See QUINOLONE ANTIBIOTICS.

MPA MYCOPHENOLIC ACID.

***mpl* gene** In *Escherichia coli*: the gene encoding a ligase involved in the recycling of tripeptide units during turnover of the cell wall polymer peptidoglycan.

M_r RELATIVE MOLECULAR MASS.

MreB protein See NUCLEOID.

mRFP1 See MONOMERIC RED FLUORESCENT PROTEIN.

MRI (magnetic resonance imaging) A non-invasive method for monitoring gene expression *in vitro* and *in vivo*. MRI is based on the phenomenon of *nuclear magnetic resonance* in which certain types of atomic nuclei, when placed in a strong magnetic field and exposed to suitable radio-frequency electromagnetic radiation, emit characteristic, informative signals; the nature of the signals varies according e.g. to the particular molecular environment in which the nuclei occur, and also according to the concentration of the given nuclei.

MRI was used e.g. for monitoring gene expression in the yeast *Saccharomyces cerevisiae* [Nucleic Acids Res (2006) 34:e51].

***mrr* gene** In *Escherichia coli*: a gene which encodes a type IV RESTRICTION ENDONUCLEASE that cleaves DNA at the sequences 5′-C^mAG-3′ and 5′-G^mAC-3′ (in which the adenine residue is methylated).

Inactivation of *mrr* is reported to permit greater efficiency when cloning DNA containing methylated adenine residues in the above sequences.

(See also ESCHERICHIA COLI (table).)

MRSA Methicillin-resistant *Staphylococcus aureus*: various strains of *S. aureus* which are resistant to (at least) METHICILLIN – and are generally resistant to a range of other antibiotics (in some cases including vancomycin); MRSA causes problems in a clinical setting owing to the reduced range of effective chemotherapeutic agents that are available for the treatment of infections involving these strains. [Evolutionary history of MRSA: Proc Natl Acad Sci USA (2002) 99(11):7687–7692.]

In *S. aureus*, resistance to methicillin can arise in different ways. Most attention has been paid to resistance conferred by the MECA GENE; *mecA* encodes a penicillin-binding protein (PBP 2a) with low affinity for methicillin (and other β-lactam antibiotics), allowing ongoing synthesis of the cell wall polymer peptidoglycan (and hence, growth) in otherwise inhibitory concentrations of these antibiotics.

The resistance encoded by *mecA* depends on the formation of normal products from the *fem* genes (*fem* refers to *f*actor *e*ssential for *m*ethicillin resistance). Mutations in the *femAB* operon can result in the formation of abnormal cross-links in peptidoglycan; these abnormal cross-links are poor substrates for the enzymic role of PBP 2a but are better substrates for the normal, methicillin-sensitive PBPs – so that cells with the mutant *fem* genes are sensitive to methicillin.

(See also GISA, PFGE and SCCMEC.)

MRSE Methicillin-resistant *Staphylococcus epidermidis*.

MSBE See METHYLATION-SPECIFIC SINGLE-BASE EXTENSION.

msDNA See RETRON.

MSP See METHYLATION-SPECIFIC PCR.

MSRE Methylation-sensitive restriction enzyme.

MSSA Methicillin-sensitive *Staphylococcus aureus*.

MTase DNA METHYLTRANSFERASE.

mtDNA MITOCHONDRIAL DNA.

mtDNA Popstats Population Database See entry FORENSIC APPLICATIONS.

mucolytic agent Any agent used for liquefying specimens of (mucoid) sputum. Mucolysis facilitates manipulation of the specimen and also serves to expose cells, including bacteria. Some mucolytic agents – e.g. *N*-acetyl-L-cysteine and dithiothreitol – are used e.g. to prepare samples of sputum for nucleic-acid-based tests for *Mycobacterium tuberculosis*.

mucopolysaccharidosis type IH (Hurler's syndrome) An autosomal recessive disease resulting from a mutant allele in the *IDUA* gene, encoding the lysosomal enzyme α-L-iduronidase. The disease affects various organs, including the heart; death sometimes results from congestive heart failure.

(See also GENETIC DISEASE (table).)

multicopy inhibition (Tn*10*) The increased level of inhibition of transposition in the presence of multiple copies of Tn*10*. It is due to the regulatory influence of the IS*10* element which forms part of the transposon (see TN10). Thus, transposition of IS*10* is regulated by a (stable) ANTISENSE RNA molecule which binds to the transposase-encoding mRNA and inhibits translation. The promoter of the sequence encoding the antisense RNA is somewhat stronger than the promoter of the transposase gene. With a higher copy number of the transposon, the concentrations of both mRNA and the antisense molecule increase, apparently enhancing the effectiveness of the control mechanism.

multicopy plasmid Any PLASMID whose COPY NUMBER (in a given type of cell) – e.g. >10 copies per cell – is in contrast to that of low-copy-number plasmids (such as the F PLASMID).

Examples of multicopy plasmids include ColE1 (typically 10–30 copies per cell) and the PUC PLASMIDS.

The copy number of ColE1 was reported to be decreased in *Escherichia coli* host cells with a mutant *pcnB* gene – which encodes poly(A)polymerase I (PAP I); in these cells, the absence of polyadenylation of the (ColE1-encoded) antisense molecule RNA I has the effect of stabilizing this molecule, enhancing its inhibitory action on RNA II and thus inhibiting replication of the plasmid.

multicopy single-stranded DNA (msDNA) See RETRON.

multilocus sequence typing See MLST.

multilocus VNTR analysis *Syn.* multiple loci VNTR analysis: see MLVA.

multiple cloning site (MCS) *Syn.* POLYLINKER.

multiple displacement amplification Isothermal replication of DNA (30°C) in WHOLE-GENOME AMPLIFICATION. Multiple sites are primed by random (exonuclease-resistant) hexamers, and replication is mediated by the highly processive DNA polymerase from bacteriophage φ29 (omitting an initial stage of heat denaturation) [Proc Natl Acad Sci USA (2002) 99: 5261–5266]; average product length: >10 kb. Amplification bias is less than that reported in PCR-based methods, and the products are said to be useful for genomic studies and for SNP analysis.

Under-representation of terminal sequences in linear DNA may be overcome by ligation (forming a circular template) [BioTechniques (2005) 39(2):174–180].

Multiple displacement amplification (MDA) has been used for amplifying DNA in low-level sources: samples of plasm a stored at −40°C for ~10 years [BioTechniques (2005) 39(4): 511–515].

multiple loci VNTR analysis   See MLVA.

multiplex amplifiable probe hybridization (MAPH)   A technique used for assessing the copy number of target sequences and detecting deletion mutations. Essentially, genomic DNA is denatured and exposed to a range of probes; the probes are complementary to various target sequences in the genome, but all the probes have the same terminal 5′ and 3′ primer-binding sites. The probes are allowed to hybridize with the genomic DNA (which is immobilized on a filter), following which any unbound probes are removed by washing. Bound probes are then recovered (separated from genomic DNA) and amplified by PCR using a primer pair which is common to all the probes. The quantity of PCR product obtained from a given type of probe is assumed to correlate with the number of such probes present in the reaction mixture. A probe that is complementary to a deleted sequence in the genome is likely to yield no product by PCR.

multiplex ligation-dependent probe amplification (MLPA)   A technique used for *relative* quantitation of specific sequences of nucleotides; the applications of MLPA include detection of, for example, Down's syndrome (trisomy 21), gene duplications, exon deletions and SNPs.

Probes are added to a sample, each probe consisting of two oligonucleotides that bind *adjacently* on the target sequence. If both oligonucleotides hybridize correctly on the target sequence they can be *ligated* and the (now complete) probe can be amplified by PCR (each probe includes two primer-binding sites). Quantitation of the PCR products can be facilitated by using labeled primers in the PCR reaction. Products obtained from the target sequence in a given sample can be compared, quantitatively, with products obtained from the corresponding target sequence in other samples.

[Examples of multiplex ligation-dependent probe amplification: Nucleic Acids Res (2005) 33(14):e128 and PLoS Med (2006) 3(10):e431.]

(cf. COMPARATIVE GENOMIC HYBRIDIZATION.)

multiplex PCR   A form of PCR for simultaneously amplifying two or more target sequences *in the same assay*; the reaction mixture contains primers for each target. PCR with several targets can be monitored by (target-specific) probes labeled with different types of fluorescent dye (i.e. dyes with differ-

ent emission spectra).

As multiple primers are used, extra care is required in order to prevent the formation of PRIMER–DIMERS.

In some cases, one primer can be shared by two targets. For example, a sequence in the 16S rRNA gene in *Bacteroides forsythus* and *Prevotella intermedia* has been amplified with one FORWARD PRIMER (a BROAD-RANGE PRIMER common to both species) and two species-specific reverse primers.

Multiplex PCR has been used e.g. for detecting *mecA* and *coa* genes in *Staphylococcus aureus* [J Med Microbiol (1997) 46:773–778]; for diagnostic virology [Clin Microbiol Rev (2000) 13:559–570]; for detecting toxin genes in *Clostridium difficile* [J Clin Microbiol (2004) 42:5710–5714] and for subspeciation of *Campylobacter jejuni* isolates [BMC Microbiol (2007) 7:11].

Multiplex PCR is also used e.g. for amplification of STRs in human DNA profiling (e.g. CODIS).

An alternative approach is SELECTOR-BASED MULTIPLEX PCR.

multiplex QEXT   See QEXT.

multiplex real-time PCR   REAL-TIME PCR (q.v.) in which more than one target sequence is amplified in a given assay.

multiplicity of infection (MOI)   (1) In any given system: the ratio of infectious virions to susceptible cells.

(2) The number of viral genomes per infected cell.

MultiSite Gateway® technology   A GATEWAY SITE-SPECIFIC RECOMBINATION SYSTEM in which a range of vector molecules, each having *att* sites with distinct, modified sequences and specificities, offers the choice of diverse recombination partners and directional insertion of the sequence of interest.

Example of use

MultiSite technology was used e.g. for inserting a sequence (simultaneously) into two different locations in one plasmid. Initially, a target site was introduced into the plasmid at each of the two locations. Each target site contained a copy of the *ccdB* gene (see entry CCD MECHANISM) flanked by a pair of asymmetric *att*P sequences; the pair of asymmetric sequences flanking one target site was different to the asymmetric pair flanking the other target site.

Copies of the sequence to be inserted were prepared by PCR.

One PCR reaction used primers that introduced terminal *att*B sequences corresponding to one pair of asymmetric *att*P sites.

A separate PCR used primers that introduced terminal *att*B sequences corresponding to the other pair of asymmetric *att*P sites.

Thus, as a result of the two PCR reactions, there were two sets of inserts, each prepared for introduction into one of the two target sites.

The (recipient) plasmid was then incubated with the two sets of inserts (for 1 hour at 25°C) together with the Int and IHF proteins. During incubation, each insert was exchanged, by site-specific recombination, with its corresponding target sequence in the plasmid. (Note that elimination of each target sequence from the plasmid resulted in the removal of a *ccdB* gene from the plasmid.)

All the above steps were carried out *in vitro*.

The recombinant plasmids were then used to transform a CcdB-sensitive strain of bacteria. As the plasmid included an ampicillin-resistance gene, positive selection of the (dual) recombinants was obtained by using an ampicillin-containing medium. Any cell containing a plasmid in which *both* (CcdB-encoding) target sites had not been exchanged for inserts was killed by the CcdB toxin.

In this experiment, all copies of the insert were identical, except for their *att* sites, but it seems likely that this protocol can be easily adapted for the insertion of non-identical donor sequences at required sites.

[Approach used in the above experiment: BioTechniques (2005) 39(4):553–557.]

[Conversion of Gateway® vectors to MultiSite Gateway® vectors by means of a single recombination event: BMC Mol Biol (2006) 7:46.]

mung bean nuclease A SINGLE-STRAND-SPECIFIC NUCLEASE. Mung bean nuclease differs from e.g. endonuclease S_1 in that it cannot cleave the DNA strand opposite a nick in a DNA duplex.

(See also RIBONUCLEASE PROTECTION ASSAY.)

mutagen Any physical or chemical agent which can promote MUTAGENESIS. Some mutagens are CARCINOGENS.

Mutagens typically interact with, and alter/damage, nucleic acid. In some cases a mutagen may alter a base such that, in a subsequent round of replication, incorrect base-pairing leads to the insertion of a different nucleotide.

Some mutagens are more effective with ssDNA than with dsDNA.

Physical mutagens include ionizing radiations and ULTRA-VIOLET RADIATION. Heat apparently increases the level of spontaneous mutation.

Chemical mutagens include compounds of a wide range of types – alkylating agents, base analogs, bisulfite, hydroxyl-amine, nitrous acid etc. Others include e.g. the AFLATOXINS (associated with some instances of hepatocellular carcinoma) and β-naphthylamine (implicated in bladder cancer).

mutagenesis (*in vitro*) The creation of mutation(s) in one or more target sequences of nucleic acid. Mutations are created for various reasons: e.g. (i) to inactivate a gene, (ii) to modify the coding sequence of a gene, (iii) to modify the regulation of a gene's expression. A gene may be inactivated e.g. to in-vestigate its involvement (or otherwise) in a given function – cells with an inactivated gene being compared to those with a normal, wild-type gene. Modification of a gene's coding sequence, or its regulation, has widespread applications in medicine and industry as well as in biological research.

There are two basic approaches to mutagenesis: (i) random mutagenesis (i.e. creating mutation(s) at random sites within a given target sequence) and (ii) site-directed (= site-specific) mutagenesis – in which mutations are created at known, pre-determined sites.

Random mutagenesis

Random mutagenesis may be carried out in order to produce specific types of mutant (e.g. temperature-sensitive mutants) for use in various types of study; such mutants are recovered by the use of selective procedures.

Random, transposon-mediated mutagenesis has been used for the detection of virulence-associated genes in pathogenic bacteria: see e.g. SIGNATURE-TAGGED MUTAGENESIS.

Transposition with Tn5 can be carried out in wholly *in vitro* systems, insertions occurring randomly in e.g. a population of plasmid vectors (see TN5-TYPE TRANSPOSITION).

Random mutations in bacteria can be created by exposing the cells to a *mutagen*, i.e. a physical or chemical agent such as ultraviolet radiation, X-rays, alkylating agents, bisulfite or hydroxylamine. Mutations develop in different genes (and/or non-coding sequences) in different cells. Those cells which have developed the required type of mutation may be isolated by using appropriate *selective* conditions – such as particular types of selective medium (see e.g. AUXOTROPHIC MUTANT for some approaches to methodology).

Random mutations can be introduced into an insert/gene in a vector molecule by replicating the vector within a so-called MUTATOR STRAIN; one advantage of this is that mutagenesis can be achieved without the use of mutagens.

Random mutations can be introduced into a target sequence *in vitro* by a PCR-based method involving the use of an error-prone DNA polymerase (see e.g. GENEMORPH PCR MUTA-GENESIS KIT).

Site-directed mutagenesis (site-specific mutagenesis)

Mutation at specific site(s) is used e.g. for studies on gene expression, and also for modifying the products encoded by genes – for example, increasing the efficiency of an enzyme used in an industrial process by changing specific nucleotides in the coding region of the gene.

(See also SITE-DIRECTED MUTAGENESIS.)

Site-directed mutations can be single-nucleotide mutations (point mutations) or may involve insertion/deletion of short or long sequences of nuleotides.

For examples of methods used in site-directed mutagenesis see entries EXSITE PCR-BASED SITE-DIRECTED MUTAGENESIS KIT, GENETAILOR SITE-DIRECTED MUTAGENESIS SYSTEM and QUIKCHANGE SITE-DIRECTED MUTAGENESIS KIT.

(See also CHIMERAPLAST.)

mutagenic repair See SOS SYSTEM.

mutasynthesis The synthesis of new type(s) of end-product by a mutant organism in which a normal biosynthetic pathway is blocked and the pathway is completed by an abnormal sub-strate. Mutasynthesis has been exploited e.g. for synthesizing novel products.

Mutatest *Syn.* AMES TEST.

mutator strain Any strain of bacteria that is deficient in DNA repair function(s) and which is used e.g. for creating random mutations (see MUTAGENESIS) in target sequences replicated within such strains.

One advantage of using a mutator strain is that mutagenesis can be achieved without the use of mutagens.

An example of a mutator strain is the XL1-Red strain of *Escherichia coli* (Stratagene, La Jolla CA); this strain lacks several of the normal repair functions and is reported to generate mutations at a rate which is several thousand times higher than is possible with a corresponding wild-type strain. The genotype of XL1-Red is *endA1, gyrA96, thi-1, hsdR17, supE44, relA1, lac, mutD5, mutS, mutT*, Tn*10* (Tet^r).

Examples of use of XL1-Red: generation of mutations in the *lolC* gene of *Escherichia coli* [J Bacteriol (2006) 188(8): 2856–2864] and investigation of the effect of mutation in the *RPB1* gene of *Saccharomyces cerevisiae* [Genetics (2006) 172(4):2201–2209].

A derivative of XL1-Red, containing the *lacI*^{q} element, was used in studies on the *E. coli* ribonuclease E gene to control expression of *rne* [Genetics (2006) 172(1):7–15].

Mutazyme®   See GENEMORPH and COMPETENT CELLS.

MutH   See MISMATCH REPAIR.

MutL   See MISMATCH REPAIR.

MutM   See 8-OXOG.

MutS   See MISMATCH REPAIR.

MutT   See 8-OXOG.

MutY   See 8-OXOG.

Mx162   See RETRON.

myb (*MYB*)   An ONCOGENE first identified in avian myeloblastosis virus (AMV). AMV causes rapidly fatal leukemia in chickens. The product of v-*myb* occurs in the nucleus. The c-*myb* product is a transcription factor that has roles e.g. in cell proliferation and apoptosis; it is strongly expressed e.g. in *immature* hemopoietic cells – but expression falls markedly during differentiation.

In chickens, insertional activation of c-*myb* is seen e.g. in lymphomas and myeloid leukemias.

myc (*MYC*)   An ONCOGENE first detected in avian myelocytomatosis virus. The v-*myc* product (found in the nucleus) is a *gag*–*myc* fusion protein which has no protein kinase activity. Human c-*myc* normally occurs on chromosome 8; it encodes a transcription factor which may regulate activities such as e.g. proliferation, differentiation and apoptosis. Translocation of c-*myc* may be causally connected with Burkitt's lymphoma.

The oncogenic activity of c-*myc* appears to arise mainly by overexpression.

In mice, experimental expression of c-*myc* results in the formation of tumors.

Mycobacterium tuberculosis   A species of Gram-positive, acid-fast bacteria; a causal agent of tuberculosis. [Genome: Nature (1998) 393:537–544.] Detection of *M. tuberculosis* in smear-positive sputa may be achieved e.g. by the AMTDT; typing: e.g. by SPOLIGOTYPING. Some typing schemes have been based on the insertion sequence IS*6110*, which appears to be specific to members of the '*M. tuberculosis* complex' (which includes *M. tuberculosis*, *M. bovis* and *M. africanum*). The number of copies of IS*6110*, per genome, varies according to strain, some strains apparently containing none; H37rv, the reference strain of *M. tuberculosis*, contains 16 copies. In at least some strains of *M. tuberculosis* the value of long-term IS*6110*-based typing may be compromised by a high rate of transposition of the element within the genome.

The detection of antibiotic resistance in clinical isolates of *M. tuberculosis* can be achieved e.g. by several commercial PROBE-based assay systems: see e.g. LINE PROBE ASSAY.

(See also W-BEIJING STRAIN.)

mycophenolate mofetil (MMF)   A prodrug which is converted, intracellularly, to the active agent MYCOPHENOLIC ACID.

mycophenolic acid   An agent with antitumor and antimicrobial activity synthesized e.g. by the fungus *Penicillium brevicompactum*; it inhibits the synthesis of guanosine monophosphate by inhibiting the formation of xanthosine monophosphate from inosine monophosphate – thus depleting the pool of guanine nucleotides.

The prodrug, mycophenolate mofetil (MMF), is converted, intracellularly, to mycophenolic acid.

Examples of use: a pilot study in which MMF was used for treating HIV-positive patients [AIDS Res Ther (2006) 3:16], and studies on the accumulation of RNAs of hepatitis delta virus (HDV) [J Virol (2006) 80(7):3205–3214].

mycovirus   Any (commonly dsRNA) virus which can infect one or more species of fungus; in at least some cases mycoviruses encode an RNA-dependent RNA polymerase.

Transmissibility of mycoviruses seems to depend primarily on processes such as hyphal fusion and mating (as opposed to the passage of virions from one individual to another via an extracellular route).

Some mycoviruses do not form conventional virions, their nucleic acid being encapsulated in host-encoded vesicles.

myeloid lineage   Cells that include e.g. monocytes and macrophages, granulocytes (e.g. neutrophils, basophils and eosinophils) and erythrocytes (red blood cells).

(See also LYMPHOID LINEAGE.)

myristylation membrane localization signal   A function used e.g. in the CYTOTRAP TWO-HYBRID SYSTEM.

myxophage   Any bacteriophage that infects one or more species of gliding bacteria (bacteria of the order Myxobacterales).

N (1) An indicator of ambiguity in the recognition sequence of a RESTRICTION ENDONUCLEASE (or in any other sequence of nucleic acid); 'N' indicates A or C or G or T (in RNA: A or C or G or U), i.e. any nucleotide.

(2) L-Asparagine (alternative to Asn).

N-acetyl-L-cysteine   See MUCOLYTIC AGENT.

N-acetylmuramidase   See LYSOZYME.

N-acyl-homocysteine thiolactone   See QUORUM SENSING.

N-acyl-L-homoserine lactone   See QUORUM SENSING.

N-degron   See N-END RULE.

N-end rule   The observed rule that the half-life of a given protein is influenced by the identity of its N-terminal amino acid. The N-end rule applies in prokaryotes and eukaryotes.

The features which determine early degradation are signals (*degrons*) that are incorporated in the protein itself. One of these is the *N-degron*: a destabilizing N-terminal amino acid recognized by the cell's specific degradation machinery. For example, in *Escherichia coli*, proteins with arginine or lysine at the N-terminal have characteristically short half-lives (see AAT GENE).

The eukaryotic signals for protein degradation include not only an N-terminal amino acid residue but also internal lysine residue(s). A protein with the appropriate degradation signals binds a polyubiquitin chain (through multi-enzyme activity) as a prerequisite to degradation in a 26S PROTEASOME.

N15 phage   See PHAGE N15.

NAAT   Nucleic-acid-amplification test: any of various types of test (involving e.g. PCR) used in a clinical diagnostic setting.

NAD (former names: coenzyme I; cozymase; diphosphopyridine nucleotide, DPN)   Nicotine adenine dinucleotide: a carrier of energy (and hydrogen) in many reactions; it is also involved in ADP-RIBOSYLATION. The oxidized form is written NAD^+, the reduced form is written NADH.

NAD⁺-dependent ligase   See DNA LIGASE.

nalidixic acid   See QUINOLONE ANTIBIOTICS.

nano-   A prefix meaning 10^{-9}.

nanocircle DNA   See DNA NANOCIRCLE.

nanopore (experimental)   A nanometer-scale pore prepared e.g. from certain proteins or by a synthetic process. Movement of a DNA molecule through a nanopore, under appropriate control, may offer the possibility of using a nanopore device for sequencing the molecule. [Kinetics of translocation of DNA through synthetic nanopores: Biophys J (2004) 87(3):2086–2097.]

NASBA   Nucleic acid sequence-based amplification: a method used primarily for the isothermal amplification of specific sequences in RNA (at a temperature of e.g. 41°C/42°C).

Amplification of an RNA target sequence by NASBA is shown diagrammatically in the figure.

(For isothermal amplification of DNA see e.g. MOLECULAR ZIPPER and SDA.)

NASBA and TMA both reflect an earlier technique used for the *in vitro* amplification of nucleic acids: see entry SELF-SUSTAINED SEQUENCE REPLICATION.

The use of an RNA target sequence (as compared to DNA targets) is an advantage in some circumstances. For example, in a diagnostic assay of cellular pathogens, the abundance of rRNA molecules in every cell – as compared e.g. to (single-copy) genes – increases the chances of detecting small numbers of pathogens in a clinical sample. Additionally, certain short-lived bacterial mRNAs are useful targets for detecting *viable* cells.

In the context of virology, NASBA has been useful e.g. for assaying genomic RNA of the retrovirus HIV-1 in a range of clinical specimens – including plasma, CSF (cerebrospinal fluid) and brain tissue.

NASBA is also useful for monitoring the appearance of transcriptional activity in latent DNA viruses. For example, transcripts of the late genes of cytomegalovirus (CMV) have been used as targets for monitoring patients at risk from CMV-related conditions. Recipients of transplants have been monitored by assaying transcripts of the CMV gene *UL65*, which encodes protein pp67.

The products of a NASBA assay can be detected in various ways. In one approach, products are examined by agarose gel electrophoresis, and blotting, followed by hybridization of a biotinylated probe and detection by an alkaline phosphatase–streptavidin conjugate and a chemiluminescent substrate.

A system involving electrochemiluminescence is available commercially (NucliSens™, bioMérieux, Boxtel, Holland).

Real-time detection of NASBA products can be achieved e.g. with MOLECULAR BEACON PROBES.

Quantitation of NASBA products has been achieved e.g. by using several internal 'calibrators', i.e. RNA molecules which are co-amplified and co-extracted with target RNA; because the initial concentration of each of the calibrators is known accurately, the initial concentration of the target sequence can be calculated.

Examples of the use of NASBA include measurement of plasma levels of RNA from human immunodeficiency virus (HIV) [Clin Vaccine Immunol (2006) 13(4):511–519], and detection of 16S rRNA from *Chlamydophila pneumoniae* in respiratory specimens [J Clin Microbiol (2006) 44(4):1241–1244]. NASBA was also reported to be useful for assaying noroviruses (common causal agents of viral gastroenteritis) in environmental waters – factors causing inhibition of reverse transcriptase PCR had little or no inhibitory effect on a real-time NASBA assay [Appl Environ Microbiol (2006) 72(8): 5349 5358]

National Bioforensics Analysis Center   See NBFAC.

NBFAC   National Bioforensics Analysis Center: the microbial forensics laboratory which forms part of the Department of Homeland Security in the USA; it works closely with the FBI (Federal Bureau of Investigation) and is a center specializing in the examination and analysis of material evidence in cases of actual or suspected criminal/terrorist activity.

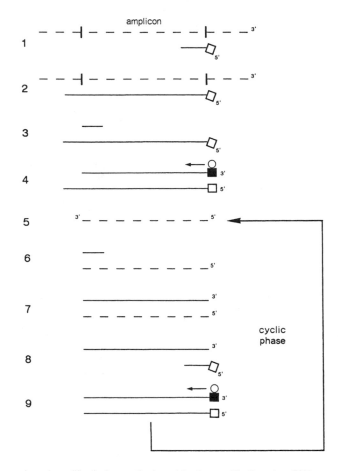

NASBA (nucleic acid sequence-based amplification): a method used for the amplification of an RNA sequence (diagrammatic, to show principle). The dashed lines are strands of RNA. The solid lines are strands of DNA. The following is an outline of the stages involved.

1. A strand of RNA showing the target sequence (the amplicon) delimited by the two, short vertical bars. A primer (primer 1) has bound to the 3′ end of the amplicon. The 5′ end of the primer has an extension (tag) which includes a short sequence (□) corresponding to the promoter of an RNA polymerase; the tag itself does not bind to the target RNA.
2. The enzyme reverse transcriptase has extended the primer to form a strand of cDNA.
3. The enzyme RNase H has degraded (removed) the strand of RNA, and a different primer (primer 2) has bound to the amplicon sequence in cDNA.
4. Reverse transcriptase (which can also synthesize DNA on a DNA template) has extended primer 2 to form double-stranded cDNA; note that primer 2 has been fully extended to form the complementary strand (■) of the promoter – so that a functional (double-stranded) promoter is now present. An RNA polymerase (○) has bound to the promoter and will synthesize a strand of RNA in the direction of the arrow, i.e. 5′-to-3′.
5. The newly synthesized strand of RNA. Note the polarity of the strand: it is *complementary* to the amplicon in the sample RNA (compare 5 with 1).
6. Primer 2 has bound to the strand of RNA.
7. Reverse transcriptase has synthesized cDNA on the strand of RNA.

158

(See also FORENSIC APPLICATIONS.)

negative control (in operons) See OPERON.

negative selection In general, selection based on the absence of a given feature, function or reaction.

(cf. POSITIVE SELECTION.)

neighbor exclusion principle See INTERCALATING AGENT.

nelfinavir See PROTEASE INHIBITORS.

neomycin See AMINOGLYCOSIDE ANTIBIOTICS.

neoplasia Progressive, uncontrolled division of cells, resulting e.g. in a solid tumor or in leukemia.

(See also ONCOGENESIS.)

neoplasm A tumor.

neoschizomer See ISOSCHIZOMER.

nested deletions Any process in which segments are progressively removed from the end of a DNA molecule. This type of procedure can be used e.g. when sequencing a long (>500-nucleotide) molecule of DNA. Thus, the initial ~500-nucleotide length of the sample DNA may be sequenced (by the DIDEOXY METHOD) from the first primer-binding site. Further sequencing of the molecule can be achieved by (i) removing that part of the (double-stranded) sample DNA which has already been sequenced, and (ii) sequencing the next section of single-stranded template from a new primer-binding site. This procedure is then repeated, so that sequencing of the entire molecule is achieved in a series of consecutive steps along the length of the sample DNA.

Unidirectional nested deletions in a cloned fragment within a circular vector can be prepared by first cutting the vector, with appropriate RESTRICTION ENDONUCLEASES, *at two sites close to one end of the insert*: (i) one enzyme to produce a 5′ overhang adjacent to the insert, and (ii) another enzyme to produce a 3′ overhang at the other end of the cleaved vector. The digested vector is then incubated with EXONUCLEASE III, and aliquots of the mixture are removed at intervals of time. Exonuclease III digests the 3′ end recessed under the 5′ overhang (but not the 3′ overhang at the other end of the cleaved vector). Increasing lengths of incubation with exonuclease III result in progressively greater digestion of the recessed 3′ end i.e. increasing the extent of deletion of the insert – so that aliquots removed later from the incubation will contain molecules in which more of the insert sequence has been deleted.

The 5′ single-stranded sequences (resulting from digestion by exonuclease III) – and the 3′ overhangs at the other end of the molecule – are removed by incubation with e.g. mung bean nuclease or ENDONUCLEASE S1. The resulting blunt-ended products can be ligated e.g. with T4 DNA ligase to re-form vector molecules containing inserts with a range of deletions.

neu In the rat: an ONCOGENE whose product is related to members of the EPIDERMAL GROWTH FACTOR RECEPTOR FAMILY; this product has TYROSINE KINASE activity associated with the intracellular domain.

Neu In the rat: the product of the *neu* gene (a homolog of the human HER2 protein).

Neulasta® See BIOPHARMACEUTICAL (table).

Neupogen® See BIOPHARMACEUTICAL (table).

nevirapine A NON-NUCLEOSIDE REVERSE TRANSCRIPTASE INHIBITOR.

Newcombe experiment An early (1949) classic experiment in which Newcombe demonstrated that *pre-existing* mutants are selected when a population of bacteria appears to adapt to a change in the environment.

A number of plates, containing nutrient agar, are each inoculated from a culture of phage-sensitive bacteria and are then incubated for a few hours. During the incubation period each viable cell gives rise to a number of progeny cells (a clone), forming a colony.

At this stage, the plates are divided into two groups: group A and group B.

In group A plates the bacterial growth is re-distributed over the surface of each plate by means of a sterile glass spreader. As a result, the cells of each clone (colony) are dispersed over the surface of the agar.

In group B plates the growth is left undisturbed.

Every plate (in both groups, A and B) is then sprayed with a suspension of virulent phage and re-incubated.

During the period of re-incubation all phage-sensitive cells are lysed. Any colonies that form on the plates necessarily arise from phage-resistant cells.

If resistance to phage developed adaptively (as a response to the presence of phage) it would be observed only *after* the cells had been exposed to phage. Were this the case, then re-distribution of growth on group A plates should be irrelevant

NASBA (*continued*)

8. RNase H has removed the strand of RNA, and primer 1 has bound to the amplicon sequence in cDNA.

9. Reverse transcriptase has synthesized a complementary strand of cDNA; note that the 3′ end of the template strand of cDNA has also been extended to form a functional (double stranded) promoter for the RNA polymerase. RNA polymerase has bound to this promoter and will (repeatedly) synthesize strands of RNA identical to the one shown at stage 5; these strands can participate in the cyclic phase, leading to high-level amplification of the target.

The double-stranded molecules of cDNA in stage 9 are permanent products which are continually transcribed by the RNA polymerase. Operation of the cyclic phase produces many copies of the amplicon in the form of (i) *complementary* RNA and (ii) cDNA.

Reproduced from *Bacteria in Biology, Biotechnology and Medicine*, 6th edition, Figure 8.25, pages 264–265, Paul Singleton (2004) John Wiley & Sons Ltd, UK [ISBN 0-470-09027-8] with permission from the publisher.

because it was done before the cells were exposed to phage. Hence, if resistance to phage developed adaptively, similar numbers of phage-resistant colonies should develop on all the plates (in groups A and B).

If, however, phage-resistant cells had been present *before* exposure to phage (on both the A and B plates), then each phage-resistant cell (mutant) would form a clone of cells (i.e. a single colony) before exposure to phage. In this case, the re-distribution of growth on group A plates would spread the cells of each (phage-resistant) colony – so that each of these cells would itself give rise to a separate colony. By contrast, any colony of (phage-resistant) cells on group B plates would remain as a single colony because growth on these plates had not been re-distributed.

In practice, many more (phage-resistant) colonies are found on the group A plates, indicating the presence of pre-existing phage-resistant mutant cells in the original culture.

(cf. FLUCTUATION TEST.)

NF-κB Nuclear factor κB: a major transcription factor found in mammalian cells. An inactive form of NF-κB, complexed with the inhibitory factor IκB, is found in the cytoplasm. On activation, NF-κB (no longer complexed with IκB) can enter the nucleus and regulate expression of various genes.

[An assay of NF-κB–DNA binding: BioTechniques (2006) 41(1):79–90.]

(See also PATHDETECT SYSTEMS.)

NHGRI National Human Genome Research Institute.

nick In dsDNA: a break in one strand of the duplex at a particular phosphodiester bond.

(cf. GAP.)

nick-closing enzyme See TOPOISOMERASE (type I).

nick translation A technique for labeling DNA (for example, cloned fragments) by replacing the existing nucleotides with nucleotides carrying a radioactive or other label. Essentially, the (ds) DNA is exposed to an endonuclease which makes a number of (random) nicks. Using each of the nicks as a starting point, DNA polymerase I extends the 3′ terminus – the newly synthesized strand incorporating labeled dNTPs (that are abundant in the reaction mixture); during synthesis, the polymerase exerts 5′-to-3′ exonucleolytic activity, i.e. it progressively removes nucleotides from the nick's 5′ terminus.

nickel-charged affinity resin A resin (charged with nickel ions, Ni^{2+}) which can bind proteins that have an (accessible) sequence of six consecutive histidine residues; it is used e.g. for the purification of 6xHis-tagged recombinant proteins – including those produced by expression vectors such as the CHAMPION PET SUMO VECTOR and the VOYAGER VECTORS. Elution of proteins bound to the resin can be achieved e.g. by using a low-pH buffer or by histidine competition.

(See also PROBOND NICKEL-CHELATING RESIN.)

nicking enzyme See RESTRICTION ENDONUCLEASE.

nicotine adenine dinucleotide See NAD.

Niemann–Pick disease See GENETIC DISEASE (table).

nisin See LANTIBIOTIC.

nitrocefin An agent used, *in vitro*, to test for β-LACTAMASES;

nitrocefin is a CEPHALOSPORIN which changes from red to yellow when cleaved by a β-lactamase.

(See also PADAC.)

nitrous acid (as a mutagen) Nitrous acid (HNO_2) brings about oxidative deamination of guanine (to xanthine), cytosine (to uracil) and adenine (to hypoxanthine). Replication of nitrous acid-treated DNA can lead to GC→AT mutation (deaminated cytosine) and AT→GC mutation (deaminated adenine).

(See also HYDROXYLAMINE.)

NMR Nuclear magnetic resonance, a phenomenon which has been exploited e.g. for monitoring gene expression *in vitro* and *in vivo*: see MRI.

NNRTIs NON-NUCLEOSIDE REVERSE TRANSCRIPTASE INHIBITORS (q.v.).

non-coding strand (of a gene) See CODING STRAND.

non-isotopic labeling (of probes) See PROBE LABELING.

non-Mendelian inheritance CYTOPLASMIC INHERITANCE.

non-nucleoside reverse transcriptase inhibitors (NNRTIs) A structurally diverse group of ANTIRETROVIRAL AGENTS that inhibit viral reverse transcriptase; they include delavirdine, efavirenz, GW678248 and nevirapine (see also SURAMIN).

(See also HAART.)

non-ribosomal peptide synthetase (NRPS) Any of a range of multisubunit enzymes which mediate ribosome-independent synthesis of peptides [e.g. NRPS from the bacterium *Pseudomonas aeruginosa*: J Bacteriol (2003) 185(9):2848–2855].

NRPSs have been genetically modified in order to generate new types of product; these and other advances have allowed the synthesis of e.g. various peptide antibiotics and integrin receptors.

[Chemoenzymatic and template-directed synthesis of bioactive macrocyclic peptides: Microbiol Mol Biol Rev (2006) 70(1):121–146.]

nonsense-associated disease Any of various diseases (such as Duchenne muscular dystrophy) which may develop through a NONSENSE MUTATION that affects a specific protein.

nonsense codon (chain-terminating codon, stop codon, termination codon) Any of the three codons – UAA (*ochre* codon), UAG (*amber* codon) and UGA (*opal* codon or *umber* codon) – which usually specify termination of polypeptide synthesis during translation.

nonsense mutation Any mutation that produces a NONSENSE CODON from a codon previously specifying a product.

nonsense suppressor See SUPPRESSOR MUTATION.

nopaline See CROWN GALL.

norfloxacin See QUINOLONE ANTIBIOTICS.

noroviruses See NASBA (uses).

Northern blotting A form of BLOTTING in which RNA is transferred from gel to matrix. (cf. SOUTHERN BLOTTING.) A Northern blot may be probed e.g. by labeled DNA.

(See also WESTERN BLOTTING.)

NotI A RARE-CUTTING RESTRICTION ENDONUCLEASE.

(See also GC% (figure).)

Novex® gels A range of gels (Invitrogen, Carlsbad CA) used in gel electrophoresis of nucleic acids and proteins.

Novex® TBE (Tris, boric acid, EDTA) gels are used for the separation of fragments of DNA of a wide range of sizes.

Novex® TBE-urea gels are optimized for fragments of DNA in the range ~20–800 bp.

novobiocin A coumarin derivative that binds to the B subunit of bacterial gyrase, blocking the enzyme's ATPase activity and, hence, blocking DNA synthesis. (See also QUINOLONE ANTIBIOTICS.) Novobiocin is less effective against topoisomerase IV – apparently because of a one-residue difference in the target sequence [Antimicrob Agents Chemother (2004) 48:1856–1864].

A mutation in the B subunit of gyrase, causing *hypersensitivity* to novobiocin, was found to be partly suppressed by a further mutation in the A subunit [J Bacteriol (2005) 187 (19):6841–6844].

NovoRapid® See BIOPHARMACEUTICAL (table).

NovoSeven® See BIOPHARMACEUTICAL (table).

NPVs NUCLEAR POLYHEDROSIS VIRUSES.

nrdA **gene** (*dnaF* gene) In *Escherichia coli*: a gene encoding the enzyme ribonucleotide reductase (which converts ribonucleotides to deoxyribonucleotides).

NRPS NON-RIBOSOMAL PEPTIDE SYNTHETASE.

NRTIs NUCLEOSIDE REVERSE TRANSCRIPTASE INHIBITORS.

nuclear magnetic resonance (NMR) See e.g. MRI.

nuclear polyhedrosis viruses (NPVs) A category of baculoviruses which are distinguished from GRANULOSIS VIRUSES e.g. on the basis of characteristics of their occlusion bodies: see BACULOVIRIDAE. Those NPVs in which a single nucleocapsid is enveloped have been designated *S*NPV, while those in which multiple nucleocapsids are enveloped have been designated *M*NPV.

Unlike granulosis viruses, NPVs occur in various orders of arthropods, including Coleoptera, Diptera and Hymenoptera as well as Lepidoptera.

The type species of NPVs is *Autographa californica* NPV (Ac*M*NPV) (genome: ~135 kb) which infects insects of the Lepidoptera. Other viruses in this group include the silkworm pathogen *Bombyx mori* NPV (Bm*S*NPV) and the Douglas Fir tussock moth virus *Orygia pseudotsugata* NPV (Op*M*NPV).

5′-nuclease PCR Any of various forms of PCR in which the 5′-exonuclease activity of the polymerase is used to degrade a labeled probe which is bound to an amplicon; the signal (for example, fluorescence) generated by degradation of the probe is monitored.

nuclease protection assay See e.g. RIBONUCLEASE PROTECTION ASSAY.

nuclease S1 *Syn.* ENDONUCLEASE S1.

nucleic acid A single- or double stranded (hetero)polymer of NUCLEOTIDES in which adjacent nucleotides in a given strand are linked by a phosphodiester bond between the 5′ and 3′ positions of their pentose residues.

In a double-stranded nucleic acid the two strands are held together by base-pairing between *complementary* bases (i.e. between A in one strand and T (U in RNA) in the other, and between G in one strand and C in the other).

A nucleic acid molecule may be linear (with free 5′ and 3′ ends) or covalently closed circular (ccc) with no free 5′ or 3′ ends. (A 'nicked' molecule is a double-stranded molecule that contains one or more nicks – see NICK.)

Information is encoded in the *sequence* of the nucleotides in the polymer. In all organisms, the genome is composed of one or more molecules of nucleic acid.

DNA is a nucleic acid consisting of *deoxy*ribonucleotides (in which the pentose residues carry –H, rather than –OH, at the 2′-position).

RNA is a nucleic acid consisting of ribonucleotides.

nucleic acid amplification (*in vitro*) Any of various methods used for the amplification (i.e. repeated copying) of specific sequences of nucleotides in RNA or DNA.

Some examples are listed in the table.

nucleic acid enzyme Any nucleic acid molecule (either RNA or DNA) which has enzymic capability – e.g. as a nuclease or a ligase. See e.g. RIBOZYME and DEOXYRIBOZYME.

nucleic acid isolation (nucleic acid extraction) Any procedure which is used for removing and concentrating DNA or RNA from cells or tissues: see e.g. DNA ISOLATION, RNAQUEOUS TECHNOLOGY and PAXGENE BLOOD RNA KIT.

Reagents commonly used in the isolation of nucleic acids are listed in the table. Note that some of these reagents may inhibit amplification in processes such as PCR – indicating the need for a pre-amplification clean-up. For example, lysozyme and proteinase K have both been reported as inhibitors of PCR.

nucleic acid sequence-based amplification See NASBA.

nucleic acid staining See DNA STAINING and RIBOGREEN.

(See also ULTRAVIOLET ABSORBANCE.)

nucleocapsid A composite structure, consisting of nucleic acid and protein, that forms part, or all, of certain virions.

nucleoid In a prokaryotic cell: the body consisting mainly of genomic DNA (one or more chromosomes) and NUCLEOID-ASSOCIATED PROTEINS. The DNA in a nucleoid is highly compacted.

(See also A-TRACT and CHROMOSOME.)

The *toroidal* form of the nucleoid in *Deinococcus radiodurans* may contribute to this organism's unusual resistance to ionizing radiation [Science (2003) 299:254–256].

Segregation of genetic material to daughter cells during cell division may require a force-generating system involving e.g. the actin-like cytoskeletal protein MreB and RNA polymerase in *Escherichia coli* [Genes Dev (2006) 20(1):113–124]. An alternative view is that segregation occurs in an entropy-driven (i.e. spontaneous) manner due to the tendency of two nucleoids to exhibit mutual repulsion in order to maximize the conformational entropy [Proc Natl Acad Sci USA (2006) 103(33):12388–12393]. Whatever the mechanism, studies on segregation of the (paired) chromosomes in *Vibrio cholerae* have suggested the possibility of coordination between these chromosomes in order to ensure their correct transmission to daughter cells [J Bacteriol (2006) 188(3):1060–1070].

Note. The term *nucleoid* is also used to refer to the DNA–

NUCLEIC ACID AMPLIFICATION (summary of *in vitro* methods)[a]

Method	Targets in[b]	Temperature	Basis
cHDA[c]	DNA	Isothermal	Amplification of *circular* dsDNA templates by helicase-dependent strand separation followed by a rolling circle mechanism to produce concatemeric products; the helicase, DNA polymerase and single-strand binding proteins from bacteriophage T7 are key components
HDA[d]	DNA	Isothermal	Strands of (double-stranded) sample DNA are separated by helicase activity rather than by heat or recombinase activity (as in other methods)
LCR[e]	DNA	Cycling	Use of a binary probe (two oligonuleotides) binding specifically to two closely adjacent regions in the target sequence; closure of the gap between the two bound oligonucleotides by a DNA polymerase is followed by ligation and then temperature-based release of the newly formed amplicon – the newly formed and pre-existing amplicons then acting as templates for the next round of amplification. Thermostable enzymes (i.e. polymerase and ligase) are required. *Product detection.* One approach uses gel electrophoresis. A commercial system uses a microparticle enzyme immunoassay in which immobilized ligated probes are detected by an antibody–enzyme conjugate
MDA[f]	DNA	Isothermal	A form of WGA (whole-genome amplification) in which multiple sites are primed by random, exonuclease-resistant hexamers, and DNA synthesis is mediated by the highly processive DNA polymerase derived from bacteriophage φ29
Molecular zipper[g]	DNA	Isothermal	The target sequence is initially in the form of an ssDNA circle. A single primer is extended (by the rolling circle mechanism), yielding an ssDNA multimer of the target. The multimer binds many molecular zippers (each a composite, labeled probe) which, when extended via their 3′ ends, displace the downstream (bound and extended) zippers. Primers bind to the displaced zippers and are extended to form dsDNA products; extension of these primers displaces a quencher-labeled oligonucleotide hybridized to the original zipper, permitting detection of products via the zippers' fluorophore label
NASBA[h]	RNA	Isothermal	Initially, primer 1 is extended, by reverse transcription on the RNA target sequence, forming a strand of cDNA as part of an RNA/DNA hybrid duplex; primer 1 carries a 5′ tag containing the promoter sequence of an RNA polymerase. The RNA strand of the duplex is degraded, and primer 2 binds to the first strand of cDNA; primer 2 is extended to form the second strand of duplex cDNA – thus creating a functional promoter. Transcription of the duplex cDNA forms single-stranded RNA products (complementary to the target sequence). Amplification of these products, first by primer 2 then by primer 1, yields further copies of the double-stranded cDNA which, as before, are transcribed into RNA products; this process constitutes a cyclic phase in which the products are (i) ssRNA amplicons (complementary to the target sequence) and (ii) dsDNA amplicons. *Product detection.* Gel electrophoresis (e.g. to compare size of amplicons with target sequence). Also, real-time monitoring e.g. with molecular beacon probes. In a commercial system: probe-based monitoring involving generation of an electrochemiluminescent signal
PAP[i]	DNA	Cycling	Pyrophosphorolysis-activated polymerization: a form of amplification used for high-level specificity (owing to minimal non-specific priming); it is employed e.g. for allele-specific amplification. Initially, primer extension is blocked because the 3′ terminal nucleotide of each primer is a dideoxyribonucleotide monophosphate (ddNMP); given correct hybridization to the target sequence, and the presence of pyrophosphate, the ddNMP is excised – so that primer extension can occur
PCR[j]	DNA	Cycling	Extension of primers on opposite strands of the target sequence following heat denaturation of double-stranded sample DNA, the two primer-binding sites delimiting the target sequence to be amplified. Temperature-based release of newly formed amplicons from the templates and subsequent binding of primers to newly formed and pre-existing target sequences for the next round of amplification. (See entry PCR for a detailed descripiton of the process.) *Product detection.* Gel electrophoresis (e.g. to compare the size of amplicons with expected size – as may be required in diagnostic tests). Monitoring with a dsDNA-binding fluorophore (such as SYBR® Green I). Quantitation of target sequences in the original sample by use of TaqMan® probes or by the LightCycler™ system. Monitoring by a combined probe–dye approach: see REAL-TIME PCR for details

(*continued*)

Method	Targets in[b]	Temperature	Basis
Rolling circle	DNA	Isothermal	Ongoing synthesis on a *circular* template, with concurrent displacement of the strand bound to the template strand (in a circular dsDNA target molecule). The target molecule may also be single-stranded; in some cases an RNA polymerase may be able to initiate synthesis on an ssDNA strand with GTP (see e.g. entry DNA NANOCIRCLE). (See also entry for ROLLING CIRCLE.) The product may be a concatemeric form of the target molecule; however, a double-stranded product can be produced if primers bind to this strand and undergo extension and ligation
RPA[k]	DNA	Isothermal	In this method, the binding of primers does not involve initial separation of the strands in sample dsDNA by heat or helicase activity (as in other methods). Instead, primer binding is mediated by a recombinase following the formation of primer–recombinase complexes. Extension of primers by a strand-displacing DNA polymerase produces a growing loop of ssDNA (from the target duplex) which is stabilized by single-strand binding proteins. Various factors within the reaction mixture are required to bring about a balance between development and disassembly of the primer–recombinase complexes. *Product detection.* Probe-based detection in which a bound probe with an abasic-site mimic is cleaved by an endonuclease, releasing a fluorophore from the influence of a quencher
SDA[l]	DNA	Isothermal	Two phases: target generation and amplification. In target generation, primers – 5′-tagged with the recognition sequence of HincII RESTRICTION ENDONUCLEASE – are extended, and the newly formed strands are displaced through extension of bumper primers. As the reaction mixture contains α-thiophosphoryl dATP (dATPαS) in place of normal dATP, the ongoing reaction sequence leads to the formation of double-stranded intermediates having two terminal HincII recognition sites that are hemi-modified asymmetrically – i.e. both recognition sites contain one modified strand and one unmodified strand but the modified/unmodified nucleotides are in different strands at the two sites (see figure in SDA). Nicking of a recognition site (in the unmodified strand), and extension of the 3′ end of the nick, displaces a strand with one terminal modified site; a primer extended on this strand yields a double-stranded product that feeds into the amplification phase (see figure in SDA). Amplification is based essentially on the nicking of a hemi-modified site (in the unmodified strand) and the displacement of a sense or antisense strand by extension of the 3′ end of the nick – such extension regenerating a new amplicon in readiness for the next round of nicking. *Product detection.* Various ways, including gel electrophoresis and probe-based approaches
TMA[m]	RNA	Isothermal	Similar to NASBA. Commercial TMA-based diagnostic tests have been used for detecting pathogens such as *Chlamydia trachomatis* and *Mycobacterium tuberculosis* in clinical specimens. *Product detection.* In a commercial system: probe-based monitoring involving generation of a chemiluminescent signal
WGA[n]	DNA	Isothermal	Whole-genome amplification: any of several techniques in which multiple regions of a sample of genomic DNA are amplified simultaneously by either random-sequence primers or e.g. bioinformatically optimized primers

[a]For further information see separate entries.
[b]Some methods can be adapted to amplify either DNA or RNA targets.
[c]Circular helicase-dependent amplification: see entry CHDA.
[d]Helicase-dependent amplification: see entry HELICASE-DEPENDENT AMPLIFICATION.
[e]Ligase chain reaction: see entry LCR.
[f]Multiple displacement amplification: see entry MULTIPLE DISPLACEMENT AMPLIFICATION.
[g]See entry MOLECULAR ZIPPER.
[h]Nucleic acid sequence-based amplification: see entry NASBA.
[i]See entry PYROPHOSPHOROLYSIS-ACTIVATED POLYMERIZATION.
[j]Polymerase chain reaction: see entry PCR.
[k]Recombinase polymerase amplification: see entry RPA.
[l]Strand displacement amplification: see entry SDA.
[m]Transcription-mediated amplification: see entry TMA.
[n]Whole-genome amplification: see entry WHOLE-GENOME AMPLIFICATION.

NUCLEIC ACID ISOLATION: some of the reagents commonly used in the isolation of nucleic acids from cells and tissues

Reagent	Function (e.g.)
EDTA (ethylenediaminetetra-acetic acid)	Destabilizes the cell envelope (outer membrane) of Gram-negative bacteria by chelating those ions (e.g. Mg^{2+}) which confer stability
Guanidinium isothiocyanate	Cell lysis and inactivation of nucleases
Lysostaphin	Cleaves peptide cross-links in the cell-wall polymer peptidoglycan in *Staphylococcus aureus* (a Gram-positive bacterium), weakening the wall and thus promoting cell lysis
Lysozyme	Cleaves the glycan backbone chains in the bacterial cell-wall polymer peptidoglycan, promoting cell lysis by weakening the cell wall
Phenol–chloroform–isoamyl alcohol	Promotes partitioning of DNA in the upper layer; the DNA can be precipitated e.g. by ethanol or by isopropanol
Proteinase K	Non-specific digestion of proteins. It is also useful e.g. as an inactivator of nucleases
RNase A	Elimination of RNA from isolated DNA (used e.g. in plasmid preparations)
RNase inhibitors	Protection of RNA from RNA-degrading enzymes (see e.g. RNA*secure*™ in the entry RIBONUCLEASE)
Sodium hydroxide–sodium dodecyl sulfate	Disrupts cell membranes, allowing leakage
Tris (tris(hydroxymethyl)-aminomethane	As a hydrochloride: a buffering system which is used (e.g.) with EDTA
TRIzol®	Constituents: phenol and guanidine isothiocyanate. Used e.g. for the isolation of total RNA from cells. The integrity of the RNA is maintained during homogenization/lysis of the cells

protein complex in a mitochondrion and to the electron-dense core of a peroxisome.

nucleoid-associated proteins Certain small proteins, such as H-NS PROTEIN and HU PROTEIN, which are generally found to be abundant in the (prokaryotic) nucleoid.

nucleolar phosphoprotein B23 *Syn.* NUCLEOPHOSMIN.

nucleophosmin (nucleolar phosphoprotein B23; numatrin) A multifunctional nuclear phosphoprotein with roles e.g. in ribosome synthesis and cell proliferation (see also histone ACETYLATION). It apparently regulates/stabilizes the tumor suppressors P53 and p19^Arf [Mol Cell Biol (2005) 25(20): 8874–8886], and is formed in response to chemotherapy of lung cancer [Exp Cell Res (2007) 313(1):65–76].

nucleoprotein filament See HOMOLOGOUS RECOMBINATION.

nucleoside A compound consisting of the residue of a purine or pyrimidine base linked covalently to a pentose (i.e. 5-carbon sugar) – commonly ribose (in *ribo*nucleosides) or 2′-deoxyribose in *deoxyribo*nucleosides. A pyrimidine is linked via its 1-position to the sugar, a purine is linked via its 9-position.

A ribonucleoside which incorporates a residue of adenine, guanine, cytosine, uracil, thymine or hypoxanthine is called (respectively) adenosine, guanosine, cytidine, uridine, thymidine (or *ribo*thymidine) or inosine. Corresponding *deoxy*-

*ribo*nucleosides are deoxyadenosine, deoxyguanosine etc. In general, 'thymidine' is used to refer to deoxythymidine.

(cf. NUCLEOTIDE.)

nucleoside reverse transcriptase inhibitors (NRTIs) A class of synthetic nucleoside analogs used in antiretroviral therapy, e.g. anti-AIDS therapy; in cells, an NRTI is phosphorylated (to the triphosphate) and, when incorporated into DNA by the (viral) reverse transcriptase (RT), it blocks chain elongation by blocking formation of the next phosphodiester bond. All NRTIs have a similar mode of action. The NRTIs include e.g. ABACAVIR, adefovir, didanosine, LAMIVUDINE, stavudine, tenofovir, zalcitabine and ZIDOVUDINE.

The anti-HIV activity of an NRTI *in vivo* may be raised by raising the ratio of the NRTI to the cell's own dNTPs; this can be done e.g. by using hydroxyurea to inhibit the host's enzyme ribonucleotide reductase (thereby causing a decrease in endogenous dNTPs). This approach gave clinical benefit e.g. when used in combination with didanosine.

Resistance to NRTIs can be due to a mutant RT gene. In one *in vitro* study of the activity of various NRTIs against a mutant (K65R) strain of HIV-1, all NRTIs except those with a 3′-azido moiety were less active against the mutant virus, indicating the value of including AZT in drug combinations

[Antimicrob Agents Chemother (2005) 49(3):1139–1144].

Some NRTIs are also useful against DNA viruses: see e.g. LAMIVUDINE.

nucleosome See CHROMATIN.

nucleotide A NUCLEOSIDE that carries one or more phosphate groups at the 5′ position of the sugar residue.

Nucleotides are subunits of the NUCLEIC ACIDS DNA and RNA.

Certain nucleotides, e.g. adenosine triphosphate (ATP) and guanosine triphosphate (GTP), have an important function in energy-transfer reactions.

Biosynthesis of nucleotides in microbial and/or tumor cells may be inhibited by various agents such as AZASERINE, DON, HADACIDIN, MYCOPHENOLIC ACID and PSICOFURANINE.

(See also UNIVERSAL NUCLEOTIDE.)

nucleotide excision repair *Syn.* UVRABC-MEDIATED REPAIR.

NucliSens™ See NASBA.

numatrin *Syn.* NUCLEOPHOSMIN.

numts Nuclear mitochondria-like sequences: those mtDNA-like sequences ('mitochondrial pseudogenes') which occur in nuclear (chromosomal) DNA. Numts are a possible source of contamination when mtDNA *specifically* is being targeted for amplification by PCR (e.g. in certain forensic investigations).

A total of 46 fragments of nuclear DNA, representing the entire (human) mitochondrial genome, have been sequenced [BMC Genomics (2006) 7:185].

nutrient agar A general-purpose bacteriological MEDIUM that contains peptone, sodium chloride, beef extract and 1.5–2% agar. It supports the growth of various types of nutritionally undemanding heterotrophic bacteria such as *Escherichia coli*; many species of bacteria will not grow on such (*basal*) media unless they are supplemented with serum or other forms of enrichment.

O

o^c **mutant** See LAC OPERON.

O^6-**alkylguanine-DNA alkyltransferase** (AGT) See 'Uses of gene fusion' in the entry GENE FUSION.

OB Occlusion body: see BACULOVIRIDAE.

occlusion body (OB) See BACULOVIRIDAE.

occlusion-derived virions (ODVs) See BACULOVIRIDAE.

ochre codon See NONSENSE MUTATION.

ochre suppressor See SUPPRESSOR MUTATION.

OCT plasmid A large (~500 kb) plasmid, found in strains of *Pseudomonas*, which confers the ability to metabolize octane and decane.

octopine See CROWN GALL.

ODVs Occlusion-derived virions: see BACULOVIRIDAE.

OFAGE Orthogonal-field-alternation gel electrophoresis: one of a number of variant forms of PFGE which is used for the separation of large pieces of nucleic acid.

ofloxacin See QUINOLONE ANTIBIOTICS.

Okayama–Berg method An early method used for obtaining a full-length cDNA – in a known orientation within a vector – from an mRNA molecule with a poly(A) tail. Essentially, the vector was built around the mRNA in sequential steps. The initial step involved base-pairing between the poly(A) of the mRNA and a poly(T) overhang present on an added fragment of dsDNA. The FIRST STRAND was subjected to 3' homopolymer tailing to enable base-pairing with (another) segment of dsDNA having a complementary 3' overhang; the other end of this (second) segment was cut with a restriction endonuclease, enabling its ligation to the free end of the first fragment.

Okazaki fragment One of a large number of short, discontinuous sequences of deoxyribonucleotides synthesized during the formation of the lagging strand in DNA replication; each fragment is about 100–200 nt in eukaryotes (but reported to be ~1000–2000 nt in *Escherichia coli*). These fragments are joined together to form the lagging strand.

In a current model, the formation of an Okazaki fragment (in eukaryotes) begins with a hybrid RNA/DNA primer that is synthesized by the complex primase–DNA polymerase α. This primer consists of ~10 nt RNA and ~20 nt DNA (and has been referred to as iRNA/DNA); it is extended with deoxyribonucleotides, by DNA polymerase δ (pol δ), until it reaches the 5' terminal of the last Okazaki fragment. Pol δ continues DNA synthesis, its strand-displacement activity displacing the iRNA/DNA as a 5' 'flap'; the flap is excised before the newly synthesized Okazaki fragment is joined to the previous one. In the yeast *Saccharomyces cerevisiae*, excision of the flap may involve mainly *flap endonuclease 1* (FEN1) [J Biol Chem (2004) 279(15):15014–15024]; in a supplementary mechanism for flap removal in this yeast, the flap is coated with *replication protein A* (RPA), promoting flap cleavage by the Dna2p helicase/nuclease protein.

(See also IDLING.)

oligo Abbreviation for 'oligonucleotide' (used only when the meaning is clear).

OliGreen® A fluorescent dye (Molecular Probes Inc., Eugene OR/Invitrogen, Carlsbad CA) used e.g. for the quantitation of ssDNA in solution. The sensitivity of the method is reported to be ~10000-fold greater than that obtainable with measurements made by the ULTRAVIOLET ABSORBANCE method.

(See also DNA STAINING and PICOGREEN ASSAY.)

omega (ω) **protein** See TOPOISOMERASE (type I).

OMIM See ONLINE MENDELIAN INHERITANCE IN MAN.

ompT **gene** In *Escherichia coli*: a gene encoding a protease, OmpT, which is part of the (wild-type) cell's *outer membrane* – i.e. the outermost structure of the cell wall.

Some of the proteins secreted by *E. coli* consist of two parts, one of which forms a channel in the outer membrane through which the other part is translocated to the cell's surface. This type of protein secretion mechanism is referred to as an *autotransporter* system (also called type IV secretion by some authors and type V secretion by different authors). The surface-exposed part of a secreted protein may be cleaved by OmpT and released into the environment [Autotransporters in *E. coli*: Appl Environ Microbiol (2007) 73(5):1553–1562; EMBO J (2007) 26:1942–1952.]

on-chip PCR See SOLID-PHASE PCR.

on-chip synthesis See MICROARRAY.

oncogene A gene which, if aberrantly expressed, may cause neoplastic transformation ('cancer'). Oncogenes were initially found in acutely oncogenic retroviruses; subsequently, highly conserved homologs were found in a wide range of normal eukaryotic cells, including human, fruitfly (*Drosophila*) and yeast (*Saccharomyces cerevisiae*) cells. Retroviral oncogenes appear to have derived from cellular genes.

An oncogene is usually given a three-letter designation that is based on the name of the retrovirus in which it was first identified. Two examples of *viral* oncogenes are: v-*fes* from the feline sarcoma virus and v-*myc* from myelocytomatosis virus; the corresponding *cellular* homologs of these genes are designated, respectively, c-*fes* (or proto-*fes*) and c-*myc* (or proto-*myc*).

At least some oncogenes have role(s) in the regulation and/or development of normal (i.e. non-neoplastic) cells (see e.g. MYB). Oncogenesis may arise as a result of dysregulation of these genes; it may occur e.g. through mutation, insertional activation, or chromosome rearrangements (e.g. ABL).

Viral oncogenes can cause cancer in various ways. In some cases the product of a viral gene may interfere with the cell's growth related reactions which normally involve factors such as epidermal growth factor (EGF) or platelet-derived growth factor (PDGF). The v-*sis* product is almost identical to the B chain of PDGF. Other products may be active in the cell's nucleus.

(See also entries for individual oncogenes: ABL, FES, FPS, KIT, MYB, MYC, RAS, SIS, SRC.)

Cancers resulting from dysregulated tyrosine kinase activity have been treated with specific drugs, but resistance to these agents can arise through mutation in the oncogene. The problem of drug-resistance (similar to antibiotic-resistance in bacteria) requires the ongoing development of new drugs; a fruitful approach has been to screen *existing* clinically useful drugs for agents that are active against newly mutant targets [Proc Natl Acad Sci USA (2005) 102 (31):11011–11016].

Oncogenes also occur in certain DNA viruses (e.g. mastadenoviruses, polyomaviruses), although these genes appear to have no cellular homologs.

oncogenesis The development of a neoplastic condition such as a tumor or leukemia.

(See also NEOPLASIA.)

oncornaviruses The former name of viruses of the subfamily ONCOVIRINAE.

Oncovirinae A subfamily of viruses of the family Retroviridae (see RETROVIRUSES) that includes all the oncogenic viruses in this family; some – apparently non-oncogenic but related – viruses have also been included in the subfamily. Members of the Oncovirinae were divided into types B, C and D on the basis of e.g. morphology and mode of development.

Online Mendelian Inheritance in Man (OMIM) A database of human genes and genetic disorders [see Nucleic Acids Res (2005) 33(Database Issue):D514–D517] accessible at: http://www.ncbi.nlm.nih.gov/omim/

ONPG The compound *o*-nitrophenyl-β-D-galactopyranoside; it is hydrolyzed by the enzyme β-galactosidase to galactose and the (yellow) compound *o*-nitrophenol.

ONPG is used e.g. as an indicator for the presence of β-galactosidase in the SOS CHROMOTEST and in other tests. In some species (e.g. *Escherichia coli*) ONPG can pass through the cell envelope (i.e. it can enter cells) without the need for a specific permease.

opa **genes** (of *Neisseria*) See OPA PROTEINS.

(See also PHASE VARIATION.)

Opa proteins Cell-surface antigens encoded by the *opa* genes in pathogenic strains of *Neisseria*; they affect the opacity and color of the bacterial colonies and bind to epithelial cells and polymorphonuclear leukocytes (e.g. via eukaryotic CD66a, c, d or e adhesins).

opal codon See NONSENSE MUTATION.

open reading frame (ORF) A sequence of nucleotides, starting with an initiator codon and ending with a stop codon, which encodes an actual or potential polypeptide/protein or an RNA product. A reading frame is 'blocked' if it contains a stop codon close to the initiator codon.

Adjacent ORFs (which may be separated by a gap) may *jointly* encode a polypeptide; in such cases, translation of the polypeptide requires a mechanism for coupling the two ORFs [see e.g. EMBO J (2000) 19:2671–2680].

operon Two or more contiguous genes coordinately expressed from a common promoter and transcribed as a polycistronic mRNA (see e.g. LAC OPERON).

The operon is sometimes regarded as a regulatory system specific to prokaryotic gene organization but a similar type of organization is also found in trypanosomes and (in some instances) in genes of the nematode *Caenorhabditis elegans* (see also TRANS SPLICING).

The following refers to operons in *bacteria*.

The control mechanism varies according to operon. Some operons are controlled at the level of transcription, and some are controlled at the level of translation.

Some operons are regulated by CATABOLITE REPRESSION.

Promoter control. This involves the synthesis of a regulator protein, which may be produced constitutively. One example of promoter control is the LAC OPERON of *Escherichia coli*; this operon is under *negative control* – meaning that the regulator protein inhibits or blocks expression of the operon. In the *lac* operon, the repressor protein binds to the operator region immediately downstream of the binding site of RNA polymerase, thus inhibiting transcription of the operon.

An example of *positive control* is found in the *araBAD* operon of *E. coli* which encodes enzymes involved in the metabolism of L-arabinose to D-xylulose 5′-phosphate. In the presence of arabinose the regulator protein, AraC (encoded by gene *araC*), acts as an *activator* of the *araBAD* operon – i.e. positive control. In the absence of arabinose (metabolic enzymes not needed) the regulator protein acts as a repressor (negative control).

Attenuator control. Operons under attenuator control are typically involved in the synthesis of amino acids. The upstream sequence of nucleotides in the mRNA transcript (the *leader sequence*) encodes a short *leader peptide* which is rich in the given amino acid whose synthesis is regulated by the operon. The leader sequence also includes a so-called *attenuator*: a rho-dependent terminator situated between the first gene of the operon and the sequence encoding the leader peptide.

Given adequate levels of the relevant amino acid (synthesis not required), transcription stops at the attenuator. If the level of amino acid is inadequate (synthesis needed), the ribosome stalls when it reaches that part of the transcript containing codons of the given amino acid within the leader peptide sequence; this permits downstream regions of the transcript to base-pair, preventing formation of the attenuator and, hence, permitting transcription of the genes.

Attenuator control is found e.g. in the *his* operon of *E. coli* – which regulates synthesis of histidine. This operon contains nine structural genes. The mRNA sequence that encodes the leader peptide includes a run of seven successive histidine codons.

The *trp* operon of *E. coli* (synthesis of tryptophan) is under both attenuator and (negative) promoter control. This operon may be more stable than other operons which have a less complex regulatory system [Microbiol Mol Biol Rev (2003) 67:303–342].

Translational control. In *E. coli* the genes *infC–rpmI–rplT* form an operon which encodes, respectively, the translation initiation factor IF3 and the two ribosomal proteins L35 and L20. High levels of L20 repress translation of both L35 and L20. L20 appears to bind to the mRNA upstream of the *rpmI* region, and it has been suggested that it stabilizes an RNA pseudoknot that includes the initiator codon, thus inhibiting the translation of both *rpmI* and *rplT*.

operon fusion The engineered fusion of two operons such that genes of both operons are controlled by regulatory regions (promoter, operator etc.) of one of the operons.

opine See CROWN GALL.

Op*M*NPV See NUCLEAR POLYHEDROSIS VIRUSES.

Orc1–6 proteins See DNAA GENE.

ORF OPEN READING FRAME.

ORFeome A set of open reading frames (see ORF), representing many, most or all ORFs from a given species, that are stored as inserts in a collection of plasmid vectors. An ORFeome can be used as a source of material for functional analysis; thus, for example, a given ORF may be inserted into a protein expression vector or used to generate fusion products.

To facilitate use, ORFs may be made more accessible for transfer to other plasmids by using a protocol involving e.g. the GATEWAY SITE-SPECIFIC RECOMBINATION SYSTEM.

ORFmer sets Commercially available (Sigma-Genosys) sets of primer pairs designed to enable the PCR-based amplification of sequences from most or all ORFs (open reading frames) in the genomic DNA of a particular organism. The primers contain ORF-specific sequences.

The 5′ terminus of each primer consists of an *adaptamer*: a sequence incorporating the recognition site of a particular restriction endonuclease; this facilitates insertion of a given PCR-amplified product (amplicon) into a cloning vector for re-amplification, if required.

orientation (*DNA technol.*) The *direction* in which a given sequence is found, or inserted, in relation to other sequence(s) or in relation to the other parts of a sequence.

For example, when using FLP recombinase (q.v.), a target fragment which is bracketed by two recognition sequences (FRT sites) that are in the same orientation will be excised; however, the target will be inverted if the two FRT sites are in opposite orientation.

oriT The origin of transfer (in a conjugative plasmid): see CONJUGATION.

orthologous genes Functionally analogous genes in different species.

orthomere See MACRONUCLEUS.

Orygia pseudotsugata NPV A baculovirus within the category NUCLEAR POLYHEDROSIS VIRUSES.

overexpression (of proteins) (*syn.* overproduction) Synthesis of high concentrations of a given protein, usually a heterologous ('foreign') protein, in a recombinant organism – either a prokaryotic or a eukaryotic organism; this procedure is used e.g. for manufacturing various products, especially for therapeutic or diagnostic use but also for research purposes (see e.g. BIO-PHARMACEUTICAL).

Proteins are synthesized in cells from bacteria (particularly the Gram-negative species ESCHERICHIA COLI), yeasts (such as *Pichia pastoris*, *Saccharomyces cerevisiae*), insects (such as *Bombyx mori*, *Spodoptera frugiperda*) and mammals (such

as hamster: CHO (Chinese hamster ovary) and BHK (baby hamster kidney) cells).

Choice of cells

The choice of cells is influenced by factors such as the need for specific type(s) of post-translational modification in the recombinant product, and/or the preferred secretion of the recombinant protein by the producing cells (rather than intracellular accumulation) in order to facilitate the recovery and purification of the product.

For proteins produced on an industrial scale, the important factors include e.g. the need to maximize the yield and the ease of downstream processing of the product. Downstream processing may be simplified by choosing cells which secrete the recombinant protein (see below). Other considerations include e.g. the safety of the product; thus, for example, if recombinant proteins are synthesized in *E. coli*, or in other Gram-negative bacteria, there is a need for rigorous exclusion of endotoxin (see PYROGEN). Additionally, agents used for induction of transcription in the producing cells should not be associated with a risk of toxicity if the recombinant products are intended for therapeutic use.

Optimization of transcription

One obvious requirement is a strong promoter to control the expression of the target gene. Moreover, transcription should be *tightly regulated* – meaning that the target gene should not be expressed prior to the time of its intended induction or derepression. One reason for this is that the cells are commonly grown to high density before expression of the target gene in order to maximize the yield of product. Were the gene to be expressed before the appropriate time then there may be a depression in the growth rate with a possible decrease in the final yield of recombinant protein.

Another reason for tight regulation is found in the case in which the recombinant protein is toxic to the producing cells. In this case, early expression of the recombinant protein can be expected to decrease final cell density and, hence, yield.

Optimization of translation

In designing a recombinant gene there is a need to ensure that the characteristics of the *transcript* are optimal for the given translation system. Thus for example, the efficient translation of mRNA in *Escherichia coli* demands attention to factors such as the precise composition of the (ribosome-binding) Shine–Dalgarno (SD) sequence, and the number of nucleotides between the SD sequence and the start codon. Moreover, optimal translation may depend on the provision of a translational enhancer ('downstream box') located close to the start codon. Failure to optimize these features may result in a marked reduction in the yield of recombinant protein.

Codon bias

The synthesis of a heterologous protein (for example, when a mammalian gene is expressed in *E. coli*) may be inefficient owing to CODON BIAS (q.v.).

(See also CODON OPTIMIZATION.)

Inclusion bodies

Inclusion bodies are insoluble aggregates of the unfolded, or incorrectly folded, heterologous protein which may develop within the cytoplasm of overexpressing cells. In *E. coli*, the formation of inclusion bodies can sometimes be inhibited e.g. by using a lower growth temperature (say, 30°C instead of 37°C) or by using the 'thiofusion' procedure (see below).

Another approach to the problem of inclusion bodies is to co-express *chaperone* proteins in overexpressing cells. These are normal constituents of cells that promote correct folding of nascent proteins.

If the inclusion bodies can be correctly folded *in vitro* (i.e. after isolation from the cells) then the formation of inclusion bodies can be an advantage in that they may facilitate purification of the product, i.e. by simplifying separation of product from cell debris etc.

The problem of proteolysis
Proteolysis of recombinant proteins in the cytoplasm of *E. coli* may be minimized in several ways. Thus, for example, the given protein may be targeted to the cell's *periplasm* (i.e. the region between the cytoplasmic membrane and the cell wall) – in which there are fewer proteolytic enzymes. This is possible e.g. by fusing the gene of interest with the gene of a periplasmic protein (such as DsbA).

Alternatively, the target protein may be made secretable by fusing its gene to the gene of a secreted protein.

A further possibility is re-coding the gene to eliminate particular proteolytic sites in the protein.

Additionally, use may be made of *rpoH* mutant cells of *E. coli*. RpoH can promote synthesis of the Lon protease (which degrades abnormal proteins), and these mutants have been found to give increased yields of recombinant proteins in *E. coli*.

Post-translational modification
Many proteins (particularly those used therapeutically) are non-functional unless they have appropriate post-translational modification, such as the glycosylation of specific amino acid residues; hence, only cells that are capable of such activity are used for the synthesis of these proteins. For this reason, a number of the commercial therapeutic agents are produced in e.g. Chinese hamster ovary cells or baby hamster kidney cells – i.e. mammalian cells which can carry out the correct forms of post-translational modification.

In some cases the absence of glycosylation has little or no effect on normal biological activity; for example, unglycosylated recombinant interleukin-2 (IL-2) has essentially normal biological activity compared with the natural protein, and this agent can be produced satisfactorily in *E. coli*.

Secreted/intracellular proteins
The *secretion* of a recombinant protein can be advantageous in a production process because it tends to simplify isolation and purification of the product. Thus, if a protein remains intracellular it is necessary to lyse the cells in order to harvest the product; this entails (i) extra work to ensure efficient lysis of cells, and (ii) the need to separate the (one) target protein from the cell's own natural proteins (as well as from the other types of cell debris).

The production of recombinant proteins intracellularly can be a problem particularly in *E. coli* and insect cells.

One approach to the problem of intracellular recombinant proteins is to design the expression vector in such a way that the recombinant gene is fused to another gene, or sequence, which promotes secretion/release of the fusion protein. When isolated *in vitro*, the product can be cleaved (with a suitable protease) to release the protein of interest.

In *E. coli*, the so-called thiofusion approach can yield extracellular recombinant products. In this process, the expression vector contains the gene of interest fused with the gene of THIOREDOXIN. This protein is found normally in the cell envelope, and the fusion protein can be released from the cells simply by subjecting the cells to osmotic shock (which disrupts the outer membrane).

Detection/isolation/purification of recombinant proteins
In vitro detection, isolation and purification of recombinant proteins can be facilitated by the use of expression vectors that encode certain types of peptide/protein tag which form a fusion product with the protein of interest. For example, the LUMIO tag provides fluorescent detection of the recombinant protein, while the calmodulin-binding peptide (CBP) of the Affinity® system (from Stratagene, La Jolla CA) helps in the isolation of a recombinant protein by binding the protein to a CALMODULIN-based adsorption resin (see also SIX-HISTIDINE TAG). The KEMPTIDE SEQUENCE permits robust labeling of the protein product.

Separation of the protein of interest from its tag may be achieved e.g. by using an endopeptidase which has a known cutting site (see e.g. ENTEROKINASE; see also TEV protease in the entry TEV).

(See also RAINBOW TAG.)

Quantitation of recombinant proteins
See e.g. Q TAG.

overhang See STICKY ENDS.

overlapping genes Two or more genes that share sequence(s) of nucleotides, part (or all) of a given gene being coextensive with part of another. This arrangement serves e.g. to maximize the amount of information carried by a genome. Such genes may differ e.g. in being translated in different reading frames, or they may be translated in the same reading frame but with different start/stop signals and/or a different pattern of splicing.

[Overlapping genes in mammals: Genome Res (2004) 14 (2):280–286; in microbial genomes: Genome Res (2004) 14 (11):2268–2272.]

overproduction (of proteins) *Syn.* OVEREXPRESSION.

8-oxoG 7,8-dihydro-8-oxoguanine: a mutagenic base produced in DNA e.g. by reactive oxygen species; if unrepaired (by the BASE EXCISION REPAIR system), it may cause a GC-to-TA transversion mutation as 8-oxoG (in the template strand) may pair with adenine during DNA replication.

During DNA replication, adenine misincorporated opposite a template-strand 8-oxoG can be excised by the *Escherichia coli* MutY DNA glycosylase (or by the human homolog of

MutY, hMUTYH). In *Helicobacter pylori*, the product of a putative MutY-encoding gene was reported to be able to complement *mutY* strains of *E. coli* [J Bacteriol (2006) 188 (21):7464–7469].

In duplex DNA, 8-oxoG can be excised from 8-oxoG:C pairs by the *E. coli* DNA glycosylase MutM (= Fpg protein).

The *E. coli* MutT protein prevents the incorporation of free 8-oxoG into DNA by eliminating it from the pool of oxidized guanines.

oxolinic acid   See QUINOLONE ANTIBIOTICS.

P

p (1) A prefix often used to indicate a recombinant PLASMID (e.g. pBR322 or any of a large number of commercial vectors such as pBluescript®).

(2) An indicator of the *short arm* of a CHROMOSOME; it is used when giving a particular location on a specific chromosome – e.g. 4p16, which refers to a location (16) on the short arm of chromosome 4.

(3) A prefix used to denote a particular polypeptide product of a retroviral gene.

P Proline (alternative to Pro).

P element Any of a range of transposable elements (up to ~3 kb) found in certain strains of *Drosophila*. Excision occurs at the flanking 31-bp inverted repeats, and an 8-bp duplication is created at the insertion site. Transposition occurs in germ line cells. P elements are used e.g. for mutagenesis.

P site (of a ribosome) The 'peptidyl' site at which the initiator tRNA binds during translation.

(cf. A SITE.)

P1 plasmid The circular (extrachromosomal) form of the prophage of PHAGE P1.

pIII protein See PHAGE DISPLAY.

p21 protein See RAS.

p53 A gene (in human chromosome 17p) whose product arrests the cell cycle and induces apoptosis following damage to DNA. Loss of *p53* activity leads to genetic instability and the survival of DNA-damaged cells. *p53* is a tumor-suppressor gene; it can e.g. inhibit oncogene-mediated transformation in cultured cells. (See also NUCLEOPHOSMIN.)

p53 is frequently mutated in (human) cancers; details of mutations in *p53* are saved in several databases (for example: www-p53.iarc.fr).

[Microarray-based assay for mutations in *p53*: BioTechniques (2005) 39(4):577–582 (578–580).]

p53 protein has a short half-life – and is often undetectable immunohistochemically. Mutation may extend the half-life, so that detection of p53 may indicate a mutant allele.

A scintillation proximity assay was used to assay binding between p53 and DNA [BioTechniques (2006) 41(3):303–308].

P210 protein See ABL.

PACE PCR-assisted contig extension. Following SHOTGUN SEQUENCING and the construction of clone contigs, PACE is used for closing *gaps* (i.e. regions in the genome for which no cloned fragments of DNA are available). Essentially, PCR is used (with genomic DNA) to amplify a sequence that extends from near the end of a contig into the (unknown) gap region. The outward-facing primers bind specifically to the known region near the end of the contig. The inward-facing primers have arbitrary sequences. In some cases an arbitrary primer will bind (with mis-matches) to a sequence within the unknown region at an amplifiable distance from the specific primer; the products formed can be sequenced, thus extending the known region outwards from the end of the contig.

PACE 2C A PROBE-based test (Gen-Probe, San Diego CA) for detecting the bacterial pathogens *Chlamydia trachomatis* and *Neisseria gonorrhoeae* in clinical samples in a single assay; the probe includes sequences specific to each of these organisms, the target sequences being in rRNA. Hybridization of the probe to target(s) is indicated by a hybridization protection assay (see entry ACCUPROBE for details).

A positive PACE 2C screening test can be followed by separate tests for *C. trachomatis* and *N. gonorrhoeae*. This is a particularly useful approach because co-infection with both pathogens is quite common.

This is an example of a *combination probe test*.

packaging (of phage DNA) Insertion of genomic DNA into the phage capsid, and the formation of an infective phage virion: a process that differs in different phages and which, in some cases, is not fully understood.

In phage lambda (λ), genome-length pieces of DNA are cut from a concatemer formed by rolling circle replication. Cuts occur at the regularly repeated *cos* sites in the concatemer; a terminal *cos* site locates in the phage capsid, and DNA is fed into the capsid until the next *cos* site – when cleavage occurs. Thus, a capsid contains the DNA between two consecutive *cos* sites, and the packaged genome has terminal sticky ends.

Commercial products are available for packing the phage λ genome: see e.g. GIGAPACK.

In phage φ29, packaging is dependent on energy from ATP hydrolysis. Moreover, the mechanism of insertion involves a 'motor' which contains various phage-encoded products: (i) a *connector* (consisting of 12 subunits) with a central channel, (ii) six molecules of RNA (which are designated pRNA), and (iii) a protein (gp16) whose copy number is not known. The motor may wind DNA into the capsid rather like a bolt drawn through a rotating nut. Two models for the packaging system in phage φ29 have been suggested. In one model the pRNA molecules are attached to the capsid, forming part of the *stator*; in another model a pRNA–connector complex forms the *rotor*. Studies using photoaffinity cross-linking indicate that pRNA molecules bind to the N-terminal amino acids of proteins in the connector [Nucleic Acids Res (2005) 33(8): 2640–2649].

packaging plasmid A plasmid encoding certain component(s) of a virion (e.g. capsid proteins) which is co-transfected into cells of a 'producer cell line' together with a plasmid that encodes (i) a replication-deficient part of a viral genome and (ii) the gene/fragment of interest. The (replication-deficient) viral particles produced in these cells are used to infect *target* cells, within which the gene of interest can be expressed.

Packaging plasmids are used e.g. in certain vector systems: see e.g. the lentiviral vector in entry GATEWAY SITE-SPECIFIC RECOMBINATION SYSTEM (table).

(See also AAV HELPER-FREE SYSTEM.)

pactamycin An antibiotic which inhibits the initiation stage of translation in protein synthesis.

PADAC A violet-colored reagent (a cephalosporin derivative) which forms a yellow product when hydrolyzed e.g. by a β-lactamase.

pAd/CMV/V5-DEST™ vector A destination vector in the GATEWAY SITE-SPECIFIC RECOMBINATION SYSTEM.

padlock probe A linear ssDNA PROBE in which the two *end* sections are complementary to *adjacent regions* of the target sequence; when bound to the target, the two end sections of the probe are therefore juxtaposed and can be ligated – thus circularizing the probe. Ligation is possible only if there is appropriate probe–target complementarity. Non-circularized probes can be eliminated by exonucleases. Padlock probes can be used e.g. to detect small variations in target sequences.

The central region of each padlock probe may include a unique identification sequence (the *ZipCode* or *zipcode*); all probes with the same target specificity have the same zipcode (and different zipcodes are found on probes with different target specificities). Universal primer-binding sites (that are the same on all the probes, regardless of zipcode) permit the (circularized) probes to be amplified; target-specific products can then be detected by a MICROARRAY of probes consisting of sequences complementary to the zipcode sequences.

This method has been used e.g. for simultaneous detection of multiple plant pathogens [Nucleic Acids Res (2005) 33(8): e70].

Padlock probes have also been used for the rapid and sensitive detection of the SARS virus in clinical samples [J Clin Microbiol (2005) 43(5):2339–2344].

(See also ZIPCODE ARRAY.)

painting (chromosome) See CHROMOSOME PAINTING.

palifermin See Kepivance® in BIOPHARMACEUTICAL (table).

palindromic sequence In a double-stranded nucleic acid molecule, a pair of INVERTED REPEAT sequences such as:

$$5'.....CCATCGATGG.....3'$$
$$3'.....GGTAGCTACC.....5'$$

This region has twofold rotational symmetry; if a sequence of nucleotides separates the two inverted repeats, the region is said to have hyphenated dyad symmetry.

A palindromic sequence can exist as a linear molecule (as shown) or as a *cruciform* (cross-like) structure in which each strand forms a *hairpin* by intrastrand base-pairing.

Palindromic sequences are commonly present in various sites associated with protein–DNA binding – including e.g. operators and recognition sequences of certain RESTRICTION ENDONUCLEASES.

palindromic unit *Syn.* REP SEQUENCE.

Pan B Dynabeads See DYNABEADS.

Pan T Dynabeads See DYNABEADS.

Pandoraea apista See ERIC-PCR in the entry REP-PCR.

panning (biopanning) See PHAGE DISPLAY.

PAP PYROPHOSPHOROLYSIS-ACTIVATED POLYMERIZATION.

papillomaviruses A category of small (~55 nm), icosahedral, non-enveloped viruses (genome: ccc dsDNA) which infect epithelial cells. More than 100 types of human papillomavirus (HPV) have been identified; of these, some (e.g. HPV6) are considered low-risk (they give rise e.g. to warts) while others (such as HPV16 and HPV18) are considered high-risk because they can cause e.g. cervical cancer. These viruses (unlike the POLYOMAVIRUSES) are refractory to propagation in cultured cells. Vaccines against HPVs have been made e.g. by using virus-like particles (see VLP) composed of the major (immunogenic) capsid protein.

paramere See MACRONUCLEUS.

paranemic Refers to an unstable juxtaposition of two strands of DNA in which the strands are not wound around each other.

(cf. PLECTONEMIC.)

parC See R1 PLASMID.

parD **system** In the R1 PLASMID: a system promoting stability of COPY NUMBER. The Kid protein is a nuclease which was believed to act solely by cleaving host-encoded mRNAs in plasmid-free cells – the (plasmid-encoded) Kis protein acting as an antidote to Kid. More recently, Kid has been reported to cleave both host mRNAs *and* a plasmid mRNA (encoding a repressor of plasmid replication) in plasmid-containing cells when the copy number falls [EMBO J (2005) 24(19):3459–3469].

parenteral administration Administered by a non-oral route.

ParR See R1 PLASMID.

partial fill-in See e.g. LAMBDA FIX II VECTOR.

particle gun *Syn.* GENE GUN.

partition (of plasmids) (syn. segregation) See PLASMID.

partitioning complex See R1 PLASMID.

partner gene See GENE FUSION and GENE FUSION VECTOR.

PathDetect® systems Reporter systems (Stratagene, La Jolla CA) used for investigating the regulatory function of a given, intracellularly expressed, gene product, or of an extracellular stimulus (e.g. a cytokine), on SIGNAL TRANSDUCTION PATHWAY(s) within mammalian cells.

There are two forms of PathDetect® system. (i) The *cis*-reporting systems can be used e.g. to determine the ability of a given (intracellularly expressed) gene product to activate a signal transduction pathway, causing a factor (such as NFκB or p53) to bind to a sequence upstream of the promoter of a reporter gene – thus promoting transcription of that gene. (ii) The *trans*-reporting systems are used e.g. to determine the ability of a given (intracellularly expressed) gene product to activate – directly or indirectly – one of certain *specific* transcription factors (such as CREB or ELK-1).

In the *cis*-reporting system, a plasmid containing the gene of interest is co-transfected into mammalian cells with a plasmid containing the *cis*-reporter gene and a regulatory region. The *cis*-reporter plasmid contains (i) a reporter gene – either a gene encoding LUCIFERASE or a gene encoding the (low-toxicity) variant of green fluorescent protein: the humanized *Renilla* GFP (see HRGFP); (ii) a promoter sequence for the reporter gene; and (iii) upstream of the promoter region, tandem repeats of a particular binding sequence (referred to as the binding element or response element). Various *cis*–reporter plasmids are available, each plasmid with a different response element; thus, for example, one type of *cis*-reporter plasmid contains a response element consisting of 5 tandem repeats of the binding site of NFκB, while another contains a response element consisting of 15 tandem repeats of the binding site of p53. (A response element of choice can be inserted into a plasmid supplied with a multiple cloning site.) If the expressed protein of interest activates a signal transduction pathway which then releases (for example) the active form of NFκB, the NFκB binds to the response element and promotes expression of the reporter gene.

The *trans*-reporting system includes a reporter plasmid and a *trans*-activator plasmid – both of which are co-transfected into cells with the expression vector encoding the protein of interest. (There are also positive and negative control plasmids.)

The reporter plasmid of the *trans*-reporting system includes (i) a reporter gene encoding e.g. luciferase or β-galactosidase; (ii) a promoter region; and (iii) upstream of the promoter, a fivefold tandem repeat of a sequence which binds the GAL4 element.

The *trans*-activator plasmid of the *trans*-reporting system includes a sequence encoding a fusion protein: GAL4 fused to a transcription factor (e.g. CREB or Elk-1); transcription of this plasmid is mediated by a CMV promoter.

If the expressed protein of interest causes phosphorylation, directly or indirectly, of the *activation domain* of the fusion protein (i.e. the fusion partner of GAL4), then the activated GAL4 fusion protein binds to the tandem repeat binding site for GAL4 on the reporter plasmid, thus promoting expression of the reporter gene.

[Example of use of PathDetect®: J Neurochem (2006) 96 (1):65–77.]

pathogenicity island (PAI) In a microbial (usually bacterial) genome: a cluster of several to many genes encoding specific determinants of pathogenicity/virulence.

Commonly, the GC% of a PAI is different from that of the organism's chromosome; this has been taken to indicate that, in general, PAIs were acquired by horizontal gene transfer, i.e. by a process such as conjugation.

Many PAIs are flanked by DIRECT REPEATS; the LEE PAI (see below) is one example of an exception. In *Moraxella bovis* (hemolytic strains) the *mbx* operon was found to be flanked by ~700-bp imperfect repeats – which, together with e.g. the GC% of *mbx* genes, suggested that this region of the genome is a PAI [J Med Microbiol (2006) 55:443–449].

[PAIs in evolution: BMC Evol Biol (2007) 7(suppl 1) S8; in *Francisella*: BMC Microbiol (2007) 7:1.]

The PAI designated LEE (*locus of enterocyte effacement*) is a 35-kb element found e.g. in all strains of enteropathogenic *Escherichia coli* (EPEC). Genes in the LEE PAI encode a so-called type III secretory system which apparently enables strains of EPEC to translocate effector proteins directly into (eukaryotic) target cells. [Type III systems and PAIs: J Med

Microbiol (2001) 50:116–126.] Proteins encoded by the LEE PAI are responsible for the typical 'attaching and effacing' lesions produced by this pathogen on intestinal epithelium. Transcription of at least some of the LEE genes is controlled from a regulatory region in the EAF plasmid (EAF = EPEC adherence factor) which occurs in all strains of EPEC.

The chromosomal site occupied by LEE is occupied by a different PAI in strains of UPEC (uropathogenic *E. coli*); the products of this 70-kb PAI include a hemolysin.

A number of distinct PAIs occur in *Salmonella* spp. One of them, SPI-1, contains the *inv–spa* genes which encode a type III secretory system involved in the invasion of intestinal epithelial cells. The PAI SPI-3 encodes the means of survival in macrophages.

In the gastric pathogen *Helicobacter pylori*, expression of the *cagA* gene (in the *cag* PAI), and the unlinked gene *vacA*, is linked to severe gastrointestinal disease. Apparently, CagA is injected into gastroepithelial cells by *H. pylori* and causes e.g. proliferation of these cells. VacA is a secreted cytotoxin (95 kDa) which, *in vitro*, blocks proliferation/activity of T cells.

The VPI pathogenicity island in *Vibrio cholerae* encodes e.g. cell-surface appendages (the so-called 'toxin co-regulated pili' – TCP) which function as receptors for phage CTXΦ – the phage whose genome encodes cholera toxin.

Certain strains of the Gram-positive pathogen *Staphylococcus aureus* contain a PAI which encodes the toxic shock syndrome toxin.

paucibacillary specimen Any specimen that contains a small number of target bacteria per unit volume. For example, a specimen may contain fewer than ~10^4 colony-forming units (cfu) per mL; such specimens usually permit detection of the target organism by culture, but nucleic-acid-based tests – which use a much smaller volume of the sample – may fail to detect the organism. Improved detection by a nucleic-acid-based test may be achieved if it is preceded by some form of concentration (such as immunomagnetic separation).

PAXgene™ blood RNA kit A product (from PreAnalytiX Hombrechtikon, Switzerland) used for the isolation of RNA from whole blood. The system was designed to avoid the problem of instability of the RNA profile *in vitro* (i.e. following collection of blood samples): during collection, storage and transport of blood – at ambient temperatures – the copy number of a given RNA species may change significantly owing to (i) degradation of the RNA, and/or (ii) the ongoing expression of genes following collection of the sample from the patient.

This approach involves collecting the blood in specialized tubes containing a mixture of reagents that stabilize the RNA profile by (i) protecting RNA from degradation by RNases and (ii) inhibiting gene expression.

Briefly, the method is as follows. The specialized collecting tube, containing sample, is centrifuged to pellet nucleic acids. The washed pellet is resuspended in buffers with the enzyme proteinase K and incubated. Following centrifugation, supernatant is transferred to a fresh tube and ethanol is added. Subsequently the supernatant is added to a PAXgene spin column for abstraction of the RNA. Following several washing steps with buffers the RNA is eluted.

The procedure generally removes most of the DNA. For a more rigorous elimination of DNA it is possible to include DNase treatment in the protocol.

Examples of use of the PAXgene™ system: studies on the time course of proinflammatory/immunomodulatory cytokine mRNAs [Infect Immun (2006) 74(7):4172–4179]; studies on expression of genes encoding e.g. the glucocorticoid receptor in children with asthma [Proc Natl Acad Sci USA (2006) 103(14):5496–5501].

(See also NUCLEIC ACID ISOLATION.)

pBAD-DEST49 vector A destination vector in the GATEWAY SITE-SPECIFIC RECOMBINATION SYSTEM.

pBLOCK-iT™3-DEST vector See table in the entry GATEWAY SITE-SPECIFIC RECOMBINATION SYSTEM.

pBluescript® Any of a set of ~3-kb PHAGEMIDS (marketed by Stratagene, La Jolla CA). Derived from plasmid pUC19, the phagemids contain: (i) the replication origin from plasmid ColE1, (ii) the replication origin from bacteriophage f1, (iii) an ampicillin-resistance gene, (iv) a sequence that encodes α-PEPTIDE (part of the *lacZ* gene), (v) the *lac* promoter, and (vi) a POLYLINKER, situated between the *lac* promoter and the α-peptide sequence. The polylinker is flanked by promoter sites for T3 and T7 RNA polymerases (allowing transcription of an insert in either direction).

The f1 origin can be inserted in either orientation – so that either the sense or antisense strand can be amplified if the host cell contains a helper phage.

These vectors can be replicated in strains of *Escherichia coli* (e.g. JM105 or JM109) which contain a chromosomal *lacZΔM15* mutation that deletes part of the N-terminal region of the enzyme β-galactosidase. Such bacteria produce inactive β-galactosidase – but *if* the (phagemid-encoded) α-peptide is synthesized it complements the mutant enzyme, by non-covalent binding, to form an active β-galactosidase; the presence of the functional enzyme can be determined e.g. by growing the bacteria on plates containing X-GAL – bacteria containing a functional enzyme form *blue* colonies.

If the phagemid contains a gene/fragment (inserted in the polylinker), the α-peptide cannot be formed and the cells will therefore lack a functional β-galactosidase; these cells form colorless (*white*) colonies on X-gal media. Hence, a colony's appearance indicates whether or not the (intracellular) phagemids are *recombinant*, that is, whether or not they contain an insert; this is *blue–white screening*. (See also BLACK–WHITE SCREENING.)

PBMCs Peripheral blood mononuclear cells.

PBP 2a (PBP 2′) See MECA GENE.

PBPs Penicillin-binding proteins: see β-LACTAM ANTIBIOTICS.

pBR322 A recombinant PLASMID (~4360 bp) constructed from several naturally occurring plasmids. Small plasmids like this are useful as VECTORS in genetic engineering; they are taken up by TRANSFORMATION more efficiently (as compared with larger plasmids) and they are also less susceptible to damage during manipulation.

pCAL vectors A set of vectors used in the AFFINITY PROTEIN EXPRESSION AND PURIFICATION system.

pcDNA™6.2/nLumio™-DEST™ A destination vector in the GATEWAY SITE-SPECIFIC RECOMBINATION SYSTEM.

***pcnB* mutant** (in *Escherichia coli*) See MULTICOPY PLASMID.

PCR Polymerase chain reaction: primarily a method for copying (amplifying) specific sequences (<100 to >1000 nucleotides) in DNA (or in RNA: REVERSE TRANSCRIPTASE PCR); millions of copies are produced within a few hours.

[The development of miniaturized on-chip PCR (review): Nucleic Acids Res (2007) 35(13) 4223–4237.]

Patents on PCR are held by Hoffmann–La Roche.

Essentially, PCR depends on the ability of a *thermostable* DNA polymerase to extend a PRIMER – bound to its target sequence (the AMPLICON) – and to do this, repeatedly, in a process involving temperature cycling: see the accompanying figure. (The use of a thermostable DNA polymerase avoids the need to add fresh polymerase to the reaction mixture after each high-temperature stage to replace the heat-inactivated enzyme.) See notes on temperature cycling (below) and also the entry THERMOCYCLER.

Alternative methods for amplifying nucleic acids include the LIGASE CHAIN REACTION (LCR) – which also involves temperature cycling. Other methods, e.g. NASBA and SDA, are conducted *isothermally*, i.e. they do not involve temperature cycling.

Volume of sample, choice of enzyme

PCR is often carried out in a total volume of approx. 25–50 μL, although smaller volumes have been used.

The choice of enzyme (i.e. DNA polymerase) depends on specific requirements; a wide range of thermostable enzymes is available from commercial sources. For example, some DNA polymerases are designed to amplify 'difficult' target sequences (e.g. GC-rich sequences: see e.g. ACCUPRIME GC-RICH DNA POLYMERASE); others are designed specifically to introduce errors into the products (in studies on mutagenesis) (see e.g. GENEMORPH).

The TAQ DNA POLYMERASE is used when the products are required for TOPOISOMERASE I CLONING.

Temperature cycling

As indicated in the figure (legend), temperature cycling often follows the pattern:

$$\rightarrow 95°C \rightarrow 45–65°C \rightarrow 72°C \rightarrow 95°C \rightarrow$$

These temperatures are designed for the cyclical repetition of (i) strand separation (denaturation of the sample dsDNA), (ii) binding (*annealing*) of primers, on opposite strands, at sites which bracket the amplicon, and (iii) extension (synthesis of DNA from the 3′ terminus of each primer) to form products – i.e. amplicons. Following the synthesis of amplicons, a rise in temperature separates the amplicons from their templates.

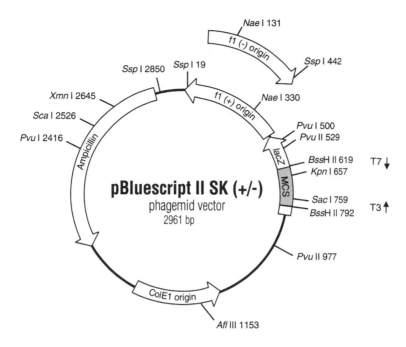

pBluescript II SK (+/−)
phagemid vector
2961 bp

Nae I 131
f1 (−) origin
Ssp I 442
Nae I 330
Pvu I 500
Pvu II 529
BssH II 619
Kpn I 657
Sac I 759
BssH II 792
Pvu II 977
Afl III 1153
ColE1 origin
Ampicillin
Pvu I 2416
Sca I 2526
Xmn I 2645
Ssp I 2850
Ssp I 19
f1 (+) origin
lacZ
MCS
T7
T3

pBluescript® II SK (+/−) PHAGEMID VECTOR One of a range of phagemid vectors in the pBluescript® series. SK indicates that the orientation of the polylinker is such that transcription of *lacZ* proceeds in the direction SacI to KpnI.

A vector containing the f1(+) origin (the origin of replication of the filamentous phage f1) permits recovery of the sense strand of the *lacZ* gene when a strain containing the pBluescript® vector is co-infected with a helper phage. The f1(−) origin permits recovery of the anti-sense strand of the *lacZ* gene.

The ColE1 origin of replication can be used in the absence of a helper phage.

The inclusion of a portion of the *lacZ* gene permits the identification of recombinant phagemids by the blue–white selection procedure (see entry for details).

Courtesy of Stratagene, La Jolla CA, USA.

Although the temperatures for denaturation and extension are usually ~94/95°C and ~72°C, respectively, the annealing temperatures reported in the literature vary significantly. One reason is that GC%-rich primers require higher annealing temperatures in order to avoid 'mispriming' – i.e. binding of primers to inappropriate (i.e. non-complementary) sequences in the template strand. (Mispriming leads to the formation of spurious products.) Optimization of the annealing temperature may be achieved e.g. by TOUCHDOWN PCR.

A different approach to avoiding mispriming is HOT-START PCR.

In some cases, depending e.g. on the primers involved, a *two-temperature protocol* has been used – e.g. 94°C for the denaturation stage and a combined annealing/extension temp-

erature of 68°C.

Theoretically, temperature cycling could be carried out by manual control, but in routine laboratory conditions it is conducted in an instrument called a THERMOCYCLER (q.v.).

Stringency

The physicochemical conditions (e.g. temperature, electrolyte concentrations) under which the primers hybridize to their respective sites on the template strands affect the accuracy (specificity) of the polymerase chain reaction. For example, if a primer is allowed to hybridize with a template strand at a temperature which is too low, binding may occur aberrantly at a site which is not complementary to the primer's sequence (and which may be outside the amplicon); thus, extension of the 3′ end of the primer may give rise to a product which is

(a)   amplicon

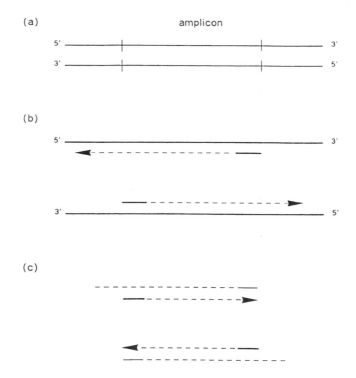

PCR (polymerase chain reaction): the basic method (principle, diagrammatic).

The reaction mixture includes: (i) The sample of (double-stranded) DNA – which may be, for example, genomic DNA or fragments of genomic DNA; (ii) millions of copies of the two types of primer, each primer being about 20–30 nucleotides in length; (iii) a thermostable DNA polymerase (e.g. the *Taq* DNA polymerase); (iv) deoxyribonuleoside triphosphates of all four types (ATP, CTP, GTP, TTP); and (v) appropriate buffer.

For PCR, the reaction mixture undergoes a cyclical series of changes in temperature, such changes being controlled automatically in an instrument called a *thermocycler*. The cycle is repeated about 20–40 times, amplification of the target sequence occurring at each cycle.

(a) Part of the sample double-stranded DNA: two antiparallel strands held together by base-pairing. The sequence to be amplified – the *amplicon* – is shown between the short vertical bars.

(b) Initial heating to about 95°C has separated the two strands of DNA. Subsequently, transient cooling to about 45–65°C has allowed the primers – shown as short, solid lines – to bind (*anneal*) to their complementary sites on the two template strands. Importantly, notice the positions of the bound primers in relation to the two ends of the amplicon. The temperature is then increased to e.g. 72°C, and DNA synthesis (mediated by the thermostable DNA polymerase, and shown here as a dashed line with an arrowhead) proceeds from the 3′ end of each primer. Each of these newly synthesized strands is longer than the amplicon.

(c) The second round of replication begins with initial heating to ~95°C – separating the new daughter strands (synthesized in the first round of replication) from their templates. Each of the new daughter strands (as well as the two parent strands) can act as a template in the next round of replication. In the diagram, a primer (short, sold line) has bound to each new daughter strand and has been extended (dashed line with arrowhead). Note that the strand synthesized on a new daughter strand is the same length as the amplicon; such strands rapidly become dominant in subsequent rounds of replication.

Reproduced from Figure 4.1 on page 57 of *DNA Methods in Clinical Microbiology* [ISBN 07923-6307-8], Paul Singleton (2000), with the kind permission of Springer Science and Business Media.

PCR (polymerase chain reaction): some of the many variant forms and their uses (see separate entries for each variant form)

Variant form	Uses (e.g.)
Allele-specific PCR	Amplification of a *particular* allele of a given gene (in the presence of other alleles of that gene)
Anchored PCR	Amplification of an unknown sequence flanking a known sequence
Asymmetric PCR	Preparation of probes and the preparation of ssDNA e.g. for sequencing
Bubble-linker PCR	See Vectorette PCR (below)
Competitive RT-PCR	Estimation of the number of RNA target sequences in a given sample
Headloop suppression PCR	Protocol arranged to promote suppression of amplification of sequences *related to* the given target sequence (without affecting the amplification of the intended target sequence)
Hot-start PCR	Cycling delayed until the temperature of the reaction mixture is sufficient to inhibit non-specific binding of the primers. The object is to increase the specificity and the sensitivity of the assay
IAN-PCR	Inverse affinity nested PCR: a modification of inverse PCR used for the recovery of flanking sequences from low-copy-number fragments: see entry METAGENOME
Immuno-PCR	Ultrasensitive detection of antigen; the antigen-binding antibody is linked to a DNA fragment containing a sequence which is amplified by PCR; the amplicons (visualized by gel electrophoresis) provide an indication of the presence of specific antigen
Inverse PCR	Amplification of a sequence that *flanks* a known sequence
Island rescue PCR	Amplification of CpG islands in cloned fragments
LMPCR	Amplification of fragments produced in an *in vivo* footprinting assay (see entry LIGATION-MEDIATED PCR)
Methylation-specific PCR	Monitoring methylation status of CpG islands in genomic DNA
Quantitative PCR (QPCR)	Absolute or relative quantitation of DNA or RNA target sequences (see entry QUANTITATIVE PCR)
Real-time PCR	Determination of the number of specific target sequences in the reaction mixture prior to cycling
Relative RT-PCR	Comparison of the numbers of RNA targets, e.g. transcripts of a given gene, in samples from different cells/tissues etc.
Sexual PCR	See entry DNA SHUFFLING.
Splice overlap extension PCR	Fusion of two sequences of DNA (present either on the same molecule or on separate molecules) without the use of restriction enzymes
Terminal transferase-dependent PCR	Detection of the presence of any obstruction or barrier to DNA polymerase during replication
Touchdown PCR	A protocol designed to optimize stringency and specificity of the assay by avoiding mispriming at the annealing stage
Vectorette (bubble-linker) PCR	Amplification of an unknown sequence adjacent to a known sequence

not the one required. Hence, such *low-stringency* conditions are not generally used – although they are used e.g. for the initial phase of AP-PCR (q.v.).

Normally, PCR uses *high-stringency* conditions (which are dictated primarily by temperature). Under such conditions the binding (annealing) of primers to the target DNA occurs only when they are exactly complementary, or very nearly so, to their appropriate binding sites; thus, the higher the stringency the greater will be the degree of matching required between primer and target sequence for successful binding and, hence, extension, to occur.

Multiplex PCR

With appropriate experimental arrangements, more than one target sequence can be amplified in a single reaction: see the entry MULTIPLEX PCR.

Contamination by extraneous DNA

Extraneous DNA that contaminates a reaction mixture may contain (i) sequence(s) to which the primers can bind, and/or (ii) sequence(s) that are able to prime irrelevant sites in the sample DNA. In either event, unwanted sequences may be amplified, resulting in a troublesome mixture of products; in addition, the efficiency of the legitimate amplification may be reduced owing to sequestration of polymerase and nucleotides.

Successful PCR needs rigorous exclusion of contaminating DNA – which may be derived from the environment and/or from the apparatus and reagents.

An important source of contaminating DNA consists of the amplicons from previous reactions in the same laboratory.

There are two basic approaches to this problem: AMPLICON CONTAINMENT and AMPLICON INACTIVATION (q.v.).

Inhibitors of PCR

In some cases the sample DNA is derived from a source that may include substance(s) inhibitory to PCR; this may give rise to a false-negative result from a sample which, in fact, contains the sequence of interest.

Inhibitors of PCR are found e.g. in various types of clinical specimen – including bone marrow aspirates, CSF (cerebrospinal fluid), feces and urine; specific inhibitory substances include hemoglobin (in red blood cells), lactoferrin (in white blood cells) and various polysaccharides (in feces).

Other inhibitors include AGAR, hemin, and the blood anticoagulants heparin and sodium polyanetholesulfonate (SPS).

Detection of inhibitors can be approached in several ways. For example, if an aliquot of the sample is 'spiked' with the target DNA, prior to assay, then failure to amplify the target in this aliquot may suggest the presence of inhibitor(s). This technique, however, increases the risk of contamination.

Alternatively, an internal control can consist of molecules of nucleic acid which (i) include binding sites for the target-specific primers, but which (ii) can be distinguished from the actual target by a unique PROBE-binding sequence. In the absence of inhibitors the control and target sequences should both be amplified; failure to obtain any amplification could indicate the presence of inhibitor(s), while amplification of the control sequence (only) would suggest the absence of the target sequence in the sample DNA.

The effects of an inhibitor may be reduced by diluting the sample, but this concomitantly reduces the number of copies of the target sequence (if present) and may therefore lower the sensitivity of the assay. An alternative approach uses a magnetic separation technique (see e.g. DYNABEADS): copies of the target sequence are captured, and held, on magnetic beads while any inhibitory substances are removed by washing.

Facilitators of PCR

Certain agents can enhance the efficiency of a PCR assay in the presence of inhibitory substances. These agents include bovine serum albumin (BSA) and betaine; for example, BSA has been reported to improve the performance of PCR in assays on fecal specimens (which characteristically contain a range of inhibitory substances). Some of these facilitators are effective against a variety of inhibitors, while others are more selective in their activity.

It was reported that the accuracy of PCR may be promoted by the presence of the RecA protein.

PCR with damaged/ancient DNA

The amplification of poor-quality DNA, for forensic or other purposes, may be facilitated by the use of DNA polymerases of the so-called Y FAMILY (q.v.). Minute quantities of DNA may be recovered e.g. by CHARGESWITCH TECHNOLOGY.

Detection of PCR products

Given that the products of PCR (amplicons) are of a *precise* length, i.e. an exact number of nucleotides delimited by the primer pair, they can be readily detected and identified by gel electrophoresis. Thus, a given product forms a single band at a precise location in the gel; the size of the product forming such a band can be verified by using a so-called DNA ladder (see entry GEL ELECTROPHORESIS). Bands of fragments in a gel may be further examined e.g. by SOUTHERN BLOTTING followed by hybridization of a target-specific, labeled PROBE.

To verify that an amplicon of a specific size and sequence has been amplified, the amplicons can be subjected to a particular RESTRICTION ENDONUCLEASE directed at a known cutting site in the amplicon; the products of restriction can then be checked by gel electrophoresis to see whether fragments of the *expected* sizes were produced.

Gel electrophoresis is a slow process. Hence, in some cases use is made of instrumentation that permits monitoring of the amplification (i.e. increase in amplicons) *during* the reaction: so-called *real-time PCR*.

Real-time PCR

Real-time detection of PCR products can be achieved with a dye-based approach, a PROBE-based approach, or a combined probe-and-dye-based approach: see the entry REAL-TIME PCR.

Quantitative PCR

PCR can be used to give an estimate of the number of copies of the target sequence which were present in the sample *prior to* amplification: see QUANTITATIVE PCR.

Some modified protocols

The flexibility of PCR can be illustrated by some examples:

- ALLELE-SPECIFIC PCR: use of an allele-specific primer (and a gene-specific primer) to amplify a particular allele among a mixture of alleles.

- ASYMMETRIC PCR: a procedure in which the concentration of one primer is much lower than that of the other; it is used for obtaining a particular strand of the template dsDNA.

- DNA SHUFFLING: a primer-less form of PCR in which fragments of DNA, in the reaction mixture, prime each other; this technique is used to promote *in vitro* recombination and the development of a product with new properties.

● EXSITE SITE-DIRECTED MUTAGENESIS KIT: a commercial system in which mutations (including point mutations, additions or deletions) can be introduced into plasmids by using appropriately designed primers in PCR.

● GENEMORPH: a commercial system in which an error-prone DNA polymerase is used for promoting mutagenesis in the amplicons.

● HEADLOOP SUPPRESSION PCR: use of modified primers that selectively suppress amplification of unwanted sequence(s) without affecting amplification of the wanted sequence.

● IMMUNO-PCR: a technique used for ultrasensitive detection of antigens.

● INVERSE PCR: used e.g. for amplifying DNA which *flanks* a known region, and for the preparation of deletion mutations.

● ISLAND RESCUE PCR: used e.g. for amplifying CpG islands from inserts in yeast artificial chromosomes.

● LIGATION-MEDIATED PCR: a procedure used for analyzing the products obtained from an *in vivo* footprinting assay.

● MEGAPRIMER MUTAGENESIS: a technique for site-directed mutagenesis.

● MULTIPLEX PCR: amplification (simultaneously, in a single assay) of more than one target sequence.

● PCR CLAMPING: use of a PNA probe to favor amplification of a given sequence by blocking amplification of other sequence(s).

● SELECTOR-BASED MULTIPLEX PCR: a procedure in which a number of different target sequences can be amplified with a single pair of primers (cf. conventional MULTIPLEX PCR).

● SOLID-PHASE PCR (on-chip PCR): the extension of primers on immobilized target sequences.

● SPLICE OVERLAP EXTENSION PCR: a procedure which can be used to fuse two sequences of DNA (either on the same molecule or on different molecules) without using restriction endonuleases.

● SUICIDE POLYMERASE ENDONUCLEASE RESTRICTION: a procedure for enhancing amplification of a low-copy-number template (in the presence of so-called dominant templates) – an alternative to PCR clamping.

● TERMINAL TRANSFERASE-DEPENDENT PCR: a procedure used for detecting an obstruction or barrier (in a sample of dsDNA) which may inhibit the activity of DNA polymerase during replication.

● VECTORETTE PCR: a modified form of ANCHORED PCR – involving a dsDNA linker with a central mismatched region – used for copying an unknown sequence adjacent to a known sequence.

PCR-assisted contig extension See PACE.

PCR clamping In a PCR reaction: an arrangement by which the amplification of one or more specific sequences is facilitated by concomitant blocking of amplification of other specific sequence(s). PCR clamping has a range of uses, one of which is the detection of rare (low-copy-number) mutant templates in the presence of a great excess of the corresponding wild-type templates; in such cases, without clamping, a dominant

template may preclude detection, or reduce the possibility of detecting, minority template(s) e.g. by the early depletion of reagents.

There are two main types of PCR clamping (see later), each of which involves the use of an oligomer of peptide nucleic acid (see PNA) as a clamp. The properties of PNA that make it particularly useful for this role are:

● duplexes formed from complementary strands of PNA and DNA have greater thermal stability than the corresponding DNA:DNA duplexes (the T_m of a PNA:DNA duplex is higher than that of the corresponding DNA:DNA duplex);

● a PNA:DNA duplex is destabilized (T_m significantly lower) by a single mismatch;

● a PNA oligomer, bound to its complementary sequence, is not extendable by any DNA polymerase and therefore cannot act as a primer.

Elongation arrest

This type of PCR clamping uses a PNA oligomer which is complementary to an internal (non-terminal) sequence in the amplicon. If the oligomer has a wild-type sequence it will hybridize strongly to its binding site in *wild-type* templates; accordingly, the wild-type templates will not be amplified because primer extension is blocked by the oligomer. Under these conditions, a *mutant* template (in which one or more mutant bases occur in the oligomer's binding site) will be amplified because the absence of a bound PNA oligomer will allow primer extension.

Primer exclusion (= competitive clamping)

In this type of PCR clamping one of the primers is targeted to a binding site that includes a particular (required) mutant sequence. If this sequence occurs in a given template then that template will be amplified (through extension of primers). If the PNA oligomer is complementary to the *wild-type version* of the primer's binding site it will block amplification of the wild-type templates but will not interfere with amplification of the mutant templates. With this scheme, point mutations at different sites in the amplicon sequence can be investigated by using primers with appropriate complementarity.

In one study, rare K-*ras* DNA was detected by a clamping procedure in which a fluorophore-labeled PNA oligomer acted as both the PCR clamp and sensor probe, the latter enabling detection of specific mutations by melting curve analyses [Nucleic Acids Res (2006) 34(2):e12].

An alternative approach to handling dominant templates is SUICIDE POLYMERASE ENDONUCLEASE RESTRICTION.

In an analogous context, dominant *RNA* templates may be dealt with e.g. by the use of COMPETIMERS.

PCR cloning See CLONING.

PCR-RFLP analysis A form of RFLP ANALYSIS in which the sample DNA is copied from genomic DNA (or from another source) by PCR. One advantage of this approach is that the amplicons (copies of the target sequence) differ from source DNA in being non-methylated; this absence of methylation permits cutting by those restriction enzymes that are inhibited by the methylation of bases in DNA isolated from cells. The

PCR-RFLP procedure is widely used e.g. for typing bacteria and for detecting mutations/polymorphisms.

PCR-ribotyping An alternative approach to the standard form of RIBOTYPING in which PCR is used to amplify the intergenic spacer region between the 16S rRNA gene and the 23S rRNA gene; one of the PCR primers is complementary to a conserved sequence in the 16S rRNA gene while the other is complementary to a conserved sequence in the gene for 23S rRNA. The amplicons are subjected to gel electrophoresis in order to generate a fingerprint.

PCR-SSCP See SSCP ANALYSIS.

pDONR™ See GATEWAY SITE-SPECIFIC RECOMBINATION SYSTEM.

PDR See DNA POLYMORPHISM DISCOVERY RESOURCE.

PEG See POLYETHYLENE GLYCOL.

PEGfilgrastim See Neulasta® in entry BIOPHARMACEUTICAL (table).

pegylated Refers to any *in vitro* construct prepared with polyethylene glycol (PEG). A molecule (e.g. an enzyme) may be conjugated to PEG in order e.g. to stabilize it.

PEI Polyethyleneimine. [Use in gene delivery: BioTechniques (2007) 42(3):285–288.] (See also MELITTIN.)

Peltier system See THERMOCYCLER.

penicillin Any of a class of β-LACTAM ANTIBIOTICS characterized by a thiazolidine ring fused to the β-lactam ring. As in all β-lactam antibiotics, the penicillins (which act only on *growing* cells) kill or inhibit bacteria by interfering with the function of the so-called *penicillin-binding proteins* (PBPs) – proteins which have enzymic roles in the synthesis of the cell wall polymer peptidoglycan (present in both Gram-positive and Gram-negative species); cells *lyse* when they are killed by penicillins (cf. STREPTOZOTOCIN).

Some penicillins, e.g. penicillin G (= benzylpenicillin), are active primarily, or solely, against Gram-positive bacteria as they cannot penetrate the outer membrane of Gram-negative species; others (e.g. ampicillin, amoxycillin and carbenicillin) have activity against both Gram-negative and Gram-positive species.

Penicillins (and cephalosporins) are synthesized by fungi; they include semi-synthetic antibiotics such as AMPICILLIN, cloxacillin, flucloxacillin, METHICILLIN and oxacillin.

Some of the other β-lactams (e.g. carbapenems and monobactams) are produced by bacteria.

In some cases, bacteria are resistant to penicillins because they produce enzymes (β-lactamases) capable of cleaving the β-lactam ring. Some bacteria contain the *mecA* gene which encodes a PBP that is resistant to the action of a number of β-lactam antibiotics.

penicillin-binding protein 2a See MECA GENE.

penicillin-binding proteins See β-LACTAM ANTIBIOTICS.

PEP Phosphoenolpyruvate.

(See also PTS.)

peplos (*virol.*) See CAPSID.

α-peptide The N-terminal 146 amino acid residues of β-galactosidase (an ezyme encoded by the *lacZ* gene in *Escherichia coli*). This peptide can complement a mutant (inactive) form of the enzyme that lacks part of the N-terminal region; that is, the α-peptide can associate (*non*-covalently) with the mutant enzyme to form an active enzyme. Such association is called *α-complementation* and is exploited in a method for selecting recombinant vectors (see e.g. PBLUESCRIPT).

(See also ENZYME FRAGMENT COMPLEMENTATION.)

peptide nucleic acid See PNA.

perfloxacin See QUINOLONE ANTIBIOTICS.

permeaplast A cell-wall-deficient cell obtained by treating a cyanobacterial cell with LYSOZYME and EDTA. Permeaplasts have been used e.g. for TRANSFORMATION in certain species.

permease See PTS.

pertussis toxin An exotoxin, formed by the Gram-negative bacterial pathogen *Bordetella pertussis*, which is a virulence factor in whooping cough (pertussis); the toxin has an AB_5 arrangement of subunits, i.e. a central A subunit surrounded by a pentameric ring of (heterogeneous) B subunits – the A subunit being to one side of the plane of the ring.

The A subunit of this toxin (~26 kDa) has ADP-ribosyltransferase activity (see ADP-RIBOSYLATION); within target cells it ADP-ribosylates the G_1 protein, thereby stimulating ADENYLATE CYCLASE and leading to an increase in the intracellular concentration of cyclic AMP (cAMP).

pESC vectors Plasmid vectors used e.g. for expression of eukaryotic genes within yeast cells (*Saccharomyces cerevisiae*); these vectors include sequences for EPITOPE TAGGING which facilitate detection/isolation of the expressed proteins.

Two different genes can be expressed in each vector (transcription occurring in opposite directions).

Four different yeast selective markers are available.

A series of pESC vectors marketed by Stratagene (La Jolla CA) contain sequences encoding FLAG and c-*myc* epitopes (used for tagging target proteins). These vectors also include GAL promoters and one of several selectable markers (see figure).

pESC vectors were used e.g. for investigations on gene regulation in yeast [Genetics (2006) 173(1):75–85] and on the suppression of viral RNA recombination by cellular exoribonuclease [J Virol (2006) 80(6):2631–2640].

Petri dish A round, shallow, flat-bottomed and vertically sided dish, made of plastic or glass, which has a flat, loosely-fitting lid.

A Petri dish is commonly about 10 cm in diameter.

(See also PLATE.)

Peutz–Jeghers syndrome (PJS) A rare autosomal dominant condition characterized by intestinal hamartomatous polyposis and pigmentation in the oro-facial region; complications include intestinal obstruction, and there is an increased risk of gastrointestinal malignancy.

Mutation in a coding region of the serine-threonine kinase gene *STK11/LKB1* (chromosomal location 19p13.3) appears to account for most – but not all – cases of PJS. A study of the promoter region of *STK11/LKB1* concluded that changes in the sequence in this region are unlikely to contribute to the

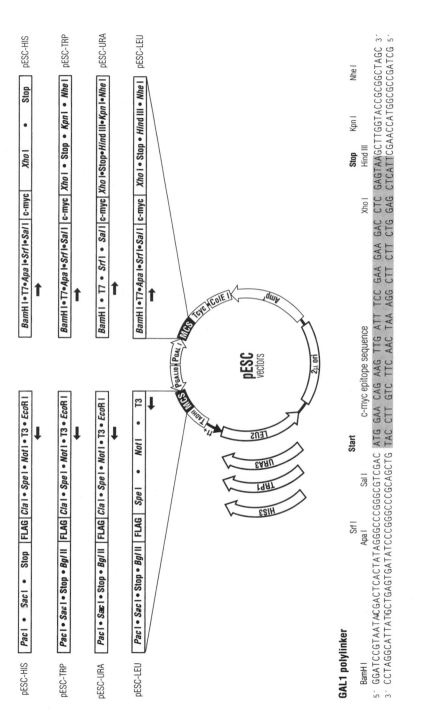

GAL1 polylinker

| | BamHI | | Apa I | Srf I | Sal I | | **Start** | c-myc epitope sequence |

5′ GGATCCGGTAATACGACTCACTATAGGGCCCGGGCGTCGAC ATG GAA CAG AAG TTG ATT TCC GAA GAC CTC GAGTAAGCTTGGTACCGGCTAGC 3′
3′ CCTAGGCCATTATGCTGAGTGATATCCCGGGCCCGCAGCTG TAC CTT GTC TTC AAC TAA AGG CTT CTG GAG CTCATTCGAACCATGGCCGATCG 5′

| | | | Xho I | **Stop** Hind III | Kpn I | Nhe I |

GAL10 polylinker

| EcoRI | Not I | Spe I | Cla I | | **Start** | FLAG epitope sequence |

5′ GAATTCAACCCTCACTAAAGGGCGGCCGCACTAGTATCG ATG GAT TAC AAG GAC GAC GAT AAG ATCTGAGCTCTTAATTAA 3′
3′ CTTAAGTTGGGAGTGATTTCCCGCCGGCGTGATCATAGC TAC CTA ATG TTC CTG CTG CTA TTC TAGACTGCAGAATTAATT 5′

| | | | Bgl II | **Stop** Sac I | Pac I |

pESC VECTORS A versatile system of vectors for expression of proteins in the yeast *Saccharomyces cerevisiae* (see entry for details). The polylinker (MCS) sequence downstream of each of the GAL promoters is shown at the bottom of the figure.

Courtesy of Stratagene, La Jolla CA, USA.

183

PJS syndrome [BMC Genomics (2005) 6:38].

pEXP-DEST vectors   See CELL-FREE PROTEIN SYNTHESIS.

pEXP3-DEST vector   A destination vector in the GATEWAY SITE-SPECIFIC RECOMBINATION SYSTEM.

(See also CELL-FREE PROTEIN SYNTHESIS.)

pEXP4-DEST vector   A destination vector in the GATEWAY SITE-SPECIFIC RECOMBINATION SYSTEM.

pFastBac™ dual vector kit   A kit (Invitrogen, Carlsbad CA) containing a vector (pFastBac™ Dual, 5.2 kb) for use in the BAC-TO-BAC expression system; the pFastBac vector contains two promoters (polyhedrin and p10), in opposite orientations (and with appropriate polylinkers), allowing the simultaneous expression of two proteins (for details of this vector see the diagram in the entry BAC-TO-BAC).

The pFastBac dual vector kit has been used e.g. in studies on generating murine heavy-chain-only antibodies [Proc Natl Acad Sci USA (2006) 103(41):15130–15135].

PFGE   Pulsed-field gel electrophoresis: a specialized form of GEL ELECTROPHORESIS which can be used to separate large pieces of nucleic acid of up to ~10–15 million base pairs. The fragments are exposed, alternately (in pulses), to two separate electric fields that are arranged at different angles to the gel.

The ability to separate fragments of linear DNA depends on several factors that include pulse time, total running time (of the experiment), the applied field strength and the positions of the electrodes. The pulse *length* affects the size range of the fragments separated: short pulses can be used to separate the relatively smaller fragments, while long pulses are needed to separate the larger fragments.

Disadvantages of PFGE include the time factor (the process may take 2–3 days) and the susceptibility of the isolated genomic DNA to endogenous nucleases.

Variant forms of PFGE differ e.g. in the arrangement of the electrodes; they include:

CHEF (*contour-clamped homogeneous electric field electrophoresis*). The electrodes are arranged on sides 2, 3, 5 and 6 of a hexagonal chamber.

Double inhomogeneous field electrophoresis. Two, long negative electrodes (cathodes) are on one side of the gel, and two short positive electrodes (anodes) are on the other side.

Field inversion electrophoresis. Two electrodes of equal size are present, one on each side of the gel; one acts as an anode, the other as a cathode – but periodically (depending on the pulse length) the polarity is switched.

PFGE has been widely used e.g. for TYPING bacteria, and is regarded by some as the 'gold standard' among molecular typing methods.

[PFGE for typing MRSA (methicillin-resistant *Staphylococcus aureus*): J Clin Microbiol (2005) 43(10):5069–5073; J Clin Microbiol (2005) 43(11):5642–5647.]

pfu   PLAQUE-FORMING UNIT.

PfuTurbo®   The trade designation (Stratagene, La Jolla CA) for certain types of DNA polymerase which are formulated for high-fidelity replication in PCR.

(See also ARCHAEMAXX.)

The enzyme *PfuTurbo®* C_x Hotstart DNA polymerase has been found useful for replicating DNA on uracil-containing templates [Nucleic Acids Res (2006) 34(18):e122].

pGEX-2T plasmid   See TEV.

Ph[1]   The Philadelphia chromosome: see ABL.

phage   A common abbreviation for BACTERIOPHAGE (q.v.); see also entries below for details of specific phages.

phage Bxb1   A BACTERIOPHAGE that infects a rapidly growing species of *Mycobacterium*: *M. smegmatis*. An integrase from phage Bxb1 (a serine recombinase) was reported to mediate efficient SITE-SPECIFIC RECOMBINATION in mammalian cells [BioTechniques (2006) 40(4):460–464].

phage conversion   See LYSOGENY.

phage CTXΦ   A filamentous BACTERIOPHAGE whose ssDNA genome encodes e.g. cholera toxin; CTXΦ infects the Gramnegative bacterium *Vibrio cholerae*. The manner of insertion of (double-stranded) versions of the phage genome into the host cell chromosome was reported to affect the ability of the prophage to give rise to phage virions [J Bacteriol (2000) 182 (24):6992–6998].

(See also (specialized) TRANSDUCTION.)

phage display   A method used for selecting a ligand that binds to a given target molecule with high-level affinity/specificity.

Initially, molecules of the given target are immobilized and exposed to a large population of recombinant phages. These phages have been genetically modified, *in vitro*, so that their coat proteins (i.e. surface proteins) differ from wild-type coat proteins; genetic modification of the phages is carried out on a random basis so that, collectively, the population of phages exhibits an enormous diversity of recombinant coat proteins, each having a potential binding site for a particular type of target molecule. This kind of genetically modified phage population is called a *phage library* (see later).

After the given target molecules have been exposed to the phage library, any phage particles which do *not* bind to the target molecules are removed, by washing, and discarded. The phages which do bind are subsequently eluted (removed from the target molecules) by physical means (e.g. adjusting the pH); these phages are used to infect their host bacteria – within which they are replicated to produce vast numbers of progeny phages. These progeny phages are therefore an expanded population of those phages which were selected from the phage library on the basis of their ability to bind to the given target molecule; they usually consist of a number of different strains with various forms of modified coat protein.

Purification of phage particles in the phage display process may be carried out by cesium chloride equilibrium density gradient centrifugation or, more easily, by chromatography with e.g. Sephacryl™ [BioTechniques (2005) 38(2): 194–198] or hydroxyapatite [BioTechniques (2005) 39(6): 879–884].

The target molecules are exposed to the progeny phages under more stringent conditions – i.e. conditions under which only those phages with the highest level of affinity/specificity will bind to target molecules. Unbound phages are removed, by washing.

The entire selective process is again repeated.

The technique described above for selecting phages from a phage library by exposing the library, and successive batches of progeny phages, to the target ligand is called *biopanning* (or simply *panning*). The basic principle involved in this process is similar to that used in the selection of aptamers by SELEX (see APTAMER).

The final batch of phages, characterized by strong, selective binding to the target molecules, are examined to determine the nature of the phage's binding site and the coding sequence of the binding site in the phage genome.

Phage display technology makes use of filamentous phages (e.g. M13) which are typically very long and thin and which (compared with e.g. phage T4) have a relatively high ratio of surface protein to nucleic acid.

Phage libraries

Phage libraries are prepared e.g. by inserting a gene library (consisting of unrelated genes/fragments) into the DNA of unmodified phages. Many of the genes/fragments will fuse with a phage gene that specifies a coat protein (e.g. protein pIII), and the resulting fusion protein will replace the phage's normal coat protein. Each hybrid gene will encode a different type of fusion protein – so that the coat proteins of the phage population, as a whole, will display a wide range of potential binding sites.

Another procedure for making a phage library involves *in vitro* randomization of a given sequence of nucleotides in the gene of a phage coat protein. The result is an immense range of different combinations of nucleotides, and the coat protein gene in a given phage particle will contain only one of these combinations; consequently, the coat proteins of the phage population collectively display an immense range of potential binding sites.

The target ligands for phage display technology include e.g. those involved in gene therapy techniques and various other mammalian cell-surface receptors (such as receptors for cytokines, and ligands relating to receptor-mediated endocytosis). The need to optimize receptor–ligand binding in the context of gene therapy is clearly important as this can help to avoid wasteful delivery of genes to untargeted cells and, therefore, help to reduce the required dosage for the patient.

Examples of use of phage display: studies on induction of an immune response by a peptide mimotope [Infect Immun (2005) 73(1):325–333]; study of *in vitro* protein evolution to optimize binding of an interleukin 13-neutralizing antibody [PNAS (2006) 103(20):7619–7624]; generating Epstein–Barr virus antigen mimotopes for diagnosis of EBV infection [J Clin Microbiol (2006) 44(3):764–771]; use of scFv antibody phage display libraries in studies on a tumor antigen [PNAS (2006) 103(4):1041–1046].

phage display-mediated immuno-PCR See IMMUNO-PCR.

phage f1 A filamentous ssDNA BACTERIOPHAGE that is related to PHAGE M13.

phage fd A filamentous ssDNA BACTERIOPHAGE that is related to PHAGE M13.

phage L54a A BACTERIOPHAGE which infects *Staphylococcus aureus*, causing phage conversion (see LYSOGENY).

phage lambda (λ) A temperate BACTERIOPHAGE of the family Styloviridae; host: *Escherichia coli*. The virion has an icosahedral head (55 nm diameter) and a non-contractile tail (~150 × 10 nm).

The genome (within the virion) is linear dsDNA (~48.5 kb) with single-stranded 12-base 5′ STICKY ENDS; circularization occurs intracellularly, the sticky ends hybridizing to form the so-called *cos* site.

During transcription of the phage early genes, the result of infection may be either lysogeny or lysis of the cell. The outcome depends e.g. on the activity of two mutually antagonistic products of the early genes: the cI protein (a repressor of transcription from certain operators) and the Cro protein – which inhibits transcription of the gene encoding cI. Factors that affect the lysogeny/lysis decision also include starvation (favoring lysogeny) and the multiplicity of infection (MOI) – a high MOI (i.e. each bacterium infected with a number of phages) favoring lysogeny.

Lysogeny involves integration of the circularized prophage into the host cell chromosome. Integration occurs by site-specific recombination between one 'attachment site' (which is designated *att*P) in the prophage and another (*att*B) in the bacterial genome (located between the *gal* gene and the *bio* gene in the chromosome).

The bacterial and phage attachment sites are not identical, although there is a central 'core' sequence (O) that is common to both sites. The bacterial (*att*B) site contains two 'arms' (B and B′) either side of the central O sequence, i.e. the structure of *att*B is BOB′. Analogously, the structure of *att*P is POP′.

Integration of the prophage into the chromosome involves a phage-encoded integrase (*int* gene product) and the bacterial INTEGRATION HOST FACTOR (IHF).

The recombination event involves strand breakage in the O region of each *att* site, strand exchange, and ligation. Hence, the integrated prophage is flanked by hybrid *att* regions BOP′ (= *att*L) and POB′ (= *att*R).

In the lytic cycle of phage λ, the prophage excises from the bacterial chromosome. This requires the product of the phage *xis* gene: an excisionase which recognizes the *att*L and *att*R sites.

The *att* sites are exploited in commercial systems: see e.g. GATEWAY SITE-SPECIFIC RECOMBINATION SYSTEM.

Phage λ also encodes another recombination system which is exploited as the LAMBDA (λ) RED RECOMBINATION system.

The phage λ *cos* site is used in COSMIDS and PHASMIDS – while modified forms of phage λ are used as cloning vectors (see e.g. LAMBDA FIX II VECTOR and ZAP EXPRESS VECTOR).

[The impact of phage lambda (from restriction to recombineering): Biochem Soc Trans (2006) 34(2):203–207.]

phage library See LIBRARY.

phage M13 A filamentous, non-lytic BACTERIOPHAGE able to infect strains of *Escherichia coli* containing an F PLASMID (or a related plasmid). When infecting cells of *E. coli*, phage

M13 initially binds to the *tips* of (plasmid-encoded) F pili or F-like pili (see PILUS); subsequently, phage DNA enters the cell.

The genome of M13 is covalently closed ssDNA.

Replication of the phage M13 genome can be divided into three stages.

In *stage I* a complementary strand (the *c* strand, or *minus* strand) is synthesized on the (circular) viral ssDNA (the *v* strand, or *plus* strand) to form the dsDNA *replicative form* (RF). When supercoiled by the cell's gyrase, RF is referred to as RFI. Phage genes are transcribed from the *c* strand of RFI. One of the early phage-encoded products is an endonuclease which initiates stage II by nicking the *v* strand at a specific site.

In *stage II*, the 3′ end of the nicked *v* strand is elongated by a rolling circle mechanism, displacing the 5′ *v* strand. Genome lengths of *v* strand are cut and circularized. Initially, the new, circularized *v* strands are converted to (double-stranded) RFs. Subsequently, a phage-encoded protein accumulates in the cell and coats the newly formed *v* strands; this prevents their conversion to RFs.

Stage III of the replication process in M13 is characterized by asymmetric DNA synthesis in which only the circularized *v* strands are formed.

The M13 coat proteins are synthesized with an N-terminal *signal sequence* that targets them to the bacterial cytoplasmic membrane. Phage virion assembly – a thioredoxin-dependent process in M13 and related phages – occurs in the bacterial cell envelope, and phage particles are extruded from (living) host cells.

The above account refers also to phages fd and f1; the other phages in this group appear to be generally similar.

Phage M13 and derivatives are used e.g. for making single-stranded copies of sample DNA and (e.g. strain M13K07) as a HELPER PHAGE for single-strand rescue from PHAGEMIDS.

phage N15 A BACTERIOPHAGE (host: *Escherichia coli*) with a linear dsDNA genome that has covalently closed (hairpin) terminal regions (*telomeres*).

The prophage of N15 does not integrate with the bacterial chromosome.

The mode of DNA replication of this phage has features in common with that of chromosomal replication in BORRELIA BURGDORFERI (q.v.).

A construct derived from phage N15 is used as a (linear) vector in the BIGEASY LINEAR CLONING SYSTEM.

DNA replication in PHAGE φ29, another phage with a linear dsDNA genome, involves a different mechanism.

phage P1 A temperate BACTERIOPHAGE of the family Myoviridae; host bacteria include *Escherichia coli*. The virion has an icosahedral head, a long contractile tail and six tail fibers.

The genome is linear dsDNA, 93.6 kb, which is circularly permuted and terminally redundant. Within the host cell, the prophage (genome) circularizes with loss of redundancy and usually remains as an extracellular low-copy-number plasmid (1 or 2 copies per chromosome) during lysogenic infection;

the plasmid is referred to as the P1 plasmid.

Within a lysogenic cell, copies of the plasmid may dimerize by homologous recombination. Nevertheless, at cell division, plasmid *monomers* are segregated to daughter cells; monomerization is mediated by a (phage-encoded) site-specific recombination system (the CRE–LOXP SYSTEM) that resolves plasmid dimers into monomers by a recombination event at the *loxP* site.

[P1 genome: J Bacteriol (2004) 186(21):7032–7068.]

phage φ29 A BACTERIOPHAGE (host: *Bacillus* species) with a linear dsDNA genome. Each of the 5′ ends of the DNA is covalently linked to a phage-encoded protein (designated TP).

DNA replication starts at both ends of the genome. DNA polymerase (encoded by the phage) forms a complex with a *free* molecule of TP and localizes at the 3′ end of each strand; a molecule of dAMP is then covalently linked to this TP – and acts as the initial nucleotide for the synthesis of the new strand. After insertion of nucleotide 10 in the new strand the polymerase dissociates from TP and continues to synthesize the remainder of the strand. TP remains bound to the 5′ end of the new strand. Such *protein priming* is one example of the strategies used for replication of linear dsDNA genomes. A different strategy is used for replicating the linear chromosomal DNA of the bacterium BORRELIA BURGDORFERI.

phage T3 A BACTERIOPHAGE (hosts: enterobacteria) which is closely related to PHAGE T7 (q.v.).

phage T4 A virulent (lytic) BACTERIOPHAGE (hosts: enterobacteria) of the family Myoviridae. The T4 genome is linear, circularly permuted and terminally redundant dsDNA (~170 kb) [T4 genome (review): Microbiol Mol Biol Rev (2003) 67:86–156]; the presence of hydroxymethylcytosine (instead of cytosine) involves the activity of phage-encoded enzymes. The virion is structurally complex; it has an elongated head (~110 × 85 nm) and a long, contractile tail.

Following infection of a bacterial cell, the phage genes are transcribed by the host cell's RNA polymerase; unlike the situation in PHAGE T7, the host's polymerase appears to be used throughout – although modified (e.g. ADP-ribosylated) in a series of phage-induced alterations.

The genome contains a number of origins of replication; replication occurs bidirectionally from a given origin. During replication, the 3′ end of a lagging strand template remains single-stranded, and this strand can displace a homologous sequence in a double-stranded region in another copy of the replicating genome. Such 3′ ends can act as primers, resulting in the formation of a complex, branching network of phage genomes.

DNA packaging occurs by the *headful mechanism*: one end of the multi-genome molecule is fed into the head until the head is full; the DNA is then cleaved.

Phage-encoded lysozyme (and a *lysis protein*) weaken the cell envelope, and the virions are released by osmotic lysis.

phage T7 A virulent (lytic) BACTERIOPHAGE (hosts: enterobacteria) of the family Podoviridae. The genome is linear ds DNA (~40 kb) with terminally redundant ends. The virion consists of an isometric head (diameter ~60 nm) and a tail with six short fibers.

Products of the early phage genes (transcribed by the host's RNA polymerase) include a protein kinase (which inactivates the host's RNA polymerase) and an RNA polymerase which transcribes the intermediate and late genes of the phage; the intermediate genes are concerned mainly with DNA replication, and late genes encode functions such as phage assembly and host cell lysis.

During DNA replication the genome remains as a linear molecule. Initiation occurs at a single site; the primers are apparently synthesized by the phage RNA polymerase, and elongation occurs bidirectionally (with leading and lagging strands) from the origin of replication. Newly formed duplexes recombine to form concatemers that are further replicated. Concatemers are cleaved into genome-length pieces, and a maturation process involves (e.g.) the formation of 160-bp terminally redundant sequences. Mature virions are released by host cell lysis.

In the initial infection of a bacterium, the phage apparently ejects channel-forming proteins which permit the transfer of DNA through the cell envelope; it was speculated that some of the ejected proteins may form components of a 'motor' that actively transports DNA into the host cell.

(See also BACTERIOPHAGE (table).)

phage typing A method for TYPING bacteria in which a given strain is exposed to a range of different phages; the strain under test is then defined in terms of the pattern of sensitivity or resistance to each of the particular set of phages used.

Essentially, a FLOOD PLATE of the test strain is prepared and excess surface moisture allowed to dry. A grid is drawn on the base of the plate, and the agar surface is inoculated with one drop of each phage suspension – each drop being placed in one of the squares of the grid. After incubation, a phage which lyses the test bacterium will form macroscopic plaques in the opaque surface layer of bacterial growth.

Certain species of bacteria, e.g. *Staphylococcus aureus* and *Yersinia enterocolitica*, are commonly typed by this method.

phagemid A circular, dsDNA hybrid VECTOR (constructed *in vitro*) which includes (i) a plasmid's origin of replication; (ii) a POLYLINKER; (iii) a marker (e.g. an antibiotic-resistance gene); and (iv) the origin of replication of an *ssDNA* bacteriophage (e.g. phage f1).

As a CLONING VECTOR, a phagemid can be used to make double-stranded copies of a gene or fragment. The DNA is inserted into the phagemid, via the polylinker, and copies of the recombinant phagemid are inserted into bacteria (e.g. by transformation); within the bacteria, the phagemids replicate as plasmids, using the plasmid origin of replication.

A phagemid can make *single-stranded* copies of the target DNA if the phagemid-carrying bacteria are infected with a *helper phage* (such as phage M13) which provides functions necessary for replication from the *phage* origin; copies of ssDNA, including the gene/fragment, are packaged in phage coat proteins (encoded by the helper phage), and phagemid particles are exported to the medium from the living bacteria. After removing the coat proteins, the ssDNA can be used e.g. for sequencing.

A phagemid can also be used as an EXPRESSION VECTOR by inserting the target DNA and also inserting an upstream, in-frame promoter of a type that functions in the host cell.

A phagemid can be used for *in vitro* transcription by including a promoter for T3 or T7 RNA polymerase (enzymes derived from phages) upstream of, and in phase with, target DNA.

Phagemid *particles* with modified coat protein have been prepared as vectors for gene delivery to eukaryotic cells (see entry GENE THERAPY).

One example of a phagemid is the PBLUESCRIPT vector.

pharmacogenomics The study of interactions between drugs and the genome, including modification of gene expression by drugs and the effect of mutation(s) in those genes whose products are involved in the response to specific drugs.

phase-shift mutation *Syn.* FRAME-SHIFT MUTATION.

phase variation ANTIGENIC VARIATION that includes on–off switching of antigen-encoding genes and changing from one antigen-encoding sequence to another.

For example, in many strains of *Salmonella* the flagellar filament is composed of one or other of two distinct types of protein (H1 and H2). Expression of the H2 gene (filament made with the H2 protein) is accompanied by production of a repressor of the H1 gene. The sequence that contains the H2 promoter is flanked by two sites which are recognized by a recombinase; SITE-SPECIFIC RECOMBINATION, mediated by the recombinase, inverts this sequence – inactivating the H2 promoter and stopping the production of the H1 repressor. Transcription of the H1 gene results in a filament made with H1 protein.

A different mechanism regulates *opa* genes in *Neisseria*. In these genes the leader region contains tandem repeats of the (pentameric) sequence CTCTT, and the *number* of repeats in a given gene may be changed through the mechanism of SLIPPED-STRAND MISPAIRING; such changes may affect the reading frame and, hence, may affect gene expression.

phasmid A construct prepared by recombination between e.g. a phage λ genome and a (modified) plasmid which includes an *att* site, to permit site-specific recombination, and a *cos* site; recombination between phage and plasmid occurs within the bacterial cell and requires e.g. the (phage-encoded) integrase. Phasmids are encapsidated in phage heads during replication of the phage – and any target DNA carried by the plasmid moiety can be inserted into other bacteria by infecting them with phasmid-containing phage particles.

(cf. COSMID and PHAGEMID.)

phenocopy (1) (*noun*) Any cell or organism that exhibits a new phenotype which mimics a phenotype that would result from a genetic change – i.e. the cell or organism *appears* to have experienced a genetic change.

One example of a phenocopy is observed when bacterial F⁺ cells are grown to high density. These cells lose their donor characteristics and mimic (transfer-deficient) F⁻ cells; however, when the F⁻ phenocopies are grown in fresh medium they revert to the F⁺ donor condition.

(2) (*verb*) To produce an effect similar to that produced by another event. For example, a null mutation in protein X may give rise to a phenotype identical to that produced by a null mutation in protein Y, one mutation being said to phenocopy the other.

phenol–chloroform–isoamyl alcohol A mixture of reagents used e.g. for isolating DNA. The DNA tends to partition in the top layer and may then be precipitated by isopropanol or ethanol.

phenotype Those characteristic(s) of a given organism which can be observed/detected/measured – manifestations of the organism's genotype; in genetics, phenotype is often used to refer to specific, designated characteristic(s).

phenotypic lag A delay in the expression of an allele which has been newly acquired e.g. by mutation or gene transfer. In bacteria, such delay may be due e.g. to SEGREGATION LAG.

phenotypic mixing A phenomenon which may occur if a cell is infected simultaneously with two genetically distinct viruses: incorporation of the genome of one virus into the capsid of the other (*transcapsidation*, *genetic masking*) or inclusion of structural components from one virus in virions of the other.

phenotypic screen Any screening process in which individuals in a given population are identified according to one or more phenotypic characteristics.

phenylketonuria An autosomal recessive disease, the classical form of which is characterized by phenylpyruvate in the urine and high levels of phenylalanine in blood and other tissues; it is caused by inadequacy of phenylalanine mono-oxygenase. The condition leads to mental retardation. Treatment includes limiting dietary phenylalanine.

(See also GENETIC DISEASE (table).)

pheromone (1) (in quorum sensing) See QUORUM SENSING. (2) (in conjugation) See CONJUGATION.

φ29 phage (phi 29 phage) See PHAGE φ29.

Philadelphia chromosome See ABL.

phleomycin D1 *Syn.* ZEOCIN.

phorbol ester (TPA) See ZEBRA.

phosphodiester bond In DNA and RNA: the bond linking the 5′-phosphate group of one sugar residue to the 3′-OH group of the next (5′) sugar residue.

(See also DNA LIGASE.)

phosphoenolpyruvate-dependent phosphotransferase system See PTS.

phosphoramidite Any of a class of compounds used e.g. in the chemical synthesis of oligonucleotides, and also for adding a group to the terminal 5′-phosphate of a pre-existing oligonucleotide.

phosphorodiamidate morpholino oligomer See MORPHOLINO ANTISENSE OLIGOMER.

photo-cross-linking assay See CROSS-LINKING ASSAY.

photolyase (DNA photolyase) In *Escherichia coli* (and some other bacteria): a flavoenzyme (product of gene *phr*) which can cleave the bonds in THYMINE DIMERS produced when DNA is damaged by ULTRAVIOLET RADIATION; this reaction (*photoreactivation*, *photorestoration*), which uses the energy in blue light, can restore a normal base sequence.

[Electrochemistry of *E. coli* photolyase action: Proc Natl Acad Sci USA (2005) 102(31):10788–10792.]

Photolyase is reported to be absent in some bacteria (e.g. *Bacillus subtilis*). It is absent in *Ehrlichia* spp but occurs in the (related) bacterium *Neorickettsia*; however, this enzyme is related more closely to the photolyase of *Coxiella burnetii* than to the *E. coli* enzyme [PLoS Genet (2006) 2(2):e21].

photoreactivation See PHOTOLYASE.

photorestoration See PHOTOLYASE.

***phr* gene** See PHOTOLYASE.

phylotype (*microbiol.*) Any hitherto uncultured species which has been defined solely on the basis of nucleic acid sequence data.

physical map (of a genome) The complete sequence of nucleotides in the genome.

When applied e.g. to a plasmid vector molecule, the term 'physical map' may refer simply to a diagram which shows the locations of e.g. specific gene(s) and restrictions sites.

phytokinins *Syn.* CYTOKININS.

Pichia A genus of budding yeasts related to *Saccharomyces*; species are widespread. The sexually derived spores (ascospores) are characteristically shaped in some species.

In DNA technology, *P. pastoris* has been used extensively for the production of a wide variety of heterologous proteins. Reasons for the choice of this organism include: (i) similarity to *Saccharomyces cerevisiae* – which has well characterized genetic and cultural properties; (ii) high-level synthesis of heterologous proteins; (iii) the ability to produce proteins intracellularly and extracellularly; (iv) the ability to carry out various types of post-translational modification – including glycosylation.

Regulated, inducible protein synthesis in *P. pastoris* can be achieved by using expression vectors that include the strong promoter of the *AOX1* gene.

For constitutive expression of a heterologous protein, use can be made of the promoter of the gene encoding glyceraldehyde 3-phosphate dehydrogenase.

(See also PPICZ VECTOR.)

pico- A prefix meaning 10^{-12}.

PicoGreen® assay An assay (Molecular Probes, Eugene OR/ Invitrogen, Carlsbad CA) for quantitating dsDNA in solution. A reagent is added and incubated for 5 minutes; when bound to dsDNA the reagent fluoresces on excitation at 480 nm. The fluorescence is linear over at least four orders of magnitude.

The assay is reported to be >10000-fold more sensitive than quantitation with ULTRAVIOLET ABSORBANCE at 260 nm.

(See also OLIGREEN and RIBOGREEN.)

pif In the F PLASMID: a locus (*pif* = phage-inhibiting function) associated with the inability of particular phages (e.g. T7) to replicate in F-plasmid-containing cells.

(See also FEMALE-SPECIFIC PHAGE.)

pilus (*bacteriol.*) (plural: pili)   An appendage that projects from the surface of those Gram-negative bacteria which contain a conjugative plasmid and in which the transfer operon of the plasmid (including pilus-encoding genes) is being expressed. These appendages are also called *conjugative pili* or *sex pili*.

Some pili are known to be essential for plasmid-mediated CONJUGATION; it is assumed that all pili play an essential role in this process.

There are morphologically and serologically distinct types of pili; different types of pili are encoded by genetically distinct plasmids.

Pili encoded by the F PLASMID are thin, flexible, protein filaments of up to several micrometers in length and ~8 nm in diameter; this type of pilus has an axial channel of ~2 nm in diameter. Other types of pilus include e.g. the short, rigid, thorn-like appendages that are encoded by plasmids of the IncN incompatibility group.

Some types of BACTERIOPHAGE infect bacteria by initially binding to specific sites on pili; infection does not occur in the absence of pili. Examples of phages that infect via F pili (encoded by the F plasmid) include e.g. phages f1, fd, M13 (and derivatives), MS2 and Qβ. (See also HELPER PHAGE.)

F-like pili (encoded e.g. by plasmids ColV and ColI-K94) resemble F pili and they bind similar types of phage.

I-like pili (encoded e.g. by plasmid ColIb-P9) are similar, morphologically, to F pili but they differ serologically; they bind a distinct range of phages – including e.g. If1 and If2.

The terms *fimbria* (plural: fimbriae) and pilus have been commonly used synonymously. This lack of discrimination is unfortunate because it is logical to distinguish between those appendages which have a specific role in conjugation (pili) and those appendages (fimbriae) which have no established role in conjugation but which have other roles (e.g. adhesion) – and which are generally distinct morphologically. In this dictionary (and in the *Dictionary of Microbiology and Molecular Biology*, revised 3rd edition, 2006) 'fimbria' and 'pilus' are *not* used synonymously.

pipemidic acid   See QUINOLONE ANTIBIOTICS.

PᵢPer™ pyrophosphate assay kit   A product from Molecular Probes Inc. (Eugene OR) used for the detection of free PYROPHOSPHATE in solution. In the assay, the enzyme inorganic pyrophosphatase initially cleaves pyrophosphate to inorganic phosphate. Catalyzed by maltose phophorylase, the inorganic phosphate then converts maltose to a mixture of glucose and glucose 1-phosphate. The resulting glucose is converted, by glucose oxidase, to gluconolactone and hydrogen peroxide. Hydrogen peroxide, in the presence of horseradish peroxidase, reacts with an added reagent to generate the compound *resorufin* whose fluorescence (maxima at approximately 563 nm and 587 nm) is monitored.

PITX2 gene   See AXENFELD–RIEGER SYNDROME.

pJAZZ-KA   See BIGEASY LINEAR CLONING SYSTEM.

pJET1/blunt   See CLONING VECTOR.

pKM101   See AMES TEST.

PKR kinase   See e.g. RNA INTERFERENCE.

plant pathogen forensics   See FORENSIC APPLICATIONS.

plaque (phage)   A usually 'circular' region in a layer of bacterial growth in which some or all of the cells are lysed, or growth-impeded, owing to phage activity.

In a PLAQUE ASSAY, on a plate which has been prepared from a high dilution of the sample, any given plaque is likely to have developed as a result of the activity of a single lytic phage; progeny phages derived from lysis of the first-infected cell diffuse outwards and progressively infect, and lyse, the neighboring cells until a visible and often 'circular' area (the plaque) is formed.

The general appearance of a plaque may indicate the nature of the infecting phage. For example, a clear plaque, in which all the cells have been lysed, is characteristic of a virulent phage. A turbid plaque, in which only a proportion of the cells are lysed, is characteristic of a temperate phage. Some non-lytic phages – e.g. filamentous phages such as f1 and M13 – may also form turbid plaques by reducing the growth rate of infected cells within the plaque.

plaque assay (of phage)   A procedure used for determining the PLAQUE TITER of a sample containing a given type of phage.

Initially, log dilutions of the sample are prepared. From a given dilution, a measured volume is added to molten, semi-solid agar (~45°C) containing an excess of phage-susceptible bacteria; the whole is well mixed and is then poured onto a plate of solid nutrient agar – forming a layer of ~1–2 mm in thickness. A similar procedure is used for each of the log dilutions, and the plates are incubated at the growth temperature of the bacteria. After incubation, the plates are examined for plaques (see PLAQUE). Assuming that each observed plaque on a given plate was caused by a single phage, the plaque titer can be calculated from the volumes and dilutions used.

An analogous procedure may be used for viruses other than phages provided that a suitable monolayer culture of susceptible cells is available. In one method, each of a set of monolayer cultures is drained of growth medium and inoculated with one of the log dilutions of the sample; after gentle rocking (to enable viral adsorption to the cells) each monolayer culture is overlaid with a buffered growth medium in semi-solid agar and is then incubated.

plaque-forming unit (pfu) (of phage)   A single bacteriophage particle which, under appropriate conditions, can give rise to a single PLAQUE in a confluent layer of susceptible bacteria.

plaque titer (of phage)   A measure of the number of PLAQUE-FORMING UNITS in a given volume of sample.

plasmid   A linear or covalently closed circular DNA molecule – distinct from chromosomal, mitochondrial, chloroplast or kinetoplast DNA – which can replicate autonomously (i.e. independently of other replicons) within a prokaryotic and/or eukaryotic cell. Plasmids are commonly dispensable, i.e. not essential to their host cells, and not all cells contain plasmids; for example, plasmids are commonly absent in bacteria of the genera *Anaplasma*, *Bartonella*, *Brucella* and *Rickettsia*.

PLASMID: a diversity of molecules (some examples)

Plasmid	Notes, context
CAM	A natural plasmid (~500 kb) present in certain strains of the Gram-negative bacterium *Pseudomonas*. It encodes the enzymic capacity that enables these organisms to metabolize the terpenoid camphor
Cit	A natural plasmid found e.g. in strains of *Escherichia coli*. It encodes a citrate transport system which confers on the host cell the ability to use citrate as the sole source of carbon and energy. Cells of *E. coli* which lack the plasmid are citrate-negative in biochemical tests
DFRS	Dual-fluorscence reporter/sensor plasmid: a type of construct which has been used e.g. to study the dynamics of microRNAs (miRNAs) in living cells. Each plasmid contains sequences that encode two different fluorophores (which have distinct emission spectra), one of the fluorophores acting as the reporter (i.e. signaling intracellular expression of the plasmid). The mRNA of the other fluorophore includes a sequence complementary to the intracellular target; if present, the intracellular target binds to this mRNA and inhibits translation – indicated by a loss of fluorescence from this (sensor) fluorophore
F	A natural, low-copy-number plasmid (~95 kb) found e.g. in strains of the Gram-negative bacterium *Escherichia coli*. The plasmid may exist as an integral part of the bacterial chromosome or as an extrachromosomal element. The presence of the plasmid confers on the host cell the ability to act as a donor of DNA (either plasmid DNA or plasmid *and* host DNA) during conjugation; for this purpose the plasmid encodes various products required for the mobilization and transfer of DNA, including a bacterial cell-surface appendage (see PILUS) required for establishment of contact between the donor and recipient cells. In DNA technology, cells containing the F plasmid are used e.g. to permit infection by certain types of bacteriophage (e.g. phage M13) which are used e.g. for the preparation of single-stranded DNA; these phages infect cells by initially binding to the pilus (cells lacking a pilus cannot be infected). The so-called *ccd* mechanism (see entry), encoded by the F plasmid, has been used to promote stable maintenance of the plasmid in populations of bacteria under experimental conditions
OCT	A natural plasmid (~500 kb), found in some strains of *Pseudomonas*, which enables these strains to metabolize octane and decane
pBR322	A small (~4.3 kb) engineered, multicopy plasmid encoding resistance to ampicillin and tetracycline. It has been widely used e.g. as a cloning vector. Many plasmids have been derived from pBR322 or from components of this plasmid
pCAL	Any of a range of engineered plasmid vectors used in the AFFINITY PROTEIN EXPRESSION AND PURIFICATION system (q.v.); each of the plasmids includes a calmodulin-binding peptide (CBP) tag to facilitate isolation/purification of the protein of interest
pCT	A natural plasmid found in most strains of the Gram-negative pathogen *Chlamydia trachomatis*. A sequence of nucleotides in this plasmid has been used as a target for a diagnostic test involving the ligase chain reaction (LCR). Rare isolates of *C. trachomatis* have been reported to lack the plasmid
pESC	Any of a range of engineered commercial plasmid vectors used e.g. for gene expression in the yeast *Saccharomyces cerevisiae*. The plasmids include sequences (e.g. FLAG) for epitope tagging; this facilitates detection/isolation of the target proteins (see entry PESC VECTORS)
pET SUMO	A small (5.6 kb) engineered plasmid used as an expression vector for high-level expression of recombinant proteins in *Escherichia coli* hosts. The plasmid encodes an 11-kDa solubility-enhancing protein that forms a fusion product with the protein of interest. This plasmid is part of a commercial protein expression system (see entry CHAMPION PET SUMO VECTOR)
pJAZZ-KA	A linear, engineered plasmid derived from the genome of a bacteriophage (coliphage N15). It replicates intracellularly as an extrachromosomal element. This plasmid is a commercial cloning vector used in the BigEasy™ linear cloning system (see entry)
pJET1/blunt	An engineered plasmid designed for cloning blunt-ended PCR products (see entry CLONING VECTOR)

(*continued*)

PLASMID: (*continued*)

Plasmid	Notes, context
pKM101	A plasmid encoding e.g. certain error-prone repair enzymes; it is used in the AMES TEST
pMG7	A plasmid (found in some strains of the Gram-negative bacterium *Pseudomonas aeruginosa*) which inhibits replication of certain phages (e.g. F116, G101)
pOG44	An engineered plasmid encoding the Flp recombinase (see FLP). It is used in conjunction with FLP-IN CELL LINES
pXO1	A natural plasmid found in virulent (anthrax-causing) strains of the Gram-positive bacterium *Bacillus anthracis*. It encodes the anthrax toxin
pXO2	A natural plasmid found in virulent (anthrax-causing) strains of the Gram-positive bacterium *Bacillus anthracis*. It encodes a poly-D-glutamic acid capsule which enables the organism to evade phagocytosis in the host
pSM19035	A natural plasmid found e.g. in strains of the Gram-positive bacterium *Streptococcus pyogenes*. It exhibits a high level of segregational stability in host cells – a feature due to the combined activity of a number of distinct mechanisms for controlling copy number
R1	A natural, low-copy-number plasmid found in strains of *Escherichia coli* and related bacteria. It encodes resistance to certain antibiotics (including ampicillin and streptomycin), and also confers on the host cell the ability to act as a donor of DNA in conjugation. During cell division, segregation of the plasmids to daughter cells appears to involve a mitosis-like process in which a plasmid-encoded protein polymerizes to form force-generating filaments that are involved in mechanical separation of the daughter plasmids
R6K	A natural multicopy plasmid (~38 kb) found in *Escherichia coli* and related bacteria. It encodes e.g. a β-lactamase (and, hence, confers resistance to certain β-lactam antibiotics) and confers on the host cell the ability to act as a DNA donor in conjugation
R100	A natural, low-copy-number plasmid found in strains of *Escherichia coli* and related bacteria. It encodes resistance to e.g. chloramphenicol, sulfonamides and mercury; a gene for tetracycline resistance is carried on transposon Tn*10*. R100 confers on the host cell the ability to act as a DNA donor in conjugation
Ti	A large plasmid found in (virulent) strains of the bacterium *Agrobacterium tumefaciens*. It encodes the means of transferring DNA into plant cells, and this is exploited in a procedure called AGROINFECTION which is used for the experimental infection of plants by viruses. In nature, DNA injected into plants by *A. tumefaciens* causes tumors (galls – see entry CROWN GALL)
TOL	A natural plasmid (~117 kb) found in strains of the Gram-negative bacterium *Pseudomonas*. The plasmid genes are arranged in two operons which jointly confer on the bacterial host the ability to metabolize toluene and xylene; these substrates are first oxidized to carboxylic acids which are then converted to pyruvate and acetaldehyde (which enter the tricarboxylic acid cycle). The availability of iron may be a factor in this metabolic activity. One isolate of a TOL plasmid was found to encode a homolog of DNA polymerase V which was reported to promote survival in DNA-damaged cells

The following account refers mainly to *bacterial* plasmids.

Features encoded by plasmids

Collectively, the plasmids encode a vast range of functions. In many cases they encode resistance to particular antibiotics or groups of antibiotics and/or to other inimical agents – such as mercury (or other heavy metal) ions. In certain pathogenic bacteria (e.g. *Bacillus anthracis*, causal agent of anthrax) the toxin(s) and/or other virulence factors are plasmid-encoded. (In some pathogens the virulence factors are phage-encoded.) Some plasmids encode products (such as particular enzymes) which enhance the metabolic potential of a cell; for example, the Cit plasmid in some strains of *Escherichia coli* enables those strains to use citrate as the sole source of carbon and energy (an ability which is lacking in wild-type strains of *E. coli*). Again, the TOL plasmid confers on certain strains of *Pseudomonas* the ability to metabolize toluene and xylene. Certain plasmids (e.g. ColE1) encode a COLICIN or other type of BACTERIOCIN. In the archaean *Halobacterium*, structural components of gas vacuoles are plasmid-encoded.

Engineered plasmids

Plasmids have been engineered in order to carry out a great diversity of functions. For example, plasmids are widely used as cloning vectors, as expression vectors and as vehicles for introducing genetic material into cells. They are also used in studies on gene expression and on the mechanisms of intracellular signaling.

A plasmid encoding a transposase may be used as a 'helper plasmid' in cells within which a specific type of transposition is required.

A plasmid may incorporate genes of the LAMBDA (λ) RED RECOMBINATION system in order to carry out an intracellular replacement of DNA (such as a gene knockout).

A plasmid may act as a PACKAGING PLASMID.

A DFRS PLASMID can be used for detecting an intracellular target sequence.

Of the enormous range of natural and engineered plasmids, only a very limited selection is shown in the table.

Size, transformability
In size, plasmids typically range from about several kilobases to several hundred kilobases. In DNA technology, the small circular plasmids can be inserted into cells by transformation more readily than large plasmids; moreover, small plasmids are less susceptible to damage by shearing forces. In general, linear plasmids are poorly transformable e.g. in normal cells of *E. coli* – although linear forms of DNA can be transformed by using a method such as the lambda (λ) red recombination system.

Circular/linear plasmids
In the literature, plasmids have been described *ad nauseam* as 'small circles of DNA'; as linear plasmids have been known for many years, this is clearly misleading. While many, even most, plasmids *are* ccc dsDNA molecules, linear plasmids (and chromosomes) occur e.g. in a number of bacteria; thus, e.g. a bacterium with one of the largest genomes (~9.7 Mbp), *Rhodococcus* sp RHA1, has three linear plasmids as well as a linear chromosome [see Proc Natl Acad Sci USA (2006) 103: 15582–15587], and linear plasmids also occur e.g. in species of *Borrelia* and *Streptomyces*.

Linear plasmids are exploited in DNA technology: see e.g. BIGEASY LINEAR CLONING SYSTEM.

Presence of transposable elements
Many plasmids contain one or more transposons or insertion sequences (see TRANSPOSABLE ELEMENT). For example, the transposon Tn*3* occurs in R1*drd*-19 while Tn*10* and Tn*21* are found e.g. in R100. The insertion sequence IS*3* is found e.g. in the F plasmid (see FINOP SYSTEM).

Copy number
The copy number is characteristic for a given plasmid, in a particular host cell, under given conditions.

Plasmids are referred to as 'low-copy-number' if they occur singly, or in a few copies, in each cell; the F PLASMID is one example.

Multicopy plasmids are normally present in appreciably higher numbers – e.g. >10 copies; the ColE1 plasmid (often 10–30 copies) is one example.

Factors which influence copy number include the plasmid's specific type of replication control system and its mode of *partition* (segregation to daughter cells during cell division). In one mechanism for maintaining copy number, encoded by the R1 plasmid, the Kid protein acts as a nuclease: if copy number falls it cleaves host-cell mRNAs and also cleaves the mRNA of a plasmid-encoded replication repressor; hence, under these conditions, the bacterial growth rate decreases and the plasmid replication rate rises, this tending to restore normal copy number and avoiding loss of plasmids from the population [EMBO J (2005) 24(19):3459–3469].

Replication of bacterial plasmids
To maintain their presence within a (growing) population of bacteria, plasmids must replicate, and the plasmid progeny must be distributed efficiently to daughter cells (see Partition, below).

Control of plasmid replication is encoded in the plasmid itself, although the cell's biosynthetic potential is an essential requirement.

The frequency with which a plasmid replicates in the host cell varies with plasmid. It is determined by the frequency at which replication is *initiated*, and this feature is regulated in a plasmid-dependent way. Early reports indicated that, in at least some plasmids (e.g. pSC101), initiation of replication involves the cell's DnaA protein (needed for *chromosomal* replication); however, it now appears that DnaA is specific for the initiation of replication of the host cell's DNA and that plasmid-encoded factors regulate the replication of plasmid DNA.

Control of plasmid replication involves different plasmid-dependent mechanisms. For example, in the ColE1 plasmid, control of replication occurs at the primer level and involves competitive interaction between two (plasmid-encoded) RNA molecules, one of which can prime replication (for details see COLE1 PLASMID).

A different mechanism operates in various small, circular plasmids found in Gram-positive bacteria. In these plasmids, replication – involving a ROLLING CIRCLE mechanism – is initiated by a plasmid-encoded Rep protein. The Rep protein nicks a specific strand of the plasmid at the origin, thus forming a free 3′ end suitable for rolling circle synthesis. A single round of replication yields a complete (circular) ssDNA copy of the plasmid that is subsequently replicated to the double-stranded state from an RNA primer. Initiation of replication may be controlled by regulating the synthesis or activity of the Rep protein. Thus, in some cases, transcription or translation of the Rep-encoding gene may be regulated by a small plasmid-encoded antisense RNA molecule which can bind to the mRNA. Alternatively, the Rep protein may be inactivated after a single use by the binding of a small plasmid-encoded oligonucleotide.

Some plasmids contain *iterons*: sequences of direct-repeats associated with their origin of replication; these regions are central to replication control. Thus, initiator proteins can bind to these regions and give rise to a nucleoprotein complex as a prerequisite to the initiation of replication. The mechanism of control may be complex, and in at least some cases initiator proteins are autoregulated at the level of transcription. Moreover, in some cases a mechanism known as HANDCUFFING appears to be involved in initiation control.

Stringent and relaxed control of replication. Plasmids whose replication depends on protein synthesis in the host cell fail to replicate if their host cells are treated with certain agents (such as the antibiotic chloramphenicol) which inhibit protein synthesis; for plasmids in this category, replication is sometimes said to be under *stringent control.*

Other plasmids, such as ColE1, can continue to replicate in the presence of agents that inhibit protein synthesis; for these plasmids, replication is sometimes said to be under *relaxed control.* Plasmids in this category can exploit pre-formed host proteins (such as polymerases). (Notice that, in the case of e.g. ColE1, the primary mode of regulation of initiation of replication involves the synthesis of oligonucleotides rather than proteins.) Given continued replication in the presence of bacteriostatic agents, plasmids such as ColE1 achieve higher-than-normal copy numbers within their host cells.

Partition (segregation) of bacterial plasmids
In certain – high-copy-number – plasmids there seems to be no special mechanism for active segregation of the plasmid progeny to daughter cells during cell division. It is generally believed that, in such cases, partition may involve a random distribution of plasmid progeny into daughter cells – the high copy number of the plasmid in the parent cell ensuring that both daughter cells will receive an appropriate complement of plasmids.

In low-copy-number plasmids there is a need for an active mechanism for partition in order to ensure that each daughter cell receives at least one copy of the plasmid – in this way achieving a stable inheritance of the plasmid in the bacterial population. In these plasmids there are specific loci (designated e.g. *par*, *sop*, *sta*) that are associated with the partition function, and in various plasmids the mechanism of partition appears to be more complex than previously understood. For example, in the R1 PLASMID (q.v.), segregation of plasmids to daughter cells seems to involve a mitosis-like process. Moreover, proteins encoded by other plasmids are also reported to polymerize, *in vitro*, into filaments that would appear to be involved in partition – e.g. the SopA protein of the F plasmid [Proc Natl Acad Sci USA (2005) 102(49):17658–17663] and the ParF protein encoded by the TP228 plasmid [EMBO J (2005) 24(7):1453–1464].

Compatibility: Inc groups
Different types of plasmid can occur in the same cell: those plasmids which have different modes of replication and partition are said to exhibit *compatibility*; such plasmids are able to co-exist – stably – within the same cell. On the other hand, plasmids with similar or identical systems of replication/partition are incompatible: they are not able to co-exist, stably, in the same cell. This is the basis of the *incompatibility groups* (the so-called Inc groups): a given Inc group consists of those plasmids which have similar or identical replication/partition systems and which cannot co-exist, stably, in the same cell.

Among enterobacteria the Inc groups include:

IncFI (e.g. the F plasmid, ColV-K94, R386)
IncFII (e.g. R1, R6)
IncIα (e.g. ColIb-P9, R64)
IncN (e.g. R46, R269N-1)
IncX (e.g. R6K)

Among *Pseudomonas* species, the Inc groups have been designated IncP-1, IncP-2 etc; for example:

IncP-2 (e.g. CAM plasmid, OCT plasmid)
IncP-9 (e.g. TOL plasmid)

Some of the enterobacterial and pseudomonad Inc groups are shared (equivalent).

Conjugative plasmids
Many bacterial plasmids encode the means for transferring a copy of the plasmid DNA to another host cell by the process of CONJUGATION – involving cell–cell contact during which donor DNA is transferred to the recipient cell; one example of such plasmids is the F PLASMID. The conjugative plasmids contain a so-called transfer operon that includes those genes required for the synthesis of products (such as the PILUS and certain enzymes) necessary for conjugative transfer of DNA.

When integrated into the chromosome, these plasmids may also be able to mobilize transfer of the chromosomal DNA during conjugation.

Plasmid persistence
In some cases, one or more mechanisms militate against the loss of a plasmid from a bacterial population: see e.g. CCD MECHANISM. The R1 mechanism involving the Kid protein (see above: Copy number) also serves to prevent plasmid loss from a bacterial population.

Experimental elimination of plasmids
In some cases there is a need for plasmid-free cells. Various approaches have been used to eliminate plasmids from a bacterial population: see e.g. CURING and SUICIDE VECTOR.

Isolation of plasmids from bacteria in the laboratory
Various commercial methods can be used for the isolation of plasmids from bacteria. For example, using the QIAGEN® plasmid mini kit, the sample undergoes controlled alkaline lysis with NaOH (sodium hydroxide) and sodium dodecyl sulfate (SDS); such treatment is designed to disrupt the cells' cytoplasmic membrane and to release e.g. RNA, proteins and plasmids. (If the procedure is carried out correctly, chromosomal DNA is trapped in the leaky cells.) Contaminating RNA is digested with RNase. The lysis period (exposure to the alkaline lysis regime) is optimized in order to promote the maximum release of plasmids and to avoid their irreversible denaturation. After neutralization of the lysate, and mixing, the whole is centrifuged to obtain a cleared lysate (containing plasmids) – which is exposed to a special QIAGEN® anion-exchange resin in a controlled electrolyte environment; after adsorption to the resin, the plasmid DNA can be eluted by

adjustment of the electrolyte/pH.

A different procedure is used in the PURELINK PLASMID PURIFICATION SYSTEMS.

plasmid profiling See REAP.

plate (1) A PETRI DISH containing a (sterile) AGAR- or gelatin-based medium (in either case, a *gel*). A plate is prepared by pouring the (molten) medium into a Petri dish and allowing it to set. A sterile plate may be *inoculated* with a given microorganism (or material containing that microorganism) and *incubated* at an appropriate temperature for a suitable period of time; if the organism grows, the result is a *plate culture*. (A plate culture may be referred to as a 'plate'.)

(2) (*verb*) To inoculate the surface of a plate (sense 1) with an *inoculum* containing (or expected to contain) a particular type (or particular types) of microorganism with the object of initiating a plate culture.

plate culture See PLATE (sense 1).

Platinum® *Taq* DNA polymerase A recombinant form of TAQ DNA POLYMERASE (marketed by Invitrogen, Carlsbad CA) designed for improved specificity in hot-start PCR; the polymerase incorporates a thermolabile inhibitor (containing an anti-*Taq* monoclonal antibody) which is degraded during the first (high-temperature) denaturation step, releasing the active *Taq* DNA polymerase.

plectonemic Refers to a (stable) arrangement of two strands of DNA in which the strands are wound around each other, each strand being base-paired to the other.

(cf. PARANEMIC.)

pleiotropic Refers e.g. to a given gene which affects multiple – apparently unrelated – phenotypic characteristics.

pleiotropic mutation Any mutation that affects multiple – apparently unrelated – targets/systems.

pLenti6/V5-DEST™ vector A destination vector in the GATEWAY SITE-SPECIFIC RECOMBINATION SYSTEM (see table).

plenum ventilation See SAFETY CABINET (class I).

ploidy The number of sets of chromosomes per cell – e.g. one set (haploid), two sets (diploid) etc. (cf. ANEUPLOID.)

In some organisms (e.g. certain algae, fungi and protozoa) the life cycle exhibits a so-called *alternation of generations* in which generation(s) or mature haploid individuals alternate with generation(s) of mature diploid individuals.

plus strand (of a gene) See CODING STRAND.

PML Progressive multifocal leukoencephalopathy: a fatal demyelinating condition caused by the JC VIRUS.

pML31 A 9-kb plasmid that was derived from the F PLASMID by digestion with the restriction endonuclease EcoRI and insertion of an antibiotic-resistance gene in a recircularized segment.

PMN (granulocyte) Polymorphonuclear leukocyte: a type of white blood cell with a lobed nucleus and granular cytoplasm which includes neutrophils, basophils and eosinophils. The term *polymorph* sometimes refers specifically to neutrophils.

PMO (phosphorodiamidate morpholino oligomer) See MORPHOLINO ANTISENSE OLIGOMER.

pMT-DEST48 vector A destination vector in the GATEWAY SITE-SPECIFIC RECOMBINATION SYSTEM.

pMT/V5-His vector See DES.

pMT/V5-His-TOPO® vector See DES.

pMyr vector See CYTOTRAP TWO-HYBRID SYSTEM.

PNA Peptide nucleic acid: a DNA analog in which the backbone chain is a modified polypeptide (rather than a chain of sugar–phosphate units).

Two strands of PNA can form a duplex that resembles the helical duplex of DNA. Moreover, a strand of PNA can bind to a strand of DNA more stably than can the complementary strand of DNA.

Unlike DNA, PNA is insensitive to the concentration of electrolyte.

PNA has been used e.g. in LIGHTUP PROBES. In a different context, an *antisense* PNA, specific for an essential gene in *Escherichia coli*, has been found to exert potent antibacterial activity and may be useful for the selection and maintenance of bacterial strains for research purposes [BioTechniques (2003) 35:1060–1064].

A microarray of PNA probes was used for the detection of specific mutations [Nucleic Acids Res (2005) 33(2):e19].

Owing to their inherent properties, oligomers of PNA are particularly useful as clamps in PCR CLAMPING. [Use of PNA as both a PCR clamp and as a sensor probe for melting curve analyses in the detection of rare mutant K-*ras* DNA: Nucleic Acids Res (2006) 34(2):e12.]

PNA-mediated PCR clamping See PCR CLAMPING.

***pncA* gene** In *Mycobacterium tuberculosis*: a gene encoding the enzyme pyrazinamidase; *in vivo*, pyrazinamidase converts the anti-tuberculosis prodrug pyrazinamide to the active form of the drug: pyrazinoic acid.

Clinical isolates of *M. tuberculosis* which are resistant to pyrazinamide are commonly found to have a mutant form of the *pncA* gene [Antimicrob Agents Chemother (2005) 49(6): 2210–2217].

PNPase POLYNUCLEOTIDE PHOSPHORYLASE.

pOG44 A plasmid encoding the Flp recombinase (see FLP). It is used in conjunction with FLP-IN CELL LINES for inserting the gene of interest into the host cell's chromosome: pOG44 is co-transfected into (engineered) host cells with an Flp-In™ vector (carrying the gene of interest) – the gene of interest then integrating into the chromosome by (Flp-mediated) site-specific recombination.

point mutation (1) Any mutation in which a single nucleotide is replaced by another type of nucleotide (see TRANSITION MUTATION and TRANSVERSION MUTATION).

In certain cases a point mutation can make the difference between a normal gene and a disease-causing gene (see e.g. RAS).

In pathogenic microorganisms, some point mutations can confer resistance to antibiotic(s).

Point mutations are detectable by a variety of procedures – such as ARMS, CLEAVASE FRAGMENT LENGTH POLYMORPHISM ANALYSIS, SINGLE-BASE EXTENSION, SSCP ANALYSIS.

Any kind of point mutation in a sample of nucleic acid can

potentially interfere with sequence-based diagnostic tests or with other procedures used for examining/amplifying specific sequences of nucleotides.

A point mutation can be inserted into a target sequence by various techniques: see, for example, RECOMBINEERING and SITE-DIRECTED MUTAGENESIS. (See also CHIMERAPLAST.)

(2) The phrase is sometimes used to include – in addition – those cases in which a single nucleotide is inserted or deleted, leading to a FRAME-SHIFT MUTATION.

poky mutant (of *Neurospora*) See MATERNAL INHERITANCE.

pol See RETROVIRUSES.

polar mutation Any mutation which affects not only the gene in which it occurs but also other gene(s) located downstream on the same operon. For example, in the LAC OPERON, a mutation in *lacY* may affect the synthesis of permease and trans-acetylase, although not the synthesis of β-galactosidase. If promoter-distal genes are strongly inhibited the mutation is said to be strongly polar.

polarity (of strands of DNA) See DNA.

polishing A non-specific term that has been used e.g. to refer to the removal of 3′ overhangs, using an exonuclease, to prepare fragments for blunt-ended ligation. [Example of use of term: Nucleic Acids Res (2005) 33(16):5172–5180; BioTechniques (2005) 38(3):451–458.]

A 'polishing kit' (marketed by Stratagene, La Jolla CA) employs the 3′ exonuclease function of *Pfu* DNA polymerase to create blunt-ended products from PCR-generated amplicons formed by *Taq* DNA polymerase (an enzyme which yields PCR products having single-stranded 3′ extensions owing to its EXTENDASE ACTIVITY).

(See also END-IT DNA END-REPAIR KIT.)

polony A 'PCR colony' formed when a target sequence of DNA is amplified by PCR within a thin film of polyacrylamide gel on a glass microscope slide [early description: Nucleic Acids Res (1999) 27(24):e34]. The purpose of the polyacrylamide is to retard diffusion of the PCR products – which therefore remain localized and accumulate to form a 'colony'. A large number of such colonies may be formed on a single slide.

It has been reported that DNA in polonies may be used for *in situ* transcription, translation and protein folding [Nucleic Acids Res (2005) 33(17):e145].

poly(A) tailing (of RNA) The process of adding a poly(A) tail to the 3′ end of RNA molecules – mediated e.g. by a poly(A)-polymerase from *Escherichia coli*.

One reason for the poly(A) tailing of RNA is to incorporate a 3′ primer-binding site to facilitate reverse transcription to cDNA and subsequent amplification of the cDNA by PCR [example: BioTechniques (2005) 39(4):519–525].

poly-MBD proteins See CPG ISLAND.

polyacrylamide A polymer of ACRYLAMIDE prepared e.g. with a chemical catalyst such as METHYLENEBISACRYLAMIDE – which promotes cross-linking (polymerization) of the acrylamide.

Polyacrylamide gels are used for separating small/ medium-sized fragments of nucleic acid by GEL ELECTROPHORESIS

(cf. AGAROSE); they are also used e.g. for separating proteins.

In polyacrylamide gels, the *pore size* depends on: (i) concentration of acrylamide, and (ii) proportion of cross-linking agent in the mixture. In the electrophoresis of nucleic acids, the ratio acrylamide: cross linker (Bis) is often ~19:1. For the electrophoresis of proteins, higher ratios – up to e.g. ~40:1 – may be used.

(See also SDS–PAGE.)

polybrene (hexadimethrine bromide) A polycationic compound used e.g. for enhancing viral infection of cells *in vitro*; polybrene is reported to enhance receptor-independent adsorption of at least some virions to the membranes of target cells.

[Use of polybrene in lentiviral and adenoviral gene transfer to human tumor cells *in vitro*: BioTechniques (2006) 40(5): 573–576.]

polycistronic mRNA A molecule of mRNA that encodes two or more gene products; polycistronic mRNAs are produced by transcription of an OPERON.

polycomb-group genes Genes, found in diverse species, whose products have an EPIGENETIC function.

In the fruit-fly *Drosophila*, polycomb-group genes encode transcriptional repressors which function via DNA elements designated polycomb-group response elements. (Trithorax-group genes of *Drosophila* encode transcriptional activators which function via trithorax-group response elements.)

In *Drosophila*, the sequence-specific DNA-binding protein Pho forms two types of complex, one of which (containing the dSfmbt protein) is involved in repression of *HOX* genes via the *HOX* gene polycomb response elements (PREs); it was proposed that this repression complex, bound to PREs, interacts selectively with methylated histones to maintain a polycomb-repressed state [Genes Dev (2006) 20:1110–1122].

In *Drosophila*, polycomb-group products have established roles in regulating homeotic genes, but they are also reported to be involved in regulating the expression of cyclin A (and, hence, having a role in the control of the cell cycle) [Genes Dev (2006) 20:501–513].

Deregulation of the human polycomb-group genes may be linked to various hematological and epithelial cancers [Hum Mol Genet (2005) 14(suppl 1):R93–R100].

The target genes of polycomb-group proteins have been mapped in a genome-wide study of human embryonic fibroblasts [Genes Dev (2006) 20:1123–1136].

polyethylene glycol (PEG) Any of a range of polymers having the general formula: $H(OCH_2.CH_2)_nOH$; those polymers with a molecular weight above ~1000 are white solids – the others are liquids.

PEG has a variety of uses. For example, it is used for CELL FUSION and as a precipitating agent in clinical chemistry. An aqueous solution of PEG is used for concentrating various solutions and suspensions (including serum); the solution or suspension is placed in a tube of semipermeable material which is partly submerged in the PEG solution – water being withdrawn from the tube by osmosis.

A brief incubation in an alkaline (pH 13.3–13.5) solution of

60% PEG 200 has been reported to allow bacteria, eukaryotic tissue, whole blood etc. to be used directly for PCR without further preparation [BioTechniques (2006) 40(4):454–458].

polyethyleneimine   See PEI.

polygenic mRNA   *Syn.* POLYCISTRONIC MRNA.

polyhedrin   A protein encoded by the NUCLEAR POLYHEDROSIS VIRUSES that forms the matrix of the intracellular *occlusion bodies* of these viruses: see BACULOVIRIDAE for details.

(cf. GRANULIN.)

The promoter of the polyhedrin-encoding gene is used e.g. in BACULOVIRUS EXPRESSION SYSTEMS because it acts as a strong promoter within insect cells.

polylinker   (MCS, multiple cloning site)   A DNA segment that contains a number of close or overlapping recognition sites for *different* types of RESTRICTION ENDONUCLEASE. A polylinker is included in a VECTOR for flexibility in manipulation (i.e. the choice of various restriction enzymes) when inserting target DNA into the vector.

The orientation of an insert within a vector can be predetermined e.g. by using a vector that includes a polylinker containing an asymmetric array of cloning sites and using fragments which are flanked by dissimilar STICKY ENDS that permit insertion in only one orientation.

polymerase chain reaction   See PCR.

polymorph   See PMN.

polymorphic   (*adj.*)   Refers to a locus, in a given sequence of nucleic acid, at which the composition varies among different samples of that sequence.

polymorphonuclear leukocyte   See PMN.

polynucleotide kinase   Any (ATP-dependent) enzyme of EC subclass 2.7 which catalyzes the addition of phosphate to the 5′-OH terminal of a nucleotide. Polynucleotide kinase is used e.g. for 5′ END LABELING using labeled phosphate.

(See also END-IT DNA END-REPAIR KIT.)

polynucleotide phosphorylase   In (e.g.) *Escherichia coli*: an enzyme that degrades RNA exonucleolytically and which can also polymerize ribonucleoside diphosphates. Another role is the addition of nucleotides to poly(A) tails [Proc Natl Acad Sci USA (2000) 97(22):11966–11971] – a role for which this enzyme appears to be relatively unimportant in the bacterium *Bacillus subtilis* [J Bacteriol (2005) 187(14):4698–4706].

Polynucleotide phosphorylase is a component of the DEGRADOSOME.

polyomaviruses   A group of small (~45 nm), icosahedral, non-enveloped viruses (genome: ccc dsDNA) which include BK virus, JC VIRUS and simian virus 40 (see SV40). These viruses appear to be common in their mammalian (including human) hosts, and – unlike PAPILLOMAVIRUSES – can be propagated readily in appropriate types of cell culture; they are resistant to lipid solvents and to low pH.

polyribosome   *Syn.* POLYSOME.

polysome   (polyribosome)   A molecule of mRNA carrying a number of ribosomes distributed along its length, the stage of translation of the mRNA-encoded polypeptide being different at each ribosome.

Polysome analysis in CELL-FREE PROTEIN SYNTHESIS systems has identified certain rate-limiting steps; for example, dilution of translation factors in the lysate is one limitation, and it was shown that the addition of purified elongation factors can increase the rate of protein synthesis [Biotechnol Bioeng (2005) 91(4):425–435].

polytene chromosome   See POLYTENIZATION.

polytenization   Repetitive replication of chromosomes in which daughter chromosomes do not separate – producing a ribbon-like *polytene* chromosome (a 'giant chromosome') consisting of many chromosomes arranged parallel to one another.

Polytenization occurs in certain ciliates – and in some of the cells in plants and insects.

polyvinylidene fluoride   See PVDF.

positive control   (in operons)   See OPERON.

positive selection   (direct selection)   Selection which is based on the presence of a given feature or the occurrence of a given reaction.

(Compare NEGATIVE SELECTION.)

post-segregational killing   Any plasmid-encoded mechanism in which, following division of the host cell, a daughter cell which lacks a plasmid is killed by a plasmid-encoded toxin; such a mechanism promotes the presence of the particular plasmid in the bacterial population by eliminating plasmid-free cells.

In one mechanism, translation of a stable, plasmid-encoded toxin is blocked in the presence of unstable plasmid-encoded antisense RNAs; in a plasmid-free daughter cell, the toxin-encoding mRNA (from the parent cell) can be translated to a lethal toxin in the absence of antisense RNA.

A further example is the CCD MECHANISM.

post-transcriptional gene silencing   See PTGS.

potyviruses   Viruses of the potato virus Y group. These viruses include potato virus Y, soybean mosaic virus and the tobacco etch virus (see TEV).

PP$_i$ See PYROPHOSPHATE.

pPICZ vector   A 3.3 kb plasmid vector (Invitrogen, Carlsbad CA) designed for high-level, inducible, intracellular expression of recombinant proteins in the yeast *Pichia pastoris* (see PICHIA). The plasmid, carrying the gene of interest, integrates stably in the *Pichia* genome.

Using the strong promoter of the *AOX1* gene, control of expression is achieved with a *lac*-based system. Subsequent purification of the isolated recombinant protein can be facilitated e.g. via a SIX-HISTIDINE TAG (encoded as a C-terminal sequence in the plasmid).

The pPICZ plasmid includes a gene encoding resistance to ZEOCIN. By using increasing concentrations of Zeocin™ it is possible to select for cells in which multiple copies of the construct have integrated in the genome; in some cases it has been found that a higher copy number results in increased levels of expression of the recombinant protein.

A related plasmid, pPICZα (3.6 kb), is designed for the production of a secreted recombinant protein. This plasmid contains an N-terminal sequence (α-factor) which functions as a secretion signal.

Prader–Willi syndrome   See GENETIC IMPRINTING.

PRD (PTS regulation domain)   See CATABOLITE REPRESSION.

pre-mRNA   See SPLIT GENE.

(See also QUADRUPLEX DNA.)

prey protein   See e.g. YEAST TWO-HYBRID SYSTEM.

primary mutation   See BACK MUTATION and SUPPRESSOR MUTATION.

primase   See RNA POLYMERASE.

prime plasmid   A (circular) plasmid which has excised from a chromosome aberrantly. During the excision process, the plasmid may have left behind a part of its sequence and taken some chromosomal DNA (type I prime plasmid). A type II prime plasmid is an *entire* excised plasmid which contains additional chromosomal DNA.

primer   An oligonucleotide, base-paired to a template sequence, which (usually) must be present before a DNA polymerase (or a reverse transcriptase) can synthesize a complementary strand on the template. The DNA polymerase, or the reverse transcriptase, *extends* a primer by sequentially adding nucleotides, as dictated by the nucleotide sequence of the template strand; nucleotides are added in a 5′-to-3′ direction from the 3′ end of the primer.

In vivo, a primer is generally a short oligonucleotide (RNA) synthesized by an RNA polymerase as an initial step in DNA synthesis – the primer being extended by a DNA polymerase and the primer itself being subsequently replaced by DNA. In at least some eukaryotes, when the DNA is synthesized dis-

PRIMER: some examples

Primer	Use (e.g.)
Anchor primer	A primer which binds to a specific *known* sequence – used when the other primer in a primer pair binds to an unknown or variable sequence (see e.g. entry ANCHORED PCR)
Arbitrary-sequence primer	A primer with a non-specific or random sequence used in certain forms of TYPING; some of these primers bind to 'best-fit' sequences in genomic DNA and may then be extended (see entry AP-PCR)
Broad-range primer	A primer which can be used to amplify DNA of a given sequence from each of a wide range of species, all the species sharing a common target sequence; broad-range primers can be used, for example, to detect the presence of *any* bacterial species by amplifying a conserved region of the 16S rRNA gene common to all bacteria
Bumper primer	A primer whose extension is used to displace a strand located downstream on the same template (see entries STRAND DISPLACEMENT and SDA)
Competimer	A *non*-extendable primer used in certain types of quantitative PCR (see entry COMPETIMER)
Degenerate primer	One of a set of primers whose binding site has been predicted e.g. on the basis of the amino acid sequence in a polypeptide (see entry DEGENERATE PRIMER)
Forward primer	A primer which binds to a non-coding strand; when extended it replicates the coding strand (see entry FORWARD PRIMER)
Inner primer	One of a pair of primers used in the second phase of nested PCR; it binds to a subterminal region of the initial amplicon
Outer primer	One of a pair of primers used in the first phase of nested PCR
PCR primer	Any primer used in PCR; PCR primers are sometimes referred to as *amplimers*
Reverse primer	A primer which binds to a coding strand; when extended it replicates the non-coding strand (see entry FORWARD PRIMER)
Self-reporting primer	A PCR primer carrying a quenched fluorophore which is activated during the formation of double-stranded amplicons (see entry SELF-REPORTING PRIMER)
T_m-shift primer	A type of primer involved in the formation of (dsDNA) products which can be identified by their melting curve characteristics (see e.g. SNP GENOTYPING)
Universal primer	A broad-range primer or, in general, any primer which anneals to a common sequence on a range of different molecules

continuously as a series of Okazaki fragments (as in lagging strand synthesis) a primer consisting of a mixture of deoxyribonucleotides and ribonucleotides is apparently synthesized to initiate each Okazaki fragment (see OKAZAKI FRAGMENT).

In some instances, an oligonucleotide primer is not a prerequisite for DNA synthesis: see e.g. *protein priming* in the entry PHAGE φ29.

In vitro, primers are normally designed for the synthesis of specific sequences of nucleotides, a given primer serving to fix the location at which synthesis begins in a template strand – i.e. primers determine that part of a template strand which is to be copied. An exception to this is the primer of arbitrary sequence: see 'Arbitrary-sequence primer' in the table.

Factors which govern the binding ('annealing') of a primer to its target sequence are the same as those which govern PROBE–target binding. Annealing of primers in PCR-based diagnostic tests is carried out under conditions of the highest stringency in order to achieve a suitable level of specificity.

The normal functioning of a primer requires that its 3'-end terminal nucleotide base-pairs with the correct (complementary) base in the template strand – even if mismatched base(s) occur elsewhere in the primer; extension from the 3' end of a primer is either significantly inhibited or blocked by a mismatch at this site.

Primer design (in terms of base sequence) reflects various requirements. In diagnostic tests, for example, primers must anneal to a highly specific target sequence. By contrast, so-called broad-range bacterial primers are designed to anneal to conserved sequences found in all bacterial 16S rRNA genes, and such primers can be used to detect *any* species of bacteria in a sample. Computer programs can assist in the design of primers for special uses [e.g. primer design for studies with bisulfite-treated genomic DNA: Nucleic Acids Res (2005) 33 (1):e9]. (See also UNIVERSAL NUCLEOTIDE.)

In addition to their main role, primers can be modified in various ways in order to fulfill extra functions. For example, primers may be labeled with a dye to facilitate detection of amplified products, or 5'-end-labeled with BIOTIN in order to immobilize a particular strand of amplified DNA. A PCR primer may carry a 5' tag (i.e. extension) that incorporates a promoter sequence so that (dsDNA) products can be transcribed; note that the *tag* does not bind to the target sequence.

PCR-generated fragments examined by DGGE (q.v.) may incorporate a 5' GC-rich tag (again, not bound by the primer-binding site) which serves to prevent unwanted *total* melting of dsDNA fragments at the concentrated end of the gradient.

A *non-extendable* primer is used in some types of quantitative PCR: see e.g. COMPETIMER.

Some examples of primers are listed in the table.

primer–dimer In PCR: an artefact formed when the 3' ends of two primers are mutually complementary; during the extension phase, each primer uses the other as a template, forming two double-stranded primers in tandem.

The formation of primer–dimers may be problematic e.g. in MULTIPLEX PCR.

primer exclusion See PCR CLAMPING.

primer-extension inhibition The principle underlying several techniques – see e.g. TERMINAL TRANSFERASE-DEPENDENT PCR and TOEPRINTING.

primer sequestration A technique (USB Corporation, Cleveland OH) used in HOT-START PCR; it involves sequestration of the primers at the lower temperatures prior to the initial stage of denaturation. In this process, the primers bind to a recombinant protein (present in the reaction mixture) which is inactivated at the initial denaturation step, following which the primers are released to function in the normal way.

primer walking The sequential use of a number of different primers which bind at successive sites along the length of a template strand, the binding sequence of a given primer being within the sequence covered by extension of the previous primer.

Primer walking can be used e.g. for solid-phase sequencing of DNA (by the DIDEOXY METHOD) in which strands of 5'-BIOTINylated template DNA (up to about 10 kb) are initially immobilized on Dynabeads® coated with streptavidin. After each sequencing reaction (with a given primer) the newly synthesized strands are eluted by formamide and examined in a sequencing gel. The immobilized template strand is then reconditioned by treatment with sodium hydroxide, washed, and used again for the next round of sequencing.

(See also DNA SEQUENCING.)

printing (*biotechnol.*) The process of adding probes to a glass or other surface – e.g. by *in situ* synthesis.

pRNA See PACKAGING (of phage DNA).

probe (*mol. biol.*) (1) Any short (single) strand of DNA, RNA or PNA which is *complementary* to a specific target sequence of nucleotides and which is used to detect, identify, amplify or monitor that target sequence by binding to it, permanently or transiently; binding, by the probe, signals the presence of the given target sequence (qualitatively or quantitatively) and is registered in various ways – usually involving the direct or indirect *labeling* of the probe (see PROBE LABELING and also UNLABELED PROBE).

(Compare BINARY PROBE; see also UNIVERSAL NUCLEOTIDE.)

(See sense (2), below, for a note on *double-stranded* DNA probes.)

Commonly, the DNA in which the *target* sequences may occur is immobilized and then exposed to many copies of one or more types of *free* probe (i.e. probes in solution) under appropriate conditions; after removal of unbound probes, by washing, the presence of (any) bound probes may be detected e.g. by their labels.

The term *probe* is also used to refer to immobilized oligonucleotides in a MICROARRAY. (See also LINE PROBE ASSAY and REVERSE HYBRIDIZATION.)

Probe–target binding is strongly influenced by factors such as electrolyte concentration and temperature. The conditions can be arranged so that probes will bind to their targets only

PROBE: some examples

Probe	Use (e.g.)
Abasic-site mimic	A (quenched) fluorescent probe used for detecting products in an isothermal method for DNA amplification (see RPA, sense 1)
bDNA probe	Quantitation of pathogens by a signal amplification process (see entry BDNA ASSAY)
Binary probe	A composite probe used e.g. in FRET-based systems and in the PYRENE BINARY PROBE approach
Capture probe	A biotinylated probe used e.g. for capturing the target sequence and linking it to streptavidin-coated DYNABEADS in a CROSS-LINKING ASSAY (also used in other procedures)
Degenerate probe	One of a set of probes used e.g. when the target sequence is not completely known but has been predicted (see the entry DEGENERATE PROBE)
End probe	See the entry CHROMOSOME WALKING
Hybridization protection probe	Detection of pathogens in clinical samples (see the entry ACCUPROBE)
LightCycler™ probe	Monitoring REAL-TIME PCR; quantitation of target sequences
LightUp® probe	Monitoring real-time PCR (see the entry LIGHTUP PROBE)
2′-O-methyl oligo probe	Probing RNA, e.g. in Northern blot analysis
Molecular beacon probe	Monitoring real-time PCR and NASBA; quantitation of target sequences (see the entry MOLECULAR BEACON PROBE)
Molecular inversion probe	SNP genotyping (see the entry MOLECULAR INVERSION PROBE GENOTYPING)
Molecular zipper	Isothermal, real-time amplification of DNA (see the entry MOLECULAR ZIPPER)
PACE 2C probe	Combination probe diagnostic test for detecting the bacterial pathogens *Chlamydia trachomatis* and *Neisseria gonorrhoeae* in clinical samples in a single assay (see the entry PACE 2C)
Padlock probe	Confirmation of sequences. Identification of variation in sequences. Detection of SARS virus in clinical samples (see the entry PADLOCK PROBE)
Pyrene binary probe	Detection of specific mRNAs (see the entry PYRENE BINARY PROBE)
Quantum dot probe	Multiplex approach in Western blot analysis (see the entry QUANTUM DOT PROBE)
Reporter probe	A probe involved e.g. in generating a fluorescent signal in a CROSS-LINKING ASSAY (q.v.)
RPA probe	Detection of products in a method for isothermal amplification of DNA: see abasic-site mimic, above
Scorpion probe	Monitoring PCR products (see the entry SCORPION PROBE)
Selector probe	Amplification of a number of specific target sequences in a single assay (see the entry SELECTOR-BASED MULTIPLEX PCR)
Smart probe	Detection of single-base mismatches, SNPs. Essentially similar in principle to the molecular beacon probe, but quenching of the fluorophore (in the unbound probe) is due to guanosine residues in the probe itself (see the entry SMART PROBE)
TaqMan® probe	Monitoring real-time PCR; quantitation of target sequences (see the entry TAQMAN PROBE)
Triple-strand probe	Detecting SNPs or e.g. single-base mismatches (see the entry TRIPLE-STRAND PROBE)

when probe and target sequences are *exactly* complementary to one another; such conditions are said to be *high-stringency* conditions and are used to promote high-level specificity in probe–target binding – necessary, for example, in diagnostic tests. Under these conditions, mismatches in base-pairing are not tolerated.

Low-stringency, in which the effect of mismatched base(s) is minimized by an appropriate choice of conditions, may be used for particular purposes (see e.g. AP-PCR).

Probe–target binding may occur (e.g.) ~25°C below the T_m (see entry THERMAL MELTING PROFILE) of the corresponding duplexed probe–target sequence. The temperature at which probe–target hybridization occurs can be manipulated by the use of agents (such as formamide) which decrease the T_m by a specified amount (depending on the concentration of agent used).

The probing of *RNA* target sequences (e.g. in Northern blot analysis) may be facilitated by using probes that consist of 2'-*O*-methyl oligoribonucleotides (instead of the usual 2'-deoxy oligoribonucleotides) [Nucleic Acids Res (1998) 26:2224–2229]. The stability of binding of these 2'-*O*-methyl oligonucleotide probes may be raised by the inclusion of LOCKED NUCLEIC ACIDS [see Nucleic Acids Res (2005) 33(16):5082–5093].

PNA is used e.g. in the LIGHTUP PROBE.

Uses of probes
The uses of probes include:
● Detection of single-base mutations/SNPs (e.g. MOLECULAR INVERSION PROBE GENOTYPING)
● Confirmation of sequence variation (e.g. PADLOCK PROBE)
● Monitoring progress in REAL-TIME PCR (q.v.)
● Quantitation of target sequences in real-time PCR
● Isothermal amplification of DNA (MOLECULAR ZIPPER)
● Amplification of specific target sequences (LIGASE CHAIN REACTION; SELECTOR-BASED MULTIPLEX PCR)
● Detection of mRNAs (e.g. PYRENE BINARY PROBE)
● Detection of pathogens in clinical samples (e.g. PACE 2C)
● Detection of toxin (or other) genes in DNA samples
● Localization of specific intracellular target sequences by *in situ* hybridization
● Identification of specific cloned sequences (e.g. COLONY HYBRIDIZATION)

Preparation of probes
Probes can be made in various ways. For example, they can be synthesized, directly, according to any required sequence of nucleotides; this option is available commercially. They can also be prepared e.g. by asymmetric PCR, the appropriate primer being used in excess, or by cloning.

(2) Any ligand used for the detection of a specific target – for example, a labeled antibody of the type used in Western blot analysis (e.g. QUANTUM DOT PROBE).

Note that a *double-stranded* DNA probe has been used to detect DNA-binding proteins (transcription factors) in the EMEA procedure.

probe labeling Any procedure in which a PROBE is modified –

either before or after binding to the target – in order to enable it to indicate the presence, quantity or location of the target.

There are many ways of labeling probes, and the following refers primarily to the labeling of oligonucleotide probes.

Labeling may be direct or indirect. In direct labeling the label is an intrinsic part of the probe. In indirect labeling the label is bound to the probe – often non-covalently – via an intermediate molecule.

Direct labeling methods
A radioactive label such as ^{32}P can be added to the terminal 5'-OH group of DNA (or RNA) by the enzyme polynucleotide kinase with [γ^{32}P]ATP, i.e. ATP labeled with ^{32}P at the terminal (γ) phosphate group; in this (end-labeling) reaction, the radioactive phosphate group is transferred to the 5'-OH terminus of the oligonucleotide.

Alternatively, a probe may be synthesized e.g. as a segment within a circular double-stranded cloning vector (such as a plasmid) and labeled by NICK TRANSLATION in a reaction mixture which includes radioactively labeled dNTPs. In this process, labeled nucleotides are incorporated randomly in the plasmid. The relevant sequence is subsequently excised and denatured to produce the single-stranded probes.

Radioactive probes can be detected by autoradiography.

Radioactive (= *isotopic*) labeling has been widely used e.g. for *in situ* hybridization. Radioactive labels are robust and are associated with good sensitivity; however, they have limited resolution. Other forms of labeling (*non-isotopic labeling*) are often preferred because of the hazards and costs that are associated with handling radioactive material.

Fluorescent labels are now popular because they are easy to handle and because there is currently an extensive range of fluorophores with diverse emission spectra, permitting multiplex working, if required.

Existing oligonucleotide probes can be labeled e.g. by a commercial process (ULYSIS®) in which a platinum–label complex forms a stable adduct at the N7 position of guanine; any of a variety of fluorescent dyes can be used as the label. This is a rapid and simple method of labeling.

As an alternative, ChromaTide™ nucleotides (marketed by Molecular Probes Inc, Eugene OR) can be incorporated into DNA or RNA during synthesis. These products consist of a nucleotide (for example, dUTP or UTP) covalently bound to a fluorescent label via a spacer link; again, any of a variety of dyes can be used as label. Depending on the particular dye–nucleotide product, incorporation may be carried out during e.g. PCR, *in vitro* transcription and/or reverse transcription; many of these products can be used for 3'-end labeling using the enzyme terminal deoxynucleotidyl transferase.

Another procedure for fluorescent labeling (ARES™, Molecular Probes) is a two-step method. Amine-modified nucleotides – 5-(3-aminoallyl)-dUTP – are first incorporated into DNA during synthesis, e.g. during reverse transcription; subsequently, an amine-reactive fluorophore binds covalently to the available amine groups in the DNA. Any of a number of amine-reactive dyes can be used – e.g. various Alexa Fluor®

dyes.

When labeling DNA probes during synthesis, the efficiency of the process can vary according e.g. to the type of DNA polymerase and to the site of labeling [BioTechniques (2005) 38(2):257–264].

(See also LIGHTUP PROBE.)

Indirect labeling methods

One common approach involves the initial insertion of a molecule of BIOTIN into the probe. This is usually achieved by incorporating covalently complexed biotin–nucleotide molecules into DNA or RNA during synthesis; this can be carried out e.g. during PCR. The probe can then be detected by using molecules of STREPTAVIDIN which are themselves linked to either a fluorophore (detected by fluorescence) or an enzyme – e.g. ALKALINE PHOSPHATASE (AP).

With an AP label the probe can be detected in several ways, depending on experimental arrangements. In some cases it may be appropriate to identify the location of a bound AP-labeled probe by a chromogenic reaction; for example, AP gives rise to a dark bluish/purple precipitate with the reagents 5-bromo-4-chloro-3-indolyl phosphate (BCIP) and nitroblue tetrazolium (NBT) – both reagents being used in the reaction.

Alternatively, AP can produce chemiluminescence (chemically generated light) with e.g. 1,2-dioxetane substrates such as AMPPD® and CSPD®.

Although the streptavidin–label complex is usually added *after* probe–target hybridization, it was reported earlier that short biotinylated probes which are *already* labeled with the streptavidin–alkaline phosphatase complex before use permit satisfactory probing [Nucleic Acids Res (1999) 27:703–705].

Indirect labeling can be carried out in a similar way using e.g. a DIGOXIGENIN tag.

ProBond™ nickel-chelating resin A (pre-charged) NICKEL-CHARGED AFFINITY RESIN (marketed by Invitrogen, Carlsbad CA) which is used e.g. for the purification of 6xHis-tagged proteins – e.g. those produced by expression vectors such as CHAMPION PET SUMO VECTOR or VOYAGER VECTORS.

[Examples of use: J Cell Physiol (2006) 206(1):103–111; Infect Immun (2006) 74(5):2676–2685; Mol Cell Biol (2006) 26 (12):4652–4663; BMC Cell Biol (2007) 8:9.]

processive enzyme Any enzyme that remains bound to the substrate as it repeatedly carries out its function.

producer cell line See e.g. PACKAGING PLASMID.

profile See e.g. DNA PROFILE.

programmable endonuclease A RESTRICTION ENDONUCLE-ASE which is linked (covalently) to a molecule that binds to a specific sequence of nucleotides in double-stranded DNA; sequence-specific binding of the latter molecule directs the activity of the restriction enzyme to a *particular* recognition (cutting) site in the region of binding.

The molecule linked to the restriction endonuclease may be e.g. a DNA-binding protein or a synthetic triplex-forming oligonucleotide (see TRIPLEX DNA). The conjugate formed between a TFO and the restriction enzyme PvuII achieved a high level of cutting specificty at a given PvuII restriction

site [Nucleic Acids Res (2005) 33(22):7039–7047].

(See also TAGM.)

programmed ribosomal frameshifting See FRAMESHIFTING.

progressive multifocal leukoencephalopathy See JC VIRUS.

prohead The precursor of a phage head (capsid) prior to the insertion of the genomic nucleic acid.

proinsulin (human, recombinant) See HUMAN INSULIN PRB.

prokaryote Any organism (limited to species of the domains Archaea and Bacteria) whose cellular structure is characterized by the absence of a nuclear membrane and the absence of organelles such as mitochondria. (cf. EUKARYOTE.) There are, in addition, many other basic differences between prokaryotes and eukaryotes – e.g. differences in ribosomes (and in translation factors etc.), in the types of enzyme which act on nucleic acids, in proteasomes, in membrane lipids, in various aspects of metabolism, and in the general organization of the genome.

The *typical* prokaryotic genome is a circular dsDNA molecule (chromosome) which may be present in more than one copy, depending e.g. on growth temperature and species. Although prokaryotes usually contain only one *type* of chromosome, the cells of e.g. *Vibrio cholerae* contain two dissimilar chromosomes which jointly constitute the bacterial genome [Nature (2000) 406:477–483]. (See also NUCLEOID.)

Some prokaryotic chromosomes are not ccc dsDNA. For example, the chromosomes are molecules of *linear* dsDNA in the bacterium BORRELIA BURGDORFERI.

promiscuous plasmid Any conjugative plasmid which is able to promote self-transmission among bacteria of widely differing species/genera.

promoter control (in operons) See OPERON.

promoter core *Syn.* CORE PROMOTER.

promoter trapping See GENE TRAPPING.

Pronase (proprietary name) A mixture of enzymes, including both exopeptidases and endopeptidases, obtained from the Gram-positive bacterium *Streptomyces griseus*. It is used for non-specific degradation of proteins.

proof reading (editing) During DNA replication: removal of an incorrectly incorporated nucleotide and its replacement with the correct nucleotide; this kind of activity is mediated only by certain types of DNA-DEPENDENT DNA POLYMERASE (i.e. those which have a 3′-to-5′ exonuclease capability).

prophage See BACTERIOPHAGE and LYSOGENY.

propidium iodide A fluorescent phenanthridinium dye which binds to DNA and RNA; it is generally excluded from living cells and is used e.g. as a stain for dead cells (see e.g. LIVE/DEAD BACLIGHT BACTERIAL VIABILITY KIT).

Compared with the related dye, ETHIDIUM BROMIDE, this dye is more water-soluble and less membrane permeant.

(See also DNA STAINING.)

protamine sulfate An agent used e.g. for the enhancement of virus-mediated transfer of genes into cells (by both retroviral and non-retroviral vectors).

[Examples of use: BioTechniques (2006) 40(5):573–576; Virol J (2006) 3:14.]

protease inhibitors (antiretroviral)   A category of ANTIRETRO-VIRAL AGENTS which inhibit *retroviral* protease: an enzyme (encoded in the *pol* region of the viral genome) that is needed for post-translational processing of viral proteins; protease inhibitors include amprenavir, indinavir, nelfinavir, ritonavir and saquinavir.

proteasome   A hollow, cylindrical, intracellular structure with internal active enzymic sites involved e.g. in the degradation of earmarked proteins and processing of exogenous antigens.

Prokaryotic proteasomes are of the 20S type while those of eukaryotes are of the 26S type. The cellular degradative pathway also differs in prokaryotes and eukaryotes in that e.g. the process is UBIQUITIN-dependent in eukaryotes.

For degradation, a given protein must initially be unfolded in order to enter the proteasome; this is an energy-dependent process, and AAA ATPASES are known to form a part of the multi-protein complex of at least some proteasomes.

Degradation of a eukaryotic protein is preceded by the sequential (cascade) binding of a number of ubiquitin molecules to the given protein; this involves three types of enzyme: an activating enzyme (E1), a ubiquitin-conjugating enzyme (E2) and a ubiquitin–protein ligase (E3). (Such ubiquitinylation is involved not only in degradative action but e.g. in regulating protein activities and influencing subcellular location.)

(See also SUMOYLATION.)

The ubiquitin-binding cascade seems to proceed as follows. In an ATP-dependent reaction, the active-site cysteine of E1 forms a thioester with ubiquitin; ubiquitin is then transferred to E2. The ubiquitin ligase (E3) then mediates attachment of ubiquitin to (usually) the ε-amino group of a lysine residue in the target protein. Some E3 enzymes form an intermediate thioester with ubiquitin before transferring it to the target protein; however, most do not form such a bond – but rather bind simultaneously to E2 and the target protein to facilitate ubiquitinylation of the protein. The way in which ubiquitin passes from E2 to the target protein is not fully understood. Some data suggest that most types of ubiquitin ligase activate E2 enzymes allosterically [Proc Natl Acad Sci USA (2005) 102(52):18890–18895].

(See also CULLIN-RING COMPLEXES and N-END RULE.)

[Proteasomes (minireview): Cell (2007) 129:659–662.]

protein A   A high-molecular-weight protein found in the cell wall in most strains of *Staphylococcus aureus*; protein A can be released, intact, from its covalent attachment to the (cell wall) polymer peptidoglycan by the enzyme LYSOSTAPHIN.

One of the domains of protein A binds with high specificity to the Fc portion of most types of IgG antibody and (via the Fab region) to immunoglobulins of other isotypes. This has been exploited in various techniques – for example, in a scintillation proximity assay for DNA binding by human p53 [BioTechniques (2006) 41(3):303–308].

Protein A has been used e.g. in affinity chromatography (for purification of IgG antibodies) and (in derivative form) in a QUANTUM DOT PROBE. (See also IMMUNO-PCR and SPA.)

(cf. PROTEIN G and SORTASE.)

protein analysis (*in vivo*)   See e.g. TEV.

protein–biotin ligase   See IN VIVO BIOTINYLATION.

protein design   The computer-aided design of synthetic (novel) proteins with the required characteristics or properties.

protein engineering   The creation of modified forms of a given protein (with required characteristics or properties) e.g. by recoding the protein's gene.

protein G   A protein, derived from group G streptococci, which apparently binds IgG of all subclasses; unlike PROTEIN A, it does not bind immunoglobulins of other isotypes.

protein kinase   Any of various ATP-dependent enzymes which phosphorylate particular residues in proteins – e.g. TYROSINE KINASE.

protein overexpression (protein overproduction)   See OVEREXPRESSION.

protein pIII   See PHAGE DISPLAY.

protein priming (of DNA replication)   See e.g. PHAGE φ29.

protein–protein interactions (detection)   See e.g. BACTERIOMATCH TWO-HYBRID SYSTEM, CYTOTRAP TWO-HYBRID SYSTEM and YEAST TWO-HYBRID SYSTEM.

protein splicing   See INTEIN.

protein synthesis (*in vitro*)   See CELL-FREE PROTEIN SYNTHESIS.

proteinase K   A non-specific serine protease which is effective over a wide range of pH.

protelomerase   An enzyme, encoded e.g. by certain bacteria and bacteriophages, which catalyzes the formation of closed (hairpin) terminal regions of genomic DNA (see TELOMERE). The target regions for protelomerase activity are reported to involve inverted repeat sequences, and the recognition of such sites may involve structure-specific as well as sequence-specific interaction.

[Mechanism of protelomerase activity: J Mol Biol (2004) 337(1):77–92.]

proto-*onc*   A *cellular* ONCOGENE.

proton PPase   See PYROPHOSPHATE.

protoplast   An osmotically sensitive structure produced *in vitro* by removal of the cell wall from a cell suspended in an isotonic or hypertonic medium; a protoplast therefore consists of the cell membrane and all that it encloses. Protoplasts can metabolize, and some are able to revert to normal cells under suitable conditions.

Bacterial protoplasts are resistant to infection by phages because phage receptors are lost with the outer layer of the cell.

(See also AUTOPLAST.)

prototroph   See AUXOTROPHIC MUTANT.

prototype (of a restriction enzyme)   See ISOSCHIZOMER.

provirus   Viral DNA integrated in the host's genome. A retroviral provirus is a reverse-transcribed viral genome.

(See also prophage in entries BACTERIOPHAGE and LYSOGENY.)

proximal box   See RNASE III.

pSC101   A ~9-kb low-copy-number mobilizable plasmid which encodes resistance to tetracycline; it has one EcoRI cleavage site. pSC101 has been used e.g. as a CLONING VECTOR.

pseudo-exons See SPLICING.

pseudo-mRNA A type of RNA molecule which resembles a normal mRNA but which has a disrupted reading frame so that it does not encode a full-length protein.

[Pseudo-mRNA: PLoS Genet (2006) 2(4):e23.]

pseudo-wild phenotype See SUPPRESSOR MUTATION.

pseudogene (truncated gene) A genomic sequence of nucleotides which may resemble an existing, functional gene but which nevertheless appears to be inactive (i.e. not expressed); failure of expression may be due e.g. to mutations affecting coding and/or control regions.

In some cases a pseudogene may resemble a DNA copy of an mRNA, with a short A–T tract corresponding to a poly(A) tail and a lack of intron-like sequences. (cf. RETROGENE.) Some pseudogenes exist in fragmented form.

Pseudogenes occur in both prokaryotes and eukaryotes. For example, truncated copies of the 5′ end of functional genes, possibly formed through duplication events, were reported in the channel catfish (*Ictalurus punctatus*) [Immunogenetics (2005) 57(5):374–383]. In the prokaryote *Mycobacterium leprae* (causal agent of leprosy) the genome was reported to contain ~27% pseudogenes [Nature (2001) 409:1007–1011], and pseudogenes have also been reported in K-12 strains of *Escherichia coli* [Nucleic Acids Res (2006) 34(1):1–9].

Pseudomonas aeruginosa A species of Gram-negative aerobic, oxidative (i.e. respiratory) bacteria which is catalase-positive and oxidase-positive, and is usually motile; it is an important opportunist pathogen in man and other animals (mucoid, i.e. alginate-producing, strains are particularly problematic e.g. in CYSTIC FIBROSIS). At least some of the organism's virulence factors are expressed via a QUORUM SENSING mechanism. *P. aeruginosa* is inherently insensitive to a number of common antibiotics.

The GC% of the genomic DNA is 67.

P. aeruginosa is the type species of the genus *Pseudomonas*.

pseudoparticle (of hepatitis C virus) An *in vitro* construct prepared by coating retroviral core particles with glycoproteins of hepatitis C virus (HCV); pseudoparticles may also include GREEN FLUORESCENT PROTEIN to facilitate the monitoring of infection.

Pseudoparticles were used e.g. in studies on the entry stage during the infection of cells by HCV [J Virol (2006) 80(10): 4940–4948].

pseudopromoter (1) Any promoter that functions *in vitro* but not *in vivo*.

(2) A promoter, constructed *in vitro*, that is able to function *in vitro* and *in vivo* [use of term (e.g.): Proc Natl Acad Sci USA (2002) 99(1):54–59].

pseudorecombination (1) During PCR cycling: the formation of hybrid products due to switching of polymerase activity from one template to another; this may occur e.g. when the reaction mixture contains different target sequences that have an appropriate level of homology. While this kind of effect is exploited in '*in vitro* evolution' (see e.g. DNA SHUFFLING), it may produce erroneous results e.g. when attempts are being made to quantitate a number of similar sequences in a multiplex PCR. One assay designed to estimate this effect reported recombination frequencies greater than 20% – with a higher rate of chimeric products apparently being produced from the longer templates [BioTechniques (2006) 40(4):499–507].

(2) In plant virology: a form of genetic change that occurs in viruses with bipartite or multipartite genomes; it is due to an exchange of (whole) sections of the genome (rather than to crossing-over).

pseudotype (*virol.*) A virion, formed by PHENOTYPIC MIXING, which contains the genome of one virus and component(s) of the co-infecting virus.

pseudotyping (*DNA technol.*) The genetic modification of a given virus which results in the surface components of the virion being replaced by those of a different virus; this is done in order to modify the range of receptors or types of cell to which the given virus can attach.

Pseudotyping is used e.g. in GENE THERAPY. For example, pseudotyping of adenovirus type 5 gave greater specificity in binding [J Virol (2001) 75:2972–2981], and cell targeting by type 41 has been modified by inserting a peptide ligand into the short-fiber knob [J Virol (2007) 81(6):2688–2699].

(See also VSV.)

pseudovirion A particle that consists of a viral capsid which encloses nucleic acid from the host cell.

ψ (psi) (1) A sequence in a retroviral genome that promotes the packaging of viral RNA during formation of virions.

(2) A symbol for pseudouridine (5-β-D-ribofuranosyluracil).

psicofuranine (9-β-D-psicofuranosyladenine) A compound that has antimicrobial and antitumor activity; it is synthesized by the (Gram-positive) bacterium *Streptomyces hygroscopicus*. This agent inhibits biosynthesis of guanosine monophosphate by inhibiting xanthosine 5′-monophosphate (XMP) aminase. *Decoyinine* has a similar action.

PSK POST-SEGREGATIONAL KILLING.

pSM19035 A PLASMID, found e.g. in strains of *Streptococcus pyogenes*, that exhibits a high level of segregational stability resulting from the combined activity of several mechanisms for controlling COPY NUMBER – e.g. resolution of multimers (promoting segregation of monomers) and post-segregational killing in which plasmid-free cells are killed. A further, novel system has been reported for plasmid segregation which is encoded by genes δ and ω [J Bacteriol (2006) 188(12):4362–4372].

psoralens (furocoumarins) Various (tricyclic) INTERCALATING AGENTS (present e.g. in certain fungi, and in tropical fruits) which can insert into dsDNA and dsRNA. After intercalation, irradiation (e.g. ~365 nm) causes the formation of covalent interstrand cross-links between pyrimidine bases.

Targeted, site-specific cross-linking with a psoralen may be achieved by means of triplex-directed methodology; in this approach, a psoralen is conjugated to a triplex-forming oligonucleotide (TFO: see TRIPLEX DNA) which is targeted to the required sequence [see e.g. Nucleic Acids Res (2005) 33(9): 2993–3001].

pSos vector See CYTOTRAP TWO-HYBRID SYSTEM.

pT-REx™-DEST31 vector A destination vector in the GATE-WAY SITE-SPECIFIC RECOMBINATION SYSTEM.

pTcINDEX See EXPRESSION VECTOR.

PTGS Post-transcriptional GENE SILENCING: in animals, plants and fungi, any of several types of phenomenon in which the transcript of a gene is either blocked (translational silencing) or degraded. One of these phenomena involves endogenous, genomically encoded molecules of RNA: see MICRORNAS. In another type of process, effector molecules are formed e.g. in response to intracellular double-stranded RNA (dsRNA) of a certain minimum length: see RNA INTERFERENCE. Both of these phenomena involve RNA processing by similar types of enzyme (see e.g. DICER). The term *co-suppression* is also used to refer to PTGS in plants.

As well as their involvement in RNA interference, siRNAs are also involved in *transcriptional gene silencing* (TGS): see SIRNA.

PTS Phosphoenolpyruvate-dependent phosphotransferase system: a transport system involved in transmembrane uptake of various substrates by bacteria; some of the components of the PTS are also involved in the regulation of (certain) catabolic OPERONS, including the LAC OPERON of *Escherichia coli* (see also CATABOLITE REPRESSION).

In all cases, the energy (for transport and phosphorylation) is derived from phosphoenolpyruvate (PEP).

The following descriptions of two examples of PTS-based transport in *E. coli* are used to illustrate various aspects of PTS involvement in the regulation of a number of catabolic operons (i.e. operons which specify enzymes etc. involved in the catabolism (breakdown) of particular types of substrate).

In each case, energy is fed into the system by the sequential transfer of phosphate, from PEP, to two soluble, cytoplasmic energy-coupling proteins: *enzyme I* (designated I) and *HPr protein* (designated H). Thus, phosphate from PEP is initially transferred to I and then from I to H. From H, phosphate is transferred to a *permease* (= *enzyme II*, designated II) in order to provide the energy for uptake of a given substrate. A cell contains a number of different permeases – a particular substrate being taken up by a particular permease; note that the molecules of I and H are not specific to any particular permease, i.e. they can be used for the phosphorylation of any of the cell's permeases.

The *E. coli* mannitol permease is a membrane-associated complex consisting of three domains: IIA, IIB and IIC. The IIC domain seems to contribute to a transmembrane channel for uptake of the substrate. It appears that the IIA domain is phosphorylated (by H) and transfers phosphate to the IIB domain – at which site the substrate is phosphorylated prior to entering the cytoplasm; phosphorylation of the substrate is an essential part of the uptake process in all types of PTS.

The *E. coli* glucose permease consists of (i) a membrane-bound complex of domains IIC and IIB and (ii) domain IIA on a separate, cytoplasmic protein. In the *presence* of glucose IIA is phosphorylated by H, and the phosphate is transferred from IIA to IIB – and thence to the substrate (glucose). In the *absence* of glucose, IIA remains in a phosphorylated state and activates the enzyme adenylate cyclase, stimulating the synthesis of cyclic AMP (cAMP). cAMP binds to the cAMP-receptor protein (CRP) and the resulting complex permits transcription of various catabolic operons in the presence of their respective inducers (see CATABOLITE REPRESSION).

Components are arranged in different ways in some of the permeases. Thus, for example, in enteric bacteria the fructose permease consists of a membrane-bound protein – which includes the IIC and IIB domains – and a cytoplasmic protein which incorporates the functions of both IIA and H. In the non-enteric species *Rhodobacter capsulatus* the functions of IIA, H and I are combined in a single, separate protein.

Note that, in catabolite repression, the IIA component of the glucose permease has a regulatory role in the typical PTS-mediated mechanism in Gram-negative bacteria, whereas the IIB and HPr~P components have a regulatory role in PRD-mediated mechanisms.

PTS regulation domain (PRD) See CATABOLITE REPRESSION.

pUC plasmids A family of small high-copy-number plasmids, derivatives of which are used e.g. as CLONING VECTORS; they contain multiple restriction sites (for inserting target DNA), and a sequence from the *lacZ* gene (encoding the α-PEPTIDE), and an ampicillin-resistance gene. When these plasmids replicate in suitable host cells, the presence of target DNA (as an insert within the plasmid) can be detected by blue–white screening (see PBLUESCRIPT for the mechanism).

pulsed-field gel electrophoresis See PFGE.

PureLink™ plasmid purification systems Systems (Invitrogen, Carlsbad CA) used for the rapid isolation of plasmids from bacteria (in about 30 minutes).

The apparatus consists of rows of cups in a 'filter plate' that are aligned vertically over cups in a 'receiver plate'; cups in the receiver plate contain isopropanol.

Bacterial (liquid) culture is added to the cups in the filter plate; lysis buffer is then added to each cup and incubation is carried out for 10 minutes. The whole is then centrifuged for 15 minutes at 3000*g* – during which plasmids (released from the cells) pass through the filter plate into the corresponding cups in the receiver plate. The filter plate is discarded, and the DNA pellets within cups in the receiver plate are washed with 70% ethanol. After discarding the supernatant the pellet is air-dried for 5 minutes and then suspended in buffer.

puromycin 6-dimethyl-3′-deoxy-3′-*p*-methoxyphenylalanyl-amino adenosine: a nucleoside antibiotic that blocks protein synthesis by entering the ribosomal A site and forming a covalent bond with the peptidyl–tRNA in the P site, thereby causing premature chain termination. Puromycin is effective against both prokaryotic and eukaryotic cells.

[Examples of use of puromycin as a selective agent: PLoS Biol (2006) 4(10): e309; Retrovirology (2006) 3:51.]

pVAX™200-DEST vector A destination vector in the GATE-

WAY SITE-SPECIFIC RECOMBINATION SYSTEM.

PVDF Polyvinylidene fluoride: a compound used for making membranes; an alternative to nitrocellulose. Membranes of PVDF have greater mechanical strength (as compared with nitrocellulose), and they are reported to have better protein-retention characteristics under chemically harsh conditions.

The FluoroTrans® PVDF membrane (Pall Life Sciences, Ann Arbor MI) is used e.g. for western blotting studies.

pXO1, pXO2 Plasmids found in virulent strains of BACILLUS ANTHRACIS (causal agent of anthrax); they encode anthrax toxin (pXO1) and the poly-D-glutamic acid bacterial cell capsule (pXO2), both of which are required for virulence of the pathogen.

Py–MS See PYROLYSIS.

pYES-DEST52 vector A destination vector in the GATEWAY SITE-SPECIFIC RECOMBINATION SYSTEM.

pyknosis (*histopathol.*) The shrinkage of a eukaryotic nucleus, forming a densely staining body.

(See also KARYOLYSIS.)

Pyr(6–4)Pyo See PYRIMIDINE DIMER.

pyrazinamidase See PNCA GENE.

pyrene binary probe A BINARY PROBE in which both of the oligonucleotides are labeled with a pyrene molecule such that these molecules are juxtaposed (and thus capable of forming an excited dimer – an *excimer*) when the probe is correctly hybridized to its target sequence. After a pulse of excitation, the lifetime of the fluorescence from the pyrene excimer is considerably longer than that of the background fluorescence which characterizes some cellular extracts; this permits the detection of fluorescence specifically from the excimer by using a *time-resolved emission spectra* (TRES) approach – in which the measurement of fluorescence begins only after the short-term background fluorescence has decayed.

Using TRES, pyrene binary probes have been useful for detecting specific mRNAs [Nucleic Acids Res (2006) 34(10): 3161–3168].

Pyrene fluorescence has also been exploited for monitoring the folding of RNA molecules [Nucleic Acids Res (2006) 34 (1):152–166].

pyrF gene (in *Escherichia coli*) See BACTERIOMATCH TWO-HYBRID SYSTEM.

pyrimidine dimer Two adjacent pyrimidine residues, in the same strand of DNA, which have become covalently cross-linked e.g. as a result of ULTRAVIOLET RADIATION; one example is the THYMINE DIMER (q.v.).

Cyclobutyl pyrimidine dimers (CPDs) may be repaired by PHOTOLYASE but this enzyme does not repair certain other products of ultraviolet radiation: the so-called (6–4) photoproducts (also referred to as Pyr(6–4)Pyo). A (6–4) photoproduct may form between a thymine residue and its adjacent (3′) cytosine residue – or between two adjacent cytosine residues – by the covalent linking of the 6-position and the 4-position of the two pyrimidines, respectively; the (6–4) photoproducts can be corrected e.g. by the excision repair system.

Pyrimidine dimers can block DNA replication. They can be detected e.g. by TERMINAL TRANSFERASE-DEPENDENT PCR.

CPDs have been reported to be an important source of UV-induced DNA breaks [EMBO J (2005) 24:3952–3962].

Pyrococcus A genus of thermophilic archaeans (see ARCHAEA). The species *P. furiosus* is the source of certain thermostable DNA polymerases used e.g. in PCR.

pyrogen Any of various, potentially lethal substances which, if introduced into the bloodstream, can affect body temperature; they typically give rise to fever if present at an appropriate concentration.

Recombinant proteins which are synthesized within Gram-negative bacteria (such as *Escherichia coli*) must be rendered free of the potent pyrogen LIPOPOLYSACCHARIDE (LPS), also called *endotoxin*, which forms a (normal) part of the Gram-negative cell envelope and which can be shed into the product.

LPS can be detected e.g. by the LAL TEST.

During the manufacture of recombinant proteins in *E. coli*, LPS can be removed from the product by appropriate downstream processing involving an efficient form of chromatographic separation such as ion-exchange or gel filtration.

pyrogram See PYROSEQUENCING.

pyrolysis Thermal degradation of a sample (*in vacuo* or in an inert gas) forming a range of (low-molecular-weight) compounds which can be analysed. Pyrolysis has been used e.g. in microbial taxonomy – the sample being a small quantity of microbial culture; in this context, the products of pyrolysis (the *pyrolysate*) are taken to be characteristic of the organism being studied and may be analyzed e.g. by pyrolysis–mass spectrometry (Py–MS).

A *filament* pyrolyser is one in which a platinum wire, coated with the sample, is heated by passing an electric current through it (cf. CURIE POINT PYROLYSIS). Pyrolysis can also be carried out in a laser-based instrument.

pyrophosphate Inorganic pyrophosphate (PP_i) or diphosphate; the ion $P_2O_7^{4-}$. Pyrophosphate is released by nucleoside triphosphates e.g. when they are incorporated (by DNA or RNA polymerase) into a growing strand of nucleic acid; the release can be monitored e.g. by the PIPER PYROPHOSPHATE ASSAY KIT.

Pyrophosphate is synthesized e.g. within animal and yeast mitochondria and in some photosynthetic bacteria; synthesis involves a proton PPase.

(See also PYROPHOSPHOROLYSIS-ACTIVATED POLYMERIZATION and PYROSEQUENCING.)

pyrophosphorolysis-activated polymerization (PAP) A form of nucleic acid amplification, involving temperature cycling, in which the extension of each primer is initially blocked by its 3′ terminal dideoxyribonucleotide (ddNMP); on annealing correctly to the template, in the presence of pyrophosphate, the ddNMP is excised (forming ddNTP) – so that the primer can be extended by DNA polymerase. Primers are used in pairs (cf. PCR) and cycling involves temperatures suitable for denaturation, annealing and extension. PAP is reported to be characterized by high-level specificity.

PAP has been used e.g. for allele-specific amplification. A multiplex form of PAP has been used to detect deletions in the human gene for factor IX [BioTechniques (2006) 40(5): 661–668].

Pyrosequencing™   A technique used for rapidly sequencing short, single-stranded fragments of DNA produced e.g. by PCR (Pyrosequencing, Uppsala, Sweden).

Target fragments are first immobilized on a solid surface.

Initially, primers bind to the immobilized target fragments. The reaction mixture includes (i) DNA polymerase, (ii) ATP sulfurylase, (iii) adenosine 5′-phosphosulfate (APS), (iv) firefly LUCIFERASE, (v) luciferin (the substrate for luciferase), and (vi) *apyrase*, an enzyme that degrades nucleotides.

Separately – at intervals of ~1 minute – the four types of deoxyribonucleoside triphosphate (dNTP) are added to the mixture, this addition being repeated cyclically; for example, the addition of [...A...T...G...C...A...T...G...C...A] takes ~9 minutes.

If a given, added nucleotide is complementary to the next free (unpaired) base in the (single-stranded) template (target), it will extend the primer strand *and release pyrophosphate*.

Pyrophosphate is converted to ATP by the enzyme ATP sulfurylase (in the presence of APS – which is present in the reaction mixture); the resulting ATP triggers the luciferase system, producing a burst of light (of intensity proportional to the amount of ATP). The light is recorded automatically as a spike on a time-based graph.

Note. If the *normal* nucleotide dATP (deoxyadenosine triphosphate) were used in this technique, the (ATP-dependent) luciferase system would generate light each time dATP was added to the reaction mixture – whether or not the nucleotide had been incorporated into the primer strand. Hence, instead of dATP, use is made of deoxyadenosine α-thiotriphosphate (dATPαS); this modified nucleotide is used as a substrate by DNA polymerase *but not* by luciferase.

If a particular, added nucleotide is complementary to the next *two* free bases, it will be incorporated into both sites, releasing a correspondingly larger amount of pyrophosphate; hence, the number of (consecutive) sites into which a given nucleotide is incorporated is signaled by the amount of light generated (shown by the height of the spike on the graph).

Apyrase continually degrades nucleotides in the reaction mixture. This enzyme acts on (i) each nucleotide added to the mixture, and (ii) the ATP derived from pyrophosphate.

If a given, added nucleotide is *not* complementary to the next free base, its degradation (by apyrase) will be complete by the time the next dNTP is due to be added; in this way, light produced at a given time can be linked to a particular dNTP.

Sequential addition of nucleotides to the primer strand is recorded as a series of spikes on the time-based graph (the *pyrogram*). Because a given spike of light (at a specific time) corresponds to the addition of a particular, known nucleotide, the final result (the series of spikes) indicates the sequence of nucleotides in the target.

A problem in the interpretation of results may arise if the target sequence contains one or more homopolymer stretches (such as TTTTT.....); this problem is due to the non-linear generation of light when more than about five nucleotides *of the same type* are incorporated consecutively.

Pyrosequencing has been used e.g. for subtyping *Helicobacter pylori* [FEMS Microbiol Lett (2001) 199:103–107]; for forensic analysis of mitochondria [BioTechniques (2002) 32:124–133]; for identifying bacterial contamination [FEMS Microbiol Lett (2003) 219:87–91]; for typing *Neisseria gonorrhoeae* (the *porB* gene) [J Clin Microbiol (2004) 42:2926–2934]; for detecting lamivudine resistance in hepatitis B virus (YMDD motif mutations) [J Clin Microbiol (2004) 42:4788–4795]; and for studying polymorphism in a malaria vaccine antigen [PLoS Med (2007) 4(3):e93].

With the use of specialized software, Pyrosequencing has been adapted to yield quantitative results and has been used e.g. for analyzing the methylation status of CpG sites in sequences of genomic DNA [BioTechniques (2003) 35:146–150; (2003) 35:152–156; (2006) 40:721–726].

With allele-specific primers, Pyrosequencing has been used in a method for determining the allele-specific methylation in samples of bisulfite-treated, PCR-amplified DNA [BioTechniques (2006) 41(6):734–739].

Q

q An indicator of the *long* arm of a CHROMOSOME; it is used when giving a particular location on a specific chromosome – e.g. 9q34, which refers to a location (34) on the long arm of chromosome 9.

Q L-Glutamine (alternative to Gln).

Q bases Certain modified forms of guanine found in molecules of tRNA. QUEUOSINE is one example.

(cf. Y BASES.)

Q-PNA Quencher-labeled PNA probe: see SELF-REPORTING PRIMER.

Q-tag A 45-amino-acid section of the enzyme β-galactosidase. Q-tags are used for the quantitative estimation of a (soluble) recombinant protein expressed from a vector; in the vector, the sequence encoding the protein and that encoding the Q-tag form a fusion gene. When expressed, the protein – which is Q-tagged at the C-terminal or the N-terminal – can interact with a non-functional form of β-galactosidase; complementation between the Q-tag and non-functional β-galactosidase produces a functional enzyme which permits quantitation of the given protein via a chemiluminescence-generating substrate. This system is marketed by Stratagene (La Jolla, CA) under the trade name VariFlex™.

(See also SOLUBILITY ENHANCEMENT TAG.)

QD QUANTUM DOT.

qdot QUANTUM DOT.

QEXT (quencher extension) A method, involving the FRET principle, which has been used e.g. for detecting SNPs; in the presence of an SNP, a probe carrying a 5′ reporter dye undergoes SINGLE-BASE EXTENSION with a TAMRA-labeled chain-terminating dideoxyribonucleotide – causing the reporter dye to either fluoresce or be quenched (according to the particular reporter used).

Multiplex QEXT uses different reporter dyes for detecting different SNPs [BioTechniques (2006) 40(3):323–329].

QIAamp® A system (QIAGEN GmbH, Hilden, Germany) that is used for rapid isolation and purification of nucleic acids (DNA or RNA) from various specimens.

Cell lysis is achieved by the use of optimized buffers, and the required nucleic acid is recovered from the lysate by adsorption to a specialized membrane in a spin column. After spin-washing, the nucleic acid is eluted from the membrane into a collecting tube.

Separate kits are available for different types of sample – e.g. one kit is designed to extract purified DNA from blood, buffy coat or body fluids etc., while another kit is used for isolating pure viral RNA from samples of plasma containing hepatitis C virus.

QIAGEN® plasmid mini kit See DNA ISOLATION.

QPCR See QUANTITATIVE PCR.

QSY dyes See FRET.

quadruplex DNA (G-quadruplex) A structure in which each of the (four) strands of DNA is associated with one of the (four) corners of a stack of G-QUARTETS; the four strands may be in parallel or antiparallel orientation relative to one another.

In vitro, quadruplex DNA may be formed by certain G-rich sequences such as those found in the (eukaryotic) TELOMERE region and those involved in the immunoglobulin switching mechanism.

[Quadruplex formation *in vivo*: see e.g. Nature Struct Mol Biol (2005) 12(10):832–833 and Nucleic Acids Res (2006) 34(3):949–954.]

It has been suggested that, at a certain site in the promoter of the KRAS proto-oncogene, quadruplex DNA (inhibiting transcription) may exist in equilibrium with double-stranded DNA (favouring transcription) [Nucleic Acids Res (2006) 34 (9):2536–2549].

Quadruplex DNA has been reported to occur in promoters throughout the (human) genome [Nucleic Acids Res (2007) 35(2):406–413].

A structure similar to that described above may be formed by RNA. [Database of quadruplex-forming G-rich sequences in alternatively processed mammalian pre-mRNAs: Nucleic Acids Res (2006) 34(Database issue):D119–D124.]

Quantiplex™ assay See BDNA ASSAY.

quantitative PCR (QPCR) Any form of PCR which is used to determine either the absolute or relative number of copies of a given target sequence in a sample.

Absolute numbers of a given sequence may be assessed by REAL-TIME PCR (real-time RT-PCR for RNA targets) or e.g. by COMPETITIVE RT-PCR.

Relative numbers of a given target sequence in two or more samples may need to be assessed e.g. when comparing the expression of a given gene in different tissues or in different individuals; such quantitation may be achieved e.g. by using RELATIVE RT-PCR.

quantum dot (QD; qdot) A nanoparticle, composed of semiconductor materials, which exhibits fluorescence on suitable excitation; while the wavelength of the fluorescence emission peak increases as the size of the QD increases, QDs of different size can be excited with a single source of light. Fluorescence from quantum dots is characterized by a large STOKES SHIFT. These properties of QDs, together with the narrow emission spectrum of a given QD, provide opportunities for a range of high-resolution *in vitro* and *in vivo* reporter systems (see e.g. QUANTUM DOT PROBE).

[Uses: Science (2005) 307:538–544; detecting single DNA molecules by QD end-labeling: Nucleic Acids Res (2005) 33 (11):e98; QD cytotoxicity: J Nanobiotechnology (2007) 5:1.]

quantum dot probe A type of PROBE in which the label is a QUANTUM DOT.

In one approach, a quantum dot probe has been developed for use in Western blot analysis. This kind of probe permits a QD (with specified characteristics) to be conjugated to the Fc portion of any of a range of IgG antibodies – i.e. antibodies with different specificities – permitting multiplex detection of proteins on a Western blot.

The probe consists essentially of a dimerized domain (that is based on the Fc-binding domain of PROTEIN A) carrying a biotinylated peptide sequence which binds a STREPTAVIDIN-coated QD; one region of the dimerized domain binds to the Fc portion of an antibody of the required specificity.

[Bioconjugation of QD probes for Western blot analysis: BioTechniques (2005) 39(4):501–506.]

quartet (G-quartet) See G-QUARTET.

quelling A form of post-transcriptional gene silencing (PTGS) in fungi.

quencher extension See QEXT.

queuosine A Q BASE (7-[4,5-*cis*-dihydroxyl-1-cyclopentene-3-aminomethyl]-7-deazaguanosine) that is found in the wobble position (see WOBBLE HYPOTHESIS) of tRNAs which carry aspartic acid, asparagine, histidine and tyrosine; this modified base is found in both eukaryotic and prokaryotic tRNAs, but apparently does not occur e.g. in *Saccharomyces cerevisiae*. Queuosine pairs with either cytosine or uracil residues.

[Functions of the *queC* gene product at an initial step in the queuosine synthesis pathway in *Escherichia coli*: J Bacteriol (2005) 187(20):6893–6901.]

QuikChange™ site-directed mutagenesis kit A kit (Stratagene, La Jolla CA) used for SITE-DIRECTED MUTAGENESIS without the need for single-stranded template DNA.

A small (<8 kb) plasmid, carrying the target DNA, is heat-denatured to expose primer-binding sites. Two primers, each containing the required mutation, are allowed to anneal – one on each strand – to target DNA; the primers bind in slightly staggered positions on the target sequence. The primers are then extended by a (thermostable) DNA polymerase, forming dsDNA copies of the plasmid with the required mutation and staggered nicks.

Ongoing thermal cycling forms many copies of the mutant plasmid (which remain unligated).

Parent template DNA is then degraded with the restriction enzyme DpnI. The parent DNA is susceptible to this (methylation-*dependent*) RESTRICTION ENDONUCLEASE because it was produced in *Escherichia coli* and will (therefore) have undergone *dam* methylation.

Because the mutant plasmids were formed *in vitro* they are non-methylated – and are therefore resistant to DpnI.

Mutant strands of the plasmid hybridize to form mutant dsDNA plasmids. Each plasmid is nicked in both strands but – because these nicks are in staggered positions (see above) – stable plasmids are formed. The nicks are repaired *in vivo* when the mutant plasmids are inserted into *E. coli* for replication.

Other versions of QuikChange™ are used e.g. to introduce mutations at multiple sites.

[Use (e.g.): BMC Struct Biol (2007) 7:6.]

quinacrine 6-Chloro-9-(4-diethylamino-1-methylbutylamino)-2-methoxyacridine: a yellow fluorescent compound that has been used e.g. for staining the DNA in chromosomes.

quinolone antibiotics Synthetic antibiotics (based on a substituted 4-quinolone ring) which target certain bacterial enzymes involved in the replication of DNA: the A subunit of gyrase, and topoisomerase IV.

Bacterial resistance to quinolone antibiotics often derives from mutation in the *gyrA* gene (gyrase subunit A), although resistance may also result e.g. from lowered permeability of the cell envelope and/or efflux mechanisms.

The early quinolone antibiotics, which were active mainly against Gram-negative bacteria (but not against e.g. *Pseudomonas aeruginosa*), included cinoxacin, nalidixic acid, oxolinic acid and pipemidic acid.

*Fluoro*quinolones such as ciprofloxacin, enoxacin, norfloxacin, ofloxacin and perfloxacin were developed later; their range of activity included *Pseudomonas aeruginosa* as well as certain Gram-positive bacteria.

A subsequent generation of the fluoroquinolones included e.g. gatifloxacin, gemifloxacin, grepafloxacin, levofloxacin, moxifloxacin and trovafloxacin.

(cf. NOVOBIOCIN.)

quinomycins See QUINOXALINE ANTIBIOTICS.

quinoxaline antibiotics A category of bifunctional INTERCALATING AGENTS that include quinomycins and triostins; the molecule is a cyclic octapeptide dilactone which links two quinoxaline 2-carboxylic acid chromophores. Some of these compounds exhibit a preference for GC-rich sequences. A synthetic member, TANDEM (des-*N*-tetramethyltriostin A), shows a preference for AT-rich regions.

Quinoxalines have antimicrobial and antitumor activity.

[The role of stacking interactions in binding sequence preferences of DNA bis-intercalators: Nucleic Acids Res (2005) 33(19):6214–6224.]

quorum sensing In certain microorganisms: the phenomenon in which a particular characteristic is expressed by cells only when their concentration (number of cells per unit volume) is higher than a certain minimum (*quorum*). Cells in a high-density population may therefore exhibit characteristics that are not exhibited when *cells of the same type* are present in low-density populations.

The archetypal presentation of quorum sensing is the BIOLUMINESCENCE exhibited by high-density populations of the bacterium *Vibrio fischeri* (= *Photobacterium fischeri*) within the light-emitting organs of certain fishes; in the free-living state (sea water: low-density populations) cells of *V. fischeri* exhibit little or no bioluminescence.

Quorum sensing involves a gene-regulatory mechanism. It is mediated by certain *secreted* low-molecular-weight molecules; in a high-density population of the secreting cells these molecules reach a threshold concentration which is sufficient to trigger activity in specific gene(s) within the cells. These low-molecular-weight signaling molecules are referred to as *autoinducer* molecules because they are synthesized by the cells themselves.

The autoinducer in many Gram-negative bacteria is an *N*-acyl-L-homoserine lactone (AHL). (In the case of *V. fischeri*, an AHL triggers activity in the *lux* operon.)

[Regulation of AHLs in *Agrobacterium vitis*: J Bacteriol

(2006) 188 (6):2173–2183.]

For Gram-positive bacteria, signaling molecules in quorum sensing are generally *peptides* (*pheromones*). The pheromone ComX, formed by *Bacillus subtilis*, promotes competence in TRANSFORMATION by activating a certain TWO-COMPONENT REGULATORY SYSTEM which, in turn, activates a transcription factor needed for competence.

In the fungus *Candida albicans*, farnesol, a sesquiterpene alcohol, was reported to act as a quorum sensing molecule and to inhibit yeast-to-mycelium transition in this organism. [Quorum sensing in fungi: Eukaryotic Cell (2006) 5(4):613–619; Appl Environ Microbiol (2006) 72:3805–3813.]

Quorum sensing is reported to regulate the expression of a wide range of characteristics in many organisms – including, for example, the formation of biofilms in *Staphylococcus aureus*, the expression of type III protein secretion systems in both EHEC and EPEC strains of *Escherichia coli*, swarming in *Burkholderia cepacia*, and the development of competence in *Bacillus subtilis* (see above). (See also CROWN GALL.)

A mutant, autoinducer-negative strain of *Chromobacterium violaceum* (CV026) produces the purple pigment *violacein* (a derivative of tryptophan) when exposed to any of a variety of exogenous inducers, including all tested AHLs – as well as AHT (*N*-acyl-homocysteine thiolactone) having *N*-acyl side-chains in the range C_4–C_8. This strain is therefore useful as a biosensor for detecting the relevant range of autoinducers.

R

R (1) A specific indicator of ambiguity in the recognition site of a RESTRICTION ENDONUCLEASE (or in any other nucleic acid sequence); for example, in GTY↓RAC (enzyme HincII) the 'R' indicates A or G. In the example, 'Y' is C or T.

(2) L-Arginine (alternative to Arg).

R loop See D LOOP.

R1 plasmid A low-copy-number conjugative PLASMID, found in strains of *Escherichia coli* and other enterobacteria, which encodes resistance to various antibiotics (e.g. ampicillin and streptomycin).

Replication of R1 DNA is controlled by the synthesis of the (plasmid-encoded) RepA protein which promotes replication of the plasmid from the origin.

RepA synthesis appears to be regulated at several different levels. When the plasmid COPY NUMBER is normal, the CopB protein (encoded by the plasmid) inhibits transcription from the *repA* gene promoter. Moreover, under these conditions, an ANTISENSE RNA molecule, *copA* (also plasmid-encoded), inhibits translation of the mRNA of gene *repA*; the inhibitory action of *copA* becomes less effective when the copy number is low. When the copy number falls, it appears that the lower concentration of CopB exerts less inhibitory action on *repA* transcription, allowing the copy number of the plasmid to recover to normal levels.

A further mechanism for maintaining a stable copy number of plasmid R1 involves the Kid protein, a component of the PARD SYSTEM. When the copy number falls, Kid, acting as a nuclease, cleaves both host-encoded mRNA (e.g. *dnaB*) and a plasmid-encoded mRNA (which encodes a repressor of R1 replication) at the specific sequence UUACU; the effects of such cleavage are to inhibit bacterial growth (thus delaying cell division) and to help restore the normal copy number of the plasmid [EMBO J (2005) 24(19):3459–3469].

Partition (that is, segregation of plasmids to daughter cells during cell division) appears to involve a remarkable mitosis-like process mediated by actin-like filaments. In this process, it appears that a pair of plasmids are linked by the (plasmid-encoded) ParR protein – which binds to the 'centromere-like' region *parC*, present in each of the plasmids, to form a so-called *partitioning complex*. (ATP-bound) ParM molecules then polymerize, forming actin-like filaments which – as they lengthen in an axial direction between the two plasmids – concurrently propel the plasmids to opposite poles of the cell. The filaments subsequently de-polymerize following hydrolysis of filament-bound ATP. Proteins encoded by some other plasmids have been reported to polymerize into filaments *in vitro* – e.g. the F plasmid [Proc Natl Acad Sci USA (2005) 102(49):17658–17663] and plasmid TP228 [EMBO J (2005) 24(7):1453–1464].

R5 strains (of HIV-1) See HIV-1.

R5X4 strains (of HIV-1) See HIV-1.

RACE Rapid amplification of cDNA ends: an approach used (i) to copy the 5′ and 3′ ends of an mRNA for which minimal sequence data are available, and/or (ii) to obtain full-length copies of the corresponding cDNA.

In the 3′ RACE procedure, an oligo(d)T-containing primer binds to the 3′ poly(A) tail of the mRNA and is extended by reverse transcriptase. After degradation of the RNA template (e.g. with RNase H), a gene-specific primer (complementary to a sequence *within* the FIRST STRAND) may be extended to form the second strand. Nested PCR may then be used to amplify smaller sections in the (part-length) double-stranded cDNA.

In the 5′ RACE procedure, a gene-specific primer (i.e. one complementary to a sequence within the mRNA) is extended with reverse transcriptase to the 5′ terminus of the mRNA template. The mRNA is then degraded (e.g. with the enzyme RNase H), and the 3′ end of the first strand is tailed with e.g. dCTP. This permits the design of a second-strand primer that includes a section: 5′.......GGG-3′. The ds cDNA may then be amplified by PCR using the two primers.

Given that the complete 3′ and 5′ ends of the mRNA have been copied it is then possible to design primers which can be used to obtain full-length copies of the corresponding cDNA.

One problem with this procedure (particularly 5′ RACE) is the formation of non-specific products; for example, in the 5′ RACE reaction the second-strand primer may base-pair with any complementary sequence (...CCC...) which happens to be available in the mixture. In one approach to this problem, use was made of a second-strand primer with an adaptor designed to suppress non-specific products [BioTechniques (2006) 40 (4):469–478].

(See also CAPFINDER and CAPSELECT.)

rad (radiation absorbed dose) A unit of the amount of radiation absorbed: 100 ergs of energy per gram (0.01 joule per kilogram).

(cf. GRAY.)

Rad51 A type of eukaryotic protein – analogous to the bacterial RecA protein and archaeal RadA protein – which is involved e.g. in strand exchange during homologous recombination. As is the case with the (*Escherichia coli*) RecA protein, and yeast (*Saccharomyces cerevisiae*) Rad51 protein, the human Rad51 protein has been reported to show a preference for binding to sequences of ssDNA that are over-represented for guanine residues and under-represented for adenine and cytosine residues [Nucleic Acids Res (2006) 34(10):2847–2852].

RadA A protein, found in members of the ARCHAEA, which is analogous to the bacterial RecA protein and to the eukaryotic Rad51 proteins; RadA is involved in strand exchange during homologous recombination.

Rainbow tag A small fusion tag, expressed as a part of a recombinant protein, which facilitates purification and quantitation of the protein by imparting *color* – thus allowing tracking during the purification process and enabling quantitation via measurement of the specific absorbance signature of the tag. [Method: BioTechniques (2005) 38(3):387–392.]

random access combinatorial chemistry   See MICROARRAY.

random amplified polymorphic DNA (RAPD)   See AP-PCR.

random match probability   See CODIS.

RAPD analysis   See AP-PCR.

rapid amplification of cDNA ends   See RACE.

rare-cutting restriction endonuclease   A RESTRICTION ENDO-
NUCLEASE whose recognition sequence generally occurs only
rarely in many or most samples of DNA.

One example is NotI. NotI has no recognition sites at all in
some AT-rich prokaryotes – such as *Staphylococcus aureus*
(GC% 32.8) and *Campylobacter jejuni* (GC% 30.5) – and it
has none in bacteriophages λ and φX174, in plasmid pBR322
or in the genome of simian virus 40 (SV40). However, NotI
has >350 sites in the genome of the archaean *Halobacterium*
(GC% 67.9) and >250 sites in *Mycobacterium tuberculosis*
(GC% 65.6).

Other rare-cutters include e.g. FseI, SfiI and SwaI (see table
in entry RESTRICTION ENDONUCLEASE).

[Engineering a rare-cutting restriction enzyme (selection of
NotI variants): Nucleic Acids Res (2006) 34(3):796–805.]

(See also the figures in the entry GC%.)

ras (*RAS*)   A family of ONCOGENES initially identified in the
Harvey and Kirsten strains of murine sarcoma virus (H-*ras* or
Ha-*ras*, K-*ras* or Ki-*ras*, respectively); c-*ras* is widespread in
eukaryotes, from humans to yeast. The *ras* protein (generic
designation p21) is located in the plasma membrane; it binds,
and hydrolyzes, GTP and is involved in the transmission of
signals that affect functions such as cell proliferation.

A transforming *ras* gene can differ by only a single point
mutation from the normal cellular *ras* – important sites for
mutation including e.g. the 12th and 61st amino acids in p21;
such mutations appear to leave the protein in a permanently
active (i.e. transforming) state.

Mutated *ras* genes are common in human tumors.

rATP   ATP that contains a ribose (rather than a deoxyribose)
residue.

RBS   (1) Ribosome-binding site.

(2) Rep-binding site.

RCA   ROLLING CIRCLE amplification.

RdDM   RNA-directed DNA methylation: a particular form of
GENE SILENCING: see e.g. SIRNA.

RDM   RIBOSOME DENSITY MAPPING.

rDNA   Genomic DNA encoding ribosomal RNA (rRNA).

RDO   RNA/DNA oligonucleotide: a CHIMERAPLAST (q.v.).

RE   RESTRICTION ENDONUCLEASE.

REA   Restriction enzyme analysis: *syn.* DNA FINGERPRINTING.

readthrough   (1) Continuation of transcription through a stop
signal.

(2) Continuation of translation through a stop codon – an
amino acid being inserted at the stop codon; the product is a
readthrough protein.

Occasional readthrough (of a UGA codon) in bacteriophage
Qβ produces the A1 protein (not the normal coat protein) –
translation continuing to the subsequent UAG stop codon.

readthrough protein   See READTHROUGH.

real-time PCR   A form of PCR in which it is possible to follow
the progress of amplification – that is, the ongoing increase in
numbers of specific amplicons in the reaction mixture – *while
it is happening*; this approach also permits estimation of the
number of specific target sequences that were present in the
reaction mixture *before* the beginning of cycling (one form of
QUANTITATIVE PCR).

The increase in numbers of amplicons in a given reaction
can be monitored in two main ways: (i) by the use of target-
specific probes (which give rise to a fluorescent signal in the
presence of specific amplicons), and (ii) by the use of certain
dyes that exhibit dsDNA-dependent fluorescence, i.e. dyes
which fluoresce when they bind to double-stranded DNA (or
which increase fluorescence from a minimal to a significant
level when they bind to dsDNA). Each of these approaches
(probe and dye) provides a type of information which is not
available from the other (see later). In both of these methods,
however, an increase in numbers of amplicons is monitored
by recording rising levels of fluorescence while the reaction
is in progress.

During the reaction, fluorescence is recorded *cycle by
cycle* – beginning at cycle 1 and continuing throughout the
reaction to the last cycle (which may be e.g. cycle ~30–40).

To estimate the number of target sequences present in the
mixture prior to cycling it is necessary to determine the so-
called *threshold cycle* (C_t, or C_T), i.e. the first cycle in which
the probe-based or dye-based fluorescence from the reaction
exceeds the background fluorescence by a specified amount.

The threshold cycle allows a quantitative estimation of the
initial number of target sequences in the reaction mixture as
there is an inverse linear relationship between (i) threshold
cycle and (ii) the logarithm of the number of target sequences
prior to cycling. That is, a linear graph is obtained – over a
range of values – if threshold cycle is plotted against the
logarithm of the initial number of target sequences in the
reaction mixture. This relationship can be understood intuit-
ively: the lower the number of target sequences present in the
reaction mixture – prior to cycling – the higher will be the
number of cycles of amplification needed to reach a level of
fluorescence corresponding to the threshold cycle (and vice
versa).

Probes used in real-time PCR

The amplification of the target sequence can be monitored by
several types of probe which differ mechanistically: see e.g.
LIGHTUP PROBE, MOLECULAR BEACON PROBE and TAQMAN
PROBE.

Probes are included in the reaction mixture prior to cycling.

Note that, in a given cycle, the time at which fluorescence
is monitored will depend on the type of probe used. Using
molecular beacon or LightUp® probes, fluorescence is monitored at the annealing stage of the PCR cycle; this is the
stage at which these probes bind to specific amplicons (their
target sequences) and fluoresce under appropriate excitation.
With this kind of probe, the level of fluorescence from the
reaction mixture increases step-wise at each annealing stage;

fluorescence is not produced at the (high-temperature) stage of denaturation because these probes are not bound to their target sequences under these conditions.

By contrast, fluorescence from TaqMan® probes increases at the primer-extension stage; the level of fluorescence from the reaction mixture increases in a step-wise fashion with each cycle – although in this case the fluorescence is not lost between cycles because the molecules of dye released from probes in previous cycles remain free (and fluorescent) in the reaction mixture.

Another type of probe is associated with the LightCycler™ instrument (Roche Diagnostics, Basel, Switzerland) used for real-time PCR. It consists of two (separate) oligonucleotides that bind adjacently on the target sequence – the 3′ end of one oligo (probe 1) binding close to the 5′ end of the other (probe 2). The 3′ end of probe 1 carries a molecule of fluorescein, and the 5′ end of probe 2 carries a molecule of the fluorophore LightCycler™ Red 640. Suitable excitation produces fluorescence from the fluorescein, but (while the two probes remain unbound) no fluorescence is produced from the molecule of LightCycler™ Red 640. If both probes are correctly bound to the target sequence, activation of the fluorescein provides excitation for the LightCycler™ Red 640 (see FRET) and the latter dye emits red light (640 nm); this emission (i.e. 640 nm) signals probe–target binding and is monitored by the instrument. Probe–target binding occurs during the *annealing* stage; subsequent extension of the primer displaces (but does not degrade) the two oligonucleotides – which can therefore function in the next cycle.

Probes used in real-time PCR may be significantly shorter if they contain LOCKED NUCLEIC ACIDS, and LNA-containing probes may be more discriminatory [BioTechniques (2005) 38(1):29–32].

Multiplex real-time PCR

Simultaneous monitoring of two or more separate reactions (in the same reaction mixture) can be achieved by the use of several fluorescent dyes that have distinct emission spectra. In this mode, probes which bind to different target sequences are labeled with different fluorophores – so that separate and distinguishable signals are produced during the amplification of each different type of target sequence.

Various types of fluorophore have been used for labeling probes – see e.g. FAM and TAMRA.

dsDNA-binding dyes used in real-time PCR

One of the most commonly used dyes is SYBR GREEN I. Dyes which fluoresce when bound to dsDNA enable progress in real-time PCR to be monitored at the end of the extension phase – i.e. when the number of (double-stranded) amplicons is at a maximum.

(See also BOXTO.)

Combined probe-based and dye-based monitoring

While a target-specific probe detects the required product, it cannot of course detect any non-specific products or primer–dimers which may be formed during the reaction. However, spurious products such as these, if formed, may interfere with the amplification of the actual target – and may reduce the yield of specific amplicons.

On the other hand, dsDNA-binding dyes signal *all* dsDNA, i.e. they do not distinguish between specific amplicons and any spurious products which may be present. However, these dyes are useful because, at the end of the reaction (i.e. after completion of cycling), it is possible to examine the products by melting curve analysis to detect any illegitimate products that may have been formed. (The basic rationale of melting curve analysis is that the temperature–fluorescence characteristics of a given dye-bound product depend on the product's length and composition; different products exhibit different characteristics, and the presence of *mixed* products may be detected in this way when only a single product is expected.)

Hence, probe-based and dye-based monitoring offer different types of information in real-time PCR. To obtain both types of information, real-time PCR can be carried out with both types of monitoring, allowing detection of the required products and also allowing detection of any non-specific and interfering products that may have been formed in the reaction mixture [BioTechniques (2006) 40(3):315–319].

real-time protein synthesis (*in vitro*) See CELL-FREE PROTEIN SYNTHESIS.

REAP Restriction endonuclease analysis of plasmid DNA (also called *plasmid profiling*).

One approach is to subject PCR-amplified plasmid DNA to restriction enzyme analysis. This approach has been used e.g. in studies on sequence variation among virulence plasmids in the equine pathogen *Rhodococcus equi* and was also used for evaluating these plasmids, as epidemiological markers, in a global surveillance program; geographic differences could be demonstrated in the distribution of these plasmids.

Some bacteria – e.g. species of *Brucella* and *Rickettsia* – normally lack plasmids, so that this method is not applicable to these organisms.

REase (RE) RESTRICTION ENDONUCLEASE.

reassortant virus A recombinant (hybrid) form of a given SEGMENTED GENOME virus: one that contains segment(s) of the genome of a genetically distinct virus (e.g. of a mutant strain of virus co-infecting the cell).

REBASE® An excellent source of regularly updated information on e.g. bacterial genomes, restriction endonucleases and methyltransferases etc. at:
http://rebase.neb.com/rebase/rebase.html

[REBASE: Nucleic Acids Res (2005) 33(Database issue): D230–D232.]

RecA The bacterial counterpart of the eukaryotic RAD51 protein and the archaeal RADA protein; the RecA protein is involved e.g. in strand exchange in HOMOLOGOUS RECOMBINATION. (See also SOS SYSTEM.)

[DNA sequence specificity of the *Escherichia coli* RecA protein: Nucleic Acids Res (2006) 34(8):2463–2471.]

The RecA protein is reported to stimulate the relaxation activity of topoisomerase I, although it is apparently without effect on the supercoiling activity of gyrase [Nucleic Acids

Res (2007) 35(1):79–86].

recA-deficient strains of bacteria are sometimes used for the stable cloning of plasmids because they tend to hinder the occurrence of homologous recombination between plasmids.

If there is a need to carry out homologous recombination in a *recA*-minus strain of bacteria it is possible to provide a *temporary* RecA function by inserting a *recA* gene on a so-called suicide plasmid – see e.g. entry SUICIDE VECTOR.

The RecA protein has various uses in DNA technology: see e.g. RECACTIVE.

RecActive™   A system (Active Motif) that was designed for rapidly isolating specific clone(s) from e.g. a cDNA library or a genomic library – avoiding the time-consuming methods often used for library screening.

To isolate a specific clone, the initial step is to prepare BIOTINylated, double-stranded probes (~200–600 bp) which represent a segment within the required clone. The probes are denatured to the single-stranded state and are then coated with RECA protein. When mixed with the library, the single-stranded, RecA-coated probes bind to homologous sequences within the required clones, forming stable hybrids. The RecA proteins are then removed by treatment with sodium dodecyl sulfate (SDS), leaving the single-stranded probes bound to their target sequences.

The probe-labeled, biotinylated clones are then bound by STREPTAVIDIN-coated magnetic beads which are held, by a magnetic field, while the remaining clones are removed by washing.

After such enrichment, molecules of the required clone can be inserted into appropriate bacteria by transformation and the colonies formed by these bacteria can be screened for the required clone.

RecBCD   See HOMOLOGOUS RECOMBINATION.

RecF   See HOMOLOGOUS RECOMBINATION.

recipient (conjugational)   See F PLASMID and CONJUGATION.

recognition site (of a restriction enzyme)   See RESTRICTION ENDONUCLEASE.

recombinant (*adj.*)   See RECOMBINATION.

recombinase   Any enzyme which, alone or in combination with other factors, can mediate CROSSING OVER (breakage and re-union) between two regions of dsDNA.

Certain recombinases mediate SITE-SPECIFIC RECOMBINATION; in such cases the enzyme has a *specific* recognition sequence of nucleotides. For example, the Int recombinase of PHAGE λ acts on *att* sites, while the Cre enzyme acts on *loxP* sites (see CRE–LOXP SYSTEM).

A recombinase from PHAGE BXB1 apparently mediates site-specific recombination efficiently in mammalian cells.

Other types of recombinase lack a specific recognition site and may mediate crossing over between any two homologous regions of dsDNA; this kind of enzyme can be useful e.g. for site-directed recombination between two suitably engineered molecules: see e.g. LAMBDA (λ) RED RECOMBINATION.

The *resolvase*-type recombinases cut all four strands concurrently, with 5′-phosphate bound to the enzyme in order to conserve energy for subsequent ligation. An example of this type of enzyme is the recombinase encoded by transposon Tn*3* (which is used to resolve the cointegrate formed during replicative transposition: see entry TRANSPOSABLE ELEMENT (figure legend)).

Integrase-type recombinases (e.g. the Int protein of phage λ, Cre protein of phage P1, and the Flp recombinase) cut and join strands in a pairwise fashion, forming an intermediate structure that is referred to as a HOLLIDAY JUNCTION (q.v.). (The λ integrase function involves the (bacterial) *integration host factor*.)

Enzymes in this category include the *serine* recombinases (encoded e.g. by phages φC31, R4) in which an N-terminal catalytic site contains a serine residue, and *tyrosine* recombinases (including the Cre and Flp enzymes – see CRE–LOXP SYSTEM and FLP) whose C-terminal catalytic site includes a tyrosine residue. A tyrosine recombinase is also encoded by transposon Tn*4655* (q.v.).

The VLF-1 (very late expression factor 1) of baculoviruses is reported to have homology with members of the tyrosine recombinase family.

recombinase-mediated cassette exchange (RMCE)   Exchange of cassettes between two regions, or molecules, of DNA in which each cassette is flanked (on both sides) by the recognition site of a given recombinase.

In one example, each cassette is flanked by one wild-type *loxP* site (see CRE–LOXP SYSTEM) and one modified *loxP* site; Cre recombinase can mediate the exchange of these two cassettes – modified *loxP* sites (one in each cassette) being used in order to maintain the cassettes' orientation following exchange.

RMCE was used e.g. to transfer a cassette from a plasmid to a *loxP*-augmented viral vector in human embryonic kidney cells that were engineered to express the Cre recombinase constitutively [Nucleic Acids Res (2005) 33(8):e76]. RMCE has also been used e.g. for carrying out genetic modification of stem cells [Nucleic Acids Res (2005) 33(4):e43; Proc Natl Acad Sci USA (2005) 102(18):6413–6418] and for studies on transcription [PLoS Genet (2007) 3(2):e27].

[RMCE: tagging genes for cassette-exchange sites: Nucleic Acids Res (2005) 33(4):e44.]

recombinase polymerase amplification   See RPA.

recombination (*DNA technol.*)   Any *in vivo* or *in vitro* process involving the re-arrangement of sequence(s) of nucleotides in one or more molecules of nucleic acid – including events such as e.g. additions, deletions, inversions, replacements and amalgamations. Any molecule which has undergone such a process is referred to by the adjective *recombinant*; this term is also employed to describe cells (and also viruses) in which recombination has occurred.

Recombination includes HOMOLOGOUS RECOMBINATION, SITE-SPECIFIC RECOMBINATION and transpositional recombination. Collectively, the various forms of recombination are involved in e.g. crossing over in meiosis; some types of DNA repair; regulation of gene expression (e.g. flagellar filament alleles in *Salmonella* – see PHASE VARIATION); and also gene inactivation through insertion of transposable elements.

recombination machine See HOMOLOGOUS RECOMBINATION.

recombineering *In vivo* production of recombinant chromosomes (or plasmids) by using certain types of phage-derived recombinase (such as the LAMBDA (λ) RED RECOMBINATION system); the molecules of DNA which are used to modify the target sequence require only short regions of homology. By using this approach, cloned DNA (within vector molecules) can be modified directly, i.e. *in vivo*.

Recombineering has been used e.g. for inserting point mutations, *loxP* sites etc. into bacterial artificial chromosomes (BACs) [Nucleic Acids Res (2005) 33(4):e36].

RecoverEase™ See DNA ISOLATION.

RED REPEAT-EXPANSION DETECTION.

Red-mediated recombination See LAMBDA (λ) RED RECOMBINATION.

reference gene *Syn.* HOUSEKEEPING GENE.

Refludan® See BIOPHARMACEUTICAL (table).

regulon A gene-regulatory system in which two or more non-contiguous genes and/or operons – each gene/operon having its own promoter – are controlled by a common regulatory molecule that is recognized by similar sequences in each of the genes/operons.

One example of a regulon is the so-called *araBAD* operon (see OPERON) which is involved in the uptake and transport of arabinose; this system includes a number of genes, several of which (*araE*, *araF*) occur at separate loci; all of the genes are controlled by the AraC protein.

relative molecular mass (M_r; 'molecular weight') Of a given molecule: the ratio of the mass of the molecule to one twelfth of the mass of a neutral ^{12}C atom (a unitless number).

relative RT-PCR A form of QUANTITATIVE PCR used for comparing the number of copies of a given target sequence in two or more samples – as, for example, when comparing the transcripts of a given gene from different cells or individuals, or from the same cells under different conditions.

Essentially, the target (in a given sample) is co-amplified with an internal control, each sequence (target and control) having its own pair of primers. The products of PCR can be separated by gel electrophoresis and scanned for quantitation.

The internal control may be a sequence of RNA encoded by a so-called housekeeping gene (= reference gene), such as the gene encoding 18S rRNA. This kind of control is expressed constitutively, but (e.g. in the case of 18S rRNA) its high level of expression means that amplification is likely to go beyond the exponential phase of PCR within a few cycles – thus failing to fulfill the requirement of an internal control; this problem may be addressed e.g. by using an appropriate COMPETIMER–primer ratio.

relaxed control (of plasmid replication) See PLASMID.

relaxed phenotype See *relA* in ESCHERICHIA COLI (table).

relaxing enzyme See TOPOISOMERASE (type I).

relaxosome See CONJUGATION.

remodeling (of chromatin) See CHROMATIN.

Renilla reniformis GFP See HRGFP.

rep-PCR A PCR-based method used for TYPING those bacteria whose chromosomes contain a repetitive sequence of nucleotides.

Repetitive sequences exploited in this method include the so-called *repetitive extragenic palindromic sequence*, which is found e.g. in *Escherichia coli* and also in other members of the family Enterobacteriaceae (see REP SEQUENCE), the ERIC SEQUENCE and SERE. (See also MIRU in the entry W-BEIJING STRAIN.)

For rep-PCR with the REP sequence (REP-PCR: compare rep-PCR), a primer is designed which binds to a consensus sequence at one end of a REP sequence. Extension from each of the primers bound to REP sequences produces fragments that reflect REP-to-REP distances, i.e. primer extension from a given REP sequence continues until the newly synthesized strand reaches the start of the next REP sequence; any further extension is blocked by the bound primer, and all the newly formed strands remain as separate entities. As REP-to-REP distances along the length of the chromosome may vary from strain to strain, analysis of PCR-generated amplicons by gel electrophoresis yields fingerprints that are characteristic of the given strains.

REP-PCR was used e.g. for typing *Klebsiella pneumoniae* [Antimicrob Agents Chemother (2006) 50(2):498–504].

SERE-PCR was used e.g. for typing *Streptococcus oralis* from dental plaque [Appl Environ Microbiol (2000) 66(8): 3330–3336].

ERIC-PCR was used e.g. for typing strains from the Greenland Glacier ice core [Appl Environ Microbiol (2005) 71(12): 7806–7818], and strains of *Pandoraea apista* [Int J Syst Evol Microbiol (2000) 50(2):887–899] isolated from patients with cystic fibrosis [J Clin Microbiol (2006) 44(3):833–836].

REP-PCR See entry above.

Rep protein See e.g. ROLLING CIRCLE.

REP sequence (palindromic unit) Repetitive extragenic palindromic sequence: a sequence of nucleotides – containing a PALINDROMIC SEQUENCE with hyphenated dyad symmetry – which is found in multiple copies (~500–1000 per chromosome) in the genomic DNA of e.g. various enterobacteria (including *Escherichia coli* and *Salmonella typhimurium*). REP sequences are located in intergenic regions (so far they have not been detected in coding sequences) and they occur e.g. in promoter-distal regions of many operons.

REP sequences have been used for TYPING various species of bacteria (see REP-PCR).

It has been suggested that the role of REP sequences *in vivo* may include a contribution to nucleoid structure.

REP sequences were reported to be targets for IS elements (insertion sequences) and 'hot spots' for transposition [BMC Genomics (2006) 7:62].

repeat-expansion detection (RED) A method for detecting an abnormally expanded series of short nucleotide repeats (e.g. repeated trinucleotide units) in a sample of genomic DNA; an abnormal increase in the number of repeated units (produced, perhaps, by the mechanism of SLIPPED-STRAND MISPAIRING) has been associated with various types of inherited neurological disease in humans. (See also MICROSATELLITE DNA.)

In this method, genomic DNA is initially heat-denatured, and *repeat-specific* oligonucleotides are allowed to anneal to one of the strands of the sample DNA. Oligonucleotides that bind adjacently (contiguously) are ligated by a (thermostable) DNA LIGASE. Ligated oligonucleotides are released from the genome by heating; they consist of a mixed population of multimers of different lengths – some containing two ligated oligonucleotides, others three, etc.

The cycle of annealing oligonucleotides, ligation, and heat-denaturation is repeated a number of times. The population of multimers is then subjected to gel electrophoresis and blotted onto a suitable membrane. The membrane is examined with labeled probes that are complementary to the given (repeat-specific) oligonucleotide. The sizes (i.e. lengths) of the multimers indicate the presence/absence of expanded repeats.

repetitive extragenic palindromic sequence   REP SEQUENCE.

replacement vector   A CLONING VECTOR containing a dispensable (non-essential) sequence (the *stuffer*) flanked by a pair of recognition sites for restriction enzymes; the stuffer region is replaced by target DNA prior to cloning.

(See also INSERTION VECTOR.)

replica plating   A technique used for the isolation of mutants which arise in a population of microorganisms grown under non-selective conditions; it can be used e.g. for the isolation of AUXOTROPHIC MUTANTS in a population of prototrophs.

For isolating auxotrophic mutants, a *master plate* is made by inoculating a complete medium with an inoculum from a population of prototrophs; when incubated, all the cells, i.e. prototrophs and any auxotrophic mutants in the inoculum, are able to grow and form individual colonies.

After incubation of the master plate, a disk of sterile velvet or similar material, fixed to one end of a cylindrical support, is lightly pressed onto the surface of the plate and then withdrawn. During contact between disk and plate a small amount of growth from each of the colonies will adhere to the velvet. The disk is then used to inoculate one (or several) plates of minimal medium (*replica plates*) – on which only the prototrophs can grow. During these procedures, it is necessary to keep a careful record of the orientation of the disk in relation to the master plate and in relation to the replica plate(s).

The replica plates are then incubated. The colonies which develop on these plates are entirely those of prototrophs – as no auxotroph is able to grow on minimal medium. Hence, by comparing the positions of colonies on the master and replica plate(s), it is possible to identify colonies on the master plate which are absent on the replica plate(s) and which are therefore those of presumptive auxotrophs.

replicase   (1) Any RNA-DEPENDENT RNA POLYMERASE.
(2) An RNA-dependent RNA polymerase used specifically for replicating a viral genome.

An RNA polymerase which synthesizes mRNA is sometimes called a TRANSCRIPTASE.

replication protein A   See e.g. OKAZAKI FRAGMENT.

repliconation   See CONJUGATION.

reporter gene   Any gene used in an experimental system for the purpose of signaling the presence (or otherwise) of specific activity or event(s), in that system, by its own expression.

In some cases a (defective) reporter gene may be included in a transfected sequence in order to signal the integration of that sequence into genomic DNA; on integration, *cis*-acting sequence(s) in the genome may supply essential function(s) (e.g. a promoter) needed for expression of the reporter gene. (In this case, the reporter gene is expressed only if the transfected sequence integrates, appropriately, in the genome.)

Examples of reporter genes include those that encode e.g. chloramphenicol acetyltransferase (CAT, an enzyme which inactivates the antibiotic chloramphenicol); β-galactosidase (an enzyme which hydrolyses lactose and X-GAL); GREEN FLUORESCENT PROTEIN; and LUCIFERASE.

A β-lactamase gene (*bla*) is used as a reporter gene in some commercial vectors: e.g. pcDNA™6.2/GeneBLAzer™ (see GATWAY SITE-SPECIFIC RECOMBINATION SYSTEM (table)).

repressor titration   A method for detecting the intracellular presence of a small, multicopy plasmid vector. The method uses an engineered strain of *Escherichia coli* that contains a kanamycin-resistance gene whose expression is *repressed* via the *lac* operator (see LAC OPERON).

The multicopy plasmid whose presence is to be detected also incorporates the *lac* operator.

Cells which lack the vector will not grow on kanamycin-containing media: in the absence of lactose (or IPTG), the *lac* promoter is blocked by the binding of LacI repressor to the *lac* operator – so that the kanamycin-resistance gene is not expressed.

Cells which contain the (multicopy) vector will have many copies of the (plasmid-borne) *lac* operator – and these extra copies of the *lac* operator compete with the chromosomal *lac* sequence for LacI repressor protein. Because so much LacI will be bound by the plasmid-borne *lac* operator sequences, insufficient LacI will be available to bind to the chromosomal *lac* sequence; hence, under these conditions, the kanamycin-resistance gene will be transcribed and the cells will be able to grow on kanamycin-containing media.

In addition to the simplicity of the method, one advantage is that the vector molecule can be *small* because there is no need for it to include an antibiotic-resistance marker gene (as is common in other methods). Moreover, small vector molecules are transformable with greater efficiency.

reptation   In gel electrophoresis: the movement of a (linear) molecule of nucleic acid in an end-on orientation (parallel to the current).

resistance integron   See INTEGRON.

resolvase   See RECOMBINASE and TRANSPOSABLE ELEMENT (figure legend).

resolving gel   See SDS-PAGE.

resorufin   A compound whose fluorescence is monitored in a commercial assay for PYROPHOSPHATE (q.v.).

respiration (*energy metab.*) A specific energy-converting process in which a substrate is metabolized with the involvement of an exogenous (i.e. external) electron acceptor such as oxygen. In this process ATP is characteristically generated by oxidative phosphorylation.

In *anaerobic* respiration (a process carried out e.g. by some bacteria in the absence of oxygen) the electron acceptor may be e.g. a substance such as fumarate, nitrate, selenate, sulfur or sulfate.

(cf. FERMENTATION.)

response regulator See TWO-COMPONENT REGULATORY SYSTEM.

restriction (*DNA technol.*) Cleavage of dsDNA by one or more types of RESTRICTION ENDONUCLEASE.

In DNA technology, one normally uses particular type(s) of restriction enzyme so that cleavage occurs at specific sites in the target molecule(s).

restriction endonuclease (restriction enzyme; REase, RE) An endonuclease which binds to dsDNA, commonly at a specific sequence of nucleotides (termed the *recognition sequence* or *recognition site*), and which typically cuts each strand once *if* certain bases are *un*methylated (for many REs) or methylated (for other REs); according to enzyme, the terminal regions at a cleaved site are STICKY ENDS or BLUNT-ENDED DNA.

Restriction endonucleases are obtained from a wide range of prokaryotic microorganisms.

The heterogeneity of REs precludes a single definition that covers all cases. Thus, some REs have no precise recognition site while others have several sites; some bind to palindromic sequences, others to asymmetric sites; some need two copies of the recognition site, to be functional, while most need only one copy; some cut within the site and others cut outside it; some REs cut on both sides of the recognition site – excising part of the target molecule; some *nicking enzymes* (see later) resemble REs but cut only one strand.

A given sequence of nucleotides may be recognized by two or more different REs, derived from different species – see ISOSCHIZOMER.

Under non-optimal conditions, the specificity of an RE, for a given recognition sequence, may become less stringent, i.e. the RE may be able to bind to certain other sequences. This phenomenon is called STAR ACTIVITY.

For some types of experiment it may be necessary to direct the activity of an RE to a *particular* recognition site, even when other copies of the given site are freely available elsewhere in the molecule: see e.g. ACHILLES' HEEL TECHNIQUE and PROGRAMMABLE ENDONUCLEASE.

The methylation of dsDNA (referred to above) is typically carried out *in vivo* by methyltransferases (= 'methylases'): enzymes which add methyl groups to specific bases (the N6 of adenine, the C5 of cytosine) in prokaryotic DNA. In many cases, restriction (cutting) and methylation can be carried out by the same enzyme, i.e. some REs have a dual role.

The nomenclature currently recommended for the REs and methyltransferases [Nucleic Acids Res (2003) 31(7):1805–1812] avoids the (former) use of italics. For example, EcoRI (instead of *Eco*RI) is used to refer to an RE from *Escherichia coli* strain R, the I indicating one particular RE from strain R. Sometimes the prefix 'R' is used – e.g. R.EcoRI, in which 'R' indicates a restriction – rather than a methylating – enzyme; enzymes which incorporate both restriction and methylating functions may have the prefix RM. Some other examples of REs are given in the table.

For online information on REs (and methyltransferases) see the entry REBASE.

REs are now classified into four main groups (types I–IV):

Type I REs. This type of RE is a multisubunit enzyme with subunits for restriction, methylation and site-specificity (the latter specifying the recognition sequence); *ATP-dependent* cleavage occurs at a non-specific site outside the recognition sequence. An example of a type I RE is EcoKI.

[New type I REs from *Escherichia coli*: Nucleic Acids Res (2005) 33(13):e114.] (See also HSD GENES.)

[Mechanism of translocation of the type IC RE EcoR124I: EMBO J (2006) 25:2230–2239.]

Type II REs. These REs typically recognize a specific sequence of nucleotides; both of the strands are cleaved in an *ATP-independent* manner, at fixed locations in or near the recognition site – leaving a 5′-phosphate terminus and a 3′-hydroxyl terminus on both sides of the cut.

Precise cutting of DNA makes the type II RE very useful in recombinant DNA technology; over 3500 type II REs have been characterized.

Subtypes of the type II RE display various characteristics. Subtype IIP includes a large number of REs that recognize symmetric (palindromic) sequences and cleave at fixed sites within, or immediately adjacent to, their recognition sites. An example of a type IIP RE is EcoRI, whose recognition and cutting ($\downarrow$) sites are:

$$5'\text{-}G\downarrow AATTC\text{-}3'$$

and 3′-CTTAA$\uparrow$G-5′ in the complementary strand. Note that the staggered cuts leave *sticky ends*: 5′-AATT overhangs on each strand.

Other subtypes of the type II RE include:

IIA. These REs recognize asymmetric sequences.

IIB. These REs cleave on both sides of the recognition site. Examples include BaeI and BcgI. The recognition and cutting sites of BaeI can be written:

$$(10/15)AC(N_4)GTAYC(12/7)$$

in which N_4 refers to four (unspecified) nucleotides and Y is either C or T. 10/15 means that the strand shown is cut 10 nucleotides upstream and the complementary strand is cut 15 nucleotides upstream. 12/7 means that the strand shown is cut 12 nucleotides downstream and the complementary strand is cut 7 nucleotides downstream.

IIC. In these REs the cutting and methylation functions are

RESTRICTION ENDONUCLEASE: some examples

Enzyme	Type	Recognition sequence (5′→3′); cutting site (↓)	Notes
AatII	IIP	GACGT↓C	
AccI	IIP	GT↓MKAC	Isoschizomers: XmiI, FblI
AccIII	IIP	T↓CCGGA	Isoschizomers: BseAI, BspEI, Kpn2I, MroI
AflII	IIP	C↓TTAAG	Isoschizomers: BfrI, BspTI
AgeI	IIP	A↓CCGGT	
AluI	IIP	AG↓CT	Blunt-ended cut Recognition sites common in genomic 'Alu sequences' Isoschizomer: MltI
AlwNI	IIP	CAGNNN↓CTG	Isoschizomer: CaiI
AocI	IIP	CC↓TNAGG	
ApaI	IIP	GGGCC↓C	Neoschizomers: Bsp120I, PspOMI
ApoI	IIP	R↓AATTY	
AscI	IIP	GG↓CGCGCC	Useful e.g. in RLGS (restriction landmark genomic scanning)
AsuNHI	IIP	G↓CTAGC	
AvaI	IIP	C↓YCGRG	Activity ~doubled at 45°C Isoschizomers: Ama87I, BsoBI, Eco88I, NspIII
AvaII	IIP	G↓GWCC	Isoschizomers: Bme18I, Eco47I, SinI
BamHI	IIP	G↓GATCC	Star activity in e.g. buffers of low strength, or >5% glycerol (v/v) Isoschizomer: BstI
BanII	IIP	GRGCY↓C	Isoschizomers: Eco24I, EcoT38I
BbeI	IIP	GGCGC↓C	
BclI	IIP	T↓GATCA	Isoschizomers: FbaI, Ksp22I
BfiI	IIS	5′-ACTGGG(5N)↓ 3′-TGACCC(4N)↑N	Cleavage site variability reported in the upper strand
BglI	IIP	GCCNNNN↓NGGC	Isoschizomer: Tsp8EI BglI was reported to generate an increased number of ribotypes in the species *Vibrio cholerae* (see entry RIBOTYPING)
BglII	IIP	A↓GATCT	
BpmI	IIG,E,S	5′-CTGGAG(16N)↓ 3′-GACCTC(14N)↑NN	
Bpu1102I	IIP	GC↓TNAGC	Isoschizomers: BlpI, Bsp1720I, CelII, EspI
BseAI	IIP	T↓CCGGA	
BsgI	IIG,E,S	5′-GTGCAG(16N)↓ 3′-CACGTC(14N)↑	
BsmI	IIS	5′-GAATGCN↓ 3′-CTTAC↑GN	Isoschizomers: BsaMI, PctI
BsmFI	IIG,S	GGGAC(10/14)	Used e.g. in serial analysis of gene expression (see entry SAGE)
Bsp106I	IIP	AT↓CGAT	
BspCI	IIP	CGAT↓CG	
BspMI	IIS	5′-ACCTGC(4N)↓NNNN 3′-TGGACG(8N)↑	
BssHII	IIP	G↓CGCGC	Used e.g. for cutting genomic DNA in CpG islands Isoschizomers: BsePI, PauI *(continued)*

RESTRICTION ENDONUCLEASE: (*continued*)

Enzyme	Type	Recognition sequence (5'→3'); cutting site (↓)	Notes
BstEII	IIP	G↓GTNACC	Isoschizomers: BstPI, Eco91I
BstNI	IIP	CC↓WGG	Isoschizomers: BptI, BseBI, BstOI, MvaI Neoschizomers: AjnI, EcoRII, Psp6I, PspGI Cleavage occurs even if the internal cytosine is methylated
BstXI	IIP	CCANNNNN↓NTGG	Isoschizomer: BstHZ55I
BstYI	IIP	R↓GATCY	Isoschizomers: MflI, XhoII
Bsu36I	IIP	CC↓TNAGG	Cutting site used e.g. in a baculovirus-related vector [BioTechniques (2006) 41(4):453–458]
CfoI	IIP	GCG↓C	Isoschizomer: HhaI Neoschizomer: Hin6I
Cfr9I	IIE,P	5'-C↓CCGGG 3'-GGGCC↑C	
Cfr10I	IIF,P	5'-R↓CCGGY 3'-YGGCC↑R	
ClaI	IIP	AT↓CGAT	Isoschizomers: BanIII, BspDI, BspXI, Bsu15I
CspI	IIP	CG↓GWCCG	
CvnI	IIP	CC↓TNAGG	Isoschizomers: AxyI, Bse21I, Bsu36I, Eco81I
DdeI	IIP	C↓TNAG	Isoschizomer: BstDEI
DpnI	IIM,P	G(m⁶A)↓TC	Activity of the enzyme *requires* methylation at the N6 position of adenine Isoschizomer: MalI
DraI	IIP	TTT↓AAA	Isoschizomers: AhaIII, SruI
DraIII	IIP	CACNNN↓GTG	
EagI	IIP	C↓GGCCG	Cutting sites e.g. in CpG islands
Eam1104I	IIS	5'-CTCTTCN↓NNN 3'-GAGAAGNNNN↓	Used e.g. in the Seamless® cloning kit
Ecl18kI	IIP	↓CCNGG	Mechanism for determining specificity: EMBO J (2006) 25:2219–2229
Eco47III	IIP	AGC↓GCT	Blunt-ended cut. Star activity in high levels of enzyme Isoschizomer: AfeI
Eco57I	IIE,G	5'-CTGAAG(16N)↓ 3'-GACTTC(14N)↑NN	
EcoKI	I	random	
EcoO109I	IIP	RG↓GNCCY	Isoschizomer: DraII Neoschizomer: PssI
EcoP15I	III	CAGCAG(25/27)	Used in superSAGE (see SAGE)
EcoRI	IIP	G↓AATTC	Star activity in e.g. buffers of low strength, >5% glycerol (v/v), pH >8 Isoschizomers: none reported See also MunI
EcoRII	IIP,E	↓CCWGG	Isoschizomers: AjnI, Psp6I Neoschizomers: BptI, BseBI, MvaI Sensitive to methylation. *Two* copies of the recognition site are needed for activity of EcoRII
EcoRII-C	IIP-type		Cleaves *single* copies of the recognition sequence in a methylation-sensitive way [BioTechniques (2005) 38(6):855–856]
EcoRV	IIP	GAT↓ATC	Blunt-ended cut. Star activity in glycerol >5% (v/v) Isoschizomer: Eco32I

(*continued*)

Enzyme	Type	Recognition sequence (5′→3′); cutting site (↓)	Notes
EcoR124I	IC	random	[Mechanism of translocation: EMBO J (2006) 25:2230–2239]
FokI	IIS	GGATG(9N)↓NNNN CCTAC(13N)↑	
FseI	IIP	GGCCGG↓CC	Rare-cutter
FspI	IIP	TGC↓GCA	Isoschizomers: AviII, NsBI
HaeII	IIP	RGCGC↓Y	Isoschizomers: Bsp143I, BstH2I
HaeIII	IIP	GG↓CC	Isoschizomers: BsnI, BsuRI, PhoI
HhaI	IIP	GCG↓C	Isoschizomer: CfoI Neoschizomers: Hin6I, HspAI
HincII	IIP	GTY↓RAC	Enzyme used in strand displacement amplification as a *nicking* enzyme (see SDA) Isoschizomer: HindII
HindIII	IIP	A↓AGCTT	
HinfI	IIP	G↓ANTC	Star activity e.g. if Mg^{2+} is replaced by Mn^{2+} or in high levels of glycerol
HinP1I	IIP	G↓CGC	Isoschizomers: Hin6I, HspAI Neoschizomers: BstHHI, CfoI, HhaI [Mechanism of action: Nucleic Acids Res (2006) 34(3):939–948]
HpaI	IIP	GTT↓AAC	Isoschizomer: KspAI
HpaII	IIE	C↓CGG	Isoschizomers: HapII, MspI
HpyHI	IIP	CTNAG	Cleavage site unknown
KpnI	IIP	GGTAC↓C	Star activity if >5% glycerol (v/v) Neoschizomers: Acc65I, Asp718I
Kpn2I	IIP	T↓CCGGA	
MboI	IIP	↓GATC	Isoschizomers: DpnII, NdeII, Sau3AI Neoschizomer: BstKTI
MboII	IIS	5′-GAAGA(8N)↓ 3′-CTTCT(7N)↑N	
MfeI	IIP	C↓AATTG	
MluI	IIP	A↓CGCGT	Isoschizomer: Bbi24I
MmeI	IIG	5′-TCCRAC(20N)↓ 3′-AGGYTG(18N)↑	Used e.g. in one method for generating shRNAs
MnlI	IIS	5′-CCTC(7N)↓ 3′-GGAG(6N)↑	Slow cleavage reported for single-stranded DNA
MroI	IIP	T↓CCGGA	
MscI	IIP	TGG↓CCA	Isoschizomers: BalI, MluNI
MseI	IIP	T↓TAA	Isoschizomer: Tru9I
MspI	IIP	C↓CGG	Isoschizomers: BsiSI, HapII, HpaII
MunI	IIP	C↓AATTG	Produces sticky ends that can hybridize with those formed by EcoRI Isoschizomer: MfeI
NaeI	IIE,P	GCC↓GGC	Blunt-ended cut. Site preference: the (single) NaeI site in phage λ DNA is reported to be cut more slowly than other NaeI sites [DNA looping dynamics: Nucleic Acids Res (2006) 34:167–174] Isoschizomer: PdiI Neoschizomers: MroNI, NgoMIV

(*continued*)

Enzyme	Type	Recognition sequence (5′→3′); cutting site (↓)	Notes
NarI	IIE	GG↓CGCC	Site preference: the (single) NarI site in phage λ DNA is reported to be cut more slowly than other NarI sites. [DNA looping dynamics: Nucleic Acids Res (2006) 34:167–174] Isoschizomer: Mly113I Neoschizomers: BbeI, DinI, EheI, KasI, SfoI
NciI	IIG,P	CC↓SGG	Isoschizomer: BcnI
NcoI	IIP	C↓CATGG	Isoschizomer: Bsp19I
NdeI	IIP	CA↓TATG	Isoschizomer: FauNDI
NdeII	IIP	↓GATC	Isoschizomers: BfuCI, BssMI, DpnII, Sau3AI Neoschizomer: BstKTI
NgoAIV	IIP	G↓CCGGC	Isoschizomer: NgoMIV Neoschizomers: NaeI, PdiI
NheI	IIP	G↓CTAGC	Isoschizomer: AsuNHI Neoschizomer: BmtI
NlaIII	IIP	CATG↓	Used e.g. in serial analysis of gene expression (see entry SAGE)
NotI	IIP	GC↓GGCCGC	'Rare-cutting' enzyme; useful e.g. for cutting genomic DNA into large fragments Used in RLGS (restriction landmark genomic scanning) Isoschizomer: CciNI
NruI	IIP	TCG↓CGA	Isoschizomers: Bsp68I, BtuMI
NsiI	IIP	ATGCA↓T	Isoschizomers: EcoT22I, Mph1103I, Zsp2I
NspI	IIP	RCATG↓Y	Isoschizomers: BstNSI, XceI
NspV	IIP	TT↓CGAA	Isoschizomers: AsuII, BstBI, Csp45I
PacI	IIP	TTAAT↓TAA	Used e.g. in the AdEasy™ adenoviral vector system
PaeI	IIP	GCATG↓C	
PalI	IIP	GG↓CC	Isoschizomers: HaeIII, BsuRI
PinAI	IIP	A↓CCGGT	Isoschizomers: AgeI, BshTI, CspAI
PmeI	IIP	GTTT↓AAAC	Isoschizomer: MssI Used e.g. in the AdEasy™ adenoviral vector system
PspAI	IIP	C↓CCGGG	Isoschizomer: XmaI Neoschizomer: SmaI
PstI	IIP	CTGCA↓G	Isoschizomer: BspMAI
PvuI	IIP	CGAT↓CG	Buffer conditions important for optimal activity. Cleavage of supercoiled plasmids may require high concentrations of enzyme Isoschizomers: BpvUI, MrvI, Ple19I
PvuII	IIP	CAG↓CTG	Star activity e.g. with >5% (v/v) glycerol and low-salt buffer Used as a programmable endonuclease when linked to a TFO (i.e. triplex-forming oligonucleotide) [see Nucleic Acids Res (2005) (22):7039–7047]
RcaI	IIP	T↓CATGA	Isoschizomers: BspHI, PagI
RsaI	IIP	GT↓AC	Isoschizomer: AfaI Neoschizomer: Csp6I
RsrII	IIP	CG↓G(A/T)CG	Isoschizomers: CpoI, CspI
SacI	IIP	GAGCT↓C	
SacII	IIE	CCGC↓GG	Reported to cleave sites in DNA of phages φX174 and λ more slowly than in other recognition sites Isoschizomers: KspI, SgrBI, SstII (*continued*)

Enzyme	Type	Recognition sequence (5′→3′); cutting site (↓)	Notes
SalI	IIP	G↓TCGAC	Star activity if glycerol is in high concentration, or with high levels of enzyme; needs salt concentration >100 mM
SanDI	IIP	GG↓GWCCC	
Sau3AI	IIE	↓GATC	Isoschizomers: DpnII, MboI, NdeII Neoschizomer: BstKTI Activity reported to be decreased when the target DNA is under mechanical tension (approx. 10-fold decrease at 0.7 pN) [Proc Natl Acad Sci USA (2006) 103(31):11555–11560]
ScaI	IIP	AGT↓ACT	Isoschizomers: AssI, BmcAI, ZrmI
SfiI	IIF,P	GGCCNNNN↓NGGCC	Rare cutter
SgrAI	IIP	5′-CR↓CCGGYG 3′-GYGGCC↑RC	
SmaI	IIP	CCC↓GGG	Neoschizomers: Cfr9I, XmaI, XmaCI
SnaBI	IIP	TAC↓GTA	Isoschizomers: BstSNI, Eco105I
SpeI	IIP	A↓CTAGT	Isoschizomers: AhlI, BcuI
SphI	IIP	GCATG↓C	Isoschizomers: BbuI, PaeI
SrfI	IIP	GCCC↓GGGC	Blunt-ended cut Ligation of SrfI-cut ends is reported to be promoted e.g. by 15% polyethylene glycol (PEG)
SspI	IIP	AAT↓ATT	Inhibited by glycerol >5%
SstI	IIP	GAGCT↓C	Isoschizomers: SacI, Psp124BI Neoschizomer: EcoICRI
SstII	IIP	CGGC↓GG	Isoschizomers: KspI, SacII, SgrBI
StuI	IIP	AGG↓CCT	Isoschizomers: AatI, Eco147I, SseBI
StyI	IIP	C↓CWWGG	Isoschizomers: Eco130I, ErhI
SuiI	IIP	G↓CWGC	
SunI	IIP	C↓GTACG	Isoschizomers: BsiWI, PspLI
SwaI	IIP	ATTT↓AAAT	Rare cutter
TaqI	IIP	T↓CGA	Isoschizomers: Tsp32I, TthHB8I
ThaI	IIP	CG↓CG	Isoschizomers: AccII, Bsh1236I, BstUI, MvnI
Tsp509I	IIP	↓AATT	Used e.g. in SUICIDE POLYMERASE ENDONUCLEASE RESTRICTION (q.v.)
TspMI			Isochizomer of XmaI (q.v.)
UbaF13I	IIS	GAG(6N)CTGG	Cleavage site unknown
UbaF14I	IIS	CCA(5N)TCG	Cleavage site unknown
VspI	IIP	AT↓TAAT	Isoschizomers: AseI, PshBI
XbaI	IIP	T↓CTAGA	Star activity with high levels of enzyme and with DMSO. Sensitive to methylation
XhoI	IIP	C↓TCGAG	Isoschizomers: StrI, TliI, PaeR7I
XhoII	IIP	R↓GATCY	
XmaI	IIP	C↓CCGGG	Isoschizomer (thermostable): TspMI [Appl Microbiol Biotechnol (2006) 72:917–923]
XmaIII	IIP	C↓GGCCG	Isoschizomers: BstZI, EclXI, Eco52I
XmnI	IIP	GAANN↓NNTTC	

combined in one polypeptide; they include members of other subtypes.

IIE. These REs cut at the recognition site but need to interact with another copy of that site for 'activation'. [DNA looping by two-site restriction enzymes: Nucleic Acids Res (2006) 34(10):2864–2877.] Studies on various 'two-site' REs have shown that these enzymes are sensitive to mechanical tension in the target DNA – enzymic activity being lost when the DNA is subjected to a few piconewtons [Proc Natl Acad Sci USA (2006) 103(31):11555–11560].

IIF. These REs interact with, and cut, two copies of the recognition site.

IIM. These REs cut at fixed locations where there is a specific pattern of *methylation*. An example is DpnI.

IIS. The type IIS REs cut one, or both, strands outside the recognition site.

Note. A given type II RE may belong to more than one subtype.

Type III REs. These REs interact with both copies of a nonpalindromic sequence that are orientated inversely; cleavage, which depends on *ATP-dependent* translocation, occurs at a specified distance from one of the sites. Examples of type III REs include EcoP1I and EcoP15I.

Type IV REs. These REs recognize a *methylated* site but, unlike the type IIM REs, their cutting sites apparently lack specificity. Example: EcoKMcrBC.

Putative REs. The existence of these REs (which have a prefix P) is inferred e.g. by comparing an open reading frame (ORF) in a sequenced genome with the sequence of a known RE.

Nicking enzymes. These are enzymes cut ('nick') only one of the strands of a DNA duplex; at least some of these enzymes resemble restriction endonucleases – e.g. BstNBI [Nucleic Acids Res (2001) 29:2492–2501].

The nicking enzymes have an 'N' prefix, e.g. N.BstNBI.

Some (normal) REs can be made to act as nicking enzymes by using DNA with chemically modified bases: see e.g. SDA. At a low pH, the type IIS restriction enzyme BfiI becomes a nicking enzyme, selectively cutting a single strand [Proc Natl Acad Sci USA (2003) 100(11):6410–6415].

restriction endonuclease analysis of plasmid DNA See REAP.

restriction enzyme *Syn*. RESTRICTION ENDONUCLEASE.

restriction enzyme analysis *Syn*. DNA FINGERPRINTING.

restriction fragment length polymorphism analysis See RFLP ANALYSIS.

restriction landmark genomic scanning (RLGS) A method used for scanning genomic DNA with the object of detecting e.g. DNA polymorphisms or altered patterns of DNA methylation.

In the original method, suitably prepared genomic DNA was initially digested with the RESTRICTION ENDONUCLEASE NotI, and the 5′ overhangs (at cleavage sites) filled in with labeled (^{32}P) nucleotides. End-labeled (^{32}P-labeled) DNA was then digested with another restriction enzyme, EcoRV, after which the first phase of gel electrophoresis was carried out.

DNA-containing gel was subsequently cut out and digested with the restriction enzyme MboI. Following this digestion with MboI the next phase of gel electrophoresis was carried out. The final bands of fragments were examined in the dried gel.

In studies on methylation patterns in genomic DNA the restriction enzyme NotI is particularly useful because its recognition site (5′-GC↓GGCCGC-3′) occurs primarily in CPG ISLANDS: >85% of NotI cutting sites within the human genome are found in CpG islands. The significance of this is that CpG islands are commonly associated with the promoter regions of genes, and aberrant patterns of methylation in such regions have been noted in cancer-related silencing of tumor-suppressor genes; hence, it is of particular interest to examine methylation patterns in fragments that include CpG islands. In this context, it is the enzyme NotI (rather than EcoRV) which determines the specific (CpG-associated) locations of the restriction fragments; hence, NotI is generally referred to as the *landmark* enzyme (or the restriction landmark) in this procedure.

Note that NotI is a methylation-sensitive enzyme, i.e. it will not cleave its recognition site if an internal cytosine residue is methylated. Consequently, an *aberrantly* methylated cutting site will not be cleaved and end-labeled – so that a particular band of RLGS fragments will be absent at the location in the gel which is normally occupied by a band.

While most RLGS studies have been carried out with the NotI landmark enzyme, it was reported that there are several advantages in complementing NotI with another restriction enzyme, AscI (cutting site: GG↓CGCGCC) [Genome Res (2002) 12(10):1591–1598].

A useful follow-up is to prepare a library by cloning the RLGS fragments, permitting further studies on particular loci of interest.

RLGS can be used not only to compare different genomes but also to compare DNA methylation patterns in different tissues within a given individual. One study found that many CpG islands are differentially methylated in a tissue-specific manner [Proc Natl Acad Sci USA (2005) 102(9):3336–3341].

restriction map In relation to a given DNA molecule or fragment: any diagram showing the positions of the recognition sequences of RESTRICTION ENDONUCLEASES; other features, e.g. origin of replication, particular genes, direction of transcription etc. may also be shown on the map in order to give orientation.

(See also FLASH CHEMILUMINESCENT GENE MAPPING KIT.)

restriction-minus cells (*DNA technol.*) Genetically engineered bacteria in which some, or all, of the restriction systems have been deleted.

An example of a restriction-minus strain is XL1-Blue MRF′ (Stratagene, La Jolla CA): Δ(*mcrA*)183, Δ(*mcrCB-hsdSMR-mrr*)173, *endA1*, *supE44*, *thi-1*, *recA1*, *gyrA96*, *relA1*, *lac*[F′ *proAB*, *lacI*^{q}*ZΔM15*, Tn*10*(Tet^r)].

Examples of the use of XL1-Blue MRF′ (e.g.): studies on MutH–MutL interaction in DNA mismatch repair [Nucleic

Acids Res (2006) 34(10):3169–3180] and on transcriptional responses to secretion stress in two species of fungi [BMC Genomics (2006) 7:32].

reticulate body (RB)   See CHLAMYDIA.

retrocopy (of a gene)   See RETROGENE.

retrogene (retrocopy)   A derivative of a normal gene formed by reverse transcription of an mRNA into DNA and subsequent insertion of the DNA into the genome (with an opportunity for expression); this type of process apparently occurs only rarely in evolution.

If the inserted sequence has no opportunity for expression, the resulting promoter-less, intron-less and function-deficient entity is referred to as a *retropseudogene*.

[Emergence of young human genes in primates: PLoS Biol (2005) 3(11):e357. Retrocopied genes in male fitness: PLoS Biol (2005) 3(11):e399. Functional displacement of a source gene by a retrocopy: Nucleic Acids Res (2005) 33(20):6654–6661.]

(See also PSEUDOGENE.)

retrohoming   See INTRON HOMING.

retron   In certain bacteria – e.g. strains of *Escherichia*, *Klebsiella*, *Proteus*, *Rhizobium*, *Salmonella*: a chromosomal sequence encoding a REVERSE TRANSCRIPTASE similar to that encoded by retroviruses. These bacteria are able to synthesize a hybrid RNA/DNA molecule – called *multicopy single-stranded DNA* (msDNA) – in which the 5′ end of ssDNA is covalently bound (via a phosphodiester linkage) to the 2′-position of a non-terminal guanosine residue in the RNA. A single cell may contain as many as 500 copies of msDNA.

Retrons have been named according to the initials of the host species and the number of bases in the DNA moiety of the corresponding msDNA; thus, for example, in *Myxococcus xanthus* the msDNA contains 162 bases, and this molecule is designated Mx162.

retroposon   *Syn.* RETROTRANSPOSON.

retropseudogene   See RETROGENE.

retroregulation   A type of post-transcriptional regulation which involves the influence of a *cis*-acting sequence downstream of the given gene. Ongoing transcription of the gene into the *cis*-acting sequence results in degradation of the transcript, thus blocking gene expression; if transcription stops before reaching the *cis*-acting sequence the transcript is available for translation.

retrotranscription   Synthesis of a strand of DNA on an RNA template.

(See also REVERSE TRANSCRIPTASE.)

retrotransfer (*bacteriol.*)   Transfer of DNA from the recipient cell, in CONJUGATION, to the donor cell.

retrotransposon (retroposon)   A TRANSPOSABLE ELEMENT that has a mode of transposition involving an RNA intermediate (and the activity of reverse transcriptase); the intermediate is reverse transcribed, and the DNA product is inserted into the target site. One example of a retrotransposon is the so-called TY ELEMENT of the yeast *Saccharomyces cerevisiae*.

(See also ALU SEQUENCES.)

Retroviridae   A family of ssRNA-containing viruses; members of this family are referred to, collectively, as RETROVIRUSES (q.v.).

retroviruses   Enveloped, ssRNA viruses (family Retroviridae) which replicate via a dsDNA intermediate.

Retroviruses are found in a wide range of species, including e.g. mammals, birds and reptiles. (See also COPIA ELEMENT.) Infection of a given host by a retrovirus may be symptomless or may be associated with any of a number of diseases which range from pneumonia and tumors to leukemia and AIDS.

Transmission of retroviruses may occur horizontally and/or vertically.

The following is a generalized account of the retroviruses.

Classification of retroviruses

The retroviruses have been placed in subfamilies on the basis of e.g. the type(s) of pathogenic effect they cause. Viruses of the LENTIVIRINAE (including HIV-1) replicate in – and kill – host cells. The subfamily ONCOVIRINAE includes oncogenic viruses, while viruses of the subfamily SPUMAVIRINAE are characteristically non-pathogenic.

The virion

The heat-sensitive and detergent-sensitive virion, 80–120 nm in diameter, consists of a nucleoprotein core (which includes the viral REVERSE TRANSCRIPTASE) and an envelope of host-derived lipid from which project virus-encoded glycoproteins that determine the types of cell which can be infected by the virus.

All the genetic information is encoded in a single-stranded, positive-sense RNA of about 3–10 kb, according to virus; the virion contains two identical (or similar) copies of this RNA linked non-covalently at the 5′ ends.

The viral RNA has regions of TERMINAL REDUNDANCY flanked, externally, by a 5′ CAP and a 3′ poly(A) tail.

U5 and U3 are sequences unique to the 5′ and 3′ regions of the RNA, respectively; each is adjacent to its corresponding region of terminal redundancy.

Coding regions of the RNA molecule include the *gag*, *pol* and *env* sequences. The *gag* region encodes proteins of the viral core. The *pol* region encodes e.g. reverse transcriptase and the viral integrase (the latter involved in integration of the dsDNA provirus into the chromosome of the host cell). The *env* region encodes e.g. major glycoprotein components of the viral envelope (gp120 and gp41). There is also e.g. a ψ (psi) sequence (which promotes packaging of viral RNA into virions).

Infection of cells

Infection of cells involves interaction between viral envelope proteins and specific type(s) of cell-surface receptor. During infection by HIV-1, the envelope glycoprotein gp120 binds to cell-surface antigen CD4; target cells for this virus therefore include e.g. the (CD4+) 'helper' subset of T lymphocytes (i.e. helper T cells). (In addition to the CD4 receptor, infection by HIV-1 is reported to depend on the presence of certain other cell-surface receptor molecules such as receptors for CXC-type and CC-type chemokines – see e.g. HIV-1.)

A PCR-based study reported that, during infection of blood leukocytes by HIV-1 *ex vivo*, blood dendritic cells were preferentially infected [J Virol (2007) 81(5):2297–2306].

(See also DC-SIGN.)

Reverse transcription and integration of provirus
Within the cell, viral RNA is converted to DNA by the viral reverse transcriptase. Priming involves a host tRNA molecule which binds at the 3′ boundary of the U5 sequence; in many cases tRNA^{pro} is used, but tRNA^{lys} is used e.g. by HIV-1.

Following extension of the (first) strand of DNA to the 5′ terminus of the RNA template, the RNA corresponding to the 5′ terminal redundancy region is degraded by RNase H. The resulting (single-stranded) sequence of DNA then hybridizes with the 3′ terminal redundancy region at the other end of the RNA template; extension of the DNA strand then continues on this end of the template.

Because synthesis of the second strand of DNA begins at a staggered site, each end of the final dsDNA product contains a so-called *long terminal repeat* (LTR) in which U3 and U5 are separated by a sequence corresponding to one copy of the terminal redundancy.

One or more copies of the dsDNA *provirus* may integrate into the host cell's DNA. Integration of the provirus DNA is mediated by retroviral integrase, a tetramer of which forms a stable complex with the two ends of the viral DNA; the two ends of the prophage are inserted, sequentially, into the host cell's chromosome [EMBO J (2006) 25(6):1295–1304].

Expression of the viral genome (the provirus)
Transcription of proviral DNA, processing of transcripts and the subsequent formation of virions are complex processes involving e.g. synthesis of polycistronic pre-mRNAs and the essential contribution of certain virus-encoded proteins. For example, the small early intronless transcripts can translocate readily from the nucleus to the cytoplasm, but larger intron-containing transcripts, formed later, require the REV PROTEIN (in HIV-1) for translocation to the cytoplasm via the CRM1 nuclear export pathway.

Other virus-encoded proteins (in HIV-1) include e.g. the transcription regulatory factor Tat, the Vif ('viral infectivity factor') protein and the Vpu protein (which promotes efficient budding of the virion during productive infection of the cell).

The maturation of retroviral RNA and post-transcriptional events leading to production of virions have been reviewed [Retrovirology (2006) 3:18].

Retroviruses in DNA technology
Recombinant (engineered) retroviral vectors have been used e.g. in clinical trials in GENE THERAPY – and also for various studies involving genetic modification of cultured cells.

Factors favorable to the use of retroviruses:
● retroviruses can effect gene transfer to (sensitive) cells with high frequency;
● once integrated in the cell's genome, the retroviral provirus can usually be expressed on a long-term basis;
● proviral DNA is transmitted to daughter cells;
● high-titer preparations of infectious, replication-deficient viral particles can be produced;
● retroviruses can be pseudotyped to control host range.

Factors unfavorable to the use of retroviruses:
● most retroviruses infect only actively dividing cells; however, lentiviruses can infect both dividing and non-dividing cells (and are used as vectors);
● the retroviral provirus integrates randomly into the DNA of the host cell – with potential lethality; thus, in a gene therapy setting, a knock-out insertion in a tumor-suppressor gene may lead e.g. to tumorigenesis;
● in a laboratory setting retroviral particles are rather labile.

Replication-*competent* retroviral vectors are currently being studied [J Virol (2007) 81(13):6973–6983].

Rett syndrome An X-linked neurodevelopmental disorder (in humans) commonly resulting from mutation in *MECP2*, a gene (Xq28) encoding methyl-CpG-binding protein 2, but it can also result from mutation in gene *CDKL5* (Xp22), which encodes a cyclin-dependent kinase.

(See also GENETIC DISEASE (table).)

Rev protein A regulatory protein encoded by human immunodeficiency virus type 1 (HIV-1). Activity of the Rev protein is essential for ongoing productive infection by HIV-1; thus, Rev is required e.g. for transporting various intron-containing mRNAs (encoding e.g. envelope and certain other proteins) from the nucleus to the cytoplasm. Rev binds to a complex secondary structure (called the Rev response element, RRE) in appropriate transcripts and mediates their transport from the nucleus.

The Rev protein itself incorporates a nuclear localization signal (NLS) and a nuclear export signal (NES).

Rev activity was found to be inhibited by a dsRNA-binding protein (nuclear factor 90) [Retrovirology (2006) 3:83].

The Rev protein has been studied in a live-cell assay for the simultaneous monitoring of expression and interaction of proteins [BioTechniques (2006) 41(6):688–692].

(See also transdominant negative proteins in the entry GENE THERAPY.)

reverse genetics Essentially: working/studying in the direction genotype → phenotype, as opposed to the usual (or 'classic') approach: phenotype → genotype. Experimental procedures used in reverse genetics include (for example) KNOCK-OUT MUTATIONS and RNAI.

reverse gyrase A hyperthermophile-specific TOPOISOMERASE, found in the archaean *Sulfolobus* and in some bacteria, which can introduce *positive* supercoiling into a ccc dsDNA molecule. It appears to have a helicase-like domain and homology with a bacterial topo I enzyme; reverse gyrase may mediate positive supercoiling in the plasmids of hyperthermophilic organisms.

This enzyme may have a supercoiling-independent, heat-protective function [Nucleic Acids Res (2004) 32(12):3537–3545]. Other studies indicate that it is not essential for growth at 90°C [J Bacteriol (2004) 186(14):4829–4833].

Selective degradation of reverse gyrase (and fragmentation of DNA) by the alkylating agent methylmethane sulfonate

(MMS) was reported in the archaean *Sulfolobus solfataricus* [Nucleic Acids Res (2006) 34(7):2098–2108].

reverse hybridization The procedure (used e.g. in some diagnostic tests) in which target sequences of nucleic acid bind to a set of *immobilized* probes, i.e. the reverse of the procedure in which the target is immobilized. (cf. REVERSE SOUTHERN HYBRIDIZATION.)

(See also LINE PROBE ASSAY.)

reverse mutation *Syn.* BACK MUTATION.

reverse primer See FORWARD PRIMER.

reverse Southern hybridization A method used to detect a specific sequence of DNA, in solution, by hybridization to a labeled probe. The probe is initially modified with a psoralen derivative such that, when bound to its target and exposed to ultraviolet radiation, the probe and target sequence become covalently cross-linked. Bound and unbound probes can then be separated e.g. by gel electrophoresis.

reverse transcriptase (RNA-dependent DNA polymerase) An enzyme which can synthesize a strand of DNA on an RNA template. Reverse transcriptases are encoded e.g. by retroviruses as an essential requirement for their intracellular development and chromosomal integration, and are also encoded by some retrovirus-like elements, such as the TY ELEMENT in the yeast *Saccharomyces cerevisiae*. Genes encoding these enzymes are found in certain bacteria, including *Escherichia coli*. (See also RETRON.) The DNA polymerase I of *E. coli* is reported to have (poorly processive) reverse transcriptase activity.

A reverse transcriptase synthesizes the DNA strand 5'-to-3' from a short RNA primer. Divalent cations are required for enzymic activity. The r*Tth* enzyme (Perkin Elmer/Applied Biosystems) can function as a reverse transcriptase in the presence of Mn^{2+}; on chelation of Mn^{2+} (with EGTA), the enzyme can behave as a DNA polymerase in the presence of Mg^{2+}. Alternatively, this enzyme can be used in a specialized single-buffer system.

The lack of 3'-to-5' exonuclease (proof-reading) activity in a reverse transcriptase results in error-prone DNA synthesis.

Some reverse transcriptases have RNase H-like activity – being able to degrade the RNA strand in a DNA/RNA hybrid.

A reverse transcriptase may be inhibited by agents such as AZT (see NUCLEOSIDE REVERSE TRANSCRIPTASE INHIBITORS) as well as NON-NUCLEOSIDE REVERSE TRANSCRIPTASE INHIBITORS. (See also SURAMIN.)

reverse transcriptase PCR (rtPCR, rt-PCR, RT-PCR; formerly RNA PCR) A PCR-based procedure for making copies of a sequence from an RNA template; rt-PCR has various uses – including studies on gene expression (e.g. detecting mRNAs that are in low concentration in cell lysates), and studies on RNA viruses.

In an early 'two-tube' protocol, a strand of DNA is initially synthesized on the RNA target by REVERSE TRANSCRIPTASE activity at ~50°C. The RNA strand is then degraded (e.g. by RNase H) and a complementary strand of DNA is synthesized on the first strand, forming a dsDNA template which is then amplified by routine PCR methodology.

The above protocol, carried out at ~50°C, can be problematic if the target RNA contains secondary structures which are stable at these temperatures and are able to inhibit DNA synthesis by physically blocking the polymerase. In a more recent protocol, RT-PCR is conducted at higher temperatures using a thermostable enzyme (e.g. RTTH POLYMERASE) that is able to act as both reverse transcriptase and DNA polymerase under appropriate conditions.

A different method for amplifying an RNA target sequence (NASBA) was found to be less inhibited by factors that were inhibitory in an RT-PCR assay of noroviruses in environmental waters [Appl Environ Microbiol (2006) 72(8):5349–5358].

RF (1) Recombination frequency.

(2) The replicative form of the genome in certain types of bacteriophage: see e.g. PHAGE M13.

RFI The *supercoiled* replicative form of the genome in certain types of bacteriophage: see e.g. PHAGE M13.

RFLP analysis Restriction fragment length polymorphism analysis: a method used for comparing *related* sequences of nucleotides (e.g. wild-type and mutant forms of a particular sequence of DNA) by comparing the subfragments produced when these molecules are cleaved by the same RESTRICTION ENDONUCLEASE; different numbers and/or sizes of fragments are produced from a given molecule if that molecule has lost or gained a restriction site (e.g. through a point mutation) or if it has undergone any insertion or deletion of nucleotides. The sets of subfragments from each sample are compared by gel electrophoresis. Differences between samples, in terms of the number and/or position of restriction sites or the existence of insertions or deletions, are manifested by the development of bands at different positions in the gel.

Various types of sample can be examined by this method – for example: viral genomes, plasmids, PCR-generated copies of particular sequences of nucleotides in bacterial and other genomes.

One factor in the sensitivity of RFLP analysis is the choice of restriction endonuclease; this, in turn, is influenced by the composition of the target sequence. Any variation among the samples is more likely to be detected if the chosen enzyme is one which has a greater number of restriction sites within the target sequence. (See also GC%.)

RFLP analysis has various uses which include the typing of bacteria (comparison of corresponding sequences of nucleotides from various strains) and the detection of mutations or polymorphisms (or methylation of specific bases) by detecting their effects on the recognition site of a given restriction enzyme.

The use of RFLP analysis for TYPING bacteria presupposes an appropriate level of stability in the target sequence. This condition may not be satisfied in some cases. Thus, in some strains of *Mycobacterium tuberculosis* the validity of results from RFLP analysis was questioned because it appeared that the target sequence was evolving too rapidly for the reliable interpretation of results on a short-term basis (a few years) [J Clin Microbiol (1999) 37:788–791].

One potential problem with this method is that samples of DNA derived directly from cells may have a pattern of modification (i.e. methylation) which is inhibitory to certain types of restriction endonuclease – thus precluding the use of these enzymes. To avoid this problem, the target sequence can be copied (from genomic DNA) by PCR and the resulting amplicons used as the sample DNA for RFLP analysis; this DNA, being synthesized *in vitro*, is non-methylated.

(See also PCR-RFLP ANALYSIS.)

RGD motif See (β₂) INTEGRIN.

rglA **gene** *Syn.* MCRA GENE.

rglB *Syn.* MCRBC.

Rh1B helicase See DEGRADOSOME.

rho-zero (ρ⁰) cells Cells which lack mitochondrial DNA; they are used e.g. in the preparation of CYBRIDS.

ribavirin 1-β-D-ribofuranosyl-1,2,4-triazole-3-carboxamide: a broad-spectrum antiviral agent which is used therapeutically against e.g. the hepatitis C, Lassa fever and SARS viruses.

Ribavirin has been reported to inhibit e.g. GTP synthesis and viral RNA-dependent RNA polymerase.

One proposal was that the activity of ribavirin mimics the 7-methylguanosine CAP region on eukaryotic mRNAs. This suggestion was tested by assessing the ability of ribavirin triphosphate to interfere with the interaction between capped mRNA and eIF4E (that part of the initiation complex which recognizes the cap region); it was concluded that ribavirin did not behave as a cap analog [RNA (2005) 11(8):1238–1244].

RibEx See RIBOSWITCH.

RiboGreen® A fluorescent dye used e.g. for quantitation of RNA in solution (Molecular Probes Inc., Eugene OR/Invitrogen, Carlsbad CA). For quantitation of RNA, the sensitivity of RiboGreen is reported to be at least 1000-fold better than that obtainable by conventional ULTRAVIOLET ABSORBANCE measurement at 260 nm.

Enhancement of fluorescence is also shown when the dye binds to DNA.

(See also DNA STAINING.)

ribonuclease Any of various enzymes which cleave RNA – see under RNASE for specific examples.

Ribonucleases that have been used for sequencing RNA are mentioned in the entry MAXAM–GILBERT METHOD.

An *endoribonuclease* acts at internal sites while an *exoribonuclease* cleaves terminal nucleotides.

Ribonucleases may need to be inactivated in solutions etc. in order to prevent loss of sample RNA. Inactivation can be achieved e.g. by DIETHYLPYROCARBONATE and by products such as RNAsecure™ (Ambion, Austin TX); this commercial product can be used for treating almost any type of solution, including those containing Tris, and there is no requirement for post-treatment autoclaving.

ribonuclease protection assay A method used e.g. for detecting a specific type of mRNA in a sample that contains total RNA. Briefly, a labeled antisense oligonucleotide is allowed

to hybridize with the required mRNA in solution. Then, the addition of RNase degrades single-stranded RNA, leaving the hybridized (double-stranded) target mRNA intact. The RNase is inactivated, and the double-stranded target molecule is precipitated and is subsequently examined e.g. in a (denaturing) polyacrylamide gel.

Nucleases used in this type of assay include e.g. mung bean nuclease and endonuclease S₁.

ribonuclease T₁ See RNASE T1.

ribonucleotide reductase An enzyme that catalyzes the conversion of ribonucleotides to deoxyribonucleotides.

RiboPrinter Microbial Characterization System™ See entry RIBOTYPING.

ribosomal frameshifting See FRAMESHIFTING.

ribosome density mapping (RDM) A method used for determining the number of ribosomes associated with particular regions of an mRNA molecule; the procedure involves site-specific cleavage of polysomal mRNAs and separation of the fractions in a sucrose density gradient; the products are then analyzed [Nucleic Acids Res (2005) 33(8):2421–2432].

riboswitch A regulatory sequence within an mRNA molecule (typically in a non-coding part); on binding a given metabolite, a riboswitch undergoes a structural change that may e.g. inhibit translation. That part of a riboswitch which binds the metabolite is called an *aptamer*; the sequence that undergoes structural change is called the *effector element* or *expression platform*.

Riboswitches are found in prokaryotes [J Bacteriol (2005) 187(2):791–794; J Bacteriol (2005) 187(23):8127–8136], and they have also been reported in some eukaryotes (e.g. fungi, plants).

[RibEx (a web server for locating riboswitches and other conserved bacterial elements): Nucleic Acids Res (2005) 33 (Web Server issue):W690–W692.]

Online source:
RibEx: http://www.ibt.unam.mx/biocomputo/ribex.html

A system analogous to the riboswitch, but engineered, has been used to regulate gene expression in mammalian cells [RNA (2006) 12:710–716].

ribothymidine See NUCLEOSIDE.

ribotype See RIBOTYPING.

ribotyping (*microbiol.*) A method for TYPING bacteria which exploits inter-strain variability in the RRN OPERON (encoding 16S, 23S and 5S rRNA).

The *rrn* operon is useful as a target in ribotyping for three main reasons:
● it is found in all bacteria;
● most species of bacteria contain more than one copy of the *rrn* operon (*Escherichia coli* has seven copies);
● the intergenic spacers are commonly of variable length.

Essentially, the genomic DNA of a given strain is cleaved by a restriction endonuclease and the fragments are separated into bands by gel electrophoresis. A labeled DNA (or RNA) probe, complementary to a sequence in the *rrn* operon, is then allowed to bind to those bands of fragments containing the target sequence. Commonly, between three and six bands are labeled by the probe. The number and position of bands produced from any given strain will depend on the following factors:

- the number of *rrn* operons in the genome;
- the lengths of the intergenic spacers;
- the precise distribution of cutting sites of the restriction endonuclease used in the procedure; loss or gain of recognition sites (e.g. through point mutations) will affect the fingerprint by altering the number/position of bands in the gel.

A strain defined by ribotyping is called a *ribotype*.

In one study on *Vibrio cholerae* the authors referred to high levels of recombination between the *rrn* operons in cells of this species (10^{-5} per cell per generation); they pointed out that any given rcombinational event could undergo reversal over extended periods of time and suggested that ribotyping may not be a suitable method for determining *evolutionary* relationships between strains. Nevertheless, in general, ribotyping is often used successfully for differentiating strains of various species of bacteria in a short-term setting.

The study on *V. cholerae* referred to above also found that recombination among *rrn* operons often resulted in a gain or loss of cutting sites for the restriction endonuclease BglI; this has suggested a reason why the range of ribotypes detected by this enzyme is often greater than that obtained with other types of restriction enzyme.

Attempts to accelerate the ribotyping procedure have lead to the development of PCR RIBOTYPING and also to an automated approach (the RiboPrinter Microbial Characterization System™, marketed by DuPont). The RiboPrinter was used e.g. in studies on *Listeria* [Appl Environ Microbiol (2005) 71 (12):8115–8122] and *Enterobacter* [BMC Microbiol (2006) 6:15].

ribozyme Any RNA molecule which has the ability to function as a catalyst, i.e. a role similar to that usually associated with a (protein) enzyme; the roles of ribozymes include nuclease and RNA–RNA ligase.

In nature, ribozymes occur in prokaryotic and eukaryotic cells and in some viruses; in cells, they carry out functions such as the processing of RNA precursor molecules (see e.g. RNASE P) and the self-splicing of introns.

Less well known are the DEOXYRIBOZYMES.

In DNA technology, ribozymes have been used in various ways, and in various types of combination, both *in vitro* and *in vivo* (see e.g. GENE THERAPY).

When complexed with polyethyleneimine (PEI), ribozymes form small particles which have been used for transfection studies. (See also MELITTIN.)

A ribozyme may also be linked to an APTAMER to form a structure in which the activity of the ribozyme is regulated by the binding of a specific molecule to the aptamer.

A functional HAMMERHEAD RIBOZYME has been expressed in cells of *Escherichia coli* from a DNA NANOCIRCLE.

Some ribozymes (e.g. one from the ciliate protozoan *Tetrahymena*) are thermostable, and there has been interest in the relationship between sequence/structure and thermostability.

In studies on stabilizing mutations in the *Tetrahymena* ribozyme, it was found that the effect on thermostability of a given mutation was highly dependent on context; thus, for example, both of the mutations A269G and A304G (close together on the ribozyme) had to be present at the same time in order to promote stability. In general, the conclusion from these studies was that mutation to stability in RNA (which may depend e.g. on the presence of rare double mutations) is less likely to occur than it is in proteins, in which stabilizing (single-site) mutations can accumulate [RNA (2006) 12(3): 387–395].

(See also ALLOSTERIC NUCLEIC ACID ENZYMES.)

rifampicin See RIFAMYCINS.

rifampin See RIFAMYCINS.

rifamycins Macrocyclic antibiotics whose target is the β subunit of (bacterial) DNA-dependent RNA polymerase – and which therefore inhibit transcription in sensitive strains. The rifamycins are active against certain Gram-positive bacteria (including mycobacteria) and some Gram-negative bacteria (e.g. strains of *Brucella*, *Chlamydia* and *Legionella*). In e.g. *Mycobacterium tuberculosis*, resistance to rifamycins may result from mutation in the *rpoB* gene (which encodes the β subunit of RNA polymerase).

The rifamycins include e.g. rifampicin (= rifampin).

(See also ANTIBIOTIC and LINE PROBE ASSAY.)

right-handed helix (of DNA) A helix which, from an axial (i.e. end-on) direction, winds away from the viewer in a clockwise fashion.

rINN Recommended international non-proprietary name.

RISC See RNA INTERFERENCE.

ritonavir See PROTEASE INHIBITORS.

RLGS RESTRICTION LANDMARK GENOMIC SCANNING.

RLU Relative light unit – see e.g. ACCUPROBE.

RMCE RECOMBINASE-MEDIATED CASSETTE EXCHANGE.

RNA amplification (*in vitro*) See NUCLEIC ACID AMPLIFICATION.

RNA chaperone See e.g. FINOP SYSTEM.

RNA degradosome *Syn.* DEGRADOSOME.

RNA-dependent DNA polymerase A DNA polymerase that is able to synthesize a strand of DNA on an RNA template: see REVERSE TRANSCRIPTASE.

RNA-dependent RNA polymerase An RNA POLYMERASE that uses an RNA template; these enzymes are encoded by some types of virus and are reported to occur in certain plants [e.g. Plant Cell (1998) 10(12):2087–2101].

In at least some cases, the role of an RNA-dependent RNA polymerase may be carried out by a cellular *DNA*-dependent RNA polymerase in association with a viral protein [J Virol (2005) 79(13):7951–7958].

(cf. REPLICASE and TRANSCRIPTASE.)

RNA-directed DNA methylation (RdDM) A particular form of GENE SILENCING: see e.g. SIRNA.

RNA-DNA chimeric oligonucleotide *Syn.* CHIMERAPLAST.

RNA editing A normal *in vivo* process (in animals, plants and some types of microorganism) in which new transcripts are generated from existing ones.

Mechanistically distinct kinds of RNA editing are carried out in different types of organism.

One example of RNA editing in mammalian cells is seen in transcripts of apolipoprotein B, a component of chylomicrons (large lipoprotein bodies produced in the intestinal mucosa). In this example, the unedited transcript encodes a protein of 4536 amino acid residues. Editing of the transcript involves an enzyme, APOBEC-1, a CYTIDINE DEAMINASE which deaminates a particular cytidine residue in the mRNA, creating a *stop codon* that reduces the length of the product to 2152 amino acid residues. Such deamination involves the mRNA-binding factor ACF/ASP (= APOBEC-1 complementation factor or APOBEC-1-stimulating protein); regulation of the editing of apolipoprotein B mRNA was reported to be associated with phosphorylation of ACF [Nucleic Acids Res (2006) 34(11):3299–3308].

The activity of the mammalian enzyme AID (ACTIVATION-INDUCED CYTIDINE DEAMINASE) may be a further example of RNA editing.

In trypanosomatids (a group of eukaryotic microorganisms) a unique type of RNA editing occurs in many or most of the mitochondrial mRNAs. This involves insertion and deletion of uridylates by a complex of proteins (see EDITOSOME) directed by small 'guide' RNA molecules (gRNAs). Most of the gRNAs are encoded by DNA minicircles which occur in the KINETOPLAST.

RNA extraction (from blood)   See e.g. PAXGENE BLOOD RNA KIT.

RNA-induced silencing complex   See RNA INTERFERENCE.

RNA interference (RNAi)   A form of post-transcriptional gene silencing (see PTGS) found in both plant and animal cells; the phenomenon appears to have evolved as a natural antiviral response which is triggered by the presence of intracellular double-stranded RNA (dsRNA). In this process, long molecules of dsRNA (more than several hundred nucleotides) are cut into regular-sized fragments by a dsRNA-specific RNase-III-like endonuclease referred to as DICER; these fragments of dsRNA, referred to as *small interfering RNA* (= siRNA: see SIRNA), are reported to be about 21–28 nucleotides in length, depending e.g. on organism. One of the strands of ds siRNA, in association with a multiprotein assembly, forms the *RNA-induced silencing complex* (RISC); among the proteins in this complex is Argonaute 2 which, guided by the single strand of siRNA, may cleave a specific (target) mRNA molecule.

Synthetic molecules of siRNA are used for experimental gene silencing, and RNAi has been used in one approach to GENE THERAPY. (See also SHORT HAIRPIN RNA.)

siRNAs are also involved in a phenomenon referred to as *transcriptional gene silencing* (TGS): see SIRNA.

Suppression of RNAi by adenovirus-associated RNA was found specifically to involve Dicer and RISC [J Virol (2005) 79(15):9556–9565].

[Therapeutic applications of RNAi: BioTechniques (2006) 40(4) supplement.]

Long dsRNA molecules also trigger the *interferon* response in mammalian cells. This response, involving the activity of a dsRNA-dependent protein kinase (known as PKR), causes generalized inhibition of viral and cellular protein synthesis.

RNA interference pathway   The gene-regulatory pathway that involves the activity of small RNA molecules such as SIRNAS (see RNA INTERFERENCE) and MICRORNAS.

RNA isolation   Separation of total RNA, or a specified fraction of RNA, from cells; thus, for example, poly(A)-tailed mRNA molecules may be isolated from a cell lysate by adsorption to a poly(T) matrix.

Isolation of RNA from blood may be carried out e.g. with the PAXGENE BLOOD RNA KIT.

The isolation of RNA from source material can be delayed, if necessary, for an extended period of time (e.g. weeks) by placing the material (e.g. tissue samples) in RNALATER and then storing at room temperature, 4°C or −20°C.

RNA modification pathways (a database)   See MODOMICS [Nucleic Acids Res (2006) 34(Database issue):D145–D149]. Data can be accessed via: http://genesilico.pl/modomics/

RNA PCR   An early name for REVERSE TRANSCRIPTASE PCR.

RNA polymerase (RPase)   Any enzyme which can polymerize ribonucleoside 5′-triphosphates on a DNA or RNA template; this term usually refers to a DNA-dependent RNA polymerase, i.e. an enzyme that uses a DNA template.

(See also RNA-DEPENDENT RNA POLYMERASE.)

In *Escherichia coli*, the bulk of RNA synthesis is carried out by a single multi-component RPase; in this enzyme, the three types of component (α, β, β'), together with a *sigma factor* protein (σ), form the functional enzyme (holoenzyme): $\alpha_2\beta\beta'\sigma$. This enzyme is sensitive to e.g. rifampicin.

The *E. coli* primase (*dnaG* gene product) is an RPase used for synthesis of the RNA primers that are extended by DNA synthesis to form the Okazaki fragments produced during the replication of DNA. Primase is resistant to rifampicin.

RPases of members of the ARCHAEA appear to resemble the eukaryotic (nuclear) RPases (see below) rather than bacterial enzymes.

In general, eukaryotes have three multi-component nuclear RPases. RPase I (= RPase A) synthesizes most rRNA in the nucleolus. RPase II (B) synthesizes pre-mRNA. RPase III (C) synthesizes e.g. tRNAs and 5S rRNA. At least one of these enzymes also synthesizes snRNAs for pre-mRNA SPLICING. These RPases are not inhibited by rifamycins.

In eukaryotes, the mitochondrial and chloroplast RPases are distinct from the nuclear enzymes.

RNA-recognition motif   See SR PROTEINS.

RNA sequencing   See e.g. MAXAM–GILBERT METHOD.

RNA splicing (pre-mRNA)   See SPLICING.

RNA staining   See e.g. RIBOGREEN.

(See also DNA STAINING and ULTRAVIOLET ABSORBANCE.)

RNAi   See RNA INTERFERENCE.

RNA*later*™   An aqueous reagent (Ambion, Austin TX) that is used for the storage of tissue samples, and other specimens, from which RNA is to be subsequently extracted.

[Use (e.g.): PLoS ONE (2007) 2(3):e281.]

In this product, the samples may be stored at 25°C (room temperature) for up to 1 week, at 4°C for up to 1 month, and at −20°C for an indefinite period.

When the RNA is required, the sample is removed from the reagent and is treated in the same way as a freshly harvested sample.

The use of this reagent has various advantages – e.g. (i) it protects the cellular RNA from endogenous RNases, (ii) it permits extraction of RNA – at a convenient time – from samples collected at different times, and (iii) it permits overnight transport of sample(s) between laboratories (at 'room temperature').

RNAqueous™ technology A commercial approach (Ambion, Austin TX) used for isolating total RNA from various types of tissue or cell without the need for phenol–chloroform extraction. Essentially, tissues are disrupted by the chaotropic agent guanidinium thiocyanate – which also inactivates the endogenous nucleases. Following dilution of the lysate with an ethanol solution, the whole is transferred to a glass-fiber filter which binds RNA; three consecutive washes are used to remove proteins and DNA etc. and the RNA is then eluted.

Various products, incorporating RNAqueous™ technology, are designed for particular applications – e.g. several kits are suitable for rt-PCR, and an automated kit is suitable for high-throughput working.

(See also NUCLEIC ACID ISOLATION.)

RNase Ribonuclease – see entries below for specific examples; see also entry RIBONUCLEASE for general information.

RNase III An endoribonuclease that cleaves double-stranded RNA (e.g. in hairpin or stem–loop structures). The enzyme is involved e.g. in the processing (maturation) of rRNA from precursor molecules (see e.g. RRN OPERON) and also in the regulation of gene expression.

The (functional) RNase III of *Escherichia coli* is a homodimer. dsRNA is cleaved into fragments with 5′-phosphate and 3′-hydroxyl termini and short 3′ overhangs. The factors which determine cleavage sites are reported to include both structure (e.g. helix length – often two helical turns) and sequence. Based on earlier observations it was suggested that the enzyme may recognize cleavage sites by the *absence* of particular base pairs within discrete regions of double-helical RNA referred to as the *proximal box* and the *distal box*. More recently, specific base pair sequence elements were reported to act as positive recognition determinants. [Characterization of RNA sequence determinants and antideterminants of processing reactivity for a minimal substrate of *Escherichia coli* RNase III: Nucleic Acids Res (2006) 34(13):3708–3721.]

(See also DICER.)

RNase Cocktail™ A product (Ambion, Austin TX) consisting of a mixture of highly purified ribonucleases: RNase A and RNase T_1; it can be used e.g. for eliminating RNA in plasmid minipreps.

RNase E See DEGRADOSOME.

(See also BL21 STAR.)

RNase H An RNase which specifically degrades a strand of RNA that is hybridized to a strand of DNA – e.g. the strand of RNA which is hybridized to FIRST STRAND cDNA. The RNase H from *Escherichia coli* is an endoribonuclease that forms products with 3′-hydroxyl and 5′-phosphate termini.

*Exo*ribonuclease activity is exhibited by the reverse transcriptase of retroviruses (but is absent e.g. in a recombinant form of the enzyme from Moloney murine leukemia virus).

RNase H is used e.g. for making cDNAs. It is also used e.g. in NASBA.

RNase P An endoribonuclease, containing protein and RNA, involved in generating 5′ termini in tRNAs; its catalytic activity is mediated by the RNA. [Human RNase P: Nucleic Acids Res (2007) 35:3519–3524.]

RNase protection assay See entry RIBONUCLEASE PROTECTION ASSAY.

RNase T_1 (RNase T1) An endoribonuclease, encoded by the fungus *Aspergillus oryzae*, which specifically cleaves single-stranded RNA 3′ of guanosine residues (Gp↓N), thus forming guanosine 3′-phosphate and oligonucleotides with 3′ terminal phosphate.

(See G-LESS CASSETTE and MAXAM–GILBERT METHOD.)

RNA*secure*™ See RIBONUCLEASE.

rne131 See BL21 STAR.

Robust-LongSAGE See SAGE.

rolling circle A mode of nucleic acid synthesis which occurs in some *circular* molecules of DNA and RNA.

In (ds) DNA molecules, the process begins with a NICK in one strand; the free 3′ end is then extended by a DNA polymerase, using the un-nicked strand as template. The 5′ end of the nicked strand is progressively displaced as polymerization continues.

Rolling circle synthesis occurs e.g. in many small circular bacterial plasmids, the nicking being mediated by a plasmid-encoded *Rep protein*; plasmid-length pieces of the displaced strand may then be circularized and then converted to dsDNA plasmids.

In bacteriophage φX174 (which has a single-stranded, ccc DNA genome), nicking of the (double-stranded) parental replicative form (RF) is followed by rolling circle synthesis (involving the bacterial DNA polymerase); genome lengths of the resulting displaced strand are excised, circularized and converted to progeny RFs.

In phage λ, rolling circle synthesis leads to the formation of a continuous multi-genome (double-stranded) CONCATEMER that is later cut at the (repeating) *cos* sites into genome-sized sections; the concatemer is double-stranded because the displaced strand is used as a template on which the complementary strand is synthesized.

Rolling circle synthesis also occurs during the replication of viroids: small plant-pathogenic circular ssRNA molecules (see VIROID).

In vitro, rolling circle synthesis has been used e.g. for the transcription of a DNA NANOCIRCLE.

Rolling circle synthesis was also used in a rapid, sensitive method for detecting SARS virus [J Clin Microbiol (2005) 43 (5):2339–2344].

The efficiency and specificity of rolling circle amplification were reported to be improved by a mutant form of the SSB (single-strand binding protein) from the bacterium *Thermus thermophilus* [Nucleic Acids Res (2006) 34(9):e69].

Rom protein   See COLE1.

Rop protein   See COLE1.

Rotor-Gene™ 6000 See HRM.

RPA   (1) Recombinase polymerase amplification: a rapid, isothermal method for amplifying specific sequences of DNA; it involves recombinase-mediated binding of primers to their target sequences coupled with strand-displacement synthesis of DNA [PLoS Biol (2006) 4(7):e204].

Essentially, in the presence of ATP, the primers form complexes with molecules of a recombinase (the UvsX enzyme of phage T4), and primer–recombinase complexes search the double-stranded sample DNA for sequences complementary to the primers. When primer-binding sites are located the recombinase mediates strand exchange: the binding of a given primer displaces a loop of ssDNA which is stabilized by the binding of single-strand binding proteins (SSBPs). The disassembly of recombinase permits the bound primer to be extended by a (strand-displacing) DNA polymerase. As primer extension continues, SSBPs stabilize the increasingly long strand of displaced DNA. Similar, repeated activity by both (opposing) primers leads to exponential amplification of the target. Ongoing activity in RPA depends on the presence of agents which mediate a balance in the development and disassembly of the primer–recombinase complexes.

Reactions in which the template is either absent or in low concentration were found to lead to primer-dependent artefacts. To combat this, the detection of products is achieved by a probe-based system. Essentially, the probe includes an abasic-site mimic flanked by a fluorophore-labeled nucleotide and a quencher-labeled nucleotide; the intact probe is associated with low-level fluorescence. Hybridization of the probe to its complementary sequence permits the abasic-site mimic to be recognized – and cleaved – by an endonuclease (*Escherichia coli* endonuclease IV; Nfo) which subsequently results in a measureable rise in fluorescence (as the fluorophore is no longer quenched). The increase in fluorescence is exploited in monitoring the products. In that cleavage by Nfo requires stable pairing between the probe and its binding site, this arrangement promotes specificity in product detection.

RPA is reported to be capable of multiplex operation, the method having been employed e.g. to amplify simultaneously targets from several different strains of methicillin-resistant *Staphylococcus aureus* (MRSA).

(2) Replication protein A (see e.g. OKAZAKI FRAGMENT).

RPase   RNA POLYMERASE.

rpmI gene   See OPERON.

rpoB gene   See RIFAMYCINS.

rpoH gene   See ESCHERICHIA COLI (table).

rpsL gene (*syn. strA* gene)   In *Escherichia coli*: a gene encoding the ribosomal protein S12; mutation in this gene may lead to resistance to the antibiotic streptomycin (for which S12 is the target protein).

RRE   Rev protein response element: see REV PROTEIN.

rrn operon (in bacteria)   An OPERON encoding the three species of rRNA (16S, 23S, 5S) which is transcribed (as a single pre-rRNA transcript) in the order 16S→23S→5S. The genes are not contiguous: a so-called *intergenic spacer region* (ISR) is found between each pair of coding sequences. The length of an ISR can vary, even in different copies of the *rrn* operon in the same chromosome, and this feature has been exploited in certain forms of TYPING (PCR-RIBOTYPING and RIBOTYPING).

Bacteria usually contain multiple copies of the *rrn* operon, but single copies are reported to occur e.g. in *Mycobacterium tuberculosis* and *Tropheryma whipplei*.

Escherichia coli contains seven copies of the *rrn* operon. The pre-rRNA molecule forms secondary structures (through base-pairing between inverted repeats) in which the 16S and 23S components form loops in separate stem–loop structures; the 16S and 23S precursor molecules are liberated by the action of an endoribonuclease (RNase III).

(See also LEUCINE-RESPONSIVE REGULATOR PROTEIN.)

RT-PCR   REVERSE TRANSCRIPTASE PCR.

rt-PCR   REVERSE TRANSCRIPTASE PCR.

Rta (*brlf-1* gene product)   See ZEBRA.

rtPCR   REVERSE TRANSCRIPTASE PCR.

rTth DNA polymerase   A 94-kDA recombinant DNA polymerase (Perkin Elmer/Applied Biosystems) that is derived from the thermophilic bacterium *Thermus thermophilus*; in a single buffer system it can act as both a reverse transcriptase and a DNA-dependent DNA polymerase.

The enzyme can function in the range 60–70°C and is used e.g. in REVERSE TRANSCRIPTASE PCR.

Examples of use: studies on the SARS virus [BMC Infect Dis (2006) 6:20] and studies on the hepatitis C virus [J Clin Microbiol (2006) 44(7):2507–2511].

S

S (1) A specific indicator of ambiguity in the recognition site of a RESTRICTION ENDONUCLEASE or in any other sequence of nucleic acid; thus, for example, in ↓GTSAC (enzyme Tsp45I) the 'S' indicates G or C.

(2) L-Serine (alternative to Ser).

S₁ nuclease *Syn.* ENDONUCLEASE S1.

Saccharomyces A genus of YEASTS; the species *S. cerevisiae* is widely used as an experimental organism (and is also used in the manufacture of alcoholic beverages and fermented products).

S. cerevisiae occurs as single cells which may be haploid or diploid, depending on the stage of the life cycle. Both haploid and diploid cells reproduce asexually by a process known as *budding* (cf. SCHIZOSACCHAROMYCES).

Sexual reproduction involves fusion of two haploid cells of appropriate MATING TYPE. The diploid zygote gives rise to diploid somatic (vegetative) cells. Diploid cells constitute a major phase in the life cycle. Diploid cells undergo meiosis to form four *ascospores* within a structure called an *ascus*; two of the ascospores are of the α mating type, and two are of the **a** mating type. Ascospores develop into haploid somatic cells.

The existence of both haploid and diploid somatic cells in the life cycle has been exploited in complementation studies in which e.g. the diploid cells can be used to study the effects of different alleles derived from parental haploids.

Cells of the AB1380 strain of *S. cerevisiae*, and derivatives, have been used e.g. as hosts for YEAST ARTIFICIAL CHROMOSOMES. These cells have mutations in genes *TRP1* and *URA3* and require both tryptophan and uracil in growth media; the corresponding (wild-type) genes in YACs are therefore useful for the selection of YAC-containing cells (in tryptophan-deficient and uracil-deficient media). The cells of this strain also have a mutation in a gene whose product is involved in adenine metabolism, leading to red pigmentation; this defect is bypassed by the suppressor gene *SUP4* which, in a YAC, is involved in a mechanism for indicating the presence/absence of an insert (see YEAST ARTIFICIAL CHROMOSOME).

S. cerevisiae is used in the YEAST TWO-HYBRID SYSTEM for studying protein–protein interactions.

(See also ARS and YEAST MARKER.)

[Yeast-based technologies in genomics and proteomics (a review): BioTechniques (2006) 40(5):625–644.]

Saccharomyces cerevisiae Genome Deletion Project See entry GENOME DELETION PROJECT.

SafeBis DNA DNA which has been treated with BISULFITE but which has not been subsequently desulfonated; it has been used e.g. in studies on DNA methylation [Nucleic Acids Res (2007) 35(1):e4].

safety cabinet (*syn.* sterile cabinet) A piece of equipment that provides a partially or totally enclosed space within which certain types of procedure can be carried out; some types of cabinet are designed specifically to provide effective containment of dangerous pathogens – with the object of protecting both laboratory staff and the environment.

Class I cabinets are accessed, for working, via an opening in the front below a glass viewing panel. A fan draws air into the cabinet, via the front opening, and air leaves the cabinet via a high-efficiency particulate air filter (a HEPA filter); the rate of airflow is such that aerosols do not leave the cabinet via the front opening.

Class I cabinets are used e.g. for work on pathogens such as *Coxiella burnetii*, *Francisella tularensis* and *Mycobacterium tuberculosis*. In addition to the use of a class I cabinet, work with this type of pathogen requires the use of gloves and also the existence of *plenum* ventilation in the laboratory – i.e. a constant inflow of air to the laboratory, with filtration of the exhausted air through a HEPA filter.

Class II cabinets are used primarily to protect materials in the cabinet from environmental contamination. Filtered air constantly flows down onto the work surface and leaves the cabinet after further filtration. Access is from the front, below a glass viewing panel. These cabinets (which are common in microbiological laboratories in universities) are used e.g. to avoid contamination when inoculating media.

Class III cabinets are high-security cabinets that are totally enclosed and gas-tight. Air is filtered before entry and before discharge. Manipulation of materials etc. within the cabinet is conducted by means of arm-length rubber gloves that are fitted securely into the front of the cabinet. The interior of the cabinet is viewed via a glass panel. Access to the cabinet is via a separate two-door sterilization/disinfection chamber.

Class III cabinets are used when handling hazardous pathogens such as the Ebola virus, Lassa fever virus and Marburg virus.

SAGE Serial analysis of gene expression: a method for detecting, identifying and quantitating genes expressed by a given type of cell, under given conditions, by analyzing a collection of short (~10-nucleotide) sequences (SAGE tags, diagnostic tags) derived from the transcript (mRNA) of each gene. This method may be used without prior knowledge of the nucleotide sequences of genes; a particular gene may be identified via its diagnostic tag.

SAGE is used for discovering new genes, for studies on the up- and down-regulation of genes under different conditions, for studies on differential expression of genes, and for establishing links between various aspects of a cell's physiology. Thus, for example, observation of the levels of transcripts has revealed a relationship between phosphate metabolism and other aspects of cell physiology in the smut fungus *Ustilago maydis* [Eukaryotic Cell (2005) 4(12):2029–2043], and the use of LongSAGE (see later) has facilitated gene discovery in a marine coccolithophorid [Appl Environ Microbiol (2006) 72:252–260].

The basic procedure for SAGE is essentially as follows.

Initially, total mRNA is isolated from the cell or tissue and is reverse transcribed, with BIOTINylated oligo(dT) primers, to cDNAs.

Double-stranded cDNA molecules are then subjected to a 'frequent-cutting' restriction endonuclease (e.g. NlaIII) which cleaves the cDNA molecules more than once. (This enzyme is sometimes called the 'anchoring enzyme'.)

The *biotinylated ends* of the cleaved cDNA molecules are then captured e.g. by STREPTAVIDIN-coated DYNABEADS.

The Dynabead-bound fragments are then separated into two subpopulations.

In one of the subpopulations, the free ends of the fragments (i.e. termini formed by cleavage with the anchoring enzyme) are ligated to a dsDNA oligonucleotide linker (linker A); this linker contains the recognition site of a type IIS RESTRICTION ENDONUCLEASE.

In the second subpopulation, the free ends are ligated to a different linker (linker B); however, this linker also contains the recognition site of the type IIS restriction enzyme.

Each subpopulation is subjected to the action of a type IIS restriction enzyme. This type of enzyme cuts some distance from its recognition site; consequently, the result of type IIS restriction is the generation of a number of free fragments (released from the Dynabeads), each of which consists of (i) the linker, and (ii) a short sequence of nucleotides (9–14 bp) derived from the (contiguous) ligated cDNA fragment. The sequence of nucleotides derived from the cDNA fragment is called the *signature tag* for the relevant gene.

Any overhang produced by type IIS restriction is filled in e.g. by the Klenow fragment.

The two subpopulations are mixed.

The tags are now ligated together by blunt-ended ligation. Structures of the following type are formed:

linker A–(signature tag)$_2$–linker B

The pair of ligated signature tags is called a *ditag*. The ditags are amplified by PCR, using primer-binding sites in each of the two types of linker.

The PCR products are subjected to the restriction enzyme used initially to cleave the cDNAs (the anchoring enzyme). This results in the excision of both (terminal) linkers, leaving a pair of ligated signature tags (a ditag).

The ditags are ligated together, serially, to form long molecules of DNA, each of these molecules containing many tags. These molecules can be cloned and sequenced.

The relative abundance of a given transcript in the original sample is reflected in the number of relevant tags in the final product. A signature tag identifies a particular gene – so that the level of expression of a given gene can be assessed by the SAGE procedure.

Computer-based analysis of the sequence data can be used to identify particular genes.

Various modifications of the basic scheme described have been devised:

MicroSAGE uses minute quantities of sample material. The principle is similar to that described, although e.g. mRNAs in the sample bind directly to oligo(dT)-coated magnetic beads (i.e. prior to reverse transcription).

LongSAGE [Nat Biotechnol (2002) 20(5):508–512] uses a longer signature tag (21 bp), and Robust-LongSAGE offers a number of improvements [Plant Physiol (2004) 134(3):890–897].

(See also 5′ LongSAGE and 3′ LongSAGE [Proc Natl Acad Sci USA (2004) 101(32):11701–11706].)

In superSAGE [Proc Natl Acad Sci USA (2003) 100(26): 15718–15723], a type III restriction endonuclease (EcoP15I) is used to increase the size of tags to 26 bp; superSAGE e.g. facilitates the identification of a gene from databases such as GenBank.

salicylate (as an inducer of gene expression)   See e.g. CASCADE EXPRESSION SYSTEM.

Salmonella   A genus of Gram-negative, rod-shaped, generally motile bacteria of the family Enterobacteriaceae (see entry ENTEROBACTERIA); the species *S. typhi* is the causal agent of typhoid.

GC% of chromosomal DNA: 50–52.

The salmonellae (i.e. members of this genus) can be grown on (e.g.) nutrient agar and MacConkey's agar; media used for enrichment include e.g. selenite broth and tetrathionate broth.

Linguistic note

The name *Salmonella* derives from the name of an American bacteriologist, D. E. Salmon; the correct pronunciation of the genus name is therefore 'Salmon-ella' – the first 'l' is silent.

***Salmonella*/microsome assay**   *Syn.* AMES TEST.

SAM   *S*-adenosyl-L-methionine (a methyl donor).

same-sense mutation   Any mutation which fails to change the identity of the amino acid that is specified by a given codon.

A same-sense mutation may not be equivalent to a SILENT MUTATION if it introduces a CODON BIAS.

SAMPL   Selective amplification of microsatellite polymorphic loci, *or* selectively amplified microsatellite polymorphic loci: a method for detecting variations (in length) of microsatellite sequences in genomic DNA. Initially – as in AFLP – genomic DNA is digested with two restriction enzymes, the fragments are ligated to adaptors, and pre-amplification is carried out by PCR with primers having a single selective 3′ nucleotide.

Another round of PCR amplification is carried out with one AFLP primer and a (labeled) SAMPL primer complementary to the particular microsatellite sequence being studied; the two primers in the second round of PCR therefore amplify those microsatellite sequences that were present in amplicons formed during pre-amplification.

sampling (DNA)   See, for example, BUCCAL CELL SAMPLING and FORENSIC APPLICATIONS.

Sandhoff disease   A GENETIC DISEASE similar to TAY–SACHS DISEASE (q.v.) but resulting from a deficiency in the activity of the β-subunit of hexosaminidase A.

Sanger's method (DNA sequencing)   See DIDEOXY METHOD.

Sapphire-II™   See CHEMILUMINESCENCE ENHANCER.

saquinavir   See PROTEASE INHIBITORS.

SARS virus (detection)   A rapid, sensitive method for detecting the SARS virus (an ssRNA coronavirus) in clinical samples has exploited (genome-specific) PADLOCK PROBES which, on circularization, act as templates for isothermal replication of target sequences by the ROLLING CIRCLE MECHANISM [J Clin Microbiol (2005) 43(5):2339–2344].

SBE   See SINGLE-BASE EXTENSION.

scaffold   In a (eukaryotic) chromosome: a central, proteinaceous structure which serves to anchor loops of DNA.

scaffolding proteins   Proteins that form a temporary (structural) framework during the assembly of (e.g.) a phage head – but which do not form part of the mature (completed) head. The scaffolding proteins may be subsequently degraded – as e.g. in phages λ and T4; they are re-cycled e.g. in phages P22 and φ29.

scanning force microscopy   *Syn.* ATOMIC FORCE MICROSCOPY.

SCC*mec*   In strains of MRSA: a mobile genetic element (name: staphylococcal cassette chromosome *mec*) which includes the MECA GENE complex and the *ccr* gene complex.

Different versions of the *mec* and *ccr* gene complexes have been found in environmental isolates of MRSA, and SCC*mec* elements have been classified into five types (I–V) on the basis of these differences; however, this classification is not ideal, and a new system of classification, which is believed to be more suitable for typing these strains, has been proposed [Antimicrob Agents Chemother (2006) 50(3):1001–1012].

SCE   Single-cell ELECTROPORATION (q.v.).

SCF (stem cell factor)   See KIT.

scFV   A SINGLE-CHAIN VARIABLE FRAGMENT.

Schizosaccharomyces   A genus of fungi in which the morphological forms are single cells that reproduce by *fission* (rather than *budding*: cf. SACCHAROMYCES) or hyphae that fragment into spores. Some strains of these fungi are homothallic (i.e. self-fertile); others are heterothallic.

Studies on the effects of mutations in replication-initiation genes and checkpoint genes in the species *S. pombe* found that the resulting replication stress, and inappropriate mitosis, resulted in the production of reactive oxygen species (ROS) and cell death [J Cell Sci (2006) 119(1):124–131].

The species of *Schizosaccharomyces* are distinguished e.g. by the number of ascospores formed in the asci and by the ability to ferment specific sugars.

schlieren system   A system used for representing a refractive index gradient.

Schneider's medium   A liquid medium used for the culture of insect cells; it includes various inorganic salts (e.g. magnesium sulfate, potassium chloride, sodium chloride), D-glucose, trehalose, malic acid, succinic acid, and a number of amino acids.

SCID   See GENETIC DISEASE (table).

SCIDX1   See GENETIC DISEASE (table).

scintillation proximity assay   See SPA.

SCNT   Somatic cell nuclear transfer: removal of the chromosomes from an unfertilized oocyte (*enucleation*) and their replacement with chromosomes from a somatic cell.

An oocyte which has undergone SCNT may be used e.g. to produce an embryonic clone which may serve as a source of embryonic stem cells (see STEM CELL). As an alternative, an SCNT-treated oocyte may be allowed to develop into a live animal (a *clone*) following appropriate follow-up procedures.

Scorpion probe   A PROBE analogous to a MOLECULAR BEACON PROBE used for monitoring the products of PCR [e.g. Nucleic Acids Res (2000) 28(19):3752–3761]. The probe resembles a molecular beacon, with fluorophore and quencher in the stem section – but it has a single-stranded 3′ extension. During the (heat) denaturation stage, both the target DNA *and* the stem section of the probe become single-stranded; on cooling, the probe's 3′ extension binds to target DNA and is subsequently extended, copying the target sequence. During the subsequent denaturation and cooling the *loop* region of the probe hybridizes with a complementary sequence in the probe's extended 3′ region; in this arrangement, the fluorophore and quencher are separated – so that the probe exhibits fluorescence under suitable excitation.

ScRad51   The RAD51 protein of *Saccharomyces cerevisiae*.

screening   Any *selective* procedure in which individual cells or molecules with given characteristics are distinguished and/or isolated from the other individuals in the same population.

For examples of screening see BLACK–WHITE SCREENING, blue–white screening (in PBLUESCRIPT), COLONY HYBRIDIZATION, ELISPOT, METAGENOME, RECACTIVE, SIGEX, SSCP ANALYSIS.

screening test (*immunol.*, *microbiol.*)   (1) Any test that is used to examine specimen(s) in order to detect a particular type of antibody, antigen or microorganism. Screening tests are often simple and inexpensive but are frequently not highly specific; as a positive result in a screening test may be followed-up by other – more specific – test(s), a proportion of false-positive results may be tolerated.

Examples of nucleic-acid-based screening tests include e.g. AMP CT and LINE PROBE ASSAY.

(2) Any test designed to assign a given, unknown organism to one of a possible range of categories or taxa.

SCS system   Separate-component-stabilization system: see CCD MECHANISM.

SDA   Strand displacement amplification: an isothermal method for copying a given sequence of nucleotides in a sample of DNA. (See also NUCLEIC ACID AMPLIFICATION.) Originally, SDA was carried out at an operating temperature of ~40°C; later, the operating temperature was raised to 50°C or above (thermophilic SDA, tSDA) with the object of improving the specificity of the method.

SDA (which is shown diagrammatically in the figure) is characterized by two distinctive features: (i) the use of a particular type of RESTRICTION ENDONUCLEASE that repeatedly *nicks* a chemically modified recognition sequence in double-stranded intermediate forms, thereby continually regenerating sense and antisense strands that are displaced from dsDNA intermediates by a strand-displacing DNA polymerase; (ii) use of a strand-displacing DNA polymerase (such as Klenow

Part I

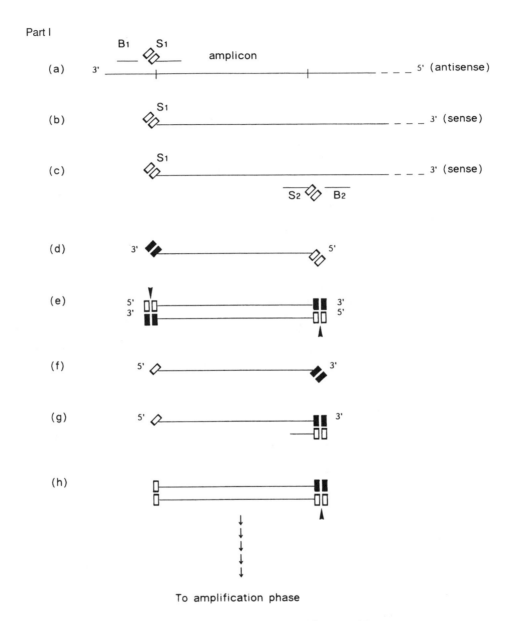

To amplification phase

SDA (strand displacement amplification) – part I: the target-generation phase (diagrammatic).

Target DNA is initially denatured to the single-stranded state prior to SDA.

(a) The antisense (3'-to-5') strand of the target duplex is shown with the amplicon (i.e. the sequence of nucleotides to be amplified) delimited by two short vertical bars. For clarity of presentation, and economy of space, only one strand of the target DNA is

236

fragment: see DNA POLYMERASE I) which is able to displace a strand from duplex DNA by extending an existing 3′ terminus at the site of a nick.

Restriction endonuclease. The restriction endonuclease used in SDA is HincII, and the specific recognition site employed is:

5′-GTT/GAC-3′
3′-CAA/CTG-5′

Normally, HincII makes a double-stranded, blunt-ended cut, as shown by the oblique (/), but this activity does not occur in SDA because, in each recognition site, one of the two strands (■ ■ in the figure) is chemically *modified* and cannot be cut; the other strand (□ □ in the figure) is *nicked* by HincII.

The *nickable* strand within a recognition site can be formed either by a primer or by regeneration of the recognition site by 3′ extension from a nick. Both primers, S_1 and S_2, have a 5′ terminal tag: 5′-GTTGAC-3′; this *unmodified* sequence, when present in a (duplex) recognition site, can be nicked by HincII between the 'T' and 'G' nucleotides.

The *un-nickable* strand in a recognition site arises because, in SDA, all strand synthesis occurs in a reaction mixture that contains a chemically modified form of deoxyadenosine triphosphate: α-thiophosphoryl dATP (dATPαS). As a consequence of the presence of dATPαS, when the complementary strand is synthesized on a template strand containing a primer sequence, the newly synthesized strand (3′-CAACTG..........) includes two modified nucleotides in the AA positions which are adjacent to the cleavage site; because of the presence of these two modified nucleotides, *this* strand cannot be cleaved by HincII. Thus the double-stranded recognition site contains a nickable site (in the primer sequence) and a non-cleavable sequence in the newly synthesized (complementary) strand. This 'hemi-modified' HincII site (= *hemiphosphorothioate* site) is therefore susceptible to nicking, only, by HincII in the primer strand between 'T' and 'G' (see e.g. (e) in part I of the figure).

A nick between the 'T' and 'G' in the primer sequence of a recognition site is followed by extension from the 3′ end of the nick – this displacing the strand downstream of the nick. Importantly, the strand which is formed by such extension (5′-GTT→→) incorporates a modified nucleotide (dATPαS) at the 'A' site within the sequence GAC. *Despite this*, the HincII site that is regenerated in the newly synthesized strand (i.e. 5′-GTTGAC....3′) is nickable because the one modified nucleotide in GAC does not interfere with nickability of the sequence GTTGAC.

SDS SODIUM DODECYL SULFATE.

SDS–PAGE (Laemmli electrophoresis) Sodium dodecyl sulfate–POLYACRYLAMIDE gel electrophoresis: a particular form of GEL ELECTROPHORESIS that is used e.g. for determining the molecular weight of a protein or separating a mixture of proteins.

SDA (*continued*)

considered here; corresponding events occur on the complementary strand. A primer (S_1) has bound at the 3′ end of the amplicon. The 5′ end of this primer carries a tag that includes one strand of the HincII recognition sequence (5′-GTTGAC-3′) (shown by the symbol □□). A bumper primer (B_1 – see entry) has bound upstream of primer S_1. Extension of S_1 will produce a sense strand on the antisense template; this sense strand will be displaced by the extension of B_1.

(b) The sense strand which has been displaced, by bumper primer B_1, from the original template strand.

(c) Primer S_2 has bound to the 3′ end of the amplicon on the sense strand. Like primer S_1, its 5′ end is tagged with the recognition sequence of HincII. The bumper primer B_2 has bound upstream of primer S_2. Extension of S_2 will produce an antisense copy of the amplicon which is tagged at both ends with a (single-stranded) HincII recognition sequence; this strand will be displaced by bumper primer B_2.

(d) The antisense strand which has been displaced from stage (c) by bumper primer B_2. Notice that the HincII sequence at the 3′ end of this strand, having been synthesized with dATPαS (see entry), is 'modified' (as indicated by the symbol ■■); this (modified) HincII sequence (when subsequently part of a double-stranded amplicon) is not susceptible to the restriction endonuclease HincII. At the other (5′) end of the strand, the HincII sequence is not modified because it originated in primer S_2 (which was synthesized with normal nucleotides). Primer S_1 (not shown) can bind at the 3′ end of this strand – the HincII sequence in S_1 hybridizing with the modified sequence in the strand. Extension of S_1 yields the double-stranded amplicon shown at (e).

(e) Each end of this amplicon has a 'hemi-modified' (hemiphosphorothioate) recognition sequence for HincII. A hemi-modified site can be nicked in the *non*-modified strand (as shown by the arrowheads). Nicking can therefore occur in the 'upper' strand or the 'lower' strand of this (double-stranded) amplicon. For clarity, nicking in only the *upper* strand is considered here. Nicking is followed by extension of the 3′ end of the nick – resulting in displacement of the nicked strand, which is shown at (f).

(f) The strand displaced from (d) following nicking and extension of the 3′ end of the nick.

(g) Primer S_2 has bound to the displaced strand and will be extended to form the double-stranded product shown at (h).

(h) This product feeds into the amplification phase (see part II of the figure).

In the above scheme, at stage (e), nicking of the *upper* strand, only, was considered. Nicking of the *lower* strand, and its displacement, produces a single-stranded product that binds primer S_1; extension of primer S_1 leads to the formation of a double-stranded product that feeds into the amplification phase.

Part II

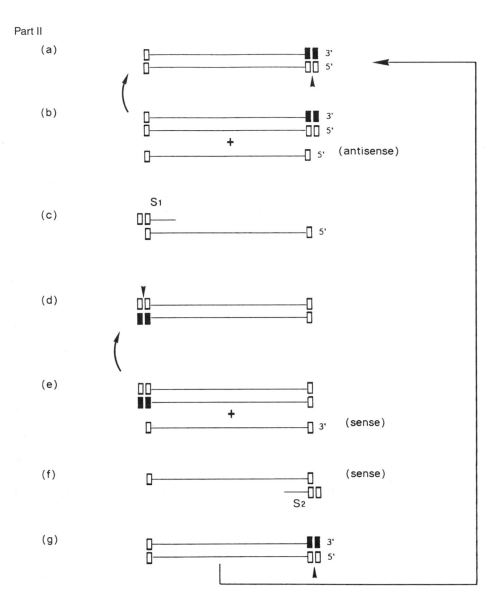

SDA (strand displacement amplification) – part II: the amplification phase (diagrammatic).

(a) A double-stranded product derived from the target-generation phase. In this product the antisense (3′-to-5′) strand contains a nick-able HincII restriction site (indicated by the arrowhead); this nickable site was derived from the tag in primer S2 (see part I (g)). When this restriction site is nicked, DNA synthesis proceeds from the 3′ end at the nick site; during synthesis, the polymerase dis-places the downstream section of the strand, producing an antisense copy of the target sequence which is flanked, on each side, by half a restriction site. Moreover, DNA synthesis from the 3′ end of the nick site regenerates the original duplex. Both of these

For the determination of molecular weights, proteins are denatured with SODIUM DODECYL SULFATE: an anionic detergent that binds cooperatively to proteins, forming rod-like SDS–polypeptide complexes in which surface charges on the protein are masked by SDS. Most proteins bind SDS in proportion to their molecular weight, so that the electrophoretic mobility of a given protein will be related to its molecular weight. Electrophoresis is carried out with the proteins under study together with one or more proteins of known molecular weight which act as standards for comparison.

For separating proteins in a mixture, maximum resolution can be achieved by using the Laemmli system in which the proteins in a sample are first compressed into a thin band by electrophoresis within a *stacking gel* before entering the so-called *resolving* (= *running* or *separating*) *gel* in which they are subjected to the sieving action of a gel structure with a smaller pore size.

Seamless® cloning kit   A kit (Stratagene, La Jolla CA) which can be used e.g. for expression cloning, for the preparation of chimeric genes, and for site-specific mutagenesis; it involves the facilitated introduction of a fragment of interest into a circular vector.

Initially, the fragment of interest, and the *functional region* of the vector, are both amplified (separately) by PCR with the use of specialized primers. Each primer's 5′ terminal region contains the recognition sequence of the (type IIS) restriction endonuclease Eam1104I (see table in the entry RESTRICTION ENDONUCLEASE); this enzyme cuts at a fixed distance from its recognition sequence – a feature that allows the fragment to be cloned without introducing additional nucleotides (see later).

The PCR reaction mixture contains a (high-fidelity) DNA polymerase which minimizes the introduction of mutations.

The final five cycles of the PCR reaction are carried out with 5-methyl-dCTP, thereby modifying, and thus protecting from subsequent cleavage, any Eam1104I sites which happen to be within the fragment or vector sequence.

After PCR the (linear) products from both the fragment and vector are mixed and digested with Eam1104I. Eam1104I binds to the termini of each product and cleaves each portion of the product derived from the 5′ flap of a primer – i.e. that part which contains the enzyme's own recognition and cutting sites; hence, these sequences are not included in the final products.

The Eam1104I-cleaved products are then ligated with T4 DNA ligase. Circularized molecules, containing both vector and fragment components, can be used to transform cells of *Escherichia coli*.

Chimeric genes may be constructed by using two different fragments, each fragment contributing to a chimeric product.

SDA (*continued*)

products – the antisense copy and the regenerated duplex – are shown at (b). Notice that the restriction site in the regenerated duplex is still nickable; this is because the regenerated site contains only one modified nucleotide (in the 5′-GAC-3′ part of site) and this does not affect nickability (see entry).

(b)   Products formed from the double-stranded structure at (a) by nicking, strand displacement and regeneration of the duplex. This process is repeated cyclically, with continual regeneration of the original duplex and the production of many copies of the antisense strand.

(c)   One of the antisense strands from (b). Each of these strands can bind primer S_1. Extension of S_1 – and of the (recessed) 3′ end of the antisense strand – produces the product shown at (d). During extension of the (recessed) 3′ end of the antisense strand, a modified, non-nickable HincII restriction site is formed (■■); the site is non-nickable because the three terminal nucleotides in this strand (3′-CAA-5′) include two modified nucleotides (dATPαS).

(d)   This product has a nickable restriction site (arrowhead) derived from primer S_1. Like the product at (a), it can undergo a cyclical process of nicking, strand displacement and regeneration of the duplex, displacing many copies of a single-stranded product. Note that this single-stranded product is a *sense* strand of the target sequence (whereas the strand formed from (a) is an antisense strand). The sense strand and regenerated duplex are shown at (e).

(e)   The products from (d). The sense strand will be able to bind primer S_2.

(f)   The sense strand from (e) has bound primer S_2. DNA synthesis (i.e. extension from S_2, and also extension from the recessed end of the sense strand) gives rise to the product shown at (g). (DNA synthesis at the 3′ end of the sense strand produces a non-nickable restriction site for the reason given under (c), above.)

(g)   This product is equivalent to the one shown at (a).

Summarizing, double-stranded products from the target-generation phase undergo cyclical nicking, strand displacement and regeneration of the original duplex, forming numerous copies of antisense and sense strands of the target duplex. Antisense strands bind primer S_1 and form the (double-stranded) products that yield sense strands; sense strands bind primer S_2 and form the (double-stranded) products that yield antisense strands. Nickable HincII restriction sites are provided by the 5′-tags on S_1 and S_2 primers (which are present in large numbers in the reaction mixture).

Parts I and II are modified from Figures 5.3 and 5.4, pages 134–137, in *DNA Methods in Clinical Microbiology* [ISBN 07923-6307-8], Paul Singleton (2000), with the kind permission of Springer Science and Business Media.

second strand (of cDNA) See FIRST STRAND.

secondary homothallism (homoheteromixis) (*fungal genetics*) In some heterothallic fungi: a seemingly homothallic state, involving a self-fertile thallus, which can occur e.g. when a given spore incorporates nuclei of two compatible mating types – leading to a self-fertile thallus. In such cases the compatibility of nuclei may be based on a one-locus two-allele system (the process then being termed *homodimixis*) or based on a one- or two-locus *multi*-allele system (*homodiaphoromixis*).

segmented genome Any *viral* genome that consists of two or more pieces of nucleic acid. Segmented genomes occur e.g. in the bunyaviruses (negative-sense/ambisense ssRNA); in the influenzaviruses A and B (negative-sense ssRNA); in reoviruses (dsRNA); and in bacteriophage φ6 (dsRNA).

segregation (of plasmids) (*syn.* partition) See PLASMID.

segregation lag A PHENOTYPIC LAG due to the time needed for segregation of a newly acquired allele. For example, a mutant allele in a bacterial cell that contains multiple chromosomes may not be expressed in the presence of the wild-type alleles; an opportunity for expression may occur when the mutant chromosome has been segregated (by cell division) to a cell which contains no wild-type alleles.

selectively amplified microsatellite polymorphic loci (selective amplification of microsatellite polymorphic loci) See SAMPL.

selector See SELECTOR-BASED MULTIPLEX PCR.

selector-based multiplex PCR A form of PCR in which a range of different target sequences can be amplified in one assay with a single pair of primers (cf. conventional MULTIPLEX PCR).

For each of the targets to be amplified the reaction mixture contains a target-specific *selector*. A selector comprises two oligonucleotides: one (the *selector probe*) of ~70 nt and the other of 34 nt; the shorter oligonucleotide is hybridized to the *central* region of the selector probe – so that the selector probe contains two terminal (~18 nt) single-stranded target-complementary regions. The central, i.e. duplex, region of the selector incorporates a primer-binding motif; this motif is the same in all the selectors (regardless of their target specificity) and is designed for a common ('universal') primer pair.

Sample DNA is first digested with appropriate restriction enzymes. Digested DNA is mixed with a pool of selectors (of different target specificities) and denatured. The subsequent circularization of target sequences with selectors is followed by ligation. (Any non-circularized DNA is degraded by exonucleolysis.) The collection of circularized templates is then amplified by PCR using the universal primer pair. [Method: Nucleic Acids Res (2005) 33(8):e71.]

SELEX See APTAMER.

self-activation (*syn.* autoactivation) (two-hybrid systems) See e.g. BACTERIOMATCH TWO-HYBRID SYSTEM.

self-reporting primer A 5′-fluorophore-labeled primer hybridized, via a 5′ tag, to a quencher-labeled PNA (Q-PNA) probe; the PNA probe is displaced when double-stranded amplicons are formed, permitting fluorescence from the primer's fluorophore [Genome Res (2001) 11(4):609–613].

self-sustained sequence replication (3SR) An early system for the *in vitro* amplification of nucleic acids; it was based on the retroviral mode of replication [see: Proc Natl Acad Sci USA (1990) 87:1874–1878].

This system is reflected in current methods such as NASBA and TMA.

SENP The designation given to a number of SUMO proteases – SENP1, SENP2, SENP3 etc. – homologous to the Ulp family of proteases: see SUMOYLATION.

sense strand (of DNA) See CODING STRAND.

separate-component-stabilization system (SCS system) See CCD MECHANISM.

Sequenase® A modified form of the DNA polymerase from bacteriophage T7 which lacks 3′→5′ exonuclease activity but which has strand-displacement activity. The processivity of the enzyme is promoted by complexing it with THIOREDOXIN from *Escherichia coli*.

sequence capture An approach used e.g. for the isolation of sequence-specific fragments of single-stranded nucleic acid in solution. In this method, a BIOTINylated probe hybridizes to the fragments; the probe is then captured by streptavidin-coated DYNABEADS that are held immobilized by a magnetic field while the other, unwanted fragments are removed by washing.

sequence conversion A phrase sometimes used to refer to the treatment of genomic DNA with BISULFITE (an initial stage in procedures used to detect methylated cytosine residues in the DNA); such treatment is used to convert non-methylated cytosine residues to uracil residues.

sequence-tagged site (STS) A unique, known sequence of nucleotides (several hundred base-pairs) in a given fragment of genomic DNA. STSs can be useful in genomic mapping; thus, for example, they may help in aligning cloned, tagged fragments into an overlapping series – e.g. if a given STS is found in two different fragments these fragments may share an overlapping sequence.

A given STS may be identified by means of an EXPRESSED SEQUENCE TAG.

sequencing (of DNA) See DNA SEQUENCING.

SEQUEROME See BLAST.

SERE *Salmonella enteritidis* repetitive element: a repetitive sequence found in the genomic DNA of *S. enteritidis*; it has been used for typing (see REP-PCR).

serial analysis of gene expression See SAGE.

serine proteinase Any proteinase which has a serine residue at the active site. Examples of serine proteinases: e.g. ENTEROKINASE and THROMBIN.

serine recombinase See RECOMBINASE.

SET SOLUBILITY ENHANCEMENT TAG.

sex chromatin *Syn.* BARR BODY.

sex determination assay See entry DNA SEX DETERMINATION ASSAY.

sex-linked chromosome *Syn.* HETEROSOME.

sex-linked disorder   *Syn.* X-LINKED DISORDER.

sex pilus   *Syn.* PILUS.

sexual PCR   *Syn.* DNA SHUFFLING.

Sf9 cells   Ovarian cells from the lepidopteran insect *Spodoptera frugiperda* which are widely used for baculovirus-mediated overexpression of recombinant proteins. These cells can be grown in monolayers or in suspension, and growth occurs in serum-free media.

(See also MIMIC SF9 INSECT CELLS.)

sfiA **gene**   See SOS SYSTEM.

SFM-adapted   Refers to any cell line which has been adapted to growth in serum-free media.

Sgal   See BLACK–WHITE SCREENING.

Shine–Dalgarno sequence   See 5′-UTR.

SHOM   Sequencing by hybridization to oligonucleotide microchips: a method used e.g. for sequencing PCR-amplified DNA by hybridization to an array of oligonucleotides immobilized on gel-based microchips.

The method was used for diagnostic investigations, e.g. the detection of mutations in chromosomal DNA of patients with β-thalassemia.

short hairpin RNA (shRNA)   A short, engineered molecule of RNA (~60 nucleotides in length) which forms a stem–loop structure and which can be cleaved *in vivo* (within cells) to an siRNA able to induce gene silencing (RNA INTERFERENCE).

shRNAs can be synthesized by *in vivo* transcription from an appropriate DNA target sequence within a plasmid or viral vector; the DNA target sequence may be synthesized chemically as two single-stranded complementary oligonucleotides that are hybridized before ligation into the vector.

In vivo transcription of shRNAs from an appropriate DNA target sequence often employs the promoter of RNA polymerase III. The use of RNA polymerase III for this purpose was reported to be advantageous in that transcription ends predictably at the second thymidine residue in a sequence of more than four thymidine residues in the template – avoiding the addition of a poly(A) tail to the transcript (which would inhibit the gene-silencing activity).

A further advantage of the RNA polymerase III promoter is that it supports transcription in many types of cell; shRNAs can be expressed constitutively in such cells. However, the RNA polymerase II promoter can also be used for expressing shRNAs, and a system based on RNA polymerase I was used for a species-specific expression vector for shRNA [Nucleic Acids Res (2007) 35(2):e10].

Once synthesized *in vivo*, an shRNA is cleaved and the product (siRNA) enters the RNA interference pathway.

A method for generating shRNA *libraries* involves random enzymatic digestion of relevant cDNA molecules by DNase I. The resulting fragments of cDNA are ligated to hairpin adaptor molecules (one adaptor at each end) which contain the recognition sequence of RESTRICTION ENDONUCLEASE MmeI. This restriction enzyme cleaves at a site 20 nt in the 3′ direction from the binding sequence (see table in the entry RESTRICTION ENDONUCLEASE), i.e. in each case it cuts the

fragment at a fixed distance from the (closed) end of the hairpin adaptor. The resulting pieces – all of the same length, and consisting of both fragment and adaptor DNA – therefore contain a hairpin adaptor at one end and a 2-nt 3′ overhang at the cut end of the fragment.

Another adaptor is then ligated to the sticky end of each fragment. PCR amplification of the resulting structure yields dsDNA containing the original hairpin sequence and flanking regions of target DNA. Appropriate target DNA is inserted into vectors at a site downstream of an RNA polymerase III promoter.

A ligand-controlled aptamer–shRNA fusion transcript has been used to regulate gene expression in mammalian cells [RNA (2006) 12:710–716].

shRNAs have been used to knock down the expression of several target genes within the same cell in an arrangement using a tetracycline-regulated RNA polymerase II promoter [BioTechniques (2006) 41(1):64–68].

[An shRNA vector for high-efficiency RNAi in embryonic stem cells: BioTechniques (2007) 42(6):738–743.]

short patch repair   *Syn.* UVRABC-MEDIATED REPAIR.

short sequence repeats (SSR)   A non-specific term that may apply e.g. to MICROSATELLITE DNA or minisatellite DNA.

(See also SNR.)

short tandem repeat   See STR.

shotgun sequencing   A method used for sequencing genomes (or large molecules of DNA). A sample of the DNA is cut extensively with a RESTRICTION ENDONUCLEASE and a large number of the fragments are cloned and sequenced. Because of overlap among the fragments, sequence data obtained from individual clones can be amalgamated to reveal long, continuous sequences within the genome. However, usually there are gaps in the genome's sequence because some parts of the genome may not have been cloned. A missing sequence may be found by using PCR to copy that sequence from genomic DNA – see e.g. PACE.

shRNA   SHORT HAIRPIN RNA.

shuffling (of DNA)   See DNA SHUFFLING.

shufflon   In e.g. the Inclα plasmid R64: a set of DNA sequences which can invert, singly or in groups, to form complex rearrangements that may influence the specificity of cell–cell contact in conjugation.

shuttle vector (bifunctional vector)   A CLONING VECTOR, or other type of vector, which is capable of replication in more than one type of organism – for example, in (the bacterium) *Escherichia coli* and (the yeast) *Saccharomyces cerevisiae*; the vector must include an appropriate origin of replication for each type of organism.

(See also BACMID.)

sickle-cell anemia   An inherited disorder involving the β-chain of hemoglobin; the mis-shaped erythrocytes (red blood cells) are eliminated, leading to (sometimes fatal) anemia.

Sickle-cell trait refers to the generally less serious condition in those heterozygous for the gene; it may be asymptomatic, and it confers a degree of resistance to falciparum malaria.

[Correction of the sickle-cell mutation in embryonic stem cells: Proc Natl Acad Sci USA (2006) 103(4):1036–1040.]
(See also THALASSEMIA.)

sickle-cell trait   See SICKLE-CELL ANEMIA.

SIDD   Stress-induced duplex destabilization: destabilization at a particular region in duplex DNA (a SIDD site), promoting strand separation, in response to a given level of superhelicity. SIDD appears to be frequently involved in the regulation of promoters and origins of replication.

In *Escherichia coli*, transcription from the *ilv*P$_G$ promoter is apparently preceded by destabilization at an upstream SIDD site; following the binding of integration host factor (a multifunctional *E. coli* heterodimeric protein) near the SIDD site, superhelical energy may be transmitted to the promoter's −10 sequence, facilitating the formation of an open complex and the initiation of transcription. In the *E. coli* genome, SIDD sites appear to be closely associated with promoters [Genome Res (2004) 14(8):1575–1584].

In *Saccharomyces cerevisiae* the autonomously replicating sequences (ARSs) appear to be much more susceptible than other regions to the influence of superhelically driven duplex destabilization [PLoS Comput Biol (2005) 1(1):e7].

SIGEX   Substrate-induced gene expression screening: a method in which induction of gene expression by substrates is used as an approach for the isolation of catabolic genes from metagenome libraries [Nat Biotechnol (2005) 23:88–93].

signal amplification   An approach used for detecting and/or quantitating a specific DNA or RNA target sequence within a given sample; essentially, each target sequence in the sample is linked to an enzyme which, with a suitable added substrate, generates an amplified signal whose intensity indicates the number and/or location of target sequences in the sample.

Signal amplification avoids a major problem associated with TARGET AMPLIFICATION methods (such as PCR), i.e. the contamination of reaction mixtures with AMPLICONS from earlier assays. One disadvantage is that this method provides no copies of the target sequence for analysis.

One example of signal amplification is the BDNA ASSAY; another is TYRAMIDE SIGNAL AMPLIFICATION.

signal peptide   *Syn.* SIGNAL SEQUENCE.

signal sequence (signal peptide)   In certain exported/secreted proteins: a specific N-terminal sequence of amino acid residues that directs the protein into, or through, the cytoplasmic membrane; typically, the signal sequence is cleaved during translocation in the membrane. Signal sequences are found in prokaryotic and eukaryotic cells, although the translocation of proteins occurs by distinct processes in the two types of cell.

In *Escherichia coli* (and in other Gram-negative bacteria) signal-sequence-dependent translocation is involved e.g. in the type II mode of export/secretion of proteins. In some cases a protein may also include other sequence(s) that help to guide it to the correct destination; for example, a protein targeted to the membrane (as opposed to a *secreted* protein) may include a *membrane anchor sequence* which binds the

mature protein on or within the membrane. In the Braun lipoprotein (which links peptidoglycan to the outer membrane in *E. coli*) the signal sequence is cleaved and replaced by a fatty acid residue; this post-translational modification appears to target the protein to its correct destination.

In the so-called Tat system, which is involved in exporting *folded* proteins across the cytoplasmic membrane, the signal sequence characteristically includes two consecutive arginine residues (hence Tat: twin arginine translocation).

Some other modes of protein export/secretion in the Gram-negative bacteria are not characterized by an N-terminal signal sequence. For example, secretion via the type I system in *E. coli* (involving a so-called ABC exporter) is characterized by a C-terminal secretion sequence.

signal transducers and activators of transduction (STATs)   In mammalian cells: a family of cytoplasmic proteins which are activated by phosphorylation when certain types of signaling molecule (e.g. interferons, interleukins) bind to cell-surface receptors. The binding of a signaling molecule initially activates a tyrosine kinase of the JAK (Janus kinase) family which then activates a STAT.

There are at least seven different types of STAT. When activated, STATs form homo- or heterodimers, according to the type of STAT, which then promote transcription of relevant gene(s).

signal transduction pathway   Any pathway which involves the sequential transmission of a signal along a series of two or more components – often involving activation of particular components e.g. by phosphorylation.

For some examples of methods used for investigating signal transduction pathways see e.g. CYTOTRAP TWO-HYBRID SYSTEM and PATHDETECT SYSTEMS.

(See also TWO-COMPONENT REGULATORY SYSTEM.)

signature-tagged mutagenesis (STM)   An approach used e.g. for detecting those genes (in a pathogen) which are essential for the pathogen's growth in a host organism.

The principle of STM is shown (diagrammatically) in the figure.

The method has been used successfully e.g. for identifying a PATHOGENICITY ISLAND in *Salmonella typhimurium*. It was also used to identify genes, in *Mycobacterium tuberculosis*, involved in parasitism of human macrophages [Infect Immun (2007) 75(1):504–507].

The possibility of a false-positive result in STM may arise e.g. if (during the *random* mutagenesis) a transposon inserts into a *non*-virulence gene in a cell which (by chance) already contains a mutation in a virulence gene; with this scenario, the given tag would be absent (or low level) in the 'recovered' pool, thus giving a false indication for the particular gene inactivated by the transposon.

STM has also been employed to generate attenuated strains of *Salmonella choleraesuis* as candidates for a live vaccine [Infect Immun (2005) 73:8194–8203].

In a non-medical context, the STM principle has been used to study the survival of certain bacteria (e.g. *Desulfovibrio*) in

SIGNATURE-TAGGED MUTAGENESIS: a method used e.g. for detecting virulence-associated genes in a bacterial pathogen. The figure shows the general principle diagrammatically.

A unique sequence ('tag'), about 40 base-pairs in length, is inserted into each of a population of transposons, i.e. the tag in a given transposon is different from that in other transposons. Each tag is flanked, on both sides, by a primer-binding site; these primer-binding sites are the same in all transposons. The transposons are used to mutagenize a population of cells of the pathogen, and they insert — randomly — into different genes in different cells.

The mutagenized cells are plated to form individual colonies. In a given colony of mutant cells, each cell contains the same uniquely tagged transposon in the same gene. A number of colonies are chosen, and an inoculum from each colony is arrayed, separately, in a anaerobic sediment [Appl Environ Micobiol (2005) 71:7064–7074].

Another method – IVET – is used e.g. to detect those genes in a pathogen which are induced (i.e. which become active) during infection of the host animal. Like STM, this method is also used in a non-medical context.

silencing (of genes)   See GENE SILENCING.

silencing (of miRNAs)   See ANTAGOMIR.

silent mutation   Any mutation lacking a phenotypic effect. (cf. SAME-SENSE MUTATION.)

Note that these mutations may not be 'silent' in DNA-based identification tests (see e.g. SSCP ANALYSIS).

silent origin   See e.g. ARS.

simian foamy virus   See SPUMAVIRINAE.

simian virus 40   See SV40.

simple sequence repeats   A non-specific term which may apply e.g. to MICROSATELLITE DNA.

The term has also been used to include single-nucleotide repeats (SNRs) [J Clin Microbiol (2006) 44(3):777–782].

simple transposon (class II transposon)   See TRANSPOSON.

SINE   Short interspersed element: any one of a number of repetitive elements, each typically <500 nt long, dispersed in the genomes of at least some mammalian species (including the human genome). The SINEs include ALU SEQUENCES.

(cf. LINE.)

single-base extension (SBE)   A method used to test for the presence of a given base at a specific location. Essentially, the presence of the base, at a specific location in a strand, is determined by hybridizing a primer (or probe) whose 3′ end *can be extended* with a nucleotide that base-pairs with the particular base in question. Extension of the primer or probe

with a known nucleotide argues for the presence of the given, complementary nucleotide at the given location. The primer or probe is extended by a single dye-linked *chain-terminating* dideoxyribonucleoside triphosphate (ddNTP); such extension is detected via the labelled product or, as in QEXT, by a FRET-based reaction.

This procedure can be used e.g. to detect a point mutation at a specific location.

(See also METHYLATION-SPECIFIC SINGLE-BASE EXTENSION.)

single-base repeat   *Syn.* single-nucleotide repeat: see SNR.

single-cell electroporation   See ELECTROPORATION.

single-cell *in vivo* fluorescence   See DFRS PLASMID.

single-chain antibody (intrabody)   See GEME THERAPY.

single-chain variable fragment (scFV)   A type of engineered antibody which has been used e.g. in IMMUNO-PCR.

[Use of scFV in phage display libraries for studying a tumor antigen: PNAS (2006) 103(4):1041–1046.]

single-nucleotide polymorphism   See SNP.

single-nucleotide repeat   See SNR.

single-strand binding protein (SSB protein; helix destabilizing protein)   Any of various proteins that bind specifically and co-operatively to single-stranded DNA in processes such as DNA replication and repair; they may stabilize and protect ssDNA but apparently do not unwind a duplex.

single-strand conformation polymorphism analysis   See SSCP ANALYSIS.

single-strand rescue   See HELPER PHAGE.

single-strand-specific nuclease   Any of a category of nucleases that degrade single-stranded DNA or single-stranded regions in double-stranded DNA; this kind of enzyme is used e.g. to

---

SIGNATURE-TAGGED MUTAGENESIS: (*continued*) microtiter dish. (The dish shown in the figure has 30 wells, but larger dishes are normally used.) Two replica 'blots' of the array are made on membranes (for subsequent DNA hybridization studies); in these blots the cells are lysed and their chromosomal DNA is exposed and fixed to the membrane.

Cells are taken from each of the wells and pooled. The pool is used in two ways. First, it provides an inoculum for infection of the test animal. Second, cells from this ('input') pool are lysed, and PCR (polymerase chain reaction) is used – with labeled primers – to amplify the unique tags of all transposons in the pool. The amplified, labeled tags are then used as probes on one of the replica blots (Replica 1); in this blot, each unique tag should hybridize with the DNA from cells containing the corresponding transposon. This 'pre-screening' process on Replica 1 checks for efficient amplification of the unique tags.

The pathogen is then recovered from the test animal by plating an appropriate specimen. The resulting colonies are pooled (forming the 'recovered' pool), and PCR is used (with labeled primers) to amplify the tag from each clone in this pool. The amplified, labeled tags are then used to probe the second replica blot (Replica 2).

Considering the original, mutagenized cells (in the 'input' pool), the cells of interest are those which, through a (transposon-mediated) mutation, are *unable* to grow within the test animal, i.e. cells whose virulence has been lowered. Such cells will be absent, or few in number, in the 'recovered' pool – compared with cells which have grown normally in the test animal. Hence, the signature tags of these 'virulence-attenuated' cells will be present in the input pool but absent (or rare) in the recovered pool; consequently, such cells can be identified by hybridization in Replica 1 but an *absence* of (or weak) hybridization in Replica 2 (see figure).

In a given, 'virulence-attenuated' clone, the relevant gene can be identified from the inserted transposon. This gene can be isolated and sequenced for further study.

Figure reproduced from *Bacteria in Biology, Biotechnology and Medicine*, 6th edition, Figure 8.22, pages 256–257, Paul Singleton (2004) John Wiley & Sons Ltd, UK [ISBN 0-470-09027-8] with permission from the publisher.

remove terminal *overhangs* in fragments of DNA which have been cut by certain types of restriction endonuclease (such removal being achieved without significantly affecting the double-stranded regions). (See also NESTED DELETIONS.)

Another useful feature of these enzymes is their ability to nick one strand at the site of a single-base-pair mismatch in (heteroduplex) DNA; this is exploited e.g. in ECOTILLING.

The category of single-strand-specific nucleases includes enzymes that have similar zinc-dependent active-site motifs; they include endonuclease CEL I (from celery), endonuclease P_1 (from the fungus *Penicillium citrinum*), ENDONUCLEASE S1 (obtained originally from the fungus *Aspergillus oryzae*), and the mung bean nuclease (from *Phaseolus aureus*).

siRNA Small interfering RNA: an effector molecule involved in RNA INTERFERENCE (q.v.).

For experimental purposes, siRNAs can be generated in a number of ways, for example:

(a) Chemical synthesis (commercially available) according to specified target sequences.

(b) *In vitro* transcription of target sequences using e.g. T3 or T7 polymerase: enzymes which can work with simple transcription signals without incorporating (an unwanted) poly(A) tail in transcripts; poly(A) tails can inhibit the silencing effect in RNAi. Relevant cDNAs can be initially amplified by PCR with primers that incorporate a T3 or a T7 promoter sequence at the 5′ end; the resulting amplicons are then transcribed.

(c) Cleavage of dsRNA with bacterial RNase III.

(d) *In vivo* transcription with cellular RNA polymerase III. By using a promoter at each end of the target sequence it is possible to obtain sense and antisense transcripts. The use of RNA polymerase III may be facilitated by means of an inducible minimal RNA polymerase III promoter activated by a transactivator in the presence of doxycycline; induction in a dose-dependent manner is achieved by the administration of doxycycline [Nucleic Acids Res (2006) 34(5):e37].

(e) RNAi may be induced in target cells by *in vivo* expression of *short hairpin RNAs* (see SHORT HAIRPIN RNA) which are then cleaved, *in situ*, to siRNAs.

Using siRNAs

siRNAs modified with 2′-deoxy-2′-fluoro-β-D-arabinonucleotide units had improved activity and serum stability, suggesting possible use in therapy [Nucleic Acids Res (2006) 34(6): 1669–1675]. [siRNAs for distinguishing between genes that differ by one nucleotide: PLoS Genetics (2006) 2(9):e140; an assessment of siRNA potency by a secreted luciferase assay: BioTechniques (2007) 42(5):599–606.]

In a novel approach to the intracellular delivery of siRNAs, an siRNA was linked, via a streptavidin bridge, to an aptamer that was known to bind to prostate tumor cells; the conjugate (i.e. siRNA plus aptamer) was taken up by cells within 30 minutes following simple addition of conjugate to the cells, and siRNA-mediated inhibition of gene expression was found to be as efficient as that produced by lipid-based internalization reagents [Nucleic Acids Res (2006) 34(10):e73].

Single-stranded siRNA molecules may also induce RNAi

but are generally less effective. However, boranophosphate-modified single-stranded siRNA was reported to have high potency [Nucleic Acids Res (2006) 34(9):2773–2781].

Transcriptional gene silencing (TGS)

siRNAs can also mediate a process known as transcriptional gene silencing (TGS) in mammalian and other cells (e.g. cells of the small plant *Arabidopsis* and the fission yeast *Schizosaccharomyces pombe*).

In some cases, TGS involves siRNA-mediated methylation of DNA as the silencing mechanism (so-called RNA-directed DNA methylation, RdDM).

In some cases the mechanism of TGS apparently involves methylation of histones.

sis (*SIS*) An ONCOGENE identified in simian sarcoma virus. The c-*sis* product is the B chain of platelet-derived growth factor (PDGF). The viral gene encodes an almost-identical B chain which is the transforming agent in virus-infected cells.

site-directed mutagenesis (or site-specific mutagenesis) (*DNA technol.*) Any form of engineered MUTAGENESIS involving change(s) in target molecules at *pre-determined* site(s). Older methods (e.g. D-loop mutagenesis) have been superseded by much simpler ones – see e.g. QUIKCHANGE SITE-DIRECTED MUTAGENESIS KIT and MEGAPRIMER MUTAGENESIS; see also EXSITE PCR-BASED SITE-DIRECTED MUTAGENESIS KIT and GENETAILOR.

A deletion can be introduced by using INVERSE PCR to copy all except an internal sequence of the target; the amplicons are ligated (making a shortened form of the target sequence), and the product is subjected to second-round amplification. This technique can also be used for making point mutations, frameshift mutations, truncations etc. [BioTechniques (2005) 38:864–868].

In PCR, insertions can be introduced e.g. via 5′ entensions on the primers.

Site-directed insertion *in vivo* (within cells) may be carried out e.g. by using a targeting vector to prepare an insertion site and subsequently using RECOMBINASE-MEDIATED CASSETTE EXCHANGE to exchange the insert for target DNA [see e.g. Figure 1 in Proc Natl Acad Sci USA (2005) 102(18):6413–6418].

site-specific biotinylation See BIOTIN.

site-specific cleavage (of proteins) Cleavage of proteins at sites between specific amino acid residues. Some of the enzymes that can carry out site-specific cleavage are exploited in DNA technology.

(See e.g. EKMAX, SUMO protease in SUMOYLATION, TEV protease in TEV; see also ENTEROKINASE and THROMBIN; see also SORTASE.)

site-specific mutagenesis *Syn.* SITE-DIRECTED MUTAGENESIS.

site-specific recombination (SSR) A form of RECOMBINATION between *specific* dsDNA sequences in the same molecule, or in different molecules, in which there is neither synthesis nor degradation of DNA; this (ATP-independent) process is mediated by a site-specific RECOMBINASE. The two sequences of dsDNA that are recognized by a given recombinase are not necessarily identical.

Examples of SSR: (i) integration of the PHAGE LAMBDA genome into the bacterial chromosome, and excision of the phage genome – the phage attachment site, *att*P, *not* being identical to the bacterial site, *att*B; (ii) PHASE VARIATION in the *Salmonella* filament protein; (iii) the CRE–LOXP SYSTEM; and (iv) insertion of a cassette into an INTEGRON.

six-histidine tag (6xHis tag) A sequence of six consecutive histidine residues, incorporated into some recombinant proteins, which facilitates detection (by anti-His antibody) or purification (by a NICKEL-CHARGED AFFINITY RESIN).

size fractionation (*DNA technol.*) Any procedure in which a population of DNA molecules/fragments – present in a range of sizes – is treated so as to obtain physical separation of the molecules/fragments according to size.

For example, a population of fragments, in a range of sizes, may be subjected to electrophoresis in an agarose gel; a particular band of fragments, of appropriate size, can be excised, purified (i.e. agar removed), and then used for the required purpose.

Size fractionation may be used e.g. for selecting fragments of appropriate size(s) from a restriction-digested genome in order to use such fragments in cloning vectors which accept inserts only within a certain range of sizes.

Skyline (DNA notation) See DNA SKYLINE.

sliding A movement made by certain DNA-binding proteins: translocation lengthwise along a DNA duplex until the appropriate binding site is reached. For example, sliding of the *lac* repressor protein along the duplex occurs until it reaches the operator.

slipped-strand mispairing (SSM) Mispairing between strands during DNA replication in susceptible regions of the genome; regions susceptible to SSM are characterized e.g. by multiple tandemly repeated short sequences of nucleotides – such as MICROSATELLITE DNA.

SSM can apparently result in an increase or a decrease in the (normal) number of repeated subunits in a given sequence of microsatellite DNA. In humans, 'microsatellite expansion' (i.e. an increase in the number of subunits at a given locus) can cause certain neurological diseases when associated with particular genes (e.g. fragile X disease, Huntington's disease).

Among bacteria, changes in such sequences are reported to have various effects. For example, they can promote PHASE VARIATION in the *opa* genes of *Neisseria*. In *Helicobacter pylori*, the *mutY* sequence (encoding a DNA excision-repair function) has a region of eight consecutive adenine residues which appears to be subject to slipped-strand mispairing – the occurrence of SSM being able to cause frameshift mutations that eliminate gene function; this has been interpreted as a mechanism which contributes to phase-variable base excision repair in *H. pylori* [J Bacteriol (2006) 188(17):6224–6234]. In *Escherichia coli* strain O157:H7, slipped-strand mispairing may be responsible for a proportion of the instability in the VNTR (variable number of tandem repeats) loci [J Bacteriol (2006) 188(12):4253–4263].

slippery sequence In an mRNA molecule: a sequence of nucleotides – downstream of the initiation codon – which causes slippage of the ribosome along the mRNA. Slippage, which may occur in an upstream (5′) or a downstream (3′) direction, is an integral part of the mechanism of FRAMESHIFTING.

slot blot See DOT BLOT.

small interfering RNA (siRNA) See RNA INTERFERENCE; see also SIRNA.

small nuclear ribonucleoprotein particles See SNRNAS.

small nuclear RNAs See SNRNAS.

small ubiquitin-like modifier See SUMOYLATION.

smart probe A (singly-labeled) PROBE based on a principle similar to that of the MOLECULAR BEACON PROBE. In this (stem–loop) probe the 5′ end carries a fluorophore that (in the unbound probe) is quenched by guanosine residues which are present in the (3′) complementary stem region.

[Example of use: Nucleic Acids Res (2006) 34(13):e90.]

smear-positive specimen See AMTDT.

Smith–Lemli–Opitz syndrome An autosomal recessive syndrome, involving (e.g.) mental retardation, reported to be due to defective cholesterol metabolism resulting from a mutation in gene *DHCR7* (encoding 3β-hydroxysterol-Δ7 reductase).

(See also GENETIC DISEASE (table).)

SMT3 The SUMO protein in *Saccharomyces cerevisiae*: see SUMOYLATION.

Smt4 (Ulp2) See SUMOYLATION.

snip-SNP Any SNP that affects RESTRICTION ENDONUCLEASE recognition site(s).

[Method for detecting snip-SNPs: BMC Genomics (2005) 6:118. Program for identifying snip-SNPs within reference sequences: BMC Genetics (2006) 7:27.]

SNP Single-nucleotide polymorphism: in the genome of an individual, a variant nucleotide which differs from that *at the corresponding site* in most other members of the population – but which occurs in at least 1% of other individuals in the population; for example, if 1% of the population has the sequence ...TTCCAT... but the majority have ...TTTCAT... then the minority group have an SNP at the third nucleotide in this sequence. SNPs are common; in the human genome they are found approximately once every 100–300 bases, making a total of several million SNPs in the whole genome. Most of the recorded SNPs in humans involve a C-to-T change.

(See also SNP GENOTYPING.)

SNPs that occur with frequencies below ~5% have been classified as 'rare' while those that occur with frequencies >5% are said to be 'common'.

SNPs are found in coding and non-coding sequences. Many SNPs have no known effect, but some may influence the response e.g. to infectious agents (bacteria, viruses etc.) and chemicals, including drugs; this characteristic is helping to shape pharmaceutical/biomedical research: the comparison of SNP patterns in groups of drug-resistant and drug-sensitive patients may reveal important links between specific SNPs and the efficacy of a given drug.

SNP patterns may also be helpful in elucidating the polygenic nature of certain diseases in which a given gene is only partly responsible for the pathology.

[Database of >1 million (human) SNPs: Nature (2005) 437: 1299–1320.]

Because of their potential uses in biomedicine, SNPs are being actively characterized and recorded in public databases by various government and commercial organizations. However, one report suggested that some of the SNPs recorded in public databases may be associated with *editing* sites rather than genuine SNPs [Nucleic Acids Res (2005) 33(14):4612–4617].

SNPs are also found in prokaryotic and eukaryotic microorganisms. For example, SNPs in the *inlB* gene of *Listeria monocytogenes* were used for classification [Appl Environ Microbiol (2001) 67(11):5339–5342], and SNP-based phylotyping has been carried out in *Escherichia coli* [Appl Environ Microbiol (2005) 71:4784–4792]. The genome of *Candida albicans* has been mapped on the basis of SNPs [Eukaryotic Cell (2004) 3(3):705–714]. SNP analysis of *Mycobacterium tuberculosis* (and other microorganisms) is reported to be facilitated by a modified ARMS assay [J Clin Microbiol (2004) 42:1236–1242]. [Global phylogeny of *Mycobacterium tuberculosis* based on SNP analysis: J Bacteriol (2006) 188 (2): 759–772.]

SNP genotyping The process of examining samples of genomic DNA with the object of detecting and recording the presence of specific SNPs. (cf. SNP MAPPING.) Large collections of validated SNPs are needed in order to facilitate so-called 'association studies' in which particular traits (such as susceptibility to a given disease, or resistance to a drug) may be linked to established patterns of SNPs.

Various methods have been proposed for the simultaneous genome-wide typing of thousands of SNPs. One such method is MOLECULAR INVERSION PROBE GENOTYPING (q.v.).

For detecting small numbers of SNPs (e.g. in studies on specific candidate genes) use can be made of a modified form of ALLELE-SPECIFIC PCR which uses T_m-shift primers. In this method [BioTechniques (2005) 39(6):885–893], the alleles of a given gene are assayed using two allele-specific forward primers, each primer containing a 3' terminal base which is complementary to a given SNP in one of two allelic variants of the gene; the same reverse primer is used with both of the forward primers.

Each of these two forward primers (one for each allelic variant) has a 5' GC-rich tag. However, the two types of primer have tags of different length; hence, the products (i.e. dsDNA amplicons) formed from one primer are characterized by a melting temperature (T_m) which differs from that of the products formed from the other primer. Consequently, the melting curve characteristics of a given product will indicate which of the two (allele-specific) primers gave rise to that product. An earlier version of this method, in which only one primer was tagged, was found to be problematic in that, in some cases, the primers were amplified unevenly.

A novel approach to the detection of SNPs was suggested

by the finding that linear dsDNA fragments and oligonucleotides form highly stable RecA-mediated terminal/subterminal triple-stranded structures specifically when the single strand is complementary to the 5'-phosphate end of a strand in the dsDNA; the stability of the structure is drastically reduced by a single mismatched base, regardless of its location. In this scheme, sample dsDNA fragments can be effectively probed by sequence-specific oligonucleotides [DNA Res (2005) 12 (6):441–449].

A number of rare SNPs have been detected by the method known as Ecotilling [Nucleic Acids Res (2006) 34(13):e99].

Detection and quantitation of SNPs can also be achieved by multiplex QEXT.

The term *call* has been used to refer to a positive identification of a specific SNP in a given sample of genomic DNA. *Call rate* was used to refer to the number of calls recorded, for a given SNP, in a range of genomic samples, divided by the total number of genomic samples examined (expressed as a percentage).

SNP mapping A phrase used to refer to a procedure in which a given gene is mapped by using SNPs as genetic markers (cf. SNP GENOTYPING). In so-called interval mapping, the object is to locate the gene of interest in the interval between two consecutive SNPs.

SNR Single-nucleotide repeat: a sequence of nucleotides *of one type*, present at a given genetic locus, which may vary in length (i.e. in number of constituent nucleotides) in different individuals; variation in length may result e.g. from SLIPPED-STRAND MISPAIRING. Mutation rates at such loci are reported to be high, apparently reflecting the ease with which events such as slipped-strand mispairing may occur.

SNRs may be found at various loci in a given genome. SNRs in the genome of *Bacillus anthracis* (causal agent of anthrax) have been exploited for the TYPING of this pathogen (an organism for which various other typing procedures have proved to be inadequately discriminatory) [J Clin Microbiol (2006) 44(3):777–782].

SNRs are also called 'mononucleotide repeats' and 'single-base repeats'.

snRNAs (small nuclear RNAs) RNA molecules, <300 nt, rich in uridylic acid residues and capped (see CAP), present in the eukaryotic nucleus. There are six types, designated U1–U6. snRNAs complex with proteins to form *small nuclear ribonucleoprotein particles* (snRNPs; snurps) which are involved in the SPLICING of pre-mRNAs; they function e.g. as *external guide sequences* (EGSs) in the (human) splicing reaction, i.e. helping to select a particular splice site.

snRNPs See SNRNAS.

snurps See SNRNAS.

SOB system The equivalent of the SOS SYSTEM in the Gram-positive bacterium *Bacillus*.

SOC medium (S.O.C. medium) A medium used for incubating bacteria following transformation. The medium contains (per liter): tryptone 20 g, yeast extract 5 g, glucose 3.6 g, together with sodium chloride (10 mM), potassium chloride (2.5 mM), magnesium chloride (10 mM), magnesium sulfate (10 mM).

sodium dodecyl sulfate (SDS) ($CH_3(CH_2)_{11}OSO_3Na$) An agent which binds co-operatively to proteins via the hydrophobic part of the molecule.

SDS is used for e.g. denaturing proteins, determining the molecular weight of proteins, and for separating components of protein–nucleic acid complexes.

(See also SDS–PAGE.)

sodium polyanetholesulfonate A blood ANTICOAGULANT; it can inhibit PCR.

SOE PCR See SPLICE OVERLAP EXTENSION PCR.

solenoid See CHROMATIN.

solid-phase PCR (on-chip PCR) A form of PCR involving the extension of primers on an immobilized complementary copy of the target sequence.

Two types of primer are used. The *immobilized* primers are covalently attached, via their 5′ termini, to a solid support. These primers are complementary to the 3′ end of the target sequence. On binding the target, these primers are extended (3′ →) using the target sequence as template; an immobilized primer therefore becomes a complementary copy of the target sequence.

The target fragment dissociates from the (extended) primer during temperature cycling.

The second type of primer is not immobilized, i.e. it is free in solution; it is labeled, and its sequence is *identical* to the 5′ end of the target sequence. This primer binds to the 3′ end of the (extended) immobilized primer and uses it as a template; extension of the labeled primer therefore forms a copy of the target – which subsequently dissociates during temperature cycling. Hence, ongoing binding and extension of the labeled primers amplifies the target.

[Use of on-chip PCR for identifying bacteria from clinical samples: J Clin Microbiol (2004) 42(3):1048–1057.]

The on-chip approach is also used for *in situ* solid-phase DNA amplification, i.e. generation of *colonies* of target DNA (each of which is a cloned product); in this context, benzene-1,3,5-triacetic acid (BTA) is useful for attaching 5′-aminated oligonucleotides to an aminosilanized glass surface [Nucleic Acids Res (2006) 34(3):e22].

solid-phase sequencing See e.g. PRIMER WALKING.

solubility enhancement tag (SET) An engineered peptide extension on a protein expressed from a vector, the purpose of the SET being to enhance the solubility of the protein; the sequences encoding the SET and the protein of interest (both on the vector) are jointly expressed as a fusion product. This system is marketed by Stratagene (La Jolla, CA) under the trade name VariFlex™.

There are a number of different SETs (e.g. SET1, SET2), each SET having a solubility-enhancing effect which may differ from that of other SETs, for a given protein. Although the solubility of many proteins can be enhanced by SETs, this is not possible for all proteins.

(See also Q-TAG.)

solution hybridization Hybridization of complementary seq-

uences wholly within the liquid phase (none of the sequences being immobilized).

somatic cell Any cell forming part of the structure, or body, of an organism.

(cf. GAMETE.)

somatic cell hybridization See CELL FUSION.

somatic cell nuclear transfer See SCNT.

SopA (in the F plasmid) See F PLASMID.

sortase An enzyme, associated with the cell envelope in the Gram-positive bacterium *Staphylococcus aureus* (and certain other bacteria), which catalyzes the site-specific cleavage of certain secreted proteins; these proteins are cleaved between a threonine residue and a glycine residue, the threonine then being bound, covalently, to the cell-wall peptidoglycan. This activity thus results in the tethering of the protein (fragment) to the cell envelope. PROTEIN A is one example of a tethered protein in *S. aureus*.

In *Bacillus anthracis*, the causal agent of anthrax, sortase is required for processing the IsdC protein to form a cell-bound fragment needed for the scavenging of heme iron [J Bacteriol (2006) 188(23):8145–8152].

Proteins that are substrates for this enzyme are characterizes by a C-terminal *cell wall sorting signal*; in *S. aureus* this is reported to include the consensus sequence LPXTG, while in *B. anthracis* it is reported as NPKTG.

Sos A guanosine nucleotide exchange factor (encoded by gene *sos*).

(See also CYTOTRAP TWO-HYBRID SYSTEM.)

SOS box See SOS SYSTEM.

SOS chromotest An assay for DNA-damaging agents (genotoxins) which uses an engineered test strain of *Escherichia coli* containing the *sulA* gene (see SOS SYSTEM) fused with the *lacZ* gene (encoding β-galactosidase); *lacZ* is thus used as a reporter gene, being expressed when the test strain of *E. coli* is exposed to any compound which triggers expression of *sulA*. Expression of *lacZ* may be registered with a substrate such as ONPG.

The strain of *E. coli* used in the SOS chromotest is deficient in DNA excision repair, and its cell envelope is made more permeable to certain chemicals. These cells also synthesize the enzyme alkaline phosphatase constitutively; this is useful for excluding the possibility that the compound under test may inhibit protein synthesis (this possibility being excluded by colorimetric assay of alkaline phosphatase).

Use of the *sulA* gene for detecting genotoxins is reported to be a less sensitive procedure than a ColD *cda* promoter-based system [Appl Environ Microbiol (2005) 71(5):2338–2346].

(See also AMES TEST.)

SOS system (in bacteria) A system which mediates the cell's response to damaged DNA, or inhibition of DNA replication, caused e.g. by ULTRAVIOLET RADIATION, QUINOLONE ANTIBIOTICS or alkylating agents.

In *Escherichia coli* the SOS system involves approximately 30 genes. The SOS response includes e.g. inhibition of cell division and an increase in the cell's capacity for DNA repair (associated with increased mutagenesis). (The SOS response also promotes induction of phages in lysogenic bacteria – see LYSOGENY.)

In *E. coli* the SOS genes are normally inhibited by LexA: a transcriptional repressor which binds to a specific consensus sequence (the *SOS box*) in the promoter region of relevant genes/operons. (Some SOS genes are expressed at low levels under normal conditions.) In the presence of damaged DNA, the RECA protein promotes autocatalytic cleavage of LexA, leading to expression of the SOS response.

The product of SOS gene *sulA* (= *sfiA*) inhibits polymerization of the FtsZ protein. FtsZ proteins normally polymerize to form a ring-shaped structure (the *Z ring*), midway in the cell, as a preliminary stage in the development of the pre-division septum. SulA therefore inhibits septum formation and, hence, inhibits cell division. (Growth may continue as septum-less *filaments*.) Resumption of normal septation takes place rapidly when repression of *sulA* is re-imposed by LexA following a return to normal conditions. Rapid resumption of septation is promoted by inactivation of SulA by the product of the *lon* gene – a heat-shock protein (a protease) whose production can be induced by some of the factors that trigger the SOS response. SulA is more stable in *lon* mutants, and even low-level induction of the SOS response in these cells may lead to lethal filamentation.

Various DNA repair systems are enhanced/expressed in the SOS response. One of these systems is an error-prone process (= *mutagenic repair*) resulting in increased levels of mutation in surviving cells; this process involves certain types of DNA polymerase (induced specifically during the SOS response) which carry out so-called *translesion synthesis* in which there is a loss of base-pairing specificity at lesions in the DNA.

In *Staphylococcus aureus* the SOS response is reported to be triggered by the quinolone antibiotic ciprofloxacin, with concomitant derepression of 16 genes [J Bacteriol (2007) 189 (2):531–539].

Southern blotting Following electrophoresis of fragments of DNA in a gel strip: transfer of the fragments from the gel to a sheet of nitrocellulose (or to another type of membrane) by capillary action; after transfer, the fragments have the same relative positions as they had in the gel strip.

First, dsDNA fragments in the gel are denatured to ssDNA by exposure to alkali. The gel is then placed onto an (absorptive) wick in contact with a neutral buffer. A nitrocellulose sheet is placed over the gel strip; this is overlaid by a stack of (absorptive) paper towels pressed onto the nitrocellulose by a weight.

Buffer rises, via the wick, and passes into, and through, the gel and then through the (permeable) nitrocellulose filter into the paper towels; this upward flow of buffer transports the fragments from the gel to the surface of the nitrocellulose filter. The filter is removed and then 'baked' (~70°C) under a vacuum to bind the DNA.

The bound fragments can be probed, probe–fragment binding (*Southern hybridization*) indicating the presence of a given sequence in a particular band of fragments in the original gel strip.

APT paper can be used instead of the nitrocellulose. This incorporates 2-aminophenylthioether which, prior to use, is modified to a reactive diazo derivative that binds ssDNA *covalently* to the paper (avoiding the need for baking). The probes can be removed from APT paper and a different set of probes used on the same sheet.

Southern hybridization See SOUTHERN BLOTTING.
   (See also REVERSE SOUTHERN HYBRIDIZATION.)

Southwestern blotting A procedure used e.g. for detecting the presence of DNA-binding proteins in a cell lysate and identifying their binding sites in genomic DNA.

The sample is first subjected to gel electrophoresis, and the *proteins* in the gel are transferred to a matrix. Proteins on the matrix are probed with specific, labeled DNA sequences, and protein–DNA binding is detected via the label. Any protein, and/or the DNA attached to it, can be isolated and analyzed.

(See also CHROMATIN IMMUNOPRECIPITATION.)

SpA *Syn.* PROTEIN A.

SPA Scintillation proximity assay: a method used for detecting binding between two molecules, or other entities, one being radioactively labeled and the other having the properties of a *scintillant* (a scintillant being a substance that produces light when in close proximity to a source of radioactivity); detection of a light signal is regarded as an indication of binding. (The principle of SPA is thus similar to that of fluorescence resonance energy transfer (FRET), although the mechanism is different.)

SPA has a range of uses, and commercial kits are available for particular applications. The procedure has been used e.g. to assay the binding of human tumor suppressor protein p53 to DNA; in this assay, the binding of p53 to radioactively (^{3}H) labeled DNA was detected by (i) an anti-p53 antibody and then (ii) PROTEIN A linked to scintillant-containing beads [BioTechniques (2006) 41(3):303–308].

SPA has also been used for studies on a phage [J Bacteriol (2006) 188(4):1643–1647] and on the lysosome/phagosome targeting process [Mol Biol Cell (2006) 17(4):1697–1710].

spacer arm See e.g. BIOTIN. A spacer arm is sometimes called a 'linker'. (cf. LINKER.)

specialized transducing particle (STP) See TRANSDUCTION.

specialized transduction See TRANSDUCTION.

spheroplast An osmotically sensitive entity which is prepared from a cell by removal of its cell-wall materials.

Spheroplasts of Gram-positive bacteria can be prepared e.g. by incubating the cells in a solution containing EDTA, LYSOZYME and Tris buffer.

Spheroplasts of the yeast *Saccharomyces cerevisiae* can be prepared e.g. by treating the cells with ZYMOLYASE.

spinning-disk microscopy See IN VIVO FLUORESCENCE.

spinoculation Centrifugally assisted viral infection of cells.

splice overlap extension PCR (SOE PCR) A form of PCR that can be used to fuse two sequences of DNA – present on the same molecule or on separate molecules – without the use of restriction endonucleases; in order to be fused by SOE PCR, the 3′ end of one sequence must have a short region of homology with the 5′ end of the other sequence.

Initially, each of the two sequences is amplified, separately, by PCR; in each case the amplicons include the homologous region referred to.

Amplicons from both reactions are mixed and subjected to a further round of PCR. In this case the primers are designed to bind to the *non*-homologous end of each of the two sequences. During the reaction, hybridization (at the region of homology) occurs between single strands of the two types of amplicon; subsequently, strand synthesis copies the hybridized strand, forming a hybrid (chimeric) product that includes both of the original sequences.

If the two sequences have no common region of homology, such a region can be added by carrying out an initial stage of PCR (for each sequence) in which a region suitable for fusion is incorporated as a 5′ tag in the primers.

SOE PCR has been used e.g. to form hybrid mouse–human monoclonal antibodies by taking advantage of the homology between analogous regions of murine and human immunoglobulin genes [BioTechniques (2005) 38(2):181–182].

splice site   See ACCEPTOR SPLICE SITE, DONOR SPLICE SITE.
(See also SPLICING.)

spliced leader   See TRANS SPLICING.

spliceosome   A large, multi-component complex involved in SPLICING pre-mRNA to mature mRNA. In (human) cells it includes e.g. SR PROTEINS, snRNPs (see SNRNAS), DEAD-BOX PROTEINS, RNA helicase and other factors.

splicing (of pre-mRNA)   The process in which non-coding sequence(s) in a SPLIT GENE are excised from the primary RNA transcript of the gene during formation of the final, mature mRNA. Splicing involves cleavage of both ends of a given intron, at precise phosphodiester bonds, and the formation of a phosphodiester bond between the exon on the 5′ side of the intron and that on the 3′ side of the intron.

(See also ALTERNATIVE SPLICING, CRYPTIC SPLICING and EXON TRAPPING.)

The mechanism of splicing is different in different types of split gene.

Bacterial introns are mainly, or solely, *autocatalytic* (i.e. self-splicing) – i.e. the RNA itself has intrinsic catalytic properties.

Introns of phage T4 are autocatalytic *in vitro*. The intron in the T4 thymidylate synthase gene was reported to require a ribosomal factor for efficient intracellular splicing.

Splicing of *human* pre-mRNAs is a complex, multi-step process involving development of a SPLICEOSOME. One early requirement is the need to select an appropriate 5′ DONOR SPLICE SITE and a 3′ ACCEPTOR SPLICE SITE; this appears to be facilitated by *cis*-acting regulatory elements within the pre-mRNA: the so-called *exonic splicing enhancers* (ESEs) and *exonic splicing silencers*. Many ESEs bind to the RNA-recognition motif of SR PROTEINS; this may help to define appropriate splice sites e.g. by promoting the binding of other

components of the spliceosome to the arginine–serine region of the SR protein and/or by antagonizing the effect(s) of adjacent silencer sequences. Such positive selection of splice sites is needed in order to counteract the effect of intronic *pseudo-exons* that are flanked by potential splice sites. [The distribution of ESE motifs in human genes: Nucleic Acids Res (2005) 33(16):5053–5062.]

An early event is duplex formation between U1 SNRNA and the 5′ splice site; enhanced recognition of this site has been found to result from extending the base-pairing complementarity of this duplex [see Nucleic Acids Res (2005) 33(16): 5112–5119]. Other components, including snRNAs, join the complex – e.g. U2 binds at the *branch point* near the 3′ end of the intron. The cut 5′ end of the intron loops over and is bonded (2′-to-5′) to a nucleotide at the branch point. Overall, the process leads to excision of the intron as a tailed loop (*lariat*) and the formation of a phosphodiester bond between the 3′ end of one exon and the 5′ end of the next.

Another post-transcriptional modifications is capping (see CAP).

Mutations that cause faults in the splicing process can give rise to pathological conditions through deficiency or absence of the normal product. For example, aberrant splicing was reported to be responsible for the Axenfeld–Rieger syndrome in some patients, and variation in the severity of the splicing fault may be reflected in the range of manifestations of this syndrome [BMC Med Genet (2006) 7:59].

splicing (of proteins)   See INTEIN.

splinker (sequencing primer linker)   A synthetic oligodeoxynucleotide containing INVERTED REPEAT sequences that form a (double-stranded) hairpin structure which contains a recognition site for a RESTRICTION ENDONUCLEASE. Splinkers are used e.g. for sequence analysis of DNA restriction fragments.

Target DNA (to be sequenced) is digested with restriction enzymes, and the fragments are treated with alkaline phosphates (to de-phosphorylate their 5′ termini). The 5′ termini of the splinkers (which are phosphorylated) are then ligated to the 3′ termini of the restriction fragments. That strand of the fragment which is *not* ligated to the splinker is removed, by heating and rapid cooling, leaving the primed splinker-bound strand. The primer is extended (in a reaction mixture containing dideoxy chain-terminating nucleotides), and each of the newly synthesized strands is released from its template strand by cleavage at the splinker's internal restriction site.

This procedure avoids e.g. the need to synthesize a specific primer.

split gene (interrupted gene)   Any gene that includes one, two, several or many *non-coding* sequences of nucleotides (called *intervening sequences*, or INTRONS) which do not encode any part of the gene product. Intron sequence(s) are represented in the primary RNA transcript (the *pre-mRNA*); usually they are spliced out during formation of the mature mRNA (the *messenger* RNA) – which therefore contains the covalently linked coding sequences (*exons*) of the gene.

(See also SPLICING.)

In higher eukaryotes, many or most genes are split genes. Split genes also occur in eukaryotic microorganisms, such as *Dictyostelium* and *Saccharomyces*, and all protein-encoding genes in the slime mold *Physarum polycephalum* apparently contain introns.

Some archaeal, bacterial and viral genes are split genes.

Examples of intron-less human genes include those encoding interferons α and β. The (human) insulin gene contains a single intron. By contrast, certain genes contain 50 to 100 introns.

spoligotype See SPOLIGOTYPING.

spoligotyping A method used for simultaneous detection and TYPING of strains of the *Mycobacterium tuberculosis* complex [original description of the procedure: J Clin Microbiol (1997) 35:907–914].

Essentially, spacer sequences within the chromosomal DR (direct repeat) region of the strain under test are amplified by PCR; the amplicons are hybridized to a set of oligonucleotides that represent spacer sequences of the reference strain (i.e. *M. tuberculosis* H37Rv). (The name 'spoligotyping' is derived from a contraction of 'spacer oligotyping'.) The pattern of matching, and mis-matching, of the test strain's spacer sequences (amplicons) with the set of oligonucleotides is called the *spoligotype* of that strain.

[Genetic diversity in the *M. tuberculosis* complex: mining the fourth international spoligotyping database: BMC Microbiol (2006) 6:23.]

spoT **gene** In *Escherichia coli*: a gene that encodes an enzyme which can synthesize and degrade the alarmone ppGpp.

SPS Sodium polyanetholesulfonate: a blood ANTICOAGULANT; it inhibits PCR.

Spumavirinae A subfamily of viruses (family Retroviridae – see RETROVIRUSES) that occur in various species of mammal; these viruses are apparently non-pathogenic. In tissue culture the spumaviruses produce characteristic cytopathic effects – including the development of syncytia and the formation of a highly vacuolated ('foamy') cytoplasm within infected cells, hence the name 'foamy viruses'.

The spumaviruses include e.g. bovine syncytial virus, feline syncytial virus, and the human and simian foamy viruses; the transmission of simian foamy virus (SFV) from macaques to humans was reported some years ago.

spumaviruses Viruses of the subfamily SPUMAVIRINAE.

SR proteins In the SPLICING of pre-mRNA: certain proteins involved in the choice of splice sites. The N-terminal region contains an *RNA-recognition motif*. The C-terminal region consists largely of alternating residues of serine and arginine (the designation SR derives from the one-letter symbols for these two amino acids).

src (*SRC*) An ONCOGENE first detected in Rous sarcoma virus (RSV). RSV is an avian virus which can cause experimental tumors in some mammals. The v-*src* product exhibits TYROSINE KINASE activity.

The product of c-*src* is expressed only weakly in a normal cell.

Differences in the C-terminal regions of viral and cellular gene products may account for the transforming ability of the former.

SRF SUBTRACTED RESTRICTION FINGERPRINTING.

SSB protein SINGLE-STRAND BINDING PROTEIN.

SSCP analysis (single-strand conformation polymorphism analysis) A technique that is used for comparing single-stranded samples of *related* nucleic acid by comparing their electrophoretic speeds within a polyacrylamide gel; even a one-base difference between strands may be detectable if it affects the intra-strand base-pairing (i.e. conformation) in such a way that it causes a change in electrophoretic mobility.

Note that SSCP analysis uses a *non*-denaturing gel; this is used in order to preserve (or promote) the intra-strand base-pairing on which differentiation depends.

Samples often consist of strands ~100–300 bp in length.

Samples for use in SSCP may be conveniently prepared by ASYMMETRIC PCR. Alternatively, samples can be prepared by using a standard form of PCR, with *one* of the primers 5′-phosphorylated, and digesting the amplicons with the lambda exonuclease (see EXONUCLEASE).

PCR-SSCP can be used e.g. for detecting point mutations that confer bacterial resistance to specific antibiotics. For this purpose, PCR is used to amplify a particular region of the genome associated with resistance to a given antibiotic; the (single-stranded) amplicons are then compared with those from wild-type (antibiotic-sensitive) strains. PCR-SSCP has been used, for example, to detect strains of *Mycobacterium tuberculosis* in which mutation in the *rpoB* gene (encoding the β-subunit of RNA polymerase) confers resistance to the anti-tuberculosis drug rifampicin (rifampin); in this organism the mutation-prone region of the *rpoB* gene was amplified by PCR and the amplicons examined as described.

SSCP analysis has also been used e.g. for screening resistance to fluoroquinolone antibiotics in the bacterium *Streptococcus pneumoniae* [J Clin Microbiol (2006) 44(3):970–975].

SSCP analysis was also used for screening the *MFN2* gene in patients with a clinical diagnosis of Charcot–Marie–Tooth disease (type 2A); this resulted in the identification of novel mutations [BMC Med Genet (2006) 7:53].

Such is the specificity of this method that, in some cases, a result can indicate a particular type of mutation at a precise locus.

In studies on antibiotic resistance, one problem associated with this method is that a SILENT MUTATION in an antibiotic-sensitive strain may produce a conformation which simulates that of an antibiotic-resistant strain – yielding a false-positive result [see e.g. J Clin Microbiol (1997) 35:492–494].

(See also DGGE.)

ssDNA Single-stranded DNA.

SSM SLIPPED-STRAND MISPAIRING.

SSR (1) See SITE-SPECIFIC RECOMBINATION.

(2) See SHORT SEQUENCE REPEATS.

(3) See SIMPLE SEQUENCE REPEATS.

ssRNA Single-stranded RNA.

SssI (M.SssI) A methyltransferase from *Spiroplasma* (species MOl) that is reported to be specific for 5′-CpG-3′ sites (in purified DNA); SssI methylates the cytosine residue at the 5-position.

stacking gel See SDS–PAGE.

staining (of DNA) See DNA STAINING.

standard virus See DEFECTIVE INTERFERING PARTICLE.

staphylococcal cassette chromosome *mec* See SCCMEC.

star activity A change in the *specificity* of certain RESTRICTION ENDONUCLEASES (e.g. BamHI and EcoRI) under non-optimal conditions.

Although it is usually a disadvantage, star activity has been exploited in a method for producing vectors with unidirectional deletions [BioTechniques (2005) 38:198–204].

STATs SIGNAL TRANSDUCERS AND ACTIVATORS OF TRANSCRIPTION.

stavudine See NUCLEOSIDE REVERSE TRANSCRIPTASE INHIBITORS.

steel factor (stem cell factor) See KIT.

stem-and-loop In a molecule of nucleic acid: a structure which has been formed by base-pairing between (complementary) sequences of nucleotides, the hybridized regions forming the (double-stranded) stem and the intervening (single-stranded) region forming the loop.

stem cell A type of cell (found e.g. in bone marrow) which has the potential for unrestricted division and differentiation to a given type of cell; stem cells act as a reserve, being able e.g. to replace those cells (blood cells etc.) that are lost during the life of the individual.

The pluripotent *embryonic* stem (ES) cells from blastocyst can be cultured for long periods in the presence of LEUKEMIA INHIBITORY FACTOR and e.g. serum (cf. FEEDER CELLS); the progeny cells retain potential for multilineage differentiation. [shRNA vector for high-efficiency RNA interference (RNAi) in ES cells: BioTechniques (2007) 42(6):738–743.]

Mouse ES cells have been extensively used in studies on gene function; these cells can be genetically modified (e.g. by GENE TARGETING or GENE TRAPPING) and then inserted into an (isolated) blastocyst for re-implantation and development.

Stem cells have been exploited e.g. in GENE THERAPY (see also SICKLE-CELL ANEMIA).

(See also SCNT.)

stem cell factor (steel factor) See KIT.

sterilant Any agent used for STERILIZATION.

sterile cabinet *Syn.* SAFETY CABINET.

sterilization Any process used to ensure the death/permanent inactivation of all forms of life – including bacterial endospores – that are present on or within objects or materials, or within environments, subjected to that process.

One common method of sterilization involves treatment in an AUTOCLAVE.

Chemicals which have been used as *sterilants* (i.e. agents used for sterilization) include ethylene oxide, glutaraldehyde and β-propiolactone; in each case, physical conditions must be carefully arranged in order to achieve maximum activity of the sterilant.

Note. The phrase 'partial sterilization' is meaningless because sterility is an 'all-or-nothing' phenomenon.

Sterne strain (*Bacillus anthracis*) See BACILLUS ANTHRACIS.

sticky ends (or cohesive ends) Complementary, single-stranded terminal regions present on dsDNA molecules. For example:

```
-----NNNNNATCTG-3'        NNNNN-----
-----NNNNN        3'-TAGACNNNNN-----
```

shows a pair of sticky ends consisting of two 3′ five-base extensions; these two single-stranded regions can hybridize and, if required, the two terminal regions can be ligated.

Sticky ends can be generated e.g. by the staggered cleavage produced by *certain* types of RESTRICTION ENDONUCLEASE (e.g. EcoRI). Note that the single-stranded region may be a 3′ extension or a 5′ extension, depending on the mode of cutting of the particular enzyme used.

Single-stranded extensions are also called *overhangs*.

Some restriction enzymes form BLUNT-ENDED DNA.

(See also entry POLYLINKER.)

Compatible sticky ends can be produced (i) when DNA is cut by the same enzyme, or by an isoschizomer, or (ii) when DNA is cut by an unrelated enzyme that creates hybridizable sequences; for an example of the latter type of enzyme see MunI in the table in entry RESTRICTION ENDONUCLEASE.

stimulator sequence See FRAMESHIFTING.

STM SIGNATURE-TAGGED MUTAGENESIS.

Stoffel fragment A recombinant form (the C-terminal region) of *Taq* polymerase which has greater thermal stability than the parent enzyme; it lacks exonuclease activity. It has been used e.g. in arbitrarily primed PCR.

Stokes' shift For a given fluorescent molecule or particle: the difference between the wavelength at maximum absorbance and the wavelength at maximum emission.

A large Stokes' shift is characteristic e.g. of the QUANTUM DOT.

stop codon See NONSENSE CODON.

STP Specialized transducing particle: see TRANSDUCTION.

STR (short tandem repeat) In the human genome: one of a number of sequences of DNA containing tandem repeats of a unit that consists of 2–6 bases; for example, an STR may consist of a series of eight repeat units, each unit consisting of four bases:

....TCTATCTATCTATCTATCTATCTATCTATCTA....

STRs are common in the genome. In a given STR (i.e. one found at a specific location on a particular chromosome), the *number* of repeat units varies in different individuals; this has made STRs useful in genetic mapping and in systems for establishing human identity (e.g. CODIS).

[STR database: Nucleic Acids Res (2001) 29:320–322.]

Male-specific STRs (on the Y chromosome) are useful e.g. in sex-based forensic investigations.

strA **gene** *Syn.* RPSL GENE.

strain (*microbiol.*) Within a given species: those individuals which have certain characteristic(s) in common and which can be distinguished from all other members of that species on the basis of such characteristic(s). The existence of strains reflects the heterogeneity in a species.

(See also TYPING.)

strand A chain of ribonucleotide or deoxyribonucleotide sub-units (of no specified length). A double-stranded molecule of nucleic acid consists of two strands that are hybridized by base-pairing between bases in one strand and complementary bases in the other.

strand displacement Displacement of the existing complementary strand on a template strand by an upstream DNA polymerase which is actively synthesizing a new complementary strand on that template. Not all DNA polymerases are able to mediate strand displacement.

Strand displacement can be initiated from a NICK, the polymerase extending the 3′ terminus and simultaneously displacing the 5′ terminus.

Alternatively, strand displacement can be achieved by the use of a *bumper primer*. A bumper primer binds to a single-stranded sequence, upstream of the double-stranded region; extension of the bumper primer's 3′ terminus displaces the existing complementary strand.

(See also SDA.)

strand displacement amplification See SDA.

StrataClean™ resin Silica-based particles used e.g. for the removal of *Taq* polymerase activity following PCR, and for removing restriction endonucleases from restriction digests. It is also used for concentrating proteins.

(See also NICKEL-CHARGED AFFINITY RESIN.)

streptavidin A protein (synthesized by the bacterium *Streptomyces avidinii*) that binds strongly to BIOTIN. Its uses include the detection of biotinylated probes; for this purpose, it is labeled with an enzyme (e.g. ALKALINE PHOSPHATASE) or with a fluorophore so that, when bound to biotin, it can signal the presence of biotin by expression of the label.

Streptavidin has also been used e.g. for separating biotin-labeled, single-stranded amplicons from unlabeled amplicons following PCR (see e.g. ASYMMETRIC PCR).

The protein was involved in developing the QUANTUM DOT PROBE.

streptococcal nuclease See STREPTODORNASE.

streptodornase (streptococcal nuclease) Any of various serologically distinct forms of DNASE produced by *Streptococcus* spp. e.g. strains of Lancefield group A; the activity of these enzymes is promoted e.g. by Ca⁺ or Mg⁺, and their products (unlike those of staphylococcal thermonuclease) have terminal 5′-phosphate groups (cf. DNASE I).

Streptodornase is a *phage*-encoded virulence factor in at least certain strains of group A streptococci [Infect Immun (2003) 71(12):7079–7086].

streptolydigin A complex, heterocyclic antibiotic that inhibits bacterial RNA polymerase.

[Structural basis of activity: Molecular Cell (2005) 19(5): 655–666.]

streptomycin An AMINOGLYCOSIDE ANTIBIOTIC used e.g. as a selective agent for bacteria containing a vector which carries a streptomycin-resistance gene.

streptonigrin An (iron-dependent) antibiotic/antitumor agent reported to cause strand breakage in DNA in the presence of oxygen and a reducing agent, and to be inhibited e.g. by superoxide dismutase and other scavengers of free radicals.

streptozotocin 2-deoxy-2-(3-methyl-3-nitrosoureido)-D-glucopyranoside: an agent which is bactericidal for (certain) Gram-positive and Gram-negative bacteria that are actively growing (cf. PENICILLIN); bacterial susceptibility to this agent depends on the presence of a functional transport (uptake) system for *N*-acetylglucosamine (which is also involved in the uptake of streptozotocin). The agent is internalized as streptozotocin 6-phosphate, which is subsequently converted to diazomethane (a highly toxic and mutagenic compound).

Non-growing cells are unaffected by streptozotocin. Growing cells are killed – but are not *lysed* (so that, unlike the cells killed by penicillin, their cytoplasmic contents are not released immediately). For this reason, streptozotocin can be more useful than penicillin for the isolation of AUXOTROPHIC MUTANTS (q.v.).

Streptozotocin is also diabetogenic in laboratory animals. A study on streptozotocin-induced diabetes in female rats found that this condition is associated with changes in e.g. vaginal hemodynamics and morphology [BMC Physiol (2006) 6:4].

stress-induced duplex destabilization See SIDD.

stringency In the hybridization (annealing, base pairing) of two single strands of nucleic acid: the level of constraint imposed by factors such as temperature, concentration of electrolyte, and the presence of compounds (such as formamide) which influence base–base interaction.

High-stringency conditions (e.g. high temperatures) require that the two strands have a high degree of complementarity (i.e. few, or no, mismatched bases) in order for annealing to take place.

Low-stringency conditions (e.g. lower temperatures) may permit annealing to occur between two (partly mis-matched) strands even when such strands would not hybridize at higher temperatures.

Appropriate levels of stringency can be used e.g. to control the specificity with which probes and primers hybridize to their target sequences.

stringent control (of plasmid replication) See PLASMID.

stringent response See *relA* in ESCHERICHIA COLI (table).

stroboscopic lighting (for *in vivo* fluorescence) See IN VIVO FLUORESCENCE.

STS SEQUENCE-TAGGED SITE.

Stuart's transport medium See TRANSPORT MEDIUM.

stuffer See REPLACEMENT VECTOR.

subcloning CLONING a DNA fragment that has been cleaved, by restriction enzymes, from a larger fragment; in general, the object of subcloning is to facilitate studies on the larger fragment by examining individual, smaller pieces.

subgenomic mRNA (of an RNA virus) An mRNA, produced from the viral genome in an infected eukaryotic cell, which is shorter than the viral genome itself. The need to produce a subgenomic mRNA arises because of the general inability of eukaryotic cells to initiate translation from an *internal* site in an mRNA.

Subgenomic mRNAs may be monocistronic, bicistronic or polycistronic.

Subgenomic mRNAs are synthesized from the genomes of e.g. retroviruses and the tobacco mosaic virus.

substrate-induced gene expression screening See SIGEX.

subtracted restriction fingerprinting (SRF) A method for TYPING bacteria involving (i) digestion of genomic DNA with two types of restriction endonuclease, (ii) end-labeling, with biotin or digoxigenin, by filling in the 5′ overhangs, (iii) differential capture (and elimination) of a proportion of the fragments (those labeled with biotin), and (iv) electrophoresis and detection of the remaining fragments (those labeled with digoxigenin) in agarose gels. [Method: BioTechniques (2003) 34(2):304–313.]

subtractive hybridization A procedure for isolating particular mRNAs that are synthesized specifically in a given type of 'target' cell – e.g. during differentiation. Essentially, the procedure involves removing (subtracting) those mRNAs which are also found in other types of cell – thus leaving target-cell-specific mRNAs.

In one approach, mRNAs are first isolated from the target cells. Separately, mRNAs are isolated from other type(s) of cell (the so-called 'subtractor cells'), and *these* mRNAs are converted to first-strand cDNAs by the use of biotinylated poly(T) primers; the mRNA templates are eliminated, and the single-stranded cDNAs, bound to superparamagnetic beads (such as DYNABEADS), are allowed to hybridize to mRNAs from the target cells. The cDNA/mRNA hybrids are removed magnetically, leaving target-cell-specific mRNAs which can be used for synthesis of cDNAs and cloning etc.

suicide polymerase endonuclease restriction (SuPER) During PCR: a method for enhancing the amplification of minor (e.g. low-copy-number) templates by the elimination of dominant templates present in the same reaction mixture; this approach is thus an alternative to PCR CLAMPING.

Essentially, within the reaction mixture (containing the unwanted, dominant template as well as the required template), the following activities occur:

● annealing of PCR primers to the unwanted template under stringent conditions;

● primer elongation by DNA polymerase;

● targeted restriction of the double-stranded amplicons, thus specifically eliminating copies of the unwanted template.

These activities depend on the establishment of appropriate operational conditions (e.g. temperature) in the reaction mixture. If temperatures are too low the specificity may be lost; if too high, the efficiency of the restriction enzyme may be reduced, allowing survival of unwanted templates.

[SuPER (method): Appl Environ Microbiol (2005) 71(8): 4721–4727.]

suicide vector Any vector which encodes the mechanism for its own elimination from a population of cells after carrying out its specific function(s) in those cells.

A suicide vector may be used, for example, to introduce a mutant sequence into a bacterial gene. The vector is inserted into the cell by transformation, or electroporation, and after integration of the given sequence into the chromosome (by homologous recombination) the vector becomes superfluous. If the vector is a plasmid that exhibits temperature-sensitive replication (i.e. unable to replicate at, say, ~43–44°C), it can be easily eliminated from the cell simply by raising the temperature to the non-permissive level; ongoing growth of the cells will therefore result in a progressive loss of the plasmid. (The bacterial strain used must, of course, be able to maintain growth at the higher temperature.)

In one approach, a suicide plasmid carrying a *recA* gene (whose expression was required *temporarily* in the host cell) also carried a gene encoding a genetically modified form of the enzyme phenylalanyl-tRNA synthetase. This variant form of the enzyme has a relaxed substrate specificity in that it can mediate the incorporation into proteins of a phenylalanine analog, *p*-chlorophenylalanine, which is lethal for the cell; hence, when the plasmid has fulfilled its function, any cells in which the plasmid has *not* been lost spontaneously are killed when the cells are grown on a medium containing *p*-chlorophenylalanine. [Method: BioTechniques (2005) 38(3): 405–408.]

sulA **gene** (*sfiA* gene) See SOS SYSTEM.

sulfamethoxazole See ANTIBIOTIC (synergism).

SUMO Small ubiquitin-like modifier: see SUMOYLATION.

SUMO-1, SUMO-2 etc. See SUMOYLATION.

SUMO proteases See SUMOYLATION.

sumoylation A form of reversible, post-translational modification, analogous to ubiquitinylation, in which a UBIQUITIN-like protein (SUMO: small ubiquitin-like modifier) is covalently bound to a specific lysine residue in a target protein; as in the ubiquitinylation process, sumoylation involves three types of enzyme: E1 (activation), E2 (conjugation) and E3 (ligation) (see PROTEASOME).

The target proteins for sumoylation include certain transcription factors and also cofactors. The effect of sumoylation depends on target protein; for example, in a number of cases it represses the function of a transcriptional activator, while for some proteins it affects subcellular localization by regulating nucleocytoplasmic shuttling. (At least one sumoylated protein is located in the mitochondrion.) Indirectly, sumoylation affects the stability of IκB (a major regulatory factor of NFκB) and is involved e.g. in histone modification, DNA repair and other cellular functions.

Sumoylation may have an essential role in certain disorders (e.g. Parkinson's disease).

Many (but not all) of the sumoylation sites in proteins are associated with a consensus motif (K-X-E, or K-X-E/D), in which the lysine (K) residue is preceded by a hydrophobic amino acid residue.

Mammals have four types of SUMO, designated SUMO-1, SUMO-2, SUMO-3 and SUMO-4; there is a confusing range of synonymous designations. These four types of protein may have distinct roles as they appear to modify different sets of target proteins; the expression of SUMO-4 may be limited to the kidney. The yeast *Saccharomyces cerevisiae* has only one type of SUMO, which is designated SMT3. Various similar proteins exist in plants.

Desumoylation (i.e. reversal of sumoylation), involving the removal of the SUMO moiety, is mediated by specific types of enzyme: the SUMO proteases (also called isopeptidases or cysteine proteases). A desumoylating enzyme, Ulp1, was first isolated from *S. cerevisiae*. Another yeast protein, Ulp2 (also referred to as Smt4), and certain proteins from vertebrates (designated SENP1, SENP2, SENP3. . . .), have desumoylation activity. The Ulp1 enzyme is reported to be essential for *S. cerevisiae*, mutation causing lethal cell-cycle defects. All the known SUMO proteases contain a highly conserved sequence in the C-terminal domain, but the N-terminal domain shows little or no homology between the enzymes; the N-terminal domain may determine substrate specificity.

[SUMO (regulating the regulator): Cell Division (2006) 1: 13; SUMOsp (a web server for predicting sumoylation sites in proteins): Nucleic Acids Res (2006) 34(Web Server issue): W254–W257.]

SUMO proteins and proteases have been exploited in DNA technology. For example, a SUMO protein has been used as a fusion partner in order to increase the solubility of the target protein: see e.g. CHAMPION PET SUMO VECTOR.

SUP4 (*Saccharomyces cerevisiae*)   See SACCHAROMYCES and YEAST ARTIFICIAL CHROMOSOME.

SuPER   SUICIDE POLYMERASE ENDONUCLEASE RESTRICTION.

super-integron   See INTEGRON.

SuperCos I vector   A 7.9-kb COSMID vector (Stratagene, La Jolla CA) used e.g. for the preparation of cosmid libraries and for COSMID WALKING. It includes the ColEl (plasmid) origin of replication and an SV40 origin. The BamHI cloning site is flanked by T3 and T7 promoters which are present in opposite orientation; flanking these two promoters are NotI recognition sites, permitting excision of the promoter-flanked insert.

The SuperCos I vector can accomodate inserts of 30–42 kb.

Example of use: preparation of a cosmid library in studies on *Rhodococcus opacus* [Appl Environ Microbiol (2005) 71 (12):7705–7715]. [See also BMC Genomics (2006) 7:322.]

superfemale   See CHROMOSOME.

(See also BARR BODY.)

superintegron   See INTEGRON.

superparamagnetic   Refers to the characteristic of certain types of material in which magnetic properties are exhibited only when they are placed in a magnetic field; such materials have no residual magnetic properties after they have been removed from the magnetic field.

(See also DYNABEADS.)

SuperSAGE   See SAGE.

suppressor mutation   Any mutation which, at least to some extent, reverses the effects of an earlier (*primary*) mutation at a *different site*. (cf. BACK MUTATION.) If the original wild-type phenotype is not fully restored, the result is referred to as a *pseudo-wild* phenotype.

An *intragenic suppressor* occurs in the same gene as the primary mutation. For example, a primary frameshift mutation may be suppressed by a nucleotide insertion/deletion that restores the correct reading frame (although the nucleotide sequence between the two mutations remains mutant).

An *intergenic suppressor* occurs outside the gene containing the primary mutation. Typically, it affects the function of the tRNA that normally binds to the given wild-type codon; the mutant tRNA may e.g. insert an amino acid at the site of a nonsense mutation (a *nonsense suppressor*), or it may insert an alternative amino acid at the site of a mis-sense mutation (a *mis-sense suppressor*).

An *ochre suppressor* mutation in a tRNA gene suppresses the effects of an ochre mutation (or, less effectively, the effects of an amber mutation) by inserting an amino acid at the mutant codon.

An *amber suppressor* can suppress the effects of an amber mutation.

Indirect suppression circumvents the effects of the primary mutation by giving the cell alternative function(s) – e.g. activating an alternative metabolic pathway to replace that disabled by the primary mutation.

suramin   A drug used e.g. for the treatment of trypanosomiasis: 8-(3-benzamino-4-methyl-benzamino)naphthalene-1,3,5-trisulfonic acid; the drug is not effective in the later stages of the disease as it does not pass the blood–brain barrier.

Suramin inhibits the REVERSE TRANSCRIPTASE of various retroviruses and is also reported to affect the alternative pathway of complement fixation (apparently by altering the reactivity of component C3b).

surface-obligatory conjugation   See CONJUGATION.

SV40   Simian virus 40: a small non-enveloped icosahedral virus in which the genome is covalently closed circular dsDNA (~5.3 kbp). Within cells the viral DNA occurs in the nucleus. The virion is resistant to lipid solvents and low pH.

SV40 was first isolated from the rhesus monkey (*Macaca mulatta*) – in which it is frequently found (in latent form) in kidney cells. This virus causes a characteristic vacuolation in kidney cells from the African green monkey (*Cercopithecus aethiops*). Although commonly non-pathogenic in the natural host, SV40 can e.g. induce tumors in newborn rodents (which lack the immunocompetence of adult animals). Cells transformed by SV40 contain viral DNA integrated in the host's genome, apparently at non-specific sites.

A strong promoter sequence from the genome of SV40 is used e.g. in a variety of systems (e.g. expression vectors) in which effective transcription is required.

(See also POLYOMAVIRUSES.)

swivelase See TOPOISOMERASE (type I).

SYBR® Green I A fluorescent dye which, bound to dsDNA, has an emission maximum at 520 nm on excitation at 497 nm. (The dye also binds to single-stranded DNA, but in this case the level of fluorescence is significantly lower compared with dsDNA.)

This dye is widely used e.g. for staining DNA in gels and for monitoring the formation of products in real-time PCR.

[DNA intercalation and surface binding by SYBR Green I (determination of structure and methodological implications): Nucleic Acids Res (2004) 32(12):e103.]

SYBR Safe™ DNA gel stain A fluorescent stain (Molecular Probes/Invitrogen) which, compared with ethidium bromide, is much less mutagenic (Ames test) and more sensitive.

The bound stain has an emission maximum at ~530 nm.

symmetric methylation A term used to refer to the methylation of DNA bases when the methylated residues are present in a symmetric arrangement within the sequence recognized by the methylating enzyme. For example, the methyltransferase M.SssI (recognition sequence 5'-CG-3'; 3'-GC-5') methylates both (symmetrically placed) cytosine residues.

syn Abbreviation for SYNCLINAL.

synapsis (in homologous recombination) See HOMOLOGOUS RECOMBINATION.

synclinal (*syn*) Of a nucleotide: the conformation in which the 6-position in a purine, or the 2-position in a pyrimidine, is the shortest distance from the oxygen atom within the sugar ring. (cf. ANTICLINAL.)

synonymous codon See CODON.

syntenic genes Genes which are present on the same chromosome; the term may also have the connotation of evolutionary stability in the locations of such genes.

synthetase *Syn*. LIGASE.

systematic evolution of ligands by exponential enrichment (SELEX) See APTAMER.

SYTO® dyes An extensive family of fluorescent cyanine dyes (Molecular Probes, Eugene OR) which stain DNA and RNA; a given SYTO® dye may fluoresce e.g. blue, green orange or red.

The SYTO® dyes have a very low intrinsic fluorescence (quantum yield commonly <0.01) when not bound to nucleic acid; the quantum yield commonly increases to >0.4 when they are bound to nucleic acids.

SYTO® dyes can penetrate the cell membranes of most types of (living and dead) cell – including mammalian and both Gram-positive and Gram-negative bacterial membranes.

A given SYTO® dye may differ from others in the family e.g. in binding affinity, cell permeability and enhancement of fluorescence on binding to nucleic acids – as well as in excitation and emission spectra.

For other DNA-staining dyes see DNA STAINING (see also LIVE/DEAD BACLIGHT BACTERIAL VIABILITY KIT).

T

T L-Threonine (alternative to Thr).

T-cell-tropic strains (of HIV-1) See HIV-1.

T-DNA See CROWN GALL.

T-even phages A category of morphologically similar, virulent, enterobacterial BACTERIOPHAGES in which the genome is dsDNA; they include phages T2, T4 and T6. When present in the same host cell, the genomes of these phages can undergo recombination.

T-odd phages The phages T1, T3, T5 and T7. T3 and T7 are related dsDNA-containing enterobacterial phages.

T3 RNA polymerase A phage-derived RNA polymerase useful e.g. for *in vitro* transcription.

T7 RNA polymerase A phage-derived RNA polymerase useful e.g. for *in vitro* transcription.

TA *Taq*-amplified – referring to products formed e.g. in PCR in which the *Taq* DNA polymerase was used for amplification.
(See also EXTENDASE ACTIVITY.)

TA Cloning® kits Kits (Invitrogen, Carlsbad CA) designed for cloning PCR products which have been generated by the *Taq* DNA polymerase; *Taq*-generated products are characterized by 3′ single-base (adenosine) extensions (due to EXTENDASE ACTIVITY), and the (linearized) vectors in these kits have complementary 3′-T overhangs.

The insertion site is located within a sequence encoding the α-peptide of β-galactosidase, allowing blue–white screening. The vectors have antibiotic-resistance genes, promoter(s) and primer-binding sites appropriate for sequencing.

tag (1) A sequence of nucleotides which is used to identify a given fragment or molecule of nucleic acid and/or to assist in its isolation/purification.

(2) A 5′ extension on a PCR primer which may include e.g. a promoter sequence (permitting double-stranded amplicons to be subsequently transcribed).

(3) A specific peptide sequence in a recombinant protein that provides a site for interaction with a given entity, e.g. a site for covalent attachment of another molecule (see e.g. biotin ligase recognition peptide in IN VIVO BIOTINYLATION) or a site for non-covalent binding of a molecule/ligand involved in the isolation or purification of the given protein (see e.g. EPITOPE TAGGING, FLAG, PESC VECTORS and SIX-HISTIDINE TAG; see also AFFINITY PROTEIN EXPRESSION AND PURIFICATION).

In some cases it may be necessary to remove a tag from an expressed recombinant protein. This may be facilitated by including a short sequence of nucleotides – e.g. a sequence encoding the recognition site of the TEV protease (see TEV) – between the gene of interest and the sequence encoding the tag; following (*in vitro*) purification of the expressed protein, the tag is removed by the activity of the relevant protease.

Tag protein (in *Escherichia coli*) See DNA REPAIR.

***tagAB* operon** (also *tagDEF* operon) See TWO-COMPONENT REGULATORY SYSTEM.

TAGM (targeted gene methylation) A technique used (*in vitro*

and *in vivo*) for the methylation of *particular* bases in DNA.

In one example, a DNA METHYLTRANSFERASE, fused to a DNA-binding protein, was used to methylate the 5-position in cytosine residues at specific CG and GC sites in the yeast genome; in this case, the targeting of methylation involved binding of the fusion protein to sites in the DNA which are recognized by the ZINC FINGER motif of the DNA-binding protein [Nucleic Acids Res (2003) 31(22):6493–6501].

(See also PROGRAMMED ENDONUCLEASE.)

It was suggested that, in certain diseases, TAGM may have therapeutic potential in helping to re-establish the normal pattern of methylation.

(See also METHYLATION.)

tailing The addition of nucleotides to the 3′-end(s) of a DNA molecule using the (template-independent) enzyme *terminal deoxynucleotidyl transferase*. If nucleotides of only one type are added the result is a *homopolymer tail*.

Tailing is most efficient on 3′ overhangs of STICKY ENDS, but BLUNT-ENDED DNA can also be tailed.

(See also TERMINAL TRANSFERASE-DEPENDENT PCR.)

TAMRA Any of the isomers of carboxytetramethylrhodamine, a fluorophore used e.g. for labeling probes and in automated sequencing of DNA.

TAMRA has been used e.g. in real-time quantitative RT-PCR for studies on circadian clocks [BMC Mol Biol (2006) 7:5] and in real-time PCR for detecting and quantitating the bacterium *Coxiella burnetii* [BMC Microbiol (2006) 6:2].

TAMRA can be used as either donor or acceptor in a FRET-based system [e.g. BioTechniques (2006) 40(3):323–329].

TANDEM See QUINOXALINE ANTIBIOTICS.

tandem epitope tagging See EPITOPE TAGGING.

tandem repeat (1) A given sequence of nucleotides repeated one or more times, consecutively, in the same molecule.

(See also ITERON.)

(2) Repeated copies of gene clusters.

***Taq* DNA polymerase** A DNA-DEPENDENT DNA POLYMERASE from the thermophilic bacterium *Thermus aquaticus*; it lacks PROOF READING (i.e. 3′→5′ exonuclease) activity. *Taq* polymerase is stable at temperatures up to ~95°C.

(cf. STOFFEL FRAGMENT.)

Recombinant forms of *Taq* DNA polymerase are available commercially (see e.g. PLATINUM TAQ DNA POLYMERASE).

During PCR, *Taq* DNA polymerase can exhibit EXTENDASE ACTIVITY – which is useful, for example, in TOPOISOMERASE I CLONING.

(See also END-IT DNA END-REPAIR KIT, POLISHING and TA CLONING KITS.)

TaqMan® probe A type of commercial PROBE (Applied Biosystems) which can be used for monitoring REAL-TIME PCR and for estimating the number of specific target sequences initially present in the reaction mixture.

Each probe is a target-specific oligonucleotide that carries a covalently bound fluorophore (the reporter dye) and – closely adjacent on the oligonucleotide – a quencher of fluorescence. In this (intact) state the probe does not exhibit fluorescence (see also FRET).

TaqMan® probes are added to the reaction mixture in large numbers prior to cycling.

At the primer-binding (annealing) stage, these probes bind to their complementary sequence at a (non-terminal) site on the amplicons. Subsequently, during primer extension, the DNA polymerase exerts 5′-to-3′ exonuclease activity – which degrades the bound probe; as a consequence, the fluorophore (i.e. reporter dye) and quencher are separated, allowing the reporter to exhibit fluorescence. The intensity of fluorescence increases as the number of free (i.e. unquenched) reporter molecules increases during ongoing cycling.

In this technology, the DNA polymerase must be able to exert 5′-to-3′ exonuclease activity. A number of commercial enzymes have this ability; the Stoffel fragment does not.

target amplification An approach used for the detection and/or quantitation of a specific DNA or RNA target sequence in a sample; it involves repeated amplification (i.e. copying) of the target sequence, producing millions of copies, and the detection and/or quantition of these copies.

In practice, the production of large numbers of copies of the target sequence can be problematic: it may be difficult to prevent them from contaminating *subsequent* assays; such contamination destroys the value of an assay. This problem is avoided in SIGNAL AMPLIFICATION.

Methods involving target amplification include NASBA, PCR and SDA.

targeted gene methylation See TAGM.

targeted trapping A modification of GENE TRAPPING in which the gene-trap vector is flanked by sequences homologous to genomic sequences; this enables insertion of the vector to be directed to a precise location in the genome by homologous recombination.

[Targeted trapping and gene trapping: Proc Natl Acad Sci USA (2005) 102(37):13001–13002.]

Tat protein (of HIV-1) See RETROVIRUSES.

Tat protein export system In certain bacteria: a system used for exporting folded proteins across the cell membrane.

(See also SIGNAL SEQUENCE.)

TATA box See CORE PROMOTER.

Tay–Sachs disease An autosomal recessive neurodegenerative condition which is caused by mutation in the gene encoding the α-subunit of hexosaminidase A – see table in the entry GENETIC DISEASE for further details.

Tay–Sachs disease and related GM2 gangliosidoses (such as SANDHOFF DISEASE) are currently incurable. A study on mice with Sandhoff disease, in which adeno-associated virus vectors (see AAVS), encoding genes for the α and β subunits of hexosaminidase, were introduced by intracranial inoculation, found that the animals survived for an extended period of time (>1 year versus <20 weeks), suggesting the possibility of appropriate GENE THERAPY for treating human Tay–Sachs and related GM2 gangliosidoses [Proc Natl Acad Sci USA

(2006) 103(27):10373–10378].

TDM Tissue-specific, differentially methylated (referring to a particular region of DNA).

TE TRANSPOSABLE ELEMENT.

telomerase In eukaryotes: a composite enzyme, consisting of reverse transcriptase and an RNA moiety, whose function is to prevent reduction in the length of the telomere at each round of replication; telomerase extends the G-rich 3′ overhang of the telomere, using the RNA as template. A primer can then bind to the extended 3′ strand and begin synthesis of the complementary (C-rich) strand.

Elimination of telomerase in the protozoan *Trypanosoma brucei* was found to cause a progressive shortening of the telomere by 3–6 bp per generation [Nucleic Acids Res (2005) 33(14):4536–4543].

telomere (1) In a eukaryote: a terminal section of a chromosome – involved e.g. in maintaining chromosomal length (see TELOMERASE).

(See also QUADRUPLEX DNA.)

[Techniques in plant telomere biology (review): BioTechniques (2005) 38(2):233–243.]

(See also VSG.)

(2) In certain prokaryotes with a *linear* genome (e.g. *Borrelia burgdorferi*), and in some bacteriophages (e.g. N15, φKO2), *telomere* refers to the closed (hairpin) terminal regions of the genome.

In e.g. BORRELIA BURGDORFERI (q.v. for further details), replication of the genome involves production of a circular intermediate form consisting of a chromosome dimer. Within the dimer, the junction regions between the chromosomes undergo a process called *telomere resolution* which generates the hairpin terminal regions present in each of the daughter chromosomes; this process is mediated by an enzyme called PROTELOMERASE.

telomere resolution See TELOMERE (sense 2).

telomeric repeat amplification protocol See TRAP.

temperate phage See BACTERIOPHAGE.

template-independent polymerase activity See EXTENDASE ACTIVITY.

template strand (of a gene) See CODING STRAND.

template-switching (in cDNA synthesis) See CAPFINDER.

temporal temperature-gradient gel electrophoresis TTGE.

tenofovir See NUCLEOSIDE REVERSE TRANSCRIPTASE INHIBITORS.

terminal deoxynucleotidyl transferase See TAILING.

terminal redundancy In a linear molecule of nucleic acid: the presence of the same sequence of nucleotides at both ends.

terminal transferase-dependent PCR A method, involving PCR, which is used to examine a given sequence of dsDNA (e.g. a gene) for the presence of any obstruction or barrier which may stop the activity of DNA polymerase during DNA replication. [Original description of method: Nucleic Acids Res (1998) 26(7):1807–1811.]

Essentially, a gene-specific primer is initially extended, repeatedly, to form single-stranded products; these products are subjected to 3′ homopolymer TAILING with ribonucleotides, using the enzyme terminal deoxynucleotidyl transferase. The (tailed) ssDNA products are then ligated to a dsDNA linker which has a complementary 3′ overhang; the overhang serves to prime the complementary strand.

During the initial primer-extension phase, any barrier that arrests the DNA polymerase will give rise to prematurely terminated ssDNA products. These short products are amplified by PCR and are then displayed by gel electrophoresis; the results are compared with the corresponding normal (i.e. wild-type) sequence which gives rise to full-length products.

Obstructions which can arrest the DNA polymerase during replication include various types of PYRIMIDINE DIMER, including cyclobutyl dimers and (6–4) photoproducts.

Terminal transferase-dependent PCR has been used e.g. for detecting photodimers and strand breaks in the *p53* gene that result from exposure to ultraviolet radiation [Proc Natl Acad Sci USA (2005) 102(29):10058–10063].

termination codon   See NONSENSE CODON.

Terrific Broth   A (liquid) medium that contains peptone, yeast extract, dipotassium hydrogen phosphate and potassium dihydrogen phosphate. It is used e.g. to promote high yields of plasmid DNA in transformed cells of *Escherichia coli*.

Tetrahymena thermophila   A single-celled, free-living ciliate protozoan which has been suggested as a model organism for studies on the molecular and cellular biology of unicellular eukaryotes.

An important (ciliate) feature is the functional and physical separation of the germline and somatic aspects into a micronucleus and a macronucleus. The DNA in the macronucleus (~104 Mb) consists of ~225 chromosomes containing an estimated 27000 protein-encoding genes – of which 15000 are homologous to genes in other organisms; DNA in the macronucleus has been sequenced [see PLoS Biology (2006) 4(9): e286].

tetraplex DNA   *Syn.* QUADRUPLEX DNA.

TEV   Tobacco etch virus: a member of the potato virus Y group (the potyviruses).

The TEV protease is used in recombinant DNA technology; it cuts the sequence Glu-Asp-Leu-Tyr-Phe-Gln-Ser between the Gln and Ser residues.

The nucleotide sequence encoding the TEV protease recognition site is included in some types of engineered plasmid in order that this cleavage site be present in an expressed fusion product; this enables e.g. a particular tag to be removed from the protein of interest by cleaving the tag with TEV protease.

Sequences encoding TEV protease cleavage sites have been inserted, *in vivo*, into *various positions* within the *putA* gene of *Salmonella* in order to investigate predictions regarding domain organization in the PutA protein. Insertion of these sequences was carried out in a two-stage process involving initial insertion of a chloramphenicol-resistance gene followed by replacement of the gene with the TEV sequences. In the recombinant cells, TEV protease activity was induced (with IPTG) from a plasmid (pGEX-2T).

Three types of mutant were found to have resulted from cleavage of the PutA protein at the various TEV protease cleavage sites:

● Mutants in which no functional PutA product was formed. In these mutants, TEV protease cleavage sites were located in positions apparently important for enzymic function, and the insertion of cleavage sites in these positions may prevent normal folding of the protein.

● Mutants in which PutA was produced but was not cleaved by the TEV protease – apparently owing to a lack of accessibility of the protease cleavage sites (which were presumed not to be at the protein's surface).

● Mutants in which PutA was cleaved by the TEV protease. In the presence of proline, one of these mutants exhibited a deficiency in proline dehydrogenase activity, possibly as a result of decreased interaction between the PutA protein and the membrane (such interaction apparently promoting proline dehydrogenase activity); the location of the relevant inserted TEV protease cleavage site, residue 1224, was close to the region (residues 1204 to 1220) which may be important in membrane binding. In a different mutant (with insertion at residue 48), increased activity of proline dehydrogenase was exhibited in the absence of proline, suggesting that this lesion decreased the ability of PutA to bind to DNA (as PutA–DNA binding represses transcription of the *put* operon).

[TEV protease cleavage site insertions for probing protein structure *in vivo*: BioTechniques (2006) 41(6):721–724.]

TFIIB recognition element   See CORE PROMOTER.

TFO   Triplex-forming oligonucleotide: see TRIPLEX DNA.

TGS   Transcriptional gene silencing: see SIRNA.

thalassemia (Cooley's anemia)   Any of several types of inherited disorder, involving the α-chain or β-chain of hemoglobin, which usually result in anemia and may involve enlargement of the spleen.

(See also SICKLE-CELL ANEMIA.)

THAM   *Syn.* TRIS.

theophylline   1,3-Dimethylxanthine: a competitive inhibitor of cyclic adenosine monophosphate (cAMP) phosphodiesterase, an enzyme that cleaves cAMP to adenosine monophosphate.

Theophylline has also been used e.g. as an effector molecule in an engineered system for controlling gene expression in mammalian cells [RNA (2006) 12:710–716].

thermal cycler   *Syn.* THERMOCYCLER.

thermal melting profile (of dsDNA)   Absorption of ultraviolet radiation (260 nm) plotted against temperature for a given sample of dsDNA; absorption increases with the progressive MELTING of dsDNA molecules and the corresponding rise in the proportion of single-stranded DNA molecules present in the sample.

The temperature at which 50% of the dsDNA molecules are dissociated is designated T_m. The T_m depends e.g. on the proportion of GC pairs in a given sample: GC pairs are more stable than AT pairs and they tend to raise the T_m.

Some reagents – such as formamide – destabilize hydrogen bonding and reduce the T_m.

thermocycler (thermal cycler)   An instrument used for making the cyclical changes in temperature that are needed e.g. for certain nucleic-acid-amplification techniques (such as PCR).

In general, these instruments are designed so that any of a range of time/temperature protocols can be selected.

A number of reaction mixtures are processed simultaneously.

Heating and cooling of the reaction mixtures is achieved in either of two main ways. In one approach (the Peltier system) each reaction mixture is contained within a thin-walled tube that fits snugly inside a hole in a metal block. The block is heated and cooled according to the required protocol. In this system the permitted cycling protocol depends on the rate at which the block can undergo heating and cooling (changes in temperature of several degrees per second). Loss of sample through evaporation may be minimized e.g. with an oil overlay; another solution involves the use of a *heated-lid cycler* in which the temperature of the cover is maintained up to e.g. 120°C.

In an alternative arrangement for temperature cycling, the sample is sealed into a capillary glass tube that is heated and cooled by a forced-air current; in this procedure, the temperature of the air surrounding the capillary tube can be changed much more rapidly than is achieved with the Peltier system.

In a distinct approach to temperature cycling, heating of the reaction mixture (and monitoring of the temperature) exploits the electrolytic resistance of the mixture itself. In this method heating is accomplished by passing an alternating current of electricity through the reaction mixture, and cooling involves a forced-air flow around the capillary tube containing the mixture; the temperature of the mixture can be monitored by measuring its resistance (exploiting the correlation between resistance and temperature).

thermonuclease   See DNASE.

thermophilic SDA   See SDA.

thi-1   See ESCHERICHIA COLI (table).

thiofusion   See entry OVEREXPRESSION (*Secreted/intracellular proteins*.)

thioredoxin   A ubiquitous, heat-stable protein (~110 amino acid residues) with various roles, including e.g. hydrogen donor in the reduction of ribonucleotides (in the formation of deoxyribonucleotides).

Thioredoxin from *Escherichia coli* (encoded by the *trxA* gene) promotes processivity in the DNA polymerase from bacteriophage T7.

Thioredoxin is also required for assembly of filamentous phages such as PHAGE M13.

The thioredoxin gene is used e.g. as a fusion partner in the production of recombinant proteins in *Escherichia coli*: see entry OVEREXPRESSION (*Secreted/intracellular proteins*).

threshold cycle (C_t) (in real-time PCR)   See REAL-TIME PCR.

thrombin (*DNA technol.*)   A serine proteinase; in at least some cases it is reported to cleave proteins or peptides between arginine and glycine residues. The enzyme has been used e.g. for cleaving components of fusion proteins.

(cf. ENTEROKINASE; see also AFFINITY PROTEIN EXPRESSION AND PURIFICATION and SITE-SPECIFIC CLEAVAGE.)

thymidine   See NUCLEOSIDE.

thymidine kinase   The enzyme ATP:thymidine 5′-phosphotransferase (EC 2.7.1.21); thymidine kinase is found in both prokaryotic and eukaryotic cells and is also encoded by some DNA viruses. It catalyzes ATP-dependent phosphorylation of thymidine to thymidine 5′-monophosphate.

A virus-encoded thymidine kinase is responsible for *in vivo* activation of the antiviral agent ACYCLOVIR.

thymine dimer   A type of PYRIMIDINE DIMER which is formed by covalent cross-linking between adjacent thymine residues in the same DNA strand; thymine dimers can be produced by ULTRAVIOLET RADIATION.

A thymine dimer can occur in several isomeric forms, a major form being the *cyclobutyl dimer* (involving covalent linkage between the 5,6-positions of adjacent residues) which contains a 4-carbon cyclobutane ring $(CH_2)_4$.

A thymine dimer, which can block DNA replication, may be lethal in the absence of a suitable repair mechanism.

(See also PHOTOLYASE.)

Ti plasmid   See CROWN GALL.

TIGR   The Institute of Genomic Research.

TIGR microbial database (microbial genomes)   A source of information on whole-genome sequences of a wide range of species which is available at:

www.tigr.org/tdb/mdb/mdb.html

TILLING   An acronym for: 'targeting induced local lesions in genomes': a method devised for the detection of chemically induced point mutations. The method was subsequently used for detecting naturally occurring polymorphisms and was re-designated ECOTILLING (q.v. for principle).

time-resolved emission spectra (TRES)   An approach used to detect the fluorescence from one specific source in an experimental system containing more than one source of fluorescence.

The method depends on the difference in the rate of decay of fluorescence from the different sources following a brief (<1 nanosecond) pulse of excitation. That fluorescence which has a longer lifetime is measured only after the shorter-term fluorescence has decayed so that only the longer-term fluorescence is monitored.

[Example of use: Nucleic Acids Res (2006) 34(10):3161–3168.]

tirandamycin   An antibiotic apparently similar in activity, and structure, to STREPTOLYDIGIN.

TK   (1) THYMIDINE KINASE.

(2) TYROSINE KINASE.

T_m See THERMAL MELTING PROFILE.

T_m-**shift genotyping** (of SNPs)   See SNP GENOTYPING.

T_m-**shift primers**   Primers whose (extension) products can be identified (and differentiated from the extension products of other primers) by their melting characteristics – see e.g. SNP GENOTYPING.

TMA   Transcription-mediated amplification: a method used for the isothermal amplification of target sequences in RNA; the principle of TMA is similar to that of NASBA (q.v.). The commercial applications of TMA and NASBA differ e.g. in the way in which amplified products are detected/quantitated.

Both TMA and NASBA reflect an earlier system for the *in vitro* amplification of nucleic acids ('self-sustaining sequence replication'), described by Guatelli et al [Proc Natl Acad Sci USA (1990) 87:1874–1878], which was based on the retroviral mode of replication.

TMA is the basis of certain diagnostic tests that are used e.g. for detecting the pathogens *Mycobacterium tuberculosis* and *Chlamydia trachomatis* in clinical specimens. These tests involve amplification of conserved sequences in rRNA and use of a probe-based system (*hybridization protection assay*: see entry ACCUPROBE) for detecting the products.

TMA-based assays include AMTDT (for *M. tuberculosis*) and AMP CT (for *C. trachomatis*).

Compared with (for example) the basic PCR methodology, TMA-based assays have several advantages which include:

● theoretically, an improved capacity to detect small numbers of target organisms owing to the use of rRNA targets (which are abundant in cellular pathogens);

● isothermal amplification, avoiding the need for thermocycling equipment.

Tn Abbreviation for TRANSPOSON.

Tn1 A TN3-like TRANSPOSON that encodes a β-lactamase.

Tn2 A TN3-like TRANSPOSON that encodes a β-lactamase.

Tn3 A ~5-kb class II TRANSPOSON which includes a gene (*bla*) encoding a TEM-type β-lactamase (which inactivates certain β-LACTAM ANTIBIOTICS). The transposon has identical 38-bp terminal inverted repeats.

Insertion of Tn3 appears to occur preferentially in AT-rich regions and it gives rise to a 5-bp target-site duplication.

Transposition of Tn3, involving a replicative mechanism (see figure in TRANSPOSABLE ELEMENT), requires two transposon-encoded genes: *tnpA* and *tnpR*, which are associated, respectively, with transposase and resolvase activities. These two genes (in Tn3) are transcribed in opposite directions.

Resolution of the cointegrate involves site-specific recombination between two copies of a so-called *internal resolution site* (IRS) present in the duplicated sequences of Tn3 in the cointegrate.

The resolvase is apparently specific for two IRS sequences in the same replicon and in the same orientation; this makes the reaction irreversible.

A replicon which contains Tn3 exhibits TRANSPOSITION IMMUNITY.

A number of the transposable elements found in bacteria are related to Tn3. All of these elements have, for example, similar inverted repeats of 35–40 bp (and they also create a 5-bp target-site duplication on insertion). All transpose replicatively, with the formation of a cointegrate, and many exhibit transposition immunity. The Tn3-like elements include Tn1, Tn2, Tn4, Tn21, Tn501, Tn551, Tn1721 and Tn2603.

Collectively, Tn3 and the Tn3-like elements are sometimes referred to as TnA.

Tn4 A TN3-like TRANSPOSON encoding resistance to ampicillin and e.g. streptomycin.

Tn5 A 5818-bp class I TRANSPOSON that includes a gene which encodes aminoglycoside 5′-phosphotransferase (an enzyme that confers resistance to aminoglycoside antibiotics) as well as other antibiotic-resistance genes. These (contiguous) antibiotic-resistance genes are flanked by the insertion sequences IS50L and IS50R, which differ slightly in sequence. Each of these two insertion sequences is flanked by a pair of 19-bp sequences called the outer end (OE) and the inner end (IE); the two OE sequences form the two ends of the transposon.

IS50R encodes the transposase, Tnp, and also an inhibitor of transposase, Inh. The frequency of transposition of Tn5 (which occurs by a cut-and-paste mechanism) is regulated by the relative levels of Tnp and Inh. Another regulatory factor is the cell's Dam methylation system which tends to inhibit transcription from the promoter of the Tnp gene; accordingly, like Tn10, transposition of Tn5 is linked to DNA replication – see the entry TRANSPOSABLE ELEMENT for a rationale.

IS50L encodes two analogous, but non-functional, proteins.

The transposase Tnp can mediate transposition of *Tn5* as a whole, or it can mediate transposition of IS50; transposition of Tn5 involves both OE sequences, while transposition of IS50 involves one OE sequence and one IE sequence.

In DNA technology a system for *in vivo* and *in vitro* transposition is based on Tn5: see TN5-TYPE TRANSPOSITION.

Tn5-type transposition TRANSPOSITION that can be carried out wholly *in vitro* with a DNA fragment flanked, on both sides, by the 19-bp outer end (OE) sequences of transposon Tn5 and the enzyme transposase [J Biol Chem (1998) 273:7367–7374] – or *in vivo*, using the Transposome™ approach (see below). Insertion into target DNA occurs at random sites.

The system has a number of uses. For example, as insertion occurs at random sites in a population of plasmids, transposition can generate a range of templates (the insert providing known primer-binding sites) that can be used for sequencing the target molecule.

The system can also be used e.g. to introduce marker genes into vector molecules.

Commercially available transposon–transposase complexes (Transposome™; Epicentre Technologies, Madison WI) can be inserted into cells e.g. by ELECTROPORATION – following which the transposons insert randomly. This system has been used for making mutations in *Rickettsia prowazekii* [Appl Environ Microbiol (2004) 70:2816–2822] and *Francisella tularensis* [Appl Environ Microbiol (2004) 70:6901–6904], identifying a gene encoding resistance to capreomycin in the bacterial pathogen *Mycobacterium tuberculosis* [Antimicrob Agents Chemother (2005) 49:571–577], and for studying the production of outer membrane vesicles by *Escherichia coli* [J Bacteriol (2006) 188(15):5385–5392].

(See also GENETIC FOOTPRINTING.)

Note. The term 'transposome' has also been used e.g. to refer (apparently) to the sum total of transposable elements/targets in *Drosophila* populations [PLoS Genet (2006) 2(10):e165].

Tn7 A TRANSPOSON which is able to insert into the chromosome of *Escherichia coli* with a high degree of specificity at a target site designated *att*Tn7; insertion depends on several transposon-encoded proteins which jointly contribute transposase activity.

(See also BACMID.)

In another, distinct mode of transposition, Tn7 inserts into certain plasmids and into the *E. coli* chromosome at locations near double-stranded breaks and at the site of termination of DNA replication.

(See also INTEGRON.)

Tn10 A 9.3-kb class I TRANSPOSON found e.g. in plasmid R100 and encoding resistance to tetracycline. The two ends of the transposon consist of 1.4-kb IS*10* elements designated IS*10*R and IS*10*L; these two elements are similar, but not identical. A transposase, essential for transposition of Tn*10*, is encoded by IS*10*R.

The insertion of Tn*10* can occur at various sites, although there are apparently certain preferred sites. Insertion results in a 9-bp target-site duplication.

As in Tn5, transposition of Tn*10* is influenced by the cell's Dam methylation – see entry TRANSPOSABLE ELEMENT for a rationale. It is also influenced by copy number: see MULTI-COPY INHIBITION.

Tn21 A ~19-kb TN3-like TRANSPOSON, found e.g. in *Shigella flexneri* plasmid R100, which encodes resistance to mercury ions, streptomycin and sulfonamides.

Transposition of Tn21 is regulated by a putative *modulator protein* encoded by the *tnpM* gene; in this transposon, *tnpA*, *tnpR* and the *tnpM* sequence are all transcribed in the same direction. The modulator protein is believed to influence the activities of both the transposase and resolvase – enhancing the former and inhibiting the latter.

(See also TN2610.)

Tn501 An ~8-kb TN3-like TRANSPOSON, found e.g. in *Pseudomonas* plasmid pUS1, which encodes resistance to mercury ions; the presence of low levels of mercury is reported to enhance the frequency of transposition.

Tn551 A ~5-kb TN3-like TRANSPOSON that encodes resistance to erythromycin; it is found e.g. in a *Staphylococcus aureus* plasmid.

Tn916 See CONJUGATIVE TRANSPOSITION.

Tn1681 A TRANSPOSON containing the gene for a heat-stable enterotoxin (STa) that is produced by enterotoxigenic strains of *Escherichia coli* (ETEC).

Tn1721 An ~11-kb TN3-like TRANSPOSON encoding resistance to tetracycline.

(See also TN2610.)

Tn2410 An 18.5-kb TRANSPOSON, present e.g. in a *Salmonella typhimurium* plasmid, encoding a β-lactamase and resistance to streptomycin and mercury.

Tn2603 A ~22-kb TN3-like TRANSPOSON which encodes a β-lactamase and resistance to mercury, streptomycin and sulf-onamides.

Tn2610 A 28.8-kb TRANSPOSON, originally isolated from an *Escherichia coli* conjugative plasmid, which appears to have developed from transposons Tn*1721* and Tn*21* following extensive recombination [Antimicrob Agents Chemother (2006) 50(4):1143–1147].

Tn4655 A class II TRANSPOSON, found e.g. in *Pseudomonas* plasmid NAH7, which includes genes encoding catabolism of naphthalene. The tyrosine recombinase, TnpI, apparently catalyzes both intra- and intermolecular recombination of *att*I sites, suggesting that this recombination system may promote mobility of these catalytic genes [J Bacteriol (2006) 188(11): 4057–4067].

(See also TOL PLASMID.)

TnA A designation sometimes used to refer – collectively – to transposon Tn*3* and the Tn*3*-like elements.

TNP Transdominant negative protein: see GENE THERAPY.

***tnpA* gene** See TN3.

Tn*phoA* See TRANSPOSON MUTAGENESIS.

TnpI See TN4655.

***tnpM* gene** See TN21.

***tnpR* gene** See TN3.

Tn*YLB-1* transposon See MARINER FAMILY.

tobacco etch virus See TEV.

tobramycin See AMINOGLYCOSIDE ANTIBIOTICS.

toeprinting A procedure used for investigating the series of events that occur during *translation* (i.e. ribosomal synthesis of a polypeptide from an mRNA template). The elongation stage is halted, as required, by adding CYCLOHEXIMIDE; this stops the movement of ribosomes, leaving them at various sites along the length of the (polysomal) transcript. Reverse transcriptase is then used to copy mRNA into cDNA, using a (labeled) mRNA-specific primer; the synthesis of cDNA is blocked by the first ribosome encountered by the transcriptase ('primer-extension inhibition'), resulting in a prematurely terminated ('toeprint') fragment. The resulting products can be examined e.g. by gel electrophoresis.

In toeprinting experiments the primer is often labeled with [32]P. However, a rapid and convenient procedure has been reported with fluorescent primers [BioTechniques (2005) 38 (3):397–400].

Toeprinting has been used e.g. for studying pseudoknots in mRNA [Nucleic Acids Res (2005) 33(6):1825–1833].

TOL plasmid A large (~117 kb) plasmid, found in some strains of the Gram-negative bacterium *Pseudomonas*, that confers the ability to metabolize certain hydrocarbons.

The plasmid encodes enzymes for a two-stage catabolic pathway for the mineralization of toluene and xylene. Both of these hydrocarbons are initially oxidized to their respective carboxylic acids; this involves enzymes encoded by the so-called *upper* operon of the TOL plasmid. The *meta* operon encodes enzymes which effect aromatic ring fission and the subsequent formation of pyruvate and acetaldehyde (both of which enter the TCA cycle).

[Regulation of operons in the TOL plasmid: EMBO Journal

(2001) 20:1–11 (4–6).]

(See also TN4655.)

A TOL plasmid has been reported to encode a homolog of the error-prone DNA polymerase pol V which facilitates the survival of host bacteria when DNA damage has accumulated [J Bacteriol (2005) 187(15):5203–5213].

***tonA* gene**   In *Escherichia coli*: a gene which encodes the TonA protein (= FhuA protein), a protein component in the outer membrane (the outermost layer of the cell envelope) which acts as a receptor for certain phages, e.g. phage T1.

***tonB* gene**   In *Escherichia coli*: a gene which encodes the TonB protein, a periplasmic protein that shuttles between the outer membrane and the cytoplasmic membrane [Mol Microbiol (2003) 49:869–882]; it has various roles in transport – such as the uptake of ferric iron complexes and vitamin B_{12}. TonB is also involved e.g. in the uptake of various colicins.

topo   TOPOISOMERASE.

topo cloning   *Syn.* TOPOISOMERASE I CLONING.

TOPO® pENTR™ vector   See DIRECTIONAL TOPO PENTR VECTOR.

TOPO TA Cloning® kits   Kits from Invitrogen (Carlsbad CA) used for TOPOISOMERASE I CLONING. All (linearized) vectors in these kits include 3′ single-nucleotide thymidine overhangs which facilitate direct ligation to PCR products which have been generated with the *Taq* DNA polymerase; these *Taq*-generated products are characterized by single-nucleotide (adenosine) 3′ overhangs that arise by EXTENDASE ACTIVITY.

In one of the kits, the vector includes *att* sites to facilitate transfer of the insert to other vectors in the GATEWAY SITE-SPECIFIC RECOMBINATION SYSTEM; it also includes primer sites for sequencing. Other vectors in the series include e.g. a *lacZα* sequence permitting *blue–white screening* (see PBLUE-SCRIPT) and antibiotic-resistance genes.

topoisomer   See TOPOISOMERASE.

topoisomerase   Any enzyme which can interconvert topological isomers (*topoisomers*) of cccDNA. (The topoisomers of a given molecule differ from one another in their topological properties – e.g. a given circular dsDNA molecule may exist in a supercoiled state or in a relaxed state, both of which are topoisomers.) Interconversion involves transient breakage of one or both strands of a DNA duplex, and the reaction may be intramolecular or intermolecular.

Type I topoisomerases (nick-closing enzymes, relaxing enzymes, swivelases, untwisting enzymes). These enzymes can relax negative supercoiling; in a ccc DNA duplex, one strand is cut, the unbroken strand is passed through the gap, and the break is repaired. The type I topoisomerases (type I topos) include the *Escherichia coli* ω (omega) protein (= topo I) and *E. coli* topo III.

Type II topoisomerases relax both negative and positive supercoiling, although the latter is relaxed more efficiently [chirality sensing by topoisomerase enzymes: Proc Natl Acad Sci USA (2003) 100:8654–8659]. In a ccc DNA duplex, the type II enzyme makes a double-stranded break and passes a double-stranded segment of DNA through the gap before re-sealing the break. The type II topos include *E. coli* topo IV and *gyrase*.

Topo IV deals with unwanted entanglements during DNA replication and appears to be the sole enzyme responsible for the decatenation of replicated chromosomes.

Gyrase is a bacterial tetrameric enzyme that appears to be essential for DNA replication. It can e.g. *introduce* negative supercoiling and, in the absence of ATP, the gyrase from *E. coli* can relax negative supercoiling. The enzyme is the target of certain antibiotics such as quinolones and novobiocin.

(cf. REVERSE GYRASE.)

Topo IV and gyrase may both oppose the positive super-coiling introduced by helicase during DNA replication – gyrase by generating negative supercoiling and topo IV by relaxing positive supercoiling.

topoisomerase I cloning   A technique in which, typically, PCR fragments generated by *Taq* DNA polymerase are ligated into certain types of vector molecule by means of the enzyme topoisomerase I *in preparation for* CLONING; 'topoisomerase cloning' is therefore somewhat misleading as, in this method, only *ligation* of the fragment into the vector is mediated by topoisomerase I – in place of (the more usual) DNA ligase.

In many of the systems that employ this method, the PCR fragment is inserted into a (linearized) vector in which both terminals have a 3′ single-nucleotide (deoxythymidine monophosphate) overhang. At each end of the vector the phosphate is covalently linked to topoisomerase I; this conserves energy that is subsequently used for bond formation with the insert.

PCR-generated fragments prepared with *Taq* DNA polymerase commonly contain 3′ single-nucleotide (adenosine) overhangs due to the enzyme's EXTENDASE ACTIVITY; these fragments can thus be readily ligated into vectors which have the 3′ deoxythymidine overhangs – formation of a phosphodiester bond (at each end of the fragment) being mediated by topoisomerase I. Topoisomerase I dissociates following bond formation.

Commercial vectors using topo cloning include e.g. vectors in the TOPO TA CLONING KITS and the DIRECTIONAL TOPO PENTR VECTORS. The latter (directional) vectors differ from the typical topo vector in that they do not contain the single-nucleotide overhangs – having instead one blunt end and one four-nucleotide overhang.

Topo cloning has been used e.g. for studies on β_1 integrin homologs in zebrafish (*Danio rerio*) [BMC Cell Biol (2006) 7:24] and studies on manganese-oxidizing spores of *Bacillus* in hydrothermal sediments [Appl Environ Microbiol (2006) 72(5):3184–3190].

topological winding number   *Syn.* LINKING NUMBER.

toroidal DNA   See DNA TOROID.

touchdown PCR   A type of protocol in which a given PCR assay is repeated a number of times with a stepwise decrease in the annealing temperature. The purpose is to determine the lowest temperature at which priming occurs correctly – i.e. avoiding *mispriming*: the binding of primers to sites that are not exactly complementary to the primer. The procedure thus seeks to promote maximum specificity in primer binding and to avoid the production of non-specific products.

TP228 plasmid   See R1 PLASMID.

TPA   12-*O*-tetradecanoylphorbol-13-acetate.

(See also ZEBRA.)

***traD* gene**   A gene in the F PLASMID (within the transfer operon) which is needed for conjugative transfer.

trailer   *Syn.* 3′-UTR.

***trans*-acting element**   A discrete sequence of nucleotides which encodes a product that can act on *another* molecule; thus e.g. an extrachromosomal plasmid may encode a protein that acts on a chromosomal receptor.

***trans* splicing**   The process, found e.g. in trypanosomes and (in some cases) in the nematode worm *Caenorhabditis elegans*, in which a polycistronic transcript is spliced into a number of monocistronic units, each of which bears a short leader sequence (a so-called spliced leader, SL) which was added to the 5′ terminus. In *C. elegans* the spliced leader is derived from a separate RNA molecule (i.e. it is not copied from the gene sequence).

transcapsidation   See PHENOTYPIC MIXING.

transconjugant   See CONJUGATION.

transcriptase   (1) See REPLICASE.

(2) A (DNA-dependent) RNA POLYMERASE.

transcription-mediated amplification   See TMA.

transcription repair coupling factor (TRCF)   See MFD GENE.

transcription vector   *Syn.* EXPRESSION VECTOR.

transcriptional enhancer   See ENHANCER (transcriptional).

transcriptional fusion   See GENE FUSION.

transcriptional gene silencing (TGS)   See SIRNA.

transcriptome   The totality of transcripts in (or isolated from) a cell or tissue under given conditions.

transdominant negative protein (TNP)   See GENE THERAPY.

transductant   See TRANSDUCTION.

transduction   Bacteriophage-mediated transfer of DNA, usually chromosomal or plasmid DNA, from a bacterium to another bacterium.

Generalized transduction involves the infrequent encapsidation of bacterial DNA (instead of phage DNA) during phage assembly in a lytic infection; this could occur, for example, if chromosomal DNA has been fragmented as a consequence of phage infection. Phage capsids containing bacterial DNA can infect other cells and donate the DNA to the recipient cell (the *transductant*). In the transductant, the fate of the fragment of (bacterial) DNA may be (i) degradation by restriction enzymes; (ii) recombination with the transductant's chromosome (or plasmid), in which case the fragment's gene(s) may be stably inherited and expressed (*complete transduction*); (iii) persistence (see ABORTIVE TRANSDUCTION).

Any given bacterial gene may have a similar probability of being transduced. However, in some cases, certain bacterial genes are more likely than others to be transduced. Thus, for example, in the *Salmonella*/phage P22 system, a sequence in the bacterial chromosome resembles that part of the phage genome which is concerned with packaging of DNA into the phage head; this region of the bacterial chromosome has a greater chance of being transduced.

Specialized transduction involves the rare aberrant excision of a prophage from the bacterial chromosome following a lysogenic infection. In such an excision, the prophage takes with it some adjacent chromosomal DNA, and may leave behind (in the chromosome) some DNA from the other end of the prophage. This (recombinant) phage genome can be packaged and assembled normally; the result is a *specialized transducing particle* (STP). Even if an STP is deficient for replication (having left behind essential genes), it can nevertheless inject its DNA into a recipient cell, thus transferring specific donor DNA to a transductant.

In any given system of specialized transduction, the gene(s) transduced are those bacterial genes that flank the prophage when it is integrated in the chromosome; for example, in the *Escherichia coli*/phage λ system, the genes *gal* (encoding galactose utilization) and *bio* (encoding biotin synthesis) may be transduced as these genes flank the integrated λ prophage.

In a unique form of specialized transduction, the genomes of two phages, VGJφ and CTXΦ, join covalently within cells of the Gram-negative pathogen *Vibrio cholerae*. The resulting single-stranded hybrid genome is packaged in a VGJφ capsid to form a particle which can infect fresh cells of *V. cholerae* via receptor sites for phage VGJφ. In this way, the genes for cholera toxin (encoded by phage CTXΦ) can be transduced to *Vibrio cholerae* independently of the (normal) receptor sites for CTXΦ [J Bacteriol (2003) 185:7231–7240].

transductional shortening   A phenomenon which is sometimes observed when a *large* plasmid is transferred by transduction from one bacterium to another: the transduced plasmid is found to be smaller than the original plasmid, an effect that may be due to the encapsidation of a deletion mutant of the plasmid (which may arise spontaneously at low frequencies).

transfection   (1) Any of various procedures in which nucleic acid is introduced into cell(s) or organism(s) – e.g. within a viral vector or by methods such as LIPOFECTION and TRANSFORMATION (see also ELECTROPORATION, MAGNETOFECTION, MELITTIN, MICROINJECTION and VECTOR).

(2) As in sense (1), above, but excluding viral and bacterial vectors; hence, in this sense, the term transfection excludes AGROINFECTION (in which DNA is transferred to plant cells by a bacterium) – in addition to genetic transfer mediated by any kind of virus.

(3) The *in vitro* introduction of proteins or peptides into cells. VOYAGER VECTORS are designed to ensure that ~100% of the (mammalian) cells in a cell culture receive a recombinant *protein* encoded by the vector – including those cells which did not receive a copy of the vector; this is achieved by using a fusion partner which promotes translocation of the (fusion) protein from the cell in which it was expressed (synthesized) to an adjacent cell.

(4) Experimental infection of a vector organism with parasitic bacteria [use of term: Appl Environ Microbiol (2005)

71:3199–3204].

transformation A process in which exogenous DNA is internalized by a cell, PERMEAPLAST, SPHEROPLAST or protoplast, the process occurring under natural conditions in some cases but only under *in vitro* conditions in others.

The *transforming* or *donor* DNA may be e.g. a fragment of chromosomal DNA or a plasmid.

Transformation is one approach to TRANSFECTION and is used for various types of cell, including e.g. bacteria, yeasts (such as *Saccharomyces cerevisiae*) and mammalian cells.

Transformation in bacteria

Uptake of DNA under natural conditions can occur e.g. in the Gram-negative bacteria *Haemophilus* and *Neisseria* and the Gram-positive bacteria *Bacillus* and *Streptococcus*. Cells that are able to take up DNA are said to exhibit *competence*.

In strains of *Neisseria gonorrhoeae* competence appears to be exhibited constitutively. However, some bacteria exhibit competence transiently, and the expression of competence is influenced by factors such as the nutritional status of the cells (and/or the phase of growth in batch cultures); for example, competence in *Haemophilus influenzae* can be induced by conditions which limit growth and is promoted by high levels of intracellular cyclic AMP (cAMP).

In both *Bacillus subtilis* and *Streptococcus pneumoniae* the population density (i.e. number of cells per unit volume) is a factor in competence (a manifestation of QUORUM SENSING). Thus, when *B. subtilis* grows to a high population density, a secreted pheromone, ComX, accumulates extracellularly and, at an appropriate concentration, activates a TWO-COMPONENT REGULATORY SYSTEM in the cells; this results in activation of *comS* and other genes whose expression is needed for the development of competence. Earlier work with *Streptococcus pneumoniae* suggested that competence is associated with the transmembrane transport of calcium.

Fragments of chromosomal DNA must be double-stranded and must be above a certain minimum size to be effective in transformation. The fragments initially bind reversibly to the cell surface, but subsequently a proportion of the fragments become irreveribly bound prior to uptake. In *B. subtilis* and *S. pneumoniae* binding is non-specific (i.e. these cells can bind DNA from other species as readily as DNA from the same species). By contrast, species of *Haemophilus* and *Neisseria* bind fragments of DNA in a sequence-dependent manner; for example, *H. influenzae* was reported to internalize only those fragments containing 5′-AAGTGCGGTCA-3′ – a so-called *DNA uptake site*; this sequence occurs often in the genome of *H. influenzae*.

B. subtilis and *S. pneumoniae* take up only one strand of a dsDNA fragment; *H. influenzae* takes up both strands.

Laboratory-induced transformation

Escherichia coli apparently does not undergo transformation in nature. However, *E. coli* (and many other Gram-negative bacteria) can be made artificially competent e.g. by treatment involving chilling and heat-shock in the presence of calcium ions. Earlier studies indicated that competence acquired by *E.*

coli in an ice-cold, calcium-containing solution is associated with the presence of a high concentration of polyhydroxybutyrate/calcium polyphosphate complexes within the cytoplasmic membrane; one suggestion was that these complexes may form channels in the membrane, thus facilitating uptake of DNA.

Gram-positive bacteria may be subjected to transformation by first converting the cells to protoplasts. Protoplasts can be induced to internalize DNA e.g. by treatment with POLYETHYLENE GLYCOL (PEG); the transformed protoplasts are then used to regenerate viable cells.

Certain cyanobacteria are able to take up DNA following their conversion to permeaplasts.

Certain unicellular green algae (including *Chlamydomonas reinhardtii*) have a thin, cellulose-free, protein-rich cell wall, and these organisms can be subjected to transformation.

Certain fungi are susceptible to *in vitro* transformation. For yeasts (e.g. *S. cerevisiae*), the cells are usually converted to spheroplasts (because cell walls are inhibitory to uptake). In one approach, spheroplasts are first mixed with DNA in the presence of calcium ions, and PEG is subsequently added. In another approach whole cells are treated with lithium ions and PEG; although simpler, this method is less efficient.

Mammalian cells can internalize DNA when it is overlaid on cell monolayers in a buffered solution containing calcium chloride; the solution develops a co-precipitate – containing DNA – which facilitates uptake by the cells. The cells are incubated overnight at 37°C, washed, and incubated in fresh medium. The efficiency of the process may be raised by including a 'carrier DNA' (e.g. calf thymus DNA) with the experimental DNA; the optimal concentration of carrier DNA must be pre-established.

transgene Any gene which has been inserted by recombinant DNA technology into a different type of cell or organism and which is able to be expressed.

transition mutation Any point mutation in which a purine is replaced by a different purine, or a pyrimidine is replaced by a different pyrimidine.

(cf. TRANSVERSION MUTATION.)

translational control (in operons) See OPERON.

translational enhancer See ENHANCER (translational).

translational frameshifting See FRAMESHIFTING.

translational fusion See GENE FUSION.

translesion synthesis Error-prone synthesis (repair) of DNA on a template containing a lesion (e.g. a pyrimidine dimer). This occurs e.g. in *Escherichia coli* during the SOS response to damaged DNA or blocked DNA replication; it may involve specialized DNA polymerases (e.g. DNA polymerase V) and characteristically leads to mutagenesis.

(See also SOS SYSTEM.)

transport medium Any MEDIUM used for the transportation (or temporary storage) of material which is to be examined, later, for the presence of particular type(s) of microorganism.

The main role of a transport medium is to maintain the viability of any organisms in the sample. One common example of this kind of medium is Stuart's transport medium (which is suitable for delicate bacteria such as *Neisseria gonorrhoeae*); Stuart's transport medium contains salts, <1% agar, sodium thioglycollate and the redox indicator methylene blue.

transposable element (TE; jumping gene)   A discrete segment of DNA – usually present within a larger molecule of DNA but sometimes in isolation (i.e. excised, or in an *in vitro* preparation) – which has the ability (actually or effectively) to move from one site to another site in (i) the same replicon, (ii) another DNA molecule in the same cell, or (iii) a DNA molecule in another cell; such movement – which is termed *transposition* – does not depend on extensive sequence homology between the TE and its new location.

A TE that can transpose to a site in *another* cell is referred to as a *conjugative transposon* because it mediates a unique (plasmid-independent) form of conjugation (between a *donor* cell and a *recipient* cell) that is an essential feature of transposition in this type of TE; the conjugative transposons are considered in the entry CONJUGATIVE TRANSPOSITION.

This entry refers to TEs other than conjugative transposons.

TEs occur in both prokaryotic and eukaryotic cells and are found as normal constituents e.g. in chromosomes, plasmids and phage genomes.

All TEs encode at least one protein: transposase, an enzyme required for transposition; some TEs also encode a resolvase (see figure). As shown in the figure, there are two *main* types of transposition: (i) a conservative, cut-and-paste mechanism, and (ii) a replicative mechanism. However, these two modes of transposition are not exclusive; thus, for example, certain types of insertion sequence (see below, and e.g. entry IS*1111*) excise in a circular, intermediate form prior to insertion at the target site.

The process by which a TE inserts into a new site usually results in the development of a pair of direct repeats which flank the inserted TE; this is due to duplication of the target site – as can be seen in the figure. The figure shows a scheme for two mechanistically distinct modes of transposition: the 'cut-and-paste' and the replicative models.

Note that, in the model of replicative transposition shown in the figure, each of the two *final* molecules includes parts of the original transposon (dashed line) as well as the newly synthesized DNA (zigzag line); accordingly, it is not strictly correct to say that a *copy* of the transposon is inserted at the new site.

In certain TEs in eukaryotes transposition involves an RNA intermediate: see RETROTRANSPOSON.

If a TE encodes *only* those functions which are necessary for transposition it is referred to as an INSERTION SEQUENCE (q.v.).

If a TE encodes functions (e.g. antibiotic resistance) which are *in addition to* those necessary for transposition it is referred to as a TRANSPOSON (q.v.).

TEs differ e.g. with respect to the specificity of their *target* site, that is, the site to which a TE can re-locate. Many TEs appear to insert at new sites in a random fashion. It seems likely, however, that even when insertion appears random, a selective process of some kind is involved. By contrast, the transposon Tn*7* has a specific insertion site that is designated *att*Tn*7*, while the insertion sequence IS*5* appears to insert only at locations which contain the sequence C(T/A)A(G/A).

Transposons of the MARINER FAMILY are characterized by minimal site-specificity of their target sequences.

In some of the TEs which form a circular intermediate (see below), the target sequence is homologous to the *interstitial junction sequence*, and this has suggested that transposition of these elements may involve site-specific recombination; indeed, in the insertion sequence IS*HP608* (q.v.) transposition is reported to be site-specific (at the sequence 5′-TTAC-3′) [EMBO J (2005) 24(18):3325–3338].

At least some of the TEs that form a circular intermediate are characterized by *sub*terminal inverted repeats – unlike other TEs, which have *terminal* inverted repeats. In some cases, the production of the circular intermediate involves an inital cleavage of a strand at the 3′ end of the TE (by the TE's transposase); the 3′ end is subsequently transferred to a site a few nucleotides upstream of the 5′ end of the TE, on the same strand. This structure leads to the formation of the circular intermediate – in which the two inverted repeat sequences are separated by a short *interstitial junction sequence*. In some of these TEs this interstitial junction sequence provides a –10 box which is located correctly in respect of a –35 box present at one end of the TE. In IS*911*, development of the circular intermediate brings together a –10 box in one inverted repeat and a –35 box in the other, the distance between the two boxes being appropriate for the region to act as an efficient promoter.

Transposition occurs only rarely *in vivo*. The frequency of transposition depends e.g. on the TE and on the physiological state of the cell. It can also be affected e.g. by the methylation status of the cell's DNA. For example, transposition of the transposon Tn*10* from a chromosomal site in *Escherichia coli* tends to be linked to the cell cycle; the reason is that the (normal) Dam methylation of the *E. coli* chromosomal DNA inhibits transcription of the transposase gene of Tn*10*, and inhibition is transiently lost when the chromosome replicates (i.e. immediately after the replication fork has passed the transposase gene but before Dam methylation of the gene has occurred). In transposon Tn*10* the frequency of transposition is also affected by copy number: see MULTICOPY INHIBITION.

The effects of transposition within a cell will depend on the site of insertion. Effects may include e.g. inactivation of a structural gene, inactivation of gene(s) within an operon, or activation of an operon (e.g. when an insertion inactivates a sequence that negatively controls the operon). The presence of insertion sequence IS*3* in the F plasmid (within the *finO* gene) results in derepression of that plasmid for conjugative transfer (see FINOP SYSTEM).

Transposon-mediated mutagenesis is a useful tool in DNA technology: see TRANSPOSON MUTAGENESIS.

The presence of a TE is commonly indicated in text by a

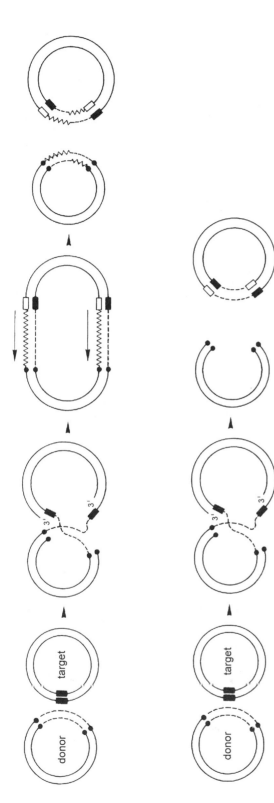

TRANSPOSABLE ELEMENT A simplified, diagrammatic scheme for the replicative transposition (top) and simple ('cut-and-paste') transposition (bottom) of a transposable element (TE).

Replicative transposition Two circular, double-stranded DNA molecules are shown at the left-hand side. The donor molecule includes a TE (dashed lines), either side of which is an old target site (●); this target site was duplicated when the TE was originally inserted into that molecule (see later). The target molecule has a single target site (■) where the TE element will be inserted.

An enzyme (*transposase* – not shown) mediates at least the initial stages of transposition. In the target molecule a staggered break has been made at the target site, leaving the 3′ ends recessed. In the donor molecule a nick has been made in each strand of the TE, at opposite ends, and the free ends have been ligated (joined) to the 5′ ends of the target molecule, as shown.

In the next stage, DNA synthesis (zigzag line) has occurred from each 3′ end in the target molecule (arrows). Such synthesis first copies the target site (□) and then continues beyond the target site – using each strand of the TE as template; that is, the TE has been replicated. The end of each newly synthesized strand has been ligated to a free strand-end in the donor molecule. The resulting structure is called a *cointegrate*.

The final stage of replicative transposition involves a *resolvase* – an enzyme, encoded by the TE, which resolves the cointegrate by mediating site-specific recombination at a site in each TE – forming the two molecules as shown.

The donor and target molecules now both contain the sequence of the TE. Note that each of these two sequences contains parts of the original TE (dashed lines) as well as newly synthesized DNA (zigzag lines). Note also that the target site in the target molecule has been duplicated – each of these target sites consisting of one newly synthesized strand (□) and one original strand (■).

Simple ('cut-and-paste') transposition. The initial stages are similar to those shown for replicative transposition. However, in this case, DNA synthesis (from the 3′ ends of the target molecule) is required simply to duplicate the target site. The remaining strand-ends of the TE have been cut and ligated to the freshly duplicated target sites, as shown. The phrase *donor suicide* is used if the remainder of the donor molecule is non-viable.

Figure reproduced from *Bacteria in Biology, Biotechnology and Medicine*, 6th edition, Figure 8.4, pages 202–203, Paul Singleton (2004) John Wiley & Sons Ltd, UK [ISBN 0-470-09027-8] with permission from the publisher.

double colon. For example, the presence of transposon Tn*3* in the genome of phage lambda (phage λ) is written λ::Tn*3*.

In addition to the main entries INSERTION SEQUENCE and TRANSPOSON, see entries for some individual TEs under 'IS' and 'Tn'.

transposase A type of enzyme required for the transposition of an INSERTION SEQUENCE or a TRANSPOSON (see TRANSPOSABLE ELEMENT).

In the *replicative* form of transposition a *resolvase* enzyme is needed in order to complete the transposition process by resolving the cointegrate.

transposition See TRANSPOSABLE ELEMENT.

Transposome™ See TN5-TYPE TRANSPOSITION.

transposon (Tn) A type of TRANSPOSABLE ELEMENT (q.v.) that encodes functions in addition to those required for transposition – functions such as antibiotic resistance (e.g. in Tn*3*, Tn*5*, Tn*10* and Tn*2410*), resistance to heavy metals (e.g. in Tn*501*) or the production of virulence factors such as toxins (e.g. in Tn*1681*) etc.

(cf. INSERTION SEQUENCE.)

As indicated above, a specific transposon is designated by the prefix 'Tn' followed by an (italic) number.

The *conjugative transposons* mediate plasmid-independent conjugation in bacteria; they differ in a number of ways from other transposons and are considered separately in the entry CONJUGATIVE TRANSPOSITION.

A *class I* (= type I, or *composite*) transposon consists of the sequence of structural genes flanked, on both sides, by an INSERTION SEQUENCE; the two insertion sequences may or may not be identical. The insertion sequences mediate transposition of the transposon as a whole. One insertion sequence may be able to transpose independently, i.e. it may be able to behave as an isolated transposable element. The class I transposons commonly transpose by a conservative, cut-and-paste mechanism (see figure in TRANSPOSABLE ELEMENT). Tn*10* is one example of a transposon that transposes by the cut-and-paste mechanism.

A *class II* (= *simple*) transposon consists of the sequence of structural genes flanked by a pair of INVERTED REPEAT sequences. The class II transposons commonly transpose in a replicative mode (see figure in TRANSPOSABLE ELEMENT). Tn*3* is one example of a transposon that transposes in the replicative mode.

The specificity with which a transposon inserts into a target sequence varies with transposon. Some transposons appear to insert more or less randomly. Others (e.g. members of the MARINER FAMILY) have minimal site specificity, while (e.g.) transposon TN7 (q.v.) has a highly specific target site.

Transposons find a number of uses in DNA technology – see e.g. TRANSPOSON MUTAGENESIS.

(See also entries for individual transposons under 'Tn'.)

transposon immunity A phenomenon in which the presence of a transposon in a given replicon inhibits the insertion of another copy of that transposon in the same replicon. Transposition immunity is exhibited by transposon Tn*3* and also by many of the Tn*3*-like transposable elements.

transposon mutagenesis MUTAGENESIS mediated by a TRANSPOSON; insertion mutations created by transposons can be readily mapped. A general requirement in this method is that the transposon used be able to insert *randomly* into the target replicon; one reason for this is that if (as in some cases) a transposon inserts primarily into certain 'hot spots' then it would be necessary to screen a large number of cells in an attempt to detect the required (rare) mutant. The transposon used is therefore one that inserts randomly, or with minimal site-specificity – e.g. a derivative of a *mariner* transposon was used in *Francisella tularensis* [Appl Environ Microbiol (2006) 72(3):1878–1885] and *Bacillus subtilis* [Appl Environ Microbiol (2006) 72(1):327–333].

In transposon mutagenesis the (known) sequence of the transposon provides information on which to base the design of primer-binding sites for investigating the sequence(s) into which the transposon has inserted. Having isolated a given mutant, it is therefore a simple procedure to identify the gene, or genes, affected by the transposon.

Transposon mutagenesis has been used to detect/identify those virulence genes (in a pathogen) which are essential for the pathogen's growth in the host organism: see SIGNATURE-TAGGED MUTAGENESIS.

The method is also used to detect/identify cell-surface or secreted proteins of pathogenic bacteria – i.e. proteins which (because of potential interaction with the host organism) *may* be associated with virulence. Cells of a given pathogen are first mutagenized with transposons containing a promoterless reporter gene encoding the enzyme ALKALINE PHOSPHATASE (AP); these transposons (designated Tn*phoA*) insert randomly into different genes in the population of cells. When plated, these (mutagenized) cells form individual colonies, i.e. each colony arises from a single cell. The colonies are tested with a substrate which is split by AP to produce a colored product. Any colony which gives a positive reaction (i.e. color) therefore indicates a secreted or cell-surface alkaline phosphatase because the substrate can be used only by an extracellular or cell-surface enzyme. As *phoA* in the transposon lacks both promoter and signal sequence, the formation of an active AP by cells of a given colony indicates that Tn*phoA* has inserted, in frame, into the gene of a secreted or cell-surface protein. If this gene is a virulence-associated gene, then the virulence of the cells in the colony may be demonstrably decreased as the gene is likely to have been inactivated by insertion of the transposon; the mutant cells in this colony can be tested for virulence and, if required, the relevant gene can be isolated and sequenced.

Transposons can be either inserted into living cells or used for *in vitro* mutagenization of e.g. a population of plasmids (see TN5-TYPE TRANSPOSITION).

(See also GENETIC FOOTPRINTING.)

transversion mutation Any point mutation in which a purine is replaced by a pyrimidine, or a pyrimidine is replaced by a purine.

(cf. TRANSITION MUTATION.)

TRAP Telomeric repeat amplification protocol: a method for gaining information on the activity of TELOMERASE.

A synthetic telomeric repeat sequence is added to a sample lysate and is extended by telomerase. The extended synthetic fragment is then amplified by PCR; on electrophoresis of the products, the extent of addition to the fragment by telomerase is reflected in the length of the PCR products.

The TRAP assay used for plants differs from human TRAP assays e.g. in temperature (room temperature, or 26°C) and in the buffers used.

trastuzumab (Herceptin®) See EPIDERMAL GROWTH FACTOR RECEPTOR FAMILY.

TRCF Transcription repair coupling factor: see MFD GENE.

TRES TIME-RESOLVED EMISSION SPECTRA.

tribrid system *Syn.* YEAST THREE-HYBRID SYSTEM.

Trichoplusia ni **GV** See GRANULOSIS VIRUSES.

trichostatin A An inhibitor of histone deacetylases (HDACs) – see ACETYLATION.

[Use (examples): Nucleic Acids Res (2006) 34(3):765–772; Nucleic Acids Res (2006) 34(5):1459–1469.]

trimethoprim See ANTIBIOTIC (synergism).

triostins See QUINOXALINE ANTIBIOTICS.

triple-strand probe A PROBE which hybridizes to a complementary sequence at the 5′ end of one strand in linear dsDNA, forming a highly stable triple-stranded structure; binding is facilitated by the RecA protein. The stability of this triple-stranded structure is greatly reduced by a single mismatched base, regardless of its location. It has been suggested that this system may be useful for the detection of SNPs [DNA Res (2005) 12(6):441–449].

triple-stranded DNA *Syn.* TRIPLEX DNA.

triplex DNA A triple-stranded helical structure in which a STRAND of nucleic acid is located in the MAJOR GROOVE of a DNA duplex – the pyrimidine or purine bases in the strand binding to purine bases in the duplex by HOOGSTEEN BASE-PAIRING.

In some cases the third strand in the triplex DNA derives from a sequence close to the acceptor region, in the same DNA molecule; in other cases it may derive from a separate DNA molecule or from a distant region of the same molecule – or it may be a synthetic strand.

The two basic triplex schemes are: (i) the purine motif (Pu) in which the third strand is A-rich or G-rich and binds in an ANTIPARALLEL fashion to the acceptor strand in the duplex; (ii) the pyrimidine motif (Py) in which the third strand is C-rich or T-rich and binds in a parallel fashion.

An intramolecular triplex may develop, for example, in a supercoiled molecule when, on separation of the two strands in a homopurine–homopyrimidine sequence (of >10 base-pairs), one of the strands forms the third strand of a triplex by binding to a given sequence via Hoogsteen base-pairing. If the third strand is pyrimidine-rich the triplex structure thus formed is called H-DNA; if purine-rich it is called H′-DNA.

Some triplex structures are stable under physiological conditions.

A triplex may be produced by a synthetic *triplex-forming oligonucleotide* (TFO). TFOs have *in vitro* applications and possibly have uses in GENE THERAPY; they can inhibit transcription and translation, and have been able to down-regulate the expression of a proto-oncogene in HeLa cells.

(See also PROGRAMMABLE ENDONUCLEASE.)

The activity of a TFO may be enhanced by using certain modified bases (see LOCKED NUCLEIC ACIDS) [*pyrimidine*: Nucleic Acids Res (2005) 33(13):4223–4234; *purine*: J Biol Chem (2005) 280(20):20076–20085].

RNA and PNA can be involved in triplex structures.

A TFO (bound e.g. to a psoralen molecule) has also been used for site-directed cross-linking of dsDNA [Nucleic Acids Res (2005) 33(9):2993–3001].

triplex-forming oligonucleotide See TRIPLEX DNA.

Tris (TRIS, tris, THAM, Tromethamine) The compound: tris (hydroxymethyl) aminomethane; with hydrochloric acid, Tris forms a (temperature-sensitive) pH buffering system which is effective between approximately pH 7 and pH 9 with a pK_a of 8 at 25°C.

(See also RIBONUCLEASE.)

trisomy (detection of) See e.g. DOWN'S SYNDROME.

(See also CHROMOSOME ABERRATION.)

trisomy 21 *Syn.* DOWN'S SYNDROME.

trithorax-group genes (*Drosophila*) See POLYCOMB-GROUP GENES.

tritium See e.g. AUTORADIOGRAPHY.

TRIzol® A reagent (Invitrogen, Carlsbad CA) used e.g. in the isolation of total RNA from cells; it consists of a monophasic solution of (i) phenol and (ii) guanidine isothiocyanate.

Tromethamine *Syn.* TRIS.

Tropheryma whipplei (former name: *Tropheryma whippelii*) A Gram-positive bacterium associated with Whipple's disease. The organism was once regarded as uncultivable but has been cultured in fibroblasts, and its complete genome sequence is known [Lancet (2003) 361:637–644].

trovafloxacin See QUINOLONE ANTIBIOTICS.

trp **operon** See OPERON.

TRP-185 protein See AAVS.

truncated gene *Syn.* PSEUDOGENE.

trxA **gene** The *Escherichia coli* gene encoding THIOREDOXIN.

trypanosomes Parasitic, flagellate protozoans of the genus *Trypanosoma* which cause diseases such as Chagas' disease and sleeping sickness in humans – and which are also responsible for e.g. dourine and nagana in animals.

In addition to their nuclear DNA, these organisms contain KINETOPLAST DNA (in the mitochondria).

The expression of protein-encoding genes in trypanosomes appears generally not to be regulated at the level of initiation of transcription; this is relevant in the design of systems for engineering gene expression in these organisms – see entry EXPRESSION VECTOR.

(See also OPERON, RNA EDITING and VSG.)

Note. The meaning of the term *trypanosomes* is sometimes

extended to include other trypanosomatids, such as species of *Leishmania*.

T-S oligo See CAPFINDER.

TSA TYRAMIDE SIGNAL AMPLIFICATION.

tSDA See SDA.

tsunami victims (identification) See FORENSIC APPLICATIONS (*Identification*).

TTGE (temporal temperature-gradient gel electrophoresis) A method – similar in principle to DGGE – in which separation of *related*, *double-stranded* fragments of DNA involves an ongoing rise in temperature (instead of a gradient of chemical denaturing agents) to achieve differential melting of sample fragments in the second phase of electrophoresis.

[TTGE compared with DGGE: Lett Appl Microbiol (2000) 30:427–431.]

TTGE has been used e.g. for investigating the microflora in Crohn's disease [J Clin Microbiol (2005) 43(9):4654–4658], for detecting particular strains of *Clostridium* [Appl Environ Microbiol (2005) 71(1):29–38], and for studying the role of mutations in mitochondrial DNA in esophageal cancer [BMC Cancer (2006) 6:93].

TTVI center The Thai Tsunami Victim Identification center: see FORENSIC APPLICATIONS.

two-component regulatory system In many bacteria (and in at least some archaeans): a system for regulating genes typically involving a histidine kinase in the cell envelope and a response regulator protein which, when phosphorylated by the kinase, regulates the expression of particular target gene(s); these two-component systems enable organisms to sense, and respond to, specific environmental factors (such as changes in extracellular osmolarity) – activation of the system occurring via a so-called *signal transduction pathway* (i.e. from the stimulated sensor to the response regulator and thence to the regulatory function).

Two-component systems are involved in the regulation of a wide range of processes. For example, they have been reported to regulate adhesion and oxygen-regulated exotoxigenesis in *Staphylococcus aureus*; uptake of potassium ions (K$^+$) in *Escherichia coli* (in hypertonic conditions); toxin production in *Clostridium perfringens*; the development of competence in transformation in *Bacillus subtilis*; and membrane permeability in *Pseudomonas aeruginosa*.

(See also CROWN GALL and QUORUM SENSING.)

In some cases the kinase itself acts as the sensor. Thus, for example, in the high-affinity transport system for K$^+$ ions in *Escherichia coli*, the sensor, KdpD, apparently responds to lowered turgor pressure in hypertonic media, phosphorylating the response regulator KdpE – which promotes expression of the *kdpABC* operon; one of the products, KdpB, a K$^+$-ATPase (potassium pump), mediates ATP-dependent uptake of K$^+$ to counteract the hypertonicity.

In other cases the sensor is distinct from the kinase. Thus, in the chemotaxis system in *E. coli*, methyl-accepting chemotaxis proteins (MCPs) in the cell envelope act as sensors to changing levels of certain chemoeffector molecules; an MCP

regulates the activity of the (physically linked) kinase, CheA, which, in turn, controls phosphorylation of the CheY protein – the response regulator which determines flagellar rotation (clockwise, counterclockwise) depending on its phosphorylation status.

Some two-component systems are *essential* for viability of the cell. In at least some cases such systems are involved in regulating gene expression in the control of the cell cycle. One example, in *Bacillus subtilis*, is the YycFG system in which YycG is the histidine kinase and YycF the response regulator. (This system is also found in other Gram-positive bacteria within the low-GC% category – e.g. *Enterococcus faecalis* and *Staphylococcus aureus*.) In *B. subtilis* YycF is reported to control genes which regulate the composition of the cell wall; these genes include those in the *tagAB* and *tagDEF* operons associated with biosynthesis of the cell wall polymer teichoic acid.

two-hybrid systems (1) (bacterial) See BACTERIOMATCH TWO-HYBRID SYSTEM.

(2) (in *Saccharomyces cerevisiae*) See YEAST TWO-HYBRID SYSTEM and CYTOTRAP TWO-HYBRID SYSTEM.

two-metal-ion catalysis (two-Mg^{2+}-ion catalysis) The proposed involvement of two metal (Mg^{2+}) ions in the substrate recognition and catalytic specificity of DNA and RNA polymerases (and of many nucleases and transposases) [Molecular Cell (2006) 22:5–13].

two-temperature protocol (in PCR) See temperature cycling in the entry PCR.

Ty element A RETROTRANSPOSON, multiple copies of which occur in the genome of *Saccharomyces cerevisiae*. At least some Ty elements resemble retroviruses; for example, the Ty3 element encodes homologs of the Gag–Pol proteins that, with genomic RNA, can assemble into virus-like particles.

Ty elements transpose to non-homologous sites, forming a 5-bp duplication at the target site; the target sites of Ty1–Ty4 elements tend to be upstream of genes transcribed by RNA polymerase III (often tRNA genes).

type I restriction endonuclease See RESTRICTION ENDONUCLEASE.

type I transposon (class I transposon) See TRANSPOSON.

type II restriction endonuclease See RESTRICTION ENDONUCLEASE.

type II transposon (class II transposon) See TRANSPOSON.

type IIA restriction endonuclease See RESTRICTION ENDONUCLEASE.

type IIB restriction endonuclease See RESTRICTION ENDONUCLEASE.

type IIE restriction endonuclease See RESTRICTION ENDONUCLEASE.

type IIM restriction endonuclease See RESTRICTION ENDONUCLEASE.

type IIP restriction endonuclease See RESTRICTION ENDONUCLEASE.

type IIS restriction endonuclease See RESTRICTION ENDONUCLEASE.

type III restriction endonuclease See RESTRICTION ENDO-NUCLEASE.

type IV restriction endonuclease See RESTRICTION ENDO-NUCLEASE.

typing (*microbiol.*) The term 'typing' has two distinct, although related, meanings. In one sense it refers to a form of *classification* in which STRAINS of a given species are categorized according to specified criteria. Thus, for example, if a large number of random clinical isolates of the pathogen *Staphylococcus aureus* are each examined for susceptibility to a range of different phages, the strains will usually be found to differ in their susceptibility to particular phages; thus, while one strain may be lysed by a certain set of phages, another strain may be lysed by a different set. The particular set of phages to which a given strain is susceptible can therefore be used to define, or classify, that strain and to distinguish it from other strains of that species; this procedure, called *phage typing*, has been used for typing *S. aureus* and certain other bacteria (e.g. *Yersinia enterocolitica*). A species typed by this method can be divided (classified) into a number of so-called 'phage types' – although not all strains of a given species may be suitable for phage typing.

The second meaning of 'typing' refers to a form of *identification*. Thus, once a species has been typed (i.e. classified) by a given typing method (such as phage typing), an *unknown* strain, isolated from a clinical or other sample, may be examined by the criteria of the given typing system to determine its relationship to other strains of the species.

Both aspects of typing – classification and identification – use similar criteria and methods.

In the context of identification, it should be appreciated that no system of typing can prove that a given unknown strain is *identical* to a particular, known strain. To obtain evidence that one strain is identical to another (a clonal relationship) it would be necessary e.g. to compare the complete genomic nucleotide sequences and to examine both strains for extrachromosomal elements etc.

Phage typing and e.g. serotyping (which is based on cell-surface antigenic differences between strains) are still viable methods, but the majority of current typing procedures are based on nucleic acid criteria (see later).

The above refers primarily to the typing of *bacteria*. Other types of microorganism, including viruses, can also be typed by appropriate methods.

The uses of typing

Some uses of typing are indicated below:

● In epidemiology, typing of strains of a pathogen isolated from a number of patients during an outbreak of disease can help to establish the *chain of infection*, i.e. the succession of patients who have been infected from the original organism. The essential premise here is that all patients in the chain of infection will have been infected by progeny of the same ancestral cell and this should be reflected in the high degree of similarity of the strains isolated from patients; a typing procedure can be used to demonstrate such a high degree of similarity.

● Typing has been useful for tracing cross-contamination of clinical specimens in the laboratory.

● Typing of isolates of *Mycobacterium tuberculosis* has been used for estimating the relative importance of new infection versus reactivation of an existing infection in tuberculosis.

● In forensic investigations, the ability to distinguish between closely related strains, and to link a particular strain with a distinct source, can be useful e.g. in providing supportive evidence in cases of sexual abuse or in cases (such as food poisoning) in which the origin of a given strain is of special relevance.

Nucleic-acid-based typing

This refers to the (many) methods in which strains are typed on the basis of sequences of nucleotides from their DNA or RNA.

In some cases typing involves comparison of the nucleic acid isolated from different strains. Alternatively, a particular sequence of DNA or RNA may be copied (by methods such as PCR) and a comparison made of the amplicons from each of the strains.

The actual process of comparison may involve e.g. direct sequencing of a specific region of DNA; digestion of samples with restriction endonucleases and comparison of the resulting fragments by gel electrophoresis; probing for specific restriction fragments; or examination of single-stranded DNA samples for strain-specific intrastrand base-pairing.

A distinct approach to typing concentrates specifically on *unstable* regions of the genome, i.e. regions that are likely to provide the maximum opportunity for detecting differences between strains. Such regions include the (many) tandemly repeated short sequences that are present in both prokaryotic and eukaryotic genomes. These regions are associated with high rates of mutation – apparently because they are more susceptible than other regions of the genome to disruptive changes due to events such as SLIPPED-STRAND MISPAIRING and recombination. Hence, selected regions of the genome, such as certain VNTRs (see VARIABLE NUMBER OF TANDEM REPEATS) can be used as a basis for comparison of isolates; thus, these regions can be amplified by PCR, with appropriate primers, and the isolates then compared by comparing the amplified products. This approach is used in methods such as MLVA.

For further details of a number of nucleic-acid-based typing procedures see individual entries for the methods listed in the table.

Conventional versus nucleic-acid-based typing

Nucleic-acid-based typing differs from 'conventional' forms of typing (such as phage typing) in various ways, not least in the type of equipment and facilities required.

● One important difference is that DNA-based typing has the potential to be carried out *directly* from a clinical or environmental specimen – i.e. without the delay involved in isolating the organism in pure culture. This has been achieved with e.g. *Mycobacterium tuberculosis* and *Neisseria gonorrhoeae* and

TYPING (*microbiol.*): some examples of methods[a]

Method	Essential features of method
AFLP	Digestion of genomic DNA with two types of restriction endonuclease followed by ligation of adaptors to fragments. PCR amplification of those fragments which have certain selective bases complementary to base(s) in the primer. Electrophoresis of amplicons to form the fingerprint
AP-PCR	Use of PCR primers of arbitrary sequence to amplify non-specific targets in genomic DNA; this is followed by gel electrophoresis of products and staining to form the fingerprint
Cleavase fragment length polymorphism analysis	Preparation of single-stranded, end-labeled samples of target DNA from each strain, heat-denaturation, and then cooling to a temperature at which intrastrand base-pairing occurs; this is followed by cleavage with a structure-dependent endonuclease (Cleavase™) and electrophoresis of products to form the fingerprint
Cleaved amplified polymorphic sequences	Comparison of strains on the basis of their CAPS markers (see entry CAPS)
DAF	See entry AP-PCR
DGGE	Comparison of DNA samples by two-phase gel electrophoresis, the samples being separated by size in the first phase and by sequence-based melting (i.e. strand separation) in the second phase
DNA fingerprinting	Restriction enzyme digestion of genomic DNA followed by gel electrophoresis and staining of bands to form the fingerprint; alternatively, blotting of gel to membrane and staining of bands on the membrane
ERIC-PCR	A particular form of rep-PCR (see entry)
MLST	Comparison of nucleotide sequences in specific alleles by direct sequencing
MLVA	Comparison on the basis of certain loci that contain tandemly repeated sequences, strains differing e.g. in the number of repeats at a given locus; relevant loci are copied by PCR, and the amplicons from different strains are compared by gel electrophoresis
PCR-RFLP analysis	RFLP analysis (see below) in which the sample DNA is copied from a primary source by PCR
PCR-ribotyping	Amplification of ISRs (intergenic spacer regions) in the 16S–23S region of the *rrn* operon by PCR and examination of products by gel electrophoresis (cf. ribotyping, below)
PFGE	Specialized electrophoresis of *large* restriction fragments of genomic DNA to form the fingerprint; large fragments are formed by so-called 'rare-cutting' restriction enzymes (such as NotI)
RAPD analysis	See entry AP-PCR
rep-PCR	PCR-based amplification in which primers bind to specific repetitive sequences found in genomic DNA (e.g. the ERIC sequence and the REP sequence) and produce amplicons that reflect the distances between consecutive target sequences; this is followed by gel electrophoresis of the amplicons to form a fingerprint
REP-PCR	A particular form of rep-PCR (see above, and entry)
RFLP analysis	Restriction digestion of DNA samples, gel electrophoresis of products, and comparison of the samples by comparing the number and sizes of fragments produced from each sample; the method detects loss/gain of recognition sites (for the given restriction endonuclease used) as well as insertions/deletions
Ribotyping	Digestion of genomic DNA with a restriction endonuclease, separation of fragments by gel electrophoresis, and then use of DNA or RNA probes, complementary to a sequence in the *rrn* operon, which label specific bands containing the target sequence, thereby generating a fingerprint

(*continued*)

Method	Essential features of method
SCC*mec* typing	A method for typing strains of MRSA (methicillin-resistant *Staphylococcus aureus*) based on strain-specific differences in the composition of the SCC*mec* element (see entry SCCMEC)
SERE-PCR	A particular form of rep-PCR (see above, and entry)
Spoligotyping	For members of the *Mycobacterium tuberculosis* complex: PCR amplification of spacers in the genomic DR region, hybridization of the amplicons to a set of oligonucleotide probes representing spacers in a reference strain, determination of the pattern of hybridization (the spoligotype)
SSCP analysis	Preparation of single-stranded samples of the given target sequence from each strain, electrophoresis under non-denaturing conditions, and comparison of strains on the basis of differences in electrophoretic mobility due to differences in the pattern of intrastrand base-pairing
Subtracted restriction fingerprinting	Restriction of genomic DNA with two types of restriction endonuclease, end-labeling of fragments with biotin and digoxigenin, selective capture and elimination of biotin-labeled fragments, and electrophoresis of the remaining fragments to form the fingerprint

[a]See individual entries for further information.

is clearly a significant advantage in the context of certain infectious diseases.

● A further difference is that, unlike conventional methods, DNA-based typing can be affected by *silent* mutations. Such mutations can affect e.g. the binding of probes and primers, and they can also affect the intrastrand base-pairing on which certain DNA-based typing methods depend.

● Another point of difference is that, with some conventional methods, certain strains do not give a result, i.e. they are *untypable* by the given procedure; for example, some strains of *Staphylococcus aureus* are not suitable for phage typing. In DNA-based methods, on the other hand, all such phenotypic aberrations are not problematic because these variations are reflected in genomic sequences. Untypability in DNA-based methods occurs if the strains under test exhibit no difference in the target sequence used for typing; this situation can be addressed by re-examining the strains with a method that involves different target sequence(s).

tyramide signal amplification (TSA) A procedure used for the ultrasensitive detection of a target nucleic acid or protein *in situ* (i.e. at its normal or relevant location within tissues or cells) – a procedure which is more sensitive than the standard form of *in situ* hybridization (FISH).

As in FISH, a probe can be synthesized as a BIOTINylated oligonucleotide. In TSA, when the probe has bound to its *in situ* target sequence it is detected by a STREPTAVIDIN-linked enzyme: horseradish peroxidase (HRP). HRP acts on (added) molecules of e.g. a fluorophore-labeled tyramide, producing highly reactive but short-lived radicals which bind covalently to local residues (particularly tyrosine residues in proteins) in the immediate vicinity of the bound enzyme, thereby deposit-

ing molecules of the label at that site. The intensity of the reaction is increased by adding an HRP-conjugated antibody which is specific for the fluorophore (or other label) already deposited at the target site; this extra HRP provides further activation of (added) labeled tyramide molecules, resulting in further deposition of the label and providing an opportunity for generating an increased level of signal.

Tyramine (*p*-(β-aminoethyl)phenol) can be substituted in a number of ways to produce a range of tyramides.

TSA is also called catalyzed reporter deposition (CARD).

[Example of TSA for the detection of specific antibodies: Mol Biol Cell (2006) 17(4):1697–1710.]

[A quantitative evaluation of peroxide inhibitors for TSA-mediated cytochemistry and histochemistry: Histochem Cell Biol (2006) 126(2):283–291.]

tyramine See TYRAMIDE SIGNAL AMPLIFICATION.

tyrosine kinase Any ATP-dependent enzyme (EC 2.7.1.112) which phosphorylates a specific tyrosine residue in a protein.

Tyrosine kinases are important factors in various forms of signal transfer in mammalian cells; they include membrane-associated enzymes, which are activated via specific signal molecules, and cytoplasmic enzymes mediating intracellular signal transfer.

(See e.g. ABL, COMPETENT CELLS, EPIDERMAL GROWTH FACTOR RECPTOR FAMILY, ERLOTINIB, FES, FPS, GEFITINIB, IMATINIB, ONCOGENE, NEU, SRC, TYRPHOSTIN.)

(See also GENISTEIN and JANUS KINASES.)

tyrosine recombinase See RECOMBINASE.

tyrphostin A synthetic monocyclic compound which strongly inhibits EGF-receptor-associated TYROSINE KINASE activity; unlike GENISTEIN, it does not inhibit the binding of ATP.

U

UAA *Ochre* codon: see NONSENSE CODON.

UAG *Amber* codon: see NONSENSE CODON.

UAS (upstream activation site) In *Saccharomyces cerevisiae*: a transcriptional ENHANCER which functions only if upstream of the promoter.

ubiquitin A polypeptide (of 76 amino acid residues) which is widely distributed in eukaryotic cells but apparently absent in prokaryotic cells.

An energy-dependent linking of ubiquitin molecules to ear-marked proteins occurs e.g. prior to degradation of a protein in the PROTEASOME (q.v.).

Ubiquitin–protein linking is involved in various types of cellular process – including regulation of a protein's function and the intracellular localization of proteins.

(See also SUMOYLATION.)

UGA *Opal* codon: see NONSENSE CODON.

Ulp1 A SUMO protease: see SUMOYLATION.

Ulp2 A SUMO protease: see SUMOYLATION.

ultraviolet absorbance In the spectrophotometric quantitation of nucleic acids in solution: absorbance measured at 260 nm (written A_{260}).

At 260 nm, 1 unit of absorbance corresponds to ~40 μg/mL of ssRNA, to ~33 μg/mL ssDNA or to ~50 μg/mL of dsDNA.

The ratio A_{260}/A_{280} can indicate the purity (homogeneity) of a sample of DNA or RNA.

(See also OLIGREEN, PICOGREEN ASSAY and RIBOGREEN.)

ultraviolet radiation (UVR) (effects on DNA) Electromagnetic radiation of wavelength ~300 nm is absorbed by bases in nucleic acids and produces a range of photoproducts; these photoproducts may be lethal to the cell (e.g. blocking DNA synthesis if the damage is not repaired) or they may give rise to MUTAGENESIS.

(See also ASEPTIC TECHNIQUE.)

The UVR-induced photoproducts include various types of dimer (see e.g. PYRIMIDINE DIMER).

In *Escherichia coli* UVR-based *mutagenesis* is promoted through the activity of the so-called SOS SYSTEM. Induction of the SOS system (by damage to DNA) leads to the activity of certain *error-prone* DNA polymerases which, when synthesizing DNA through a lesion (i.e. *translesion* synthesis), incorporate incorrect nucleotides (owing to a lack of local base-pairing specificity) and hence give rise to mutations.

(See also LYSOGENY.)

The spectrum of ultraviolet radiation has been divided into three bands, designated UV-A, UV-B and UV-C; however, the wavelengths covered by each band are defined in different ways by different authors. A brief survey of the literature shows that UV-B is defined (according to author) as: (e.g.) 280–315 nm; 280–320 nm; 290–320 nm; and 295–320 nm. Similarly, UV-A has been defined as e.g. 315–400 nm, 320–360 nm and 320–400 nm, while UV-C has been defined as e.g. 190–290 nm and <280 nm. (Some authors do not specify what they mean when using a given designation.)

The mutagenic effects of UVR which give rise to human carcinomas/melanomas have been linked primarily to wavelengths in the region 280–320 nm. Although radiation in this band represents only a small proportion of total solar UVR reaching the planet, its carcinogenic effect is much greater than that of UV-A. However, studies on the effect of 'UVA1' (defined by the authors as 340–400 nm) on cultured human fibroblasts found that radiation in these wavelengths induces pro-mutagenic CPDs (cyclobutyl pyrimidine dimers) and also oxidative damage to DNA [Proc Natl Acad Sci USA (2005) 102(29): 10058–10063].

ULYSIS® See PROBE LABELING.

umber codon See NONSENSE CODON.

umuC See DNA POLYMERASE V.

umuD See DNA POLYMERASE V.

ung gene (in *Escherichia coli*) See URACIL-N-GLYCOSYLASE.

UNG method (of decontamination in PCR) See AMPLICON INACTIVATION.

univector See VECTOR.

universal nucleotide A type of base analog that is able to 'pair' with each of the normal bases found in DNA; typically, interaction with a normal base does not involve hydrogen bonding but rather a contribution to the stability of the base stacking in dsDNA.

Universal DNA base analogs have been used e.g. at certain locations in primers; in general, they are found to be less useful in positions close to the 3′ end of a primer. These analogs have also been used in probes.

[Applications of DNA base analogs as biochemical tools: Nucleic Acids Res (2001) 29(12):2437–2447.]

universal primer *Syn.* BROAD-RANGE PRIMER.

unlabeled probe Any PROBE which lacks a label but which can nevertheless provide information on its target sequence.

Unlabeled probes can be used e.g. for detecting variation in a given target sequence – such variation being indicated by a difference in T_m (see THERMAL MELTING PROFILE) observed if different probes form different probe–target associations with variant forms of a given target sequence (for example, see T_m-shift primers in SNP GENOTYPING).

In general, a probe that is fully complementary to its target sequence will have a higher T_m when compared with the same probe bound to a variant form of the target with one or more mismatched base-pairs; the difference in T_m between a matched and a mismatched probe, for a particular target sequence, is designated ΔT_m °C.

The inclusion of LOCKED NUCLEIC ACIDS (LNAs) in an unlabeled probe is reported to increase the ability of the probe to indicate probe–target mismatches, i.e. LNAs can increase the ΔT_m [see e.g. BioTechniques (2005) 39(5):644–648].

3′-untranslated region See 3′-UTR.

5′-untranslated region See 5′-UTR.

untwisting enzyme See TOPOISOMERASE (type I).

unwinding protein Any protein which can unwind and separate the strands of dsDNA.

(See HELICASE; cf. SINGLE-STRAND BINDING PROTEIN.)

upper operon (in the TOL plasmid)   See TOL PLASMID.

upstream   See entry DOWNSTREAM.

upstream active site   See UAS.

URA3 **gene**   See SACCHAROMYCES and YEAST TWO-HYBRID SYSTEM.

uracil-containing templates (DNA synthesis)   See PFUTURBO.

uracil-DNA *N*-glycosylase   *Syn.* URACIL-N-GLYCOSYLASE.

uracil-*N*-glycosylase (UNG)   In *Escherichia coli*: an enzyme (the *ung* gene product) which cleaves uracil from an aberrant nucleotide in DNA; this is a normal repair function following the spontaneous deamination of cytosine to uracil. Complete repair of a deaminated cytosine is carried out via the BASE EXCISION REPAIR pathway.

UNG is used in one form of AMPLICON INACTIVATION in PCR (to avoid contamination with amplicons from previous assays).

Unlike uracil, 6-sulfonyluracil (formed during BISULFITE treatment of DNA) is resistant to UNG, and this sulfonated form of DNA has been used (with the UNG method of decontamination) in a PCR-based study of DNA methylation [Nucleic Acids Res (2007) 35(1):e4].

uracil-specific excision reagent cloning   See USER.

uridine   A riboNUCLEOSIDE.

USER™ cloning   Uracil-specific excision reagent cloning: a method (New England Biolabs, Ipswich MA) that is used for cloning a PCR-generated fragment by inserting the fragment, in a ligation-independent manner, into a linearized vector and then using the vector, directly, to transform the host cells.

For the initial generation of the PCR fragments, each of the primers contains one residue of uracil. The resulting blunt-ended PCR amplicons are treated with a mixture of enzymes: uracil-*N*-glycosylase (which removes the uracil residue from each strand of the (double-stranded) amplicons), and another enzyme which facilitates the release of each single-stranded fragment from its location *5′ of an abasic site*. This enzymic activity produces 8-nucleotide 3′ overhangs at both ends of each amplicon.

The linear vector is prepared as two pieces, each having one 3′ 8-nucleotide overhang complementary to *one* of the overhangs on the PCR fragment – thus ensuring directional insertion of the fragment into the vector.

Binding between the overhangs on the PCR fragment with those on the fragments of vector is sufficiently strong to permit the hybridized fragments to be inserted by transformation into appropriate cells.

One problem with the method arises during generation of the PCR fragments. Thus, the kind of (proof-reading) DNA polymerase used for error-free replication of DNA has been found to stall at uracil residues in template strands of DNA. *Taq* DNA polymerase has been used, but the absence of 3′-to-5′ exonuclease (proof-reading) activity in this enzyme precludes its use for high-fidelity cloning of DNA. More recently, a proof-reading enzyme – *PfuTurbo*® C_x Hotstart DNA polymerase (Stratagene, La Jolla CA) – has been reported to

be suitable for the USER™ methodology [Nucleic Acids Res (2006) 34(18):e122].

3′-UTR (in a eukaryotic mRNA)   The 3′-untranslated region, a sequence of nucleotides between the coding region and the poly(A) tail; it includes the signals for polyadenylation (see AAUAAA).

3′-UTRs are target sites for many, or most, of the known MICRORNAS; human microRNAs are reported preferentially to target AT-rich 3′-UTRs [Proc Natl Acad Sci USA (2005) 102(43):15557–15562].

(See also ANTISENSE RNA.)

5′-UTR (leader sequence; leader) (in mRNA)   That region of an mRNA between the 5′-terminus of the molecule and the start of the coding sequence of the first (or only) gene.

In prokaryotes, the 5′-UTR includes the *Shine–Dalgarno sequence* which base-pairs with a specific sequence in ribosomal RNA, thereby helping to locate the mRNA correctly for translation. Some 5′-UTRs specify a small peptide (the *leader peptide*) and include an *attenuator* sequence, both of which contribute to regulation of the encoded gene(s) (see OPERON).

(See also ANTISENSE RNA.)

In most eukaryotes, and in some viruses, the mRNA has a CAP at the 5′ terminus.

UV-A, UV-B, UV-C   See ULTRAVIOLET RADIATION.

UVR   ULTRAVIOLET RADIATION.

UvrABC-mediated repair (nucleotide excision repair; short patch repair)   An EXCISION REPAIR system which recognizes and repairs DNA damaged by ULTRAVIOLET RADIATION or by certain types of chemical agent; the kinds of damage repaired by this system include THYMINE DIMERS, photoproducts such as Pyr(6–4)Pyo, and some types of chemically modified nucleotide.

In *Escherichia coli*, proteins encoded by genes *uvrA*, *uvrB* and *uvrC* constitute the UvrABC enzyme system, also called *ABC excinuclease*.

UvrABC-mediated repair appears to occur in the following way. Dimerized UvrA (UvrA$_2$) interacts with either one or two molecules of UvrB, thus forming a UvrA$_2$B or UvrA$_2$B$_2$ complex. This complex apparently translocates along the helix (in an ATP-dependent manner) to the exact site of the damage. UvrA then dissociates, leaving UvrB bound to DNA. UvrC now binds to the UvrB–DNA complex, and this new complex (specifically UvrC) mediates initial cleavage of the strand at a phosphodiester bond 3 or 4 nucleotides 3′ of the damaged site. [Studies on the first incision by UvrC: EMBO J (2005) 24(5):885–894.] The next cleavage of the strand occurs 7 or 8 nucleotides 5′ of the damaged site. The sequence of nucleotides containing the lesion, together with UvrC, is displaced by UvrD (= helicase II), and the single-stranded gap is filled by DNA polymerase I, which also displaces UvrB. In *Escherichia coli* the excised region is only about 10 nucleotides in length (hence the name 'short patch repair').

UvrD (*syn.* helicase II)   See UVRABC-MEDIATED REPAIR.

UvsX enzyme (of phage T4)   See RPA (sense 1).

V

V (1) A specific indicator of ambiguity in the recognition site of a RESTRICTION ENDONUCLEASE (or in any other sequence of nucleic acid); 'V' indicates A or C or G.

(2) L-Valine (alternative to Val).

V factor A growth requirement for some species of HAEMOPHILUS: NAD⁺ or NADP⁺ (or nicotinamide mononucleotide). V factor is available in yeast extract and also in heat-lysed erythrocytes (red blood cells).

(cf. X FACTOR.)

v-*onc* An unspecified viral ONCOGENE.

v-*onc*⁺ The designation of a virus or viral genome containing an ONCOGENE.

v-*onc*⁻ The designation of a virus or viral genome which lacks an ONCOGENE.

V5 epitope A fusion tag encoded by some types of expression vector; it consists of the following sequence of amino acids: Gly-Lys-Pro-Ile-Pro-Asn-Pro-Leu-Leu-Gly-Leu-Asp-Ser-Thr (which is recognized by an anti-V5 monoclonal antibody). It facilitates detection of the fusion product by an anti-V5 mAb.

variable number of tandem repeats (VNTR) A phrase which refers to genetic loci consisting of repeated sequence(s) of nucleotides, the precise composition at a given VNTR locus varying between different individuals in the species (and/or differing from the other VNTR loci in the given genome). For many authors, VNTRs can refer to *any* type of tandemly repeated unit – e.g. MICROSATELLITE DNA or minisatellite DNA – but some authors have equated the term specifically with a particular type of repeated unit.

VNTRs are associated with high rates of mutation; this is apparently due to the relative ease with which events such as SLIPPED-STRAND MISPAIRING may occur in these sequences. Studies on 28 VNTR loci in *Escherichia coli* strain O157:H7 reported single-locus rates of up to 7×10^{-4} mutations per generation, a proportion of the observed mutations being consistent with a slipped-strand mispairing model [J Bacteriol (2006) 188(12):4253–4263].

A number of (separate) VNTRs in a particular genome – not necessarily containing the same types of repeat sequences in each VNTR – can be exploited e.g. for TYPING isolates of microorganisms and distinguishing between DNA samples from eukaryotic/mammalian individuals; this form of typing is termed *multiple loci VNTR analysis* (see MLVA). This kind of approach to typing requires prior identification of suitable VNTRs in genomic DNA [see e.g. BMC Microbiol (2006) 6:44].

VNTRs which consist of a *single type* of nucleotide (a so-called *single-nucleotide repeat*, or SNR) are associated with very high rates of mutation; they have been used for typing isolates of *Bacillus anthracis* (the causal agent of anthrax) [J Clin Microbiol (2006) 44(3):777–782].

variant antigenic type (of *Trypanosoma*) See VSG.

variant surface glycoprotein (of *Trypanosoma*) See VSG.

VariFlex™ The trade designation (Stratagene, La Jolla CA) for various products which are designed to facilitate studies on protein expression – including enhancement of solubility (see SOLUBILITY ENHANCEMENT TAG) and quantitation of soluble proteins (see Q-TAG).

vector (*mol. biol.*) Typically: a plasmid, construct or virus that incorporates the gene of interest (or other fragment of nucleic acid) and which is used for TRANSFECTION (sense 1) – often as a CLONING VECTOR or an EXPRESSION VECTOR. (See also LIPOFECTION, MAGNETOFECTION and MICROINJECTION.)

Many vectors are covalently closed (i.e. circular) molecules of DNA. *Linear* vectors are used e.g. in the BIGEASY LINEAR CLONING SYSTEM and also in the USER CLONING system.

Viral vectors incorporate target DNA in their recombinant/modified genomes; target DNA is inserted into cells following viral infection. Commercial virus-based vectors include e.g. the AAV HELPER-FREE SYSTEM, the ADEASY XL ADENOVIRAL VECTOR SYSTEM and VIRAPORT RETROVIRAL GENE EXPRESSION SYSTEM. (See also RETROVIRUSES.)

In some cases the target nucleic acid is inserted into a small intermediate vector (a *univector*) that is not *directly* used for transfection; the univector is inserted into a second vector that is inserted into host cells [see e.g. BioTechniques (2005) 39(3):301–304].

(See also BINARY VECTOR SYSTEM.)

Some vectors do not contain the insert (target nucleic acid). For example, an *insertional targeting vector* may be used to introduce an insertion site (for subsequent use) into a specific sequence of genomic DNA. Such an engineered insertion site can include e.g. recognition sequences for a given recombinase – so that target DNA (in a second vector) can be inserted into the given site by RECOMBINASE-MEDIATED CASSETTE EXCHANGE [Proc Natl Acad Sci USA (2005) 102(18):6413–6418].

Phages and phagemid particles can function as vectors in prokaryotic cells (see e.g. LAMBDA FIX II VECTOR). This kind of vector has also been used in some eukaryotic cells: see e.g. GENE THERAPY and ZAP EXPRESS VECTOR.

The Ti plasmid (see CROWN GALL) can be used as a vector for introducing DNA into plant cells (see AGROINFECTION).

In order to carry out their function, some vectors require specialized (engineered) *host cells*. For example, cells with a *lacZΔM15* mutation are used for blue–white screening of recombinant PBLUESCRIPT vectors.

Some vectors encode a peptide tag which forms a fusion product with the protein of interest; this facilitates subsequent detection or isolation of the expressed proteins (see e.g. PESC VECTORS and SOLUBILITY ENHANCEMENT TAG.)

(See also DESTINATION VECTOR, GAPPED VECTOR, GENE FUSION VECTOR, INSERTION VECTOR, REPLACEMENT VECTOR, SHUTTLE VECTOR and SUICIDE VECTOR.)

Some examples of destination vectors are given in the table in GATEWAY SITE-SPECIFIC RECOMBINATION SYSTEM.

(See also GENE-DELIVERY SYSTEM.)

Vector NTI Advance™ 9.1   Sequence analysis software: a tool for BIOINFORMATICS marketed by Invitrogen (Carlsbad CA) which is compatible with Windows® PCs.

The software includes a number of modules that permit e.g. creation, mapping and analysis of sequences; sequence alignment of nucleic acids and proteins; the analysis of genomic sequences; and motif mapping of nucleic acids and proteins, as well as annotation.

There is also a facility for Gateway® cloning *in silico*.

vectorette PCR (bubble-linker PCR)   A form of ANCHORED PCR which is used to copy an unknown sequence of nucleotides adjacent to a specific sequence.

In this technique, the double-stranded linker (*vectorette*), which contains the anchor sequence, includes a central (i.e. non-terminal) region in which the bases in the two strands are *not* complementary; the lack of hybridization between these two regions of the vectorette results in a 'bubble' that consists of the two unpaired single-stranded regions.

As in the conventional form of anchored PCR, one of the two primers (primer A) has a binding site within the known sequence of the sample DNA.

The second primer (primer B) consists of a sequence which is *identical* (not complementary) to one of the two single-stranded bubble regions in the vectorette; this primer therefore cannot bind to *any* sequence in the vectorette and, at the start of PCR, has no function as a primer.

PCR starts when DNA synthesis is initiated from primer A; the resulting strand contains a sequence complementary to one of the two 'bubble' sequences in the vectorette – and this sequence can act as a binding site for primer B. PCR then continues as normal, with primers A and B.

With this arrangement, PCR products are formed only if amplification is initiated from primer A, i.e. the occurrence of amplification requires the presence of a suitable binding site for primer A.

vertical transmission (of genes)   Transmission of gene(s) from one individual or cell to its offspring/progeny.

(cf. HORIZONTAL TRANSMISSION.)

vesiculostomatitis virus   See VSV.

Vibragen Omega   A veterinary product (used for canine parvovirus infections) synthesized as a recombinant protein within a (live) silkworm host (see BACULOVIRUS EXPRESSION SYSTEMS).

Vibrio cholerae   A species of Gram-negative bacteria; many of the (lysogenic) strains can cause cholera. The cholera toxin (genes *ctxA* and *ctxB*) is encoded by a bacteriophage (phage CTXΦ). (Genes for cholera toxin can also be acquired via the filamentous phage VGJφ through a form of specialized transduction [J Bacteriol (2003) 185:7231–7240].)

The *V. cholerae* genome consists of two dissimilar circular chromosomes that differ, slightly, in GC% (see also the table in the entry BACTERIA).

Vibrio fischeri (in quorum sensing)   See QUORUM SENSING.

Vif protein (of HIV-1)   See RETROVIRUSES.

vIL-6   A form of IL-6 (interleukin-6) encoded by HHV-8 (the human herpesvirus-8).

violacein   See QUORUM SENSING.

ViraPort® retroviral gene expression system   A commercial GENE-DELIVERY SYSTEM (Stratagene, La Jolla CA) suitable for expressing a given gene of interest in any of a wide range of target cells.

In the ViraPort® system the gene of interest is inserted into an expression vector which is based on elements of Moloney murine leukemia virus (MMLV). This gene-carrying vector is then inserted into suitable 'packaging' cells together with two other vectors: one containing a retroviral *gag–pol* region (encoding viral structural proteins and reverse transcriptase) and another containing the *env* region (encoding viral surface proteins). In these cells the transcript of the expression vector is packaged by products encoded by the other two vectors – forming infectious (but replication-deficient) particles.

Virions formed in, and released from, the packaging cells are used for transfecting *target* cells. Within the target cells the transcript is reverse transcribed (using the reverse transcriptase synthesized in the packaging cells) and the DNA is then integrated into the genome of the target cell. The gene of interest can then be transcribed and expressed in the target cell. (As target cells do not contain the viral structural genes, no virions can be produced.)

By using different *env*-containing vectors, the virions can be made suitable for transfecting different types of target cell (e.g. human, mouse, rabbit) because the products encoded by this vector affect the type(s) of cell which can be infected by the virions.

As the genes for viral components are dispersed among several vector molecules, and as there is little or no sequence overlap among the three vectors, there is minimal possibility of (undesirable) production of replication-competent virions through homologous recombination.

ViraPower™ lentiviral expression system   A system (Invitrogen, Carlsbad CA) used for gene expression in a wide range of mammalian cells – including dividing and non-dividing cells.

The plasmid vector (pLenti), into which the gene of interest is inserted, includes retroviral 5′ and 3′ LTR sequences (see RETROVIRUSES), a ψ (psi) site (which promotes packaging of viral RNA) and a gene encoding resistance to blasticidin or Zeocin™.

The retroviral *gag–pol* and *rev* sequences, and a sequence encoding the G protein of the vesiculostomatitis virus (VSV) (see PSEUDOTYPING), are provided on separate plasmids (in the 'packaging mix').

The vector (containing the insert) and the plasmids of the packaging mix are jointly used to transfect a producer cell line (293FT). The resulting infectious (replication-deficient) virions can be either stored or used to transfect target cells.

virion   A single virus particle.

viroid   Any of a variety of small, circular (covalently closed) molecules of single-stranded RNA, each of several hundred nucleotides in length, which are associated with symptomatic infection of plants; many types of viroid cause economically important diseases. Some examples of viroids include e.g. the *Citrus* exocortis viroid (CEV), coconut cadang-cadang viroid (CCCV), hop stunt viroid (HSV), potato spindle tuber viroid (PSTV), tomato bunchy top viroid (TBTV) and the tomato 'planta macho' viroid (TPMV).

Transmission of viroids may be mechanical (e.g. it may occur during grafting procedures) or it may occur via seed or pollen.

Viroid structure, apparently similar in all viroids, includes double-stranded regions (due to intramolecular base-pairing) and single-stranded (unpaired) loops.

A viroid may localize in the nucleus or in the chloroplast. In at least some cases, replication initially involves synthesis of oligomeric complementary (–) strands several times longer than the wild-type viroid.

Homology between viroids and group I introns lead to the suggestion that these agents may have derived from the (self-splicing) introns.

The viroid-pattern HAMMERHEAD RIBOZYME has been used in various genetically engineered applications.

A database for viroids (and other forms of subviral RNA) is available at:

http://subviral.med.uottawa.ca

[BMC Microbiol (2006) 6:24.]

virulent phage See BACTERIOPHAGE.

virulon In species of the Gram-negative bacterium *Yersinia*: a plasmid-encoded system which essentially comprises a range of virulence proteins and a transport channel for transferring these proteins into the cytoplasm of a eukaryotic target cell, following direct cell–cell contact.

Similar virulence systems have been found e.g. in species of *Salmonella* and *Shigella*.

virus-like particle See VLP.

visna virus See LENTIVIRINAE.

vitamin H *Syn.* BIOTIN.

Vitravene An oligonucleotide antisense therapeutic agent (ISIS Pharmaceuticals), approved by the FDA (USA) in 1998, that is used e.g. for treating cytomegalovirus (CMV) retinitis in AIDS patients; the 21-nucleotide product (administered by direct injection into the eye) binds to viral mRNA, blocking replication of the virus.

VLF-1 (in baculoviruses) Very late expression factor 1 – see BACULOVIRIDAE.

VLP Virus-like particle: any construct used as a surrogate for a virus – e.g. a VLP comprising the major capsid protein (L1) of a human papillomavirus (HPV) has been used in place of HPV in a vaccine. [Protective immunity from a VLP vaccine of influenza virus: J Virol (2007) 81(7):3514–3524.]

VNTR See VARIABLE NUMBER OF TANDEM REPEATS.

von Gierke's disease GLYCOGEN STORAGE DISORDER type Ib.

Voyager™ vectors Vectors (marketed by Invitrogen, Carlsbad

CA) with which a given target protein can be expressed in mammalian cells as a fusion product with the VP22 structural protein of herpes simplex virus type 1; the fusion protein is then able to translocate to adjacent, non-transfected cells in a cell culture – within which it localizes in the nucleus. In this way, a recombinant protein can be delivered to ~100% of cells in a culture following the initial transfection procedure; thus, the protein can be delivered to cells which had not been transfected by the vector.

The ability of the fusion protein to be translocated from the synthesizing cell to an adjacent, non-transfected cell is conferred by the VP22 partner.

The target protein can be expressed as either a C-terminal or an N-terminal fusion to the VP22 partner.

All of these vectors incorporate e.g. a T7 promoter, a CMV promoter, selectable markers and a 6xHis sequence (the latter allowing purification of the protein by a NICKEL-CHARGED AFFINITY RESIN).

Some of these vectors include a facility for topoisomerase-mediated insertion of a gene/fragment (see TOPOISOMERASE I CLONING).

VP22 A structural protein of herpes simplex virus 1 (HSV-1); it is able to translocate in a Golgi-independent, cytochalasin D-sensitive manner from a given mammalian cell to an *adjacent* cell within a cell culture. This property has been exploited by using the VP22 gene to partner the gene of a target protein in VOYAGER VECTORS; the fusion protein has the same ability as VP22 to translocate between mammalian cells.

Vpu protein (of HIV-1) See RETROVIRUSES.

VSG (variant surface glycoprotein) In some species of the protozoan *Trypanosoma*: a component of the cell-surface layer that exhibits extensive ANTIGENIC VARIATION; such variation involves periodic switching from one *VSG* gene to another of different antigenic specificity. An individual organism may encode ~1000 different VSG-specifying genes.

Only one *VSG* is expressed at any given time. Expression requires that a *VSG* be located in a specialized *expression site* situated within a telomere; the genome may contain 20 or more such expression sites. Different individuals expressing different *VSGs* are said to be different *variant antigenic types* (VATs).

The switching of *VSGs* appears to take place in at least two distinct ways. One involves transfer of transcription from one expression site to another (containing a different *VSG*); the mechanism is not understood.

The other way involves recombination between one of the (many) genomic *VSGs* and a *VSG* in an expression site; the commonest mechanism here appears to be homologous recombination and gene conversion.

Reducing the number of *VSG* transcripts to 1–2% of the normal value by RNA INTERFERENCE has been found to induce cell cycle arrest, blocking cell division; this could help to protect *the trypanosome* – i.e. preventing dilution of the protective VSG layer by blocking cell division in the absence of VSG synthesis [Proc Natl Acad Sci USA (2005) 102(24): 8716–8721].

VSV Vesiculostomatitis virus: an enveloped ssRNA-containing virus of the family Rhabdoviridae; it can infect a wide range of animals, including mammals and birds, and it can replicate in many types of cultured cell.

The G (envelope) protein of VSV has been widely used e.g. for PSEUDOTYPING because it confers on a virion the ability to infect a wide range of types of cell.

W

W (1) A specific indicator of ambiguity in the recognition site of a RESTRICTION ENDONUCLEASE (or in any other sequence of nucleic acid); for example, in C↓CWWGG (enzyme StyI), the 'W' indicates A or T. (In RNA 'W' indicates A or U.) (2) L-Tryptophan (alternative to Trp).

W-Beijing strain (also called Beijing/W) A strain of *Mycobacterium tuberculosis*, found particularly in Asia and in the former Soviet territories, associated e.g. with drug resistance and failure of anti-tuberculosis treatment. The genome of this strain is characterized by spoligotype (see SPOLIGOTYPING) and also by the presence of a copy of the insertion sequence IS*6110* in the origin of replication.

W-Beijing strains are reported to be distinguishable by a technique in which membranes from a routine IS*6110*-based RFLP typing procedure are probed with a specific 'W-Beijing polyprobe' [J Clin Microbiol (2005) 43(5):2148–2154].

Rapid PCR-based detection of this strain has been reported in which a characteristic 641-bp PCR product was obtained by amplifying a sequence at the mycobacterial interspersed repetitive unit (MIRU) locus 26 within the *M. tuberculosis* genome [J Clin Microbiol (2006) 44(1):274–277].

[Other reports of PCR-based detection: [J Clin Microbiol (2006) 44(2):302–306; (2007) 45(3):1022–1023.]

W reactivation See WEIGLE REACTIVATION.

WAS See WISKOTT–ALDRICH SYNDROME.

WASP See WISKOTT–ALDRICH SYNDROME.

Weigle mutagenesis See WEIGLE REACTIVATION.

Weigle reactivation (W reactivation) A phenomenon in which certain phages (including phage λ) which have been damaged by ULTRAVIOLET RADIATION exhibit higher rates of survival in host cells which have been irradiated with UVR prior to infection with the phage – as compared with non-irradiated host cells.

Growth of the phage in pre-irradiated cells also results in higher rates of mutagenesis in the phage (*Weigle mutagenesis*).

The phenomenon is partly explicable by the presence of repair enzymes (including error-prone DNA polymerases) in the pre-irradiated cells. However, other factor(s) appear to be involved because Weigle reactivation depends on irradiation of host cells even when they are mutant strains in which the SOS genes (including those encoding error-prone DNA polymerases) are constitutively active in the absence of UVR.

Western blot analysis Syn. IMMUNOBLOTTING.

Western blotting A procedure, analogous to SOUTHERN BLOTTING, in which *proteins* are transferred from gel to matrix using e.g. electrically driven transfer.

If the proteins on the matrix are probed by anti-protein *antibodies*, the procedure is generally referred to as *Western blot analysis* or IMMUNOBLOTTING (q.v.).

(See also NORTHERN BLOTTING.)

WGA (1) WHOLE-GENOME AMPLIFICATION.
(2) Wheat germ agglutinin.

WGD Whole-genome duplication.

Whipple's disease A malabsorption syndrome in which there is e.g. diarrhea, steatorrhea, lymphadenopathy and involvement of the central nervous system; typically there is an infiltration of the intestinal mucosa by macrophages which contain PAS-positive material (i.e. material that gives a positive test in the periodic acid–Schiff reaction).

Whipple's disease has been associated with infection by the Gram-positive pathogen TROPHERYMA WHIPPLEI.

whole-animal cloning See CLONING (whole-animal cloning).

whole-genome amplification (WGA) Any of various methods that attempt to amplify genomic DNA – typically by copying randomly primed sequences – e.g. MULTIPLE DISPLACEMENT AMPLIFICATION.

WGA with bioinformatically optimized primers is reported to give better results than MDA on degraded genomic DNA [DNA Res (2006) 13(2):77–88].

WGA of bisulfite-treated DNA has been found to be a useful approach when studying cytosine methylation in small amounts of DNA [BioTechniques (2006) 41(5):603–607].

Note. The phrase 'whole-genome amplification' is somewhat misleading. It does not mean, literally, that the entire genome is replicated (as *in vivo*). Rather, it refers to those techniques in which primers are used for the simultaneous amplification of different parts of sample DNA – (theoretically) the whole genome being available as a template.

wild-type strain Of a given organism: any strain whose characteristics are those typical of strains that are common in the natural environment.

The strains used in genetic engineering are often selected, or modified, to have specific deficiencies or other abnormal features (see e.g. COMPETENT CELLS).

Wiskott–Aldrich syndrome (WAS) An X-linked immunodeficiency disorder associated with thrombocytopenia (low levels of platelets), eczema, and a susceptibility to recurrent infection; hemorrhage is a major feature.

The WAS protein (WASP) has been reported to bind to the platelet CIB protein which normally binds Ca^{2+} and integrins [EMBO Rep (2006) 7(5):506–511].

wobble hypothesis An hypothesis (proposed by Crick) relating to the observed degeneracy of the third base of a CODON; the hypothesis provides an explanation of the way in which some tRNAs can recognize several codons that differ in their third position.

In the wobble hypothesis, base-pairing occurs normally between the first two bases in the codon (i.e. bases in positions 1 and 2, 5′ to 3′) and the corresponding bases in the anticodon (i.e. bases in positions 3 and 2, respectively, 5′-to-3′).

By contrast, the base in position 1 of the anticodon (the so-called 'wobble position') can undergo 'non-Watson–Crick' base-pairing with the base in position 3 of the codon; thus, a G in the anticodon's wobble position may pair with either C or U in the codon's position 3, and U (in the wobble position) may pair with either A or G.

Certain modified bases can occur in the wobble position of the anticodon. For example, A appears to occur invariably in a deaminated form (i.e. as inosine); in the wobble position, inosine can pair e.g. with C or U.

(See also QUEUOSINE.)

Uridine (U) residues in the wobble position may be substituted with various groups whose synthesis is reported to need genes of the so-called Elongator complex; these genes appear to encode factors involved in the elongation stage of transcription mediated by RNA polymerase II [RNA (2005) 11(4): 424–436].

While the wobble hypothesis is generally applicable, other factors (such as the conformation of the tRNA's anticodon) may influence function.

wobble position See WOBBLE HYPOTHESIS.

WRWYCR A peptide that inhibits junction-resolving enzymes at a HOLLIDAY JUNCTION (q.v.).

wyosine See Y BASES.

X

X chromatin *Syn.* BARR BODY.

X chromosome In human cells: one of the two sex chromosomes, the other being the Y chromosome; the normal female is characterized by an XX complement, while the normal male is characterized by an XY complement.

In females, in any given cell, one of the X chromosomes is inactivated; this reflects an event early in embryonic development: see X-INACTIVATION.

(See also BARR BODY.)

Genetically based disorders resulting from abnormal alleles on an X chromosome are called X-LINKED DISORDERS.

X factor A requirement for the aerobic growth of some species of HAEMOPHILUS. The requirement can be satisfied by hemin or protoporphyrin IX; the X factor is needed for the synthesis of cytochromes and catalase etc.

(cf. V FACTOR.)

X-gal 5-bromo-4-chloro-3-indolyl-β-D-galactoside: a substrate hydrolysed by the enzyme β-galactosidase to a blue-green product; bacteria forming this enzyme give rise to blue-green colonies when grown on an agar medium containing X-gal.

(See also REPORTER GENE and PBLUESCRIPT.)

Bluo-gal is a related compound that produces a darker blue; it has uses similar to those of X-gal.

Both X-gal and Bluo-gal are soluble in dimethylformamide.

X-inactivation A (normal) process that occurs in the development of embryos of female mammals in which one of the X chromosomes (i.e. from the maternal or the paternal source) is silenced, i.e. made transcriptionally inactive, in half of the cells of the embryo, and the other X chromosome is silenced in the remaining cells of the embryo.

An X chromosome destined to be silenced expresses a noncoding RNA, called Xist, that coats the chromosome and also recruits other factors; this blocks transcriptional activity of genes on that chromosome.

Following X-inactivation, the inactivated X chromosome (designated Xi) remains inactivated in successive rounds of cell division.

The active (transcribed) X chromosome is designated Xa.

X-linked disorder (sex-linked disorder) Any genetic disorder resulting from an abnormal allele on an X CHROMOSOME.

An X-linked disorder may be recessive or dominant.

Males inheriting an X-linked disorder which is recessive in the female parent exhibit the abnormal trait because (having only one X chromosome) they lack the corresponding normal X-linked allele. Females who have a single normal allele are generally asymptomatic, although they will be carriers of the condition.

In X-linked *dominant* disorders, mating between an affected male and an unaffected female will not transmit the trait to a son: male-to-male transmission does not occur because a son inherits only the Y chromosome from his father.

X4 strains (of HIV-1) See HIV-1.

Xa The designation of the *active* X chromosome in a cell of a female mammal (see X-INACTIVATION).

Xaa The designation sometimes used to indicate an unknown amino acid residue.

xanthine The product of the oxidative deamination of guanine.

Xgal See entry X-GAL (above).

Xi The *inactive* X chromosome (see X-INACTIVATION).

Xic X-inactivation center: a regulatory region on an X chromosome which is involved in X-INACTIVATION. It includes the gene for Xist.

xis **gene** (phage λ) See PHAGE LAMBDA.

Xist A non-coding RNA which is involved in silencing one of the two X chromosomes during X-INACTIVATION.

XL1-Blue MRF′ See RESTRICTION-MINUS CELLS.

XL1-Red A MUTATOR STRAIN of *Escherichia coli* (see the entry for details of genotype and examples of use).

Xpress™ A fusion tag (Invitrogen, Carlsbad CA), encoded by certain expression vectors, which facilitates detection of the fusion product; the tag, Asp-Leu-Tyr-Asp-Asp-Asp-Asp-Lys, is detected by the anti-Xpress™ monoclonal antibody.

XSCID See GENETIC DISEASE (table).

Y

Y (1) A specific indicator of ambiguity in the recognition site of a RESTRICTION ENDONUCLEASE (or in any other nucleic acid sequence); for example, in GTY↓RAC the 'Y' indicates C or T. (In RNA 'Y' indicates C or U.)

(2) L-Tyrosine (alternative to Tyr).

Y bases Certain modified forms of guanine found in molecules of tRNA; in these bases an additional ring is fused to the purine skeleton. One example is *wyosine*. Y bases occur e.g. in the tRNA for phenylalanine in bacteria and yeasts.

(cf. Q BASES.)

Y family (of DNA polymerases) DNA polymerases which can continue to synthesize DNA through lesions (e.g. THYMINE DIMERS), incorporating incorrect nucleotides. These 'error-prone polymerases' occur in all three domains of life; they include e.g. the *Escherichia coli* DNA polymerases IV and V which are active during the SOS response to DNA damage. [Structural insight into replicating damaged DNA: PLoS Biol (2006) 4(1):e32.]

Y family DNA polymerases have been found to enhance survival in *Escherichia coli* when DNA replication is inhibited by nucleotide starvation brought about by treatment with hydroxyurea; this is a role distinct from the ability of the Y family polymerases to bypass the effects of DNA damage [EMBO J (2006) 25(4):868–879].

Thermostable polymerases of the Y family were reported to be useful for PCR amplification of damaged or ancient DNA (and may have applications e.g. in forensic science) [Nucleic Acids Res (2006) 34(4):1102–1111].

(See also FORENSIC APPLICATIONS.)

One report has suggested that Y family polymerases may mediate mutagenesis by incorporating oxidized nucleotides into nucleic acids [J Bacteriol (2006) 188(13):4992–4995].

Y2H YEAST TWO-HYDRID SYSTEM.

YAC YEAST ARTIFICIAL CHROMOSOME.

yeast When used without qualification, 'yeast' generally refers specifically to the species *Saccharomyces cerevisiae* (a very common experimental organism) – cf. entry YEASTS.

yeast artificial chromosome (YAC) An *in vitro* construct that can carry a large target gene/insert (up to ~1 Mbp) and which can replicate within yeast cells (commonly *Saccharomyces cerevisiae*) in a way that generally resembles the behavior of a small chromosome (including e.g. division at mitosis and meiosis). YACs have been used for CLONING genes and other sequences of DNA that are too large for cloning in other kinds of vector, and have also been used for the expression of certain (eukaryotic) genes.

The minimal structural requirements for a YAC are: (i) an autonomous replicating sequence (see ARS) to allow ongoing autonomous intracellular replication; (ii) a centromere sequence for mediating separation of chromatids etc. during the stages of division; and (iii) TELOMERE sequences at each end of the (linear) construct.

A YAC may be constructed as a circular molecule which is subsequently cut, with RESTRICTION ENDONUCLEASES, into two separate linear pieces: the so-called left and right arms. Each arm has a telomere sequence at *one* end. The gene of interest/insert is ligated between a left arm and a right arm – leaving the telomere sequences in terminal positions. A YAC – excluding the insert – is only a few hundred base-pairs in length.

For cloning, the circular molecule is cleaved – at several sites – to form the left and right arms; during this process, a section of the circular molecule (the 'stuffer') is excised – leaving a telomeric sequence at *one* end in both the left and right arms. A mixture containing the left and right arms of the YAC, with copies of the gene/insert to be cloned, is then incubated with a ligase.

The product required from the ligation step is a construct consisting of the gene/insert of interest flanked on one side by a YAC left arm and on the other side by a YAC right arm. (The reaction mixture will include unwanted constructs – e.g. YACs containing no insert and inserts flanked by two left arms or two right arms.)

Products from the ligation step are inserted into SPHEROPLASTS of *S. cerevisiae* by transformation. (Yeast cells with intact cell walls are not used.)

YACs are designed to facilitate the selection of those yeast cells that have been transformed with the required construct (i.e. insert flanked by left and right arms). For this purpose, use is made of specific, modified strains of *S. cerevisiae*. One such strain is AB1380 (see the entry SACCHAROMYCES for details). A YAC designed for use in strain AB1380 contains a functional (wild-type) *TRP1* gene in one arm and a functional *URA3* gene in the other arm. Hence, only those cells which have received constructs containing *both* arms of the YAC will be selected (i.e. will grow) on media lacking tryptophan and uracil. However, although selecting for both arms of the YAC, this procedure does not select positively for those cells in which the construct includes an insert.

To select for the presence of an insert, the YAC is designed to include a functional *SUP4* suppressor gene which converts a mutant (red) cell to a (wild-type) colorless cell. This gene contains an EcoRI restriction site (cloning site) within which the insert can be ligated. The presence of an insert in this site inactivates the *SUP4* gene; hence, any cell which contains a complete YAC with an insert will grow with the (mutant) red coloration, while a cell containing an insert-free YAC (i.e. in which there is a functional *SUP4* gene) will form (wild-type) colorless colonies.

YACs have been used e.g. for studies on an imprinting control region [Proc Natl Acad Sci USA (2006) 103(28):10684–10689] and studies on gene transcription during fetal adrenal development [Mol Cell Biol (2006) 26(11):4111–4121].

Yeast Gene Order Browser (YGOB) An online tool used for comparative genomic studies on hemiascomycetous yeasts. [Syntenic relationships in hemiascomycetes using YGOB:

Nucleic Acids Res (2006) 34 (Database issue):D452–D455.]

yeast genetic marker See YEAST MARKER.

yeast marker (yeast genetic marker) Any chromosomal gene of a yeast which can act as a selectable marker when present in a construct (e.g. a YEAST ARTIFICIAL CHROMOSOME) used for transforming cells.

Marker genes in common use include e.g. those encoding essential products involved in amino acid biosynthesis (e.g. *HIS3*, *LEU2*) and in the biosynthesis of uracil (e.g. *URA3*). Thus, e.g. insertion of a YAC containing a functional (wild-type) *HIS3* into an auxotrophic strain of yeast – in which the corresponding gene is inactivated – will permit growth (and, hence, selection on appropriate minimal media) of those cells which have taken up the YAC.

yeast three-hybrid system (tribrid system) An experimental system, based on the YEAST TWO-HYBRID SYSTEM, which can monitor *in vivo* interactions involving three proteins.

In this system, one of the vectors encodes the extra protein – whose expression is regulated by controlling the conditions of the experiment.

When expressed, the third protein may interact with prey and/or bait proteins in various ways – for example, it may stabilize prey–bait binding or modify one (or both) proteins (e.g. by phosphorylation) to active or inactive forms, thereby promoting or inhibiting interaction. As in the two-hybrid system, suitable reporter genes signal the occurrence of specific interactions.

yeast two-hybrid system A technique used for the detection of protein–protein interaction *in vivo* (in yeast cells). (See also BACTERIOMATCH TWO-HYBRID SYSTEM and CYTOTRAP.)

This technique exploits the fact that some transcription activators can be physically split into two inactive domains: a DNA-binding domain (DBD) and an activation domain (AD) – both of which are necessary in the functional transcription activator. The DBD has a binding site for a promoter-related region, while AD is required for initiation of transcription, from that promoter, by RNA polymerase II.

A functional transcription activator can also be produced when a fusion protein (i.e. *hybrid* protein) that *includes* DBD binds to a fusion protein that *includes* AD. In this technique, combination (i.e. binding) occurs between the pair of *fusion partners* – i.e. between the protein that is fused to DBD and the protein that is fused to AD; these two fusion partner proteins (whose interaction is being studied) are referred to as the 'bait' and 'prey' proteins.

Given bait–prey binding, transcription is initiated from the corresponding promoter, which regulates a REPORTER GENE; transcription of the reporter gene indicates that a functional transcription activator is present – that is, that the two fusion partner proteins have interacted physically.

The fusion proteins are encoded on vector molecules that are introduced into cells; fusion proteins are expressed within the cells. Various reporter genes can be used.

The occurrence or otherwise of interaction between the bait and prey proteins can be indicated by either positive selection or negative selection.

For positive selection, cells of *Saccharomyces cerevisiae* can be engineered so that their growth depends, absolutely, on the occurrence of the bait–prey interaction. For example, the endogenous *HIS3* gene can be inactivated; thus, without the corresponding gene product (HIS3) the cells cannot grow on a specific selective medium. A copy of the *HIS3* gene, inserted into the cells as a reporter gene in the two-hybrid system, will therefore allow cells to grow on the selective medium *if* bait–prey interaction occurs, i.e. if the reporter gene (*HIS3*) is transcribed and expressed.

For negative selection (counterselection) in the cells of *S. cerevisiae*, the endogenous *URA3* gene can be deleted and replaced by *URA3* on a reporter cassette, expression of *UR3* then being governed by the bait–prey interaction. Bait–prey interaction promotes expression of *URA3* (which encodes orotidine-5′-phosphate decarboxylase) – with consequent activation of a functional uracil biosynthesis pathway; under these conditions, the addition of 5-fluoro-orotic acid (5-FOA) to the medium results in the formation of a suicide substrate, so that no growth occurs.

One problem that may arise is *self-activation* by the bait protein, i.e. the bait protein may trigger transcription of the reporter gene without first interacting with the prey protein, yielding a false-positive result. To address this problem, the system can be modified e.g. with a mechanism that kills a cell if self-activation occurs.

Examples of the use of yeast two-hybrid systems: checking interaction between MinC and MinD proteins (which regulate development of the septum during bacterial cell division) [J Bacteriol (2005) 187(8):2846–2857]; studies on association of odorant receptors in *Drosophila*: PLoS Biol (2006) 4(2): e20].

A yeast two-hybrid system has been devised for analysis of *competitive* binding between proteins [BioTechniques (2005) 39(2):165–168].

Comparison of the yeast two-hybrid system with the bacterial two-hybrid system found that the yeast system permitted quantitative detection of interaction over a greater range. The bacterial system, however, was found to be less susceptible to self-activation (= autoactivation) under the conditions examined. [Combined yeast/bacteria two-hybrid system: Mol Cell Proteom (2005) 4:819–826.]

yeasts A convenient (but non-taxonomic) category of fungi that includes organisms which are *typically* unicellular, fermentative and saprotrophic, and which reproduce asexually by the process of budding. *Saccharomyces cerevisiae* is an example of a typical yeast.

Many organisms that are included in the category *yeasts* do not exhibit all the typical features. For example, the species *Candida albicans* can grow in a mycelial form (as well as in a unicellular form – i.e. it is a *dimorphic* fungus); moreover, this species can also be pathogenic.

Schizosaccharomyces pombe is a 'fission yeast' – i.e. the cells divide by fission (rather than by budding).

Some yeasts (e.g. *Hansenula canadensis*, *Lipomyces* spp) are non-fermentative.

Some otherwise 'typical' yeasts (e.g. *Pichia pastoris*) can carry out a type of metabolism (methylotrophy) which is not common in this group of organisms.

The category *yeasts* is based on morphological and physiological criteria rather than on taxonomic criteria.

yellow fluorescent protein (YFP)   A (fluorescent) protein that is widely used e.g. as a partner in fusion proteins, acting as a reporter system. The YFP is also used e.g. in BIMOLECULAR FLUORESCENCE COMPLEMENTATION.

[Examples of the use of YFP: Plant Physiol (2006) 142(4): 1442–1459; PLoS Genet (2006) 2(11):e194.]

An enhanced form of YFP (eYFP, or EYFP) – analogous to the enhanced green fluorescent protein (see EGFP) – is also widely used [e.g. Plant Physiol (2006) 142(3):963–971; BMC Mol Biol (2006) 7:36; Genetics (2006) 174(1):253–263].

YFP   YELLOW FLUORESCENT PROTEIN.

YGOB   YEAST GENE ORDER BROWSER.

YTH   YEAST TWO-HYBRID SYSTEM.

YycFG system   See TWO-COMPONENT REGULATORY SYSTEM.

Z-DNA Left-handed helical dsDNA, with ~12 bases/turn, first observed in sequences such as ...GCGCGCGC... under some *in vitro* conditions (such as high concentrations of salt); the sugar–phosphate backbone forms an irregular zig-zag. Some proteins bind preferentially to Z-DNA, and this has suggested the possibility that it occurs *in vivo*.

Z ring A ring-shaped structure, composed of molecules of the FtsZ protein, which develops mid-way along the length of a dividing bacterial cell prior to the formation of the septum; it marks the plane of the forthcoming septum.

(See also GENE FUSION (uses).)

The polymerization of FtsZ proteins is inhibited in the SOS response (see SOS SYSTEM).

zalcitabine See NUCLEOSIDE REVERSE TRANSCRIPTASE INHIBITORS.

ZAP Express® vector A vector (Stratagene, La Jolla CA) that incorporates features of both phage and plasmid and which is suitable for expression in bacteria and eukaryotes. The vector can carry inserts of up to 12 kb.

Essentially, the ZAP Express® vector consists of a 4.5-kb PHAGEMID (pBK-CMV) bracketed by two PHAGE LAMBDA sequences, each having a terminal single-stranded *cos* region. One of the lambda sequences contains phage genes A→J that encode head, tail and morphogenesis. *Immediately* flanking the phagemid are two short sequences, called the initiator and terminator sequences, that are recognized by a helper phage (see later).

The phagemid includes a ColE1 (plasmid) origin of replication and an f1 (phage) origin of replication. It also includes a *lac* promoter and a CMV promoter (for gene expression in bacteria and eukaryotes, respectively). The multiple cloning site (MCS) is bracketed by T3 and T7 promoters (in opposite orientation) for *in vitro* transcription.

A sequence from the *lacZ* gene provides a facility for blue–white screening (see α-PEPTIDE).

Antibiotic-resistance genes permit the selection of vector-containing bacteria or eukaryotic cells.

The gene of interest/cDNA etc. is inserted in the MCS located in the phagemid.

The vectors, containing inserts, are packaged e.g. in GIGA-PACK components to produce complete phage particles which are used to infect an appropriate strain of *Escherichia coli*; if required, the insert can be expressed in such a strain.

Within bacterial cells the phagemid can be excised from the vector by a filamentous helper phage. A product of the helper phage recognizes the initiator and terminator sequences, and a new strand of DNA – corresponding to the sequence of the phagemid (and its insert) – is synthesized, displacing the existing strand. The displaced strand is circularized and is then packaged in products encoded by the helper phage. The (single-stranded) phagemid is secreted from the cell in the form of filamentous phage particles.

The ZAP Express® vector has been used for developing a DNA VACCINE against a bovine pathogen, *Mycoplasma mycoides* subsp *mycoides*. The approach is as follows.

Initially, a whole-genome library of *Mycoplasma mycoides* subsp *mycoides* is prepared in the ZAP Express vector. After packaging, phage particles are used to infect a plate culture of *Escherichia coli* in the presence of IPTG; IPTG promotes expression of the insert from the *lac* promoter. Thus, a given PLAQUE (one of many which develop on the phage-infected plate) will contain (i) progeny phage particles, and (ii) the protein product encoded by the insert of that particular clone.

The plaques on a given plate are transferred, by blotting, to a nitrocellulose membrane. The plaques on the membrane are probed e.g. by a hyperimmune serum (containing antibodies specific to the pathogen). Some of the plaques will contain a protein, encoded by the insert, which binds to the antibodies; any plaque that shows a strong positive reaction to the antibodies is selected for further study because the gene encoding the protein in that plaque may be a candidate gene for a DNA vaccine. The phage particles are collected from such positive plaques and are propagated further in an appropriate strain of *E. coli*; this strain is co-infected with a helper phage (see above) which excises, and packages, a single-stranded form of the phagemid (with its insert). The phage particles are then released into the medium.

The resulting phage particles, injected into the host animal, are apparently taken up by antigen-presenting cells (APCs) and then transported to the spleen and to Kuppfer cells in the liver. Following injection, the phage protein capsid appears to protect phage DNA from degradation. When intracellular, the phage DNA can be transcribed via the CMV promoter, so that protective proteins, encoded by the insert, can be synthesized in the target animal. [Screening for candidate genes for a DNA vaccine against the bovine pathogen *Mycoplasma mycoides* subsp *mycoides*: Infect Immun (2006) 74(1):167–174.]

The ZAP Express vector has also been used e.g. in studies on the biosynthesis of anandamide [Proc Natl Acad Sci USA (2006) 103(36):13345–13350].

ZBTB4 protein See KAISO PROTEIN.

ZBTB28 protein See KAISO PROTEIN.

ZEBRA (*syn.* Zta) An activator of replication of the Epstein–Barr virus (EBV): a protein, encoded by (immediate-early) viral gene *bzlf-1*, which promotes replication of EBV within latently infected B lymphocytes (B cells). In latently infected B cells, ZEBRA can be induced by treating the cells with e.g. corticosteroids, anti-immunoglobulin or the compound TPA (a phorbol ester: 12-*O*-tetradecanolyphorbol 13 acetate).

The lytic cycle of EBV is also promoted in latently infected B cells by the transcription factor Rta (encoded by the viral gene *brlf-1*); transcription of *brlf-1* was reported to be activated by acetylation of histones.

The switch from latent to lytic infection is reported to be associated with sensitization to killing by NK cells [J Virol

(2007) 81(2):474–482].

zebrafish A small teleost (bony) fish (*Danio rerio*) with a short generation time; the zebrafish is a common experimental animal. [Functional genomics research methodology for the zebrafish: BioTechniques (2005) 38(6):897–906; chromatin immunoprecipitation protocol for studying whole-embryo *in vivo* development of the zebrafish: BioTechniques (2006) 40 (1):34–40.]

The formation of microRNAs (miRNAs) in (living) cells of zebrafish was studied by dual-fluorescence reporter/sensor plasmids [BioTechniques (2006) 41(6):727–732].

(See also MITOCHONDRIAL DNA.)

Zenon® antibody-labeling reagents Products from Invitrogen (Carlsbad CA) used for the rapid (~10-minute) labeling of IgG antibodies. The reagents are labeled Fab fragments – a Fab fragment being one of the two arms of the (Y-shaped) immunoglobulin molecule; Fab fragments bind to the Fc part of an IgG antibody – the Fc region being the stem of the Y-shaped molecule. Fab fragments may be labeled e.g. with a fluorophore or with BIOTIN – or an enzyme such as HORSE-RADISH PEROXIDASE.

[Uses (e.g.): Mol Biol Cell (2006) 17(6):2722–2734; Proc Natl Acad Sci USA (2007) 104(9):3460–3465; J Clin Invest (2007) 117(1):258–269.]

Zeocin™ An antibiotic (Invitrogen, Carlsbad CA) of the bleomycin/phleomycin group which binds to DNA and cleaves it. Zeocin™ is an effective agent against eukaryotic cells (such as yeast and mammalian cells) and also against at least some types of bacteria.

Resistance to Zeocin™ can be conferred by a gene whose product binds to the antibiotic, blocking its binding to DNA.

[Examples of use of Zeocin™ as a selective agent: BMC Cancer (2006) 6:221; PLoS Medicine (2006) 3(9):e358.]

zidovudine (AZT) 3′-azido-3′-deoxythymidine, a NUCLEOSIDE REVERSE TRANSCRIPTASE INHIBITOR used e.g. in the treatment of AIDS; its mode of action is similar to that of other NRTIs.

AZT undergoes glucuronidation in the liver; drugs which inhibit glucuronidation may influence plasma levels of AZT.

Side-effects from the drug include certain types of anemia.

Ziehl–Neelsen stain A stain used for the detection of ACID-FAST BACILLI in e.g. smears of sputum.

zinc finger A type of motif which is common in DNA-binding proteins (e.g. certain transcription factors); it contains a zinc-binding site. Different families of zinc-finger proteins differ e.g. in structure and in the type(s) of zinc-binding amino acid residue; cysteine residues are commonly involved, sometimes in conjunction with histidine residues. Characteristically, an α-helix component of a zinc-finger protein binds to the major groove in DNA.

(See also METHYLATION and TAGM.)

ZIP (1) A LEUCINE ZIPPER.

(2) A sequence that binds a ZINC FINGER.

zipcode Within an mRNA molecule: a sequence of nucleotides that apparently contributes to targeting the molecule to an appropriate location in the cell; correct targeting of mRNA is necessary to ensure that the encoded polypeptide is synthesed in the right location, i.e. at or near the site of its function. Localization of an mRNA molecule to the correct site is also likely to depend on its secondary structure.

Zipcodes may differ even in functionally related molecules of mRNA. In one study on the nucleator complex involved in actin polymerization in fibroblasts, a zipcode was identified in only one of seven mRNAs encoding subunits of the given complex [J Cell Sci (2005) 118(11):2425–2433].

zipcode array An approach that avoids some of the problems inherent in a conventional MICROARRAY (q.v.). Essentially, each probe in the array has a *unique* zipcode sequence, and each of the various types of target sequence being examined carries a complementary copy of *one* of the unique zipcodes. Hence, a given probe (with its unique zipcode) will bind only those target sequences which carry a complementary copy of that particular zipcode.

All the zipcodes in the array are designed to bind optimally to their complementary sequences at a similar temperature – so that (temperature-dependent) stringency is similar for all the probe–target pairs; this is in contrast to the situation in a conventional microarray.

Another advantage of the zipcode approach is that an established zipcode array can be used for successive sets of *different* targets.

[Example of use: Nucleic Acids Res (2005) 33(2):e19.]

An analogous system, termed *barcoding*, is used e.g. in MOLECULAR INVERSION PROBE GENOTYPING.

(See also PADLOCK PROBE.)

zipper (molecular) See MOLECULAR ZIPPER.

zippering (1) Ongoing (progressive and rapid) hybridization of pairs of nucleotides in two complementary strands of nucleic acid after the initial phase of binding between a few pairs of bases.

[Kinetics of duplex formation for individual DNA strands in a single protein nanopore: Proc Natl Acad Sci USA (2001) 98(23):12996–13001.]

(2) The mode in which certain invasive bacteria attach to their (mammalian) host cells prior to internalization; zippering involves e.g. formation of multiple points of attachment between pathogen and host cell. This form of invasion occurs e.g. with *Listeria monocytogenes* and *Yersinia enterocolitica*.

zoo blot A membrane (prepared e.g. by SOUTHERN BLOTTING) containing fragments of genomic DNA from a wide range of species. Probing a zoo blot with a labeled fragment may give useful information about that fragment. Thus, for example, a fragment that hybridizes to DNA from each of a number of widely differing species may be expected to include a highly conserved coding sequence because, in general, non-coding DNA tends to be poorly conserved. In other cases, a fragment may exhibit positive hybridization to DNA of only closely related species.

Zta (*bzlf-1* gene product) See ZEBRA.

zwoegerziekte virus See LENTIVIRINAE.

zygospore A sexually derived, thick-walled resting spore which is characteristic of fungi of the subdivision Zygomycotina.

zygote A diploid cell resulting from the fusion of two (haploid) gametes.

zygotic meiosis The occurrence of meiosis in a zygote prior to the formation of haploid vegetative cells in those life cycles in which a haploid phase predominates.

zymolyase A preparation that has enzymic activity against most $(1{\rightarrow}3)$-β-glucans (found e.g. in yeast cell walls). Zymolyase is used e.g. for preparing yeast SPHEROPLASTS.

[Uses (e.g.): PLoS Genetis (2006) 2(9):e141; RNA (2006) 12(9):1721–1737; Mol Biol Cell (2007) 18(2):455–463.]

Appendix: alphabetical
list of genera

(read *across* the columns)

(A = archaean; B = bacterium; Bd = bird; C = crustacean; F = fungus (yeasts and other species); Fsh = fish; I = insect; M = mammal; N = nematode; P = plant (includes algae and higher plants); Pz = protozoan)

Abies (P)	*Acanthamoeba* (Pz)	*Acer* (P)
Acetabularia (P)	*Achlya* (F)	*Acinetobacter* (B)
Actinobacillus (B)	*Aedes* (I)	*Aeromonas* (B)
Agalliopsis (I)	*Agaricus* (F)	*Agrobacterium* (B)
Agropyron (P)	*Albugo* (F)	*Alcaligenes* (B)
Allomyces (F)	*Alnus* (P)	*Alternaria* (F)
Alteromonas (B)	*Amanita* (F)	*Anabaena* (B)
Anguina (N)	*Anopheles* (I)	*Aphelenchoides* (N)
Apis (I)	*Arabidopsis* (P)	*Arcella* (Pz)
Arcellinida (Pz)	*Armillaria* (F)	*Arthrobacter* (B)
Aschersonia (F)	*Ascosphaera* (F)	*Aspergillus* (F)
Astacus (C)	*Ateles* (M)	*Avena* (P)
Babesia (Pz)	*Bacillus* (B)	*Bacteroides* (B)
Bartonella (B)	*Bdellovibrio* (B)	*Beauveria* (F)
Beggiatoa (B)	*Belononlaimus* (N)	*Berberis* (P)
Beta (P)	*Bifidobacterium* (B)	*Bodo* (Pz)
Bodonina (Pz)	*Boletus* (F)	*Bombyx* (I)
Bordetella (B)	*Borrelia* (B)	*Bos* (M)
Botrytis (F)	*Brassica* (P)	*Bremia* (F)
Brevoortia (Fsh)	*Brochothrix* (B)	*Brucella* (B)
Bryopsis (P)	*Buchnera* (B)	*Bullera* (F)
Burkholderia (B)	*Byssochlamys* (F)	*Caedibacter* (B)
Caenorhabditis (N)	*Callithrix* (M)	*Camellia* (P)
Campylobacter (B)	*Candida* (F)	*Cantharellus* (F)
Carchesium (Pz)	*Cardiobacterium* (B)	*Carnobacterium* (B)
Caryophanon (B)	*Caseobacter* (B)	*Castanea* (P)
Caulerpa (P)	*Caulobacter* (B)	*Cellulomonas* (B)
Cephalosporium (F)	*Ceratocystis* (F)	*Cercopithecus* (M)
Chaetomium (F)	*Chenopodium* (P)	*Chionoecetes* (C)

293

Chlamydia (B)	*Chlamydomonas* (P)	*Chlorella* (P)
Chondrus (P)	*Chromobacterium* (B)	*Cicadulina* (I)
Citellus (M)	*Citeromyces* (F)	*Citrobacter* (B)
Cladophora (P)	*Cladosporium* (F)	*Claviceps* (F)
Clostridium (B)	*Cocos* (P)	*Coffea* (P)
Colletotrichum (F)	*Colpidium* (Pz)	*Colpoda* (Pz)
Coriolus (F)	*Corynebacterium* (B)	*Costia* (Pz)
Coxiella (B)	*Cricetus* (M)	*Criconemoides* (N)
Cristispira (B)	*Cryptococcus* (F)	*Cryptosporidium* (Pz)
Culicoides (I)	*Culiseta* (I)	*Curtobacterium* (B)
Cyathus (F)	*Cyclidium* (Pz)	*Cymbidium* (P)
Cyniclomyces (F)	*Cyprinus* (Fsh)	*Dacrymyces* (F)
Dactylis (P)	*Daedalea* (F)	*Daldinia* (F)
Danio (Fsh)	*Darna* (I)	*Deinococcus* (B)
Dekkera (F)	*Dendrolimus* (I)	*Desulfobacter* (B)
Desulfobulbus (B)	*Desulfococcus* (B)	*Desulfomonas* (B)
Desulfosarcina (B)	*Desulfovibrio* (B)	*Desulfurococcus* (A)
Desulfuromonas (B)	*Dictyostelium* (F)	*Dientamoeba* (Pz)
Difflugia (Pz)	*Diplocarpon* (F)	*Ditylenchus* (N)
Dolichodorus (N)	*Drosophila* (I)	*Dunaliella* (P)
Duttonella (Pz)	*Ehrlichia* (B)	*Eikenella* (B)
Eimeria (Pz)	*Elsinoë* (F)	*Emericella* (F)
Endamoeba (Pz)	*Endothia* (F)	*Ensifer* (B)
Entamoeba (Pz)	*Enterobacter* (B)	*Enterococcus* (B)
Epichloë (F)	*Erwinia* (B)	*Erysipelothrix* (B)
Erysiphe (F)	*Escherichia* (B)	*Euglena* (P)
Euplotes (Pz)	*Fagus* (P)	*Festuca* (P)
Filosea (Pz)	*Fistulina* (F)	*Fomes* (F)
Frankia (B)	*Frateuria* (B)	*Fusarium* (F)
Fusobacterium (B)	*Gaeumannomyces* (F)	*Gaffkya* (B)
Gallionella (B)	*Gallus* (Bd)	*Ganoderma* (F)
Gardnerella (B)	*Gelidium* (P)	*Giardia* (Pz)
Gigartina (P)	*Gilpinia* (I)	*Gloeobacter* (B)
Glossina (I)	*Gossypium* (P)	*Gracilaria* (P)
Graminella (I)	*Gregarina* (Pz)	*Haemophilus* (B)
Hafnia (B)	*Halimeda* (P)	*Halobacterium* (A)
Halococcus (A)	*Halomonas* (B)	*Hansenula* (F)
Helicobacter (B)	*Helicotylenchus* (N)	*Heliothis* (I)

Helvella (F)	*Hematopinus* (I)	*Hemicycliophora* (N)
Heterodera (N)	*Hexamita* (Pz)	*Histomonas* (Pz)
Histoplasma (F)	*Homo* (M)	*Hoplolaimus* (N)
Hormoconis (F)	*Humicola* (F)	*Humulus* (P)
Hydnum (F)	*Hyphomonas* (B)	*Hyposoter* (I)
Ichthyophthirius (Pz)	*Ictalurus* (Fsh)	*Inocybe* (F)
Inonotus (F)	*Ipomea* (P)	*Isospora* (Pz)
Issatchenkia (F)	*Janthinobacterium* (B)	*Juglans* (P)
Kentrophoros (Pz)	*Klebsiella* (B)	*Kloeckera* (F)
Kluyvera (B)	*Kluyveromyces* (F)	*Koserella* (B)
Kurthia (B)	*Lachnospira* (B)	*Lactobacillus* (B)
Lactococcus (B)	*Laminaria* (P)	*Legionella* (B)
Leishmania (Pz)	*Lentinula* (F)	*Lentinus* (F)
Lepista (F)	*Leptinotarsa* (I)	*Leptomis* (Fsh)
Leptomonas (Pz)	*Leptonema* (B)	*Leptospira* (B)
Leuconostoc (B)	*Limulus* (C)	*Lipomyces* (F)
Listeria (B)	*Lolium* (P)	*Longidorus* (N)
Loxodes (Pz)	*Lupinus* (P)	*Lycopersicon* (P)
Lymantria (I)	*Lyngbya* (B)	*Macaca* (M)
Malassezia (F)	*Mallomonas* (P)	*Malpighamoeba* (Pz)
Malus (P)	*Marmota* (M)	*Megasphaera* (B)
Megatrypanum (Pz)	*Meles* (M)	*Melilotus* (P)
Meloidogyne (N)	*Melopsittacus* (Bd)	*Methanobacterium* (A)
Methanococcoides (A)	*Methanococcus* (A)	*Methanosarcina* (A)
Methanospirillum (A)	*Methanothermus* (A)	*Minchinia* (Pz)
Methanothrix (A)	*Mobiluncus* (B)	*Monocystis* (Pz)
Monostroma (P)	*Moraxella* (B)	*Morchella* (F)
Morganella (B)	*Mucor* (F)	*Mus* (M)
Mustela (M)	*Mycena* (F)	*Mycobacterium* (B)
Mycoplasma (B)	*Nacobbus* (N)	*Nadsonia* (F)
Naegleria (Pz)	*Nannomonas* (Pz)	*Nectria* (F)
Neisseria (B)	*Neodiprion* (I)	*Nesoclutha* (I)
Neurospora (F)	*Nicotiana* (P)	*Nitrobacter* (B)
Nitrosococcus (B)	*Nitrospina* (B)	*Nocardia* (B)
Nosema (Pz)	*Nostoc* (B)	*Nudaurelia* (I)
Olpidium (F)	*Opalina* (Pz)	*Oryctolagus* (M)
Oryza (P)	*Oscillatoria* (B)	*Ostracoblabe* (F)
Oxalobacter (B)	*Pacifastacus* (C)	*Paramecium* (Pz)

Paratylenchus (N)	*Paspalum* (P)	*Pasteurella* (B)
Pelodictyon (B)	*Penicillium* (F)	*Penaeus* (C)
Peptostreptococcus (B)	*Peranema* (Pz)	*Perilla* (P)
Perkinsiella (I)	*Peronospora* (F)	*Petunia* (P)
Peziza (F)	*Phaffia* (F)	*Phaseolus* (P)
Phellinus (F)	*Phlebotomus* (I)	*Phleum* (P)
Phoma (F)	*Photobacterium* (B)	*Phycomyces* (F)
Phycopeltis (P)	*Physarum* (F)	*Phytolacca* (P)
Phytophthora (F)	*Pichia* (F)	*Pilobolus* (F)
Pinus (P)	*Piptoporus* (F)	*Pisum* (P)
Planktothrix (B)	*Planobispora* (B)	*Planococcus* (B)
Plantago (P)	*Plasmodiophora* (F)	*Plasmodium* (Pz)
Pleurotus (F)	*Pneumocystis* (F)	*Polyporus* (F)
Popillia (I)	*Populus* (P)	*Poria* (F)
Prevotella (B)	*Procyon* (M)	*Propionibacterium* (B)
Prorodon (Pz)	*Proteus* (B)	*Prunus* (P)
Pseudallescheria (F)	*Pseudomonas* (B)	*Psoroptes* (I)
Puccinia (F)	*Pulex* (I)	*Pyricularia* (F)
Pyrococcus (A)	*Pyrodictium* (A)	*Pyronema* (F)
Pyrus (P)	*Pythium* (F)	*Quercus* (P)
Radopholus (N)	*Rattus* (M)	*Rhipicephalus* (I)
Rhizobium (B)	*Rhizoctonia* (F)	*Rhizomucor* (F)
Rhizopus (F)	*Rhodococcus* (B)	*Rhodotorula* (F)
Rickettsia (B)	*Robinia* (P)	*Rubus* (P)
Saccharomyces (F)	*Saccharum* (P)	*Saimiri* (M)
Salix (P)	*Salmo* (Fsh)	*Salmonella* (B)
Saprolegnia (F)	*Sarcina* (B)	*Scenedesmus* (P)
Schizosaccharomyces (F)	*Sciara* (I)	*Scleroderma* (F)
Sclerotinia (F)	*Sclerotium* (F)	*Scolytus* (I)
Scutellinia (F)	*Scutellonema* (N)	*Scytonema* (B)
Selenomonas (B)	*Septoria* (F)	*Serpula* (F)
Serratia (B)	*Shigella* (B)	*Sordaria* (F)
Sorghum (P)	*Sparassis* (F)	*Spartina* (P)
Spermophilus (M)	*Sphaerotilus* (B)	*Spirillum* (B)
Spiroplasma (B)	*Spirulina* (B)	*Sporobolomyces* (F)
Sporothrix (F)	*Staphylococcus* (B)	*Stentor* (Pz)
Streptococcus (B)	*Streptomyces* (B)	*Sulfolobus* (A)
Sylvilagus (M)	*Synchytrium* (F)	*Synechococcus* (B)

Synechocystis (B)	*Tetrahymena* (Pz)	*Thea* (P)
Theileria (Pz)	*Theobroma* (P)	*Thermoplasma* (A)
Thermus (B)	*Thiobacillus* (B)	*Thomomys* (M)
Tilia (P)	*Tilletia* (F)	*Torula* (F)
Torulopsis (F)	*Toxoplasma* (Pz)	*Toxothrix* (B)
Trachelomonas (Pz)	*Trametes* (F)	*Trebouxia* (P)
Tremella (F)	*Trentepohlia* (P)	*Treponema* (B)
Trichomonas (Pz)	*Trichophyton* (F)	*Trichoplusia* (I)
Trichosporon (F)	*Triticum* (P)	*Tropheryma* (B)
Trypanosoma (Pz)	*Typhula* (F)	*Tyzzeria* (Pz)
Ulmus (P)	*Urticaria* (P)	*Ustilago* (F)
Venturia (F)	*Verpa* (F)	*Verticillium* (F)
Vibrio (B)	*Vicia* (P)	*Vigna* (P)
Volvariella (F)	*Volvox* (P)	*Vorticella* (Pz)
Wickerhamia (F)	*Wickerhamiella* (F)	*Wolbachia* (B)
Wolinella (B)	*Xanthomonas* (B)	*Xenopsylla* (I)
Xenorhabdus (B)	*Xylaria* (F)	*Yersinia* (B)
Zea (P)	*Zoogloea* (B)	*Zythia* (F)